Approximate

m	ft and in	m	ft and in
1.22	4'0"	1.69	5'6½"
1.23	4'½"	1.7	5'7"
1.24	4'1"	1.71	5'7½"
1.26	4'1½"	1.73	5'8"
1.27	4'2"	1.74	5'8½"
1.28	4'2½"	1.75	5'9"
1.29	4'3"	1.76	5'9½"
1.31	4'3½"	1.78	5'10"
1.32	4'4"	1.79	5'10½"
1.33	4'4½"	1.8	5'11"
1.35	4'5"	1.82	5'11½"
1.36	4'5½"		
1.37	4'6"	1.83	6'0"
1.38	4'6½"	1.84	6'½"
1.4	4'7"	1.85	6'1"
1.41	4'7½"	1.87	6'1½"
1.42	4'8"	1.88	6'2"
1.43	4'8½"	1.89	6'2½"
1.45	4'9"	1.9	6'3"
1.46	4'9½"	1.92	6'3½"
1.47	4'10"	1.93	6'4"
1.49	4'10½"	1.94	6'4½"
1.5	4'11"	1.96	6'5"
1.51	4'11½"	1.97	6'5½"
		1.98	6'6"
1.52	5'0"	1.99	6'6½"
1.54	5'½"	2.01	6'7"
1.55	5'1"	2.02	6'7½"
1.56	5'1½"	2.03	6'8"
1.57	5'2"	2.04	6'8½"
1.59	5'2½"	2.06	6'9"
1.6	5'3"	2.07	6'9½"
1.61	5'3½"	2.08	6'10"
1.63	5'4"	2.10	6'10½"
1.64	5'4½"	2.11	6'11"
1.65	5'5"	2.12	6'11½"
1.66	5'5½"	2.13	7'0"
1.68	5'6"		

Adapted with permission from Webster-Gandy J, Madden A, and Holdsworth M (2006). Oxford Handbook of Nutrition. Oxford University Press: Oxford.

Oxford Handbook of
Endocrinology
and Diabetes

SECOND EDITION

Edited by

Helen E. Turner

Consultant Endocrinologist,
Department of Endocrinology,
Churchill Hospital,
Oxford, UK

John A.H. Wass

Professor of Endocrinology,
Department of Endocrinology,
University of Oxford,
Churchill Hospital,
Oxford, UK

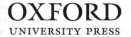

OXFORD
UNIVERSITY PRESS

OXFORD
UNIVERSITY PRESS

Great Clarendon Street, Oxford OX2 6DP

Oxford University Press is a department of the University of Oxford.
It furthers the University's objective of excellence in research, scholarship,
and education by publishing worldwide in

Oxford New York

Auckland Cape Town Dar es Salaam Hong Kong Karachi
Kuala Lumpur Madrid Melbourne Mexico City Nairobi
New Delhi Shanghai Taipei Toronto

With offices in

Argentina Austria Brazil Chile Czech Republic France Greece
Guatemala Hungary Italy Japan Poland Portugal Singapore
South Korea Switzerland Thailand Turkey Ukraine Vietnam

Oxford is a registered trade mark of Oxford University Press
in the UK and in certain other countries

Published in the United States
by Oxford University Press Inc., New York

British Library Cataloguing in Publication Data
Data available

Library Data available of Congress Cataloging-in-Publication-Data
Data available

Typeset by Cepha Imaging Private Ltd., Bangalore, India
Printed in Italy
on acid-free paper by
L.E.G.O. S.p.A. — Lavis TN

ISBN 978–0–19–856739–4

10 9 8 7 6 5 4 3 2 1

Oxford University Press makes no representation, express or implied, that the drug
dosages in this book are correct. Readers must therefore always check the product
information and clinical procedures with the most up to date published product
information and data sheets provided by the manufacturers and the most recent
codes of conduct and safety regulations. The authors and publishers do not accept
responsibility or legal liability for any errors in the text or for the misuse or misap-
plication of material in this work.

Note: This book uses international non-propriety names for medicines. Natural substances retain their traditional spelling. For example, oestrogen is spelled estrogen
when it appears as prescribed medicine.

Foreword

When prominent endocrinologists were asked for a definition of their speciality John Wass's answer was 'Endocrinologists do it with hormones'. While this statement certainly oversimplifies the complexity of endocrinology, it characterizes the approach of the editors of this handbook. On the one hand, John Wass is the co-editor of the Oxford Textbook of Endocrinology and Diabetes, a voluminous standard and reference work for the specialist, and on the other hand along with Helen Turner, he is the editor of this Handbook of Endocrinology and Diabetes for the young physician who is confronted with endocrine problems and needs quick help and guidance.

While endocrinology is a speciality, it is very much present in all fields of medicine. Hormones are everywhere and are either directly or indirectly involved in all diseases. This book provides a quick introduction for the newcomer and helps to update knowledge of the non-specialist in current diagnostic and therapeutic strategies. Of high didactic standard, this volume is well written and concisely structured. For the sake of our patients this handbook deserves a wide distribution.

Professor Dr. med. Eberhard Nieschlag, FRCP
President, European Society of Endocrinology
University Hopitals of Münster, Germany

Preface

The first edition of this handbook was well received and sold many copies. We were told by a number of specialist registrars in training and consultants that it was essential to have it in outpatients. We hope that the same will be true of the second edition.

Endocrinology remains the most exciting of specialties—enormously varied in presentation and management and with the ability to affect hugely and beneficially the quality of life over a long period of time. Our aims with this second edition remain the same, mainly to have a pocket handbook which can be easily transported in which all the pieces of information one so often needs are there as a reminder. We hope it will enable trainees to enhance their knowledge but also the older and so-called 'trained' will continue to have recourse to its pages when memory lapses occur. We regard it too as a companion to the *Oxford Textbook of Endocrinology and Diabetes*.

We are enormously indebted to our contributors who once again have provided timely texts full of practical detail. We are also hugely grateful to our external referees who have looked at all the chapters with great care and attention. Both have ensured that the text is as up-to-date as possible. As always we welcome comments for future editions and we hope this one proves as useful as the first one.

John A.H.Wass
Helen E.Turner
2009

Contents

Contributors

Julian Barth
Consultant in Chemical Pathology
and Metabolic Medicine
Leeds General Infirmary
Leeds, UK

Karin Bradley
Consultant Physician and
Endocrinologist, Bristol Royal
Infirmary
and Honorary Senior Clinical
Lecturer, University of Bristol,
Bristol, UK

Peter Clayton
Professor of Child Health and
Paediatric Endocrinology
Department of Endocrinology
Royal Manchester Children's
Hospital,
Manchester, UK

Emma Duncan
Consultant Endocrinologist
Princess Alexandra Hospital
Senior Lecturer
University of Queensland
Postdoctoral Research Fellow
UQ Diamantina Institute for
Cancer, Immunology and
Metabolic
Medicine, Australia

Pam Dyson
Research Dietician
Oxford University
Oxford, UK

Mohgah Elsheikh
Consultant Endocrinologist
Royal Berkshire Hospital
Reading, UK

Stephen Gardner
Consultant Physician
Buckinghamshire Hospitals NHS
Trust, UK

Niki Karavitaki
Locum Consultant
Oxford Centre for Diabetes
Endocrinology and Metabolism
Churchill Hospital
Oxford, UK

Niki Meston
Consultant Chemical Pathologist
and Clinical Lecturer in Clinical
Biochemistry
John Radcliffe Hospital
Oxford, UK

John Newell-Price
Senior Lecturer and Consultant
Endocrinologist
University of Sheffield
Royal Hallamshire Hospital
Sheffield, UK

Peter Selby
Consultant Physician and Senior
Lecturer in Medicine
Manchester Royal Infirmary
Manchester, UK

Kevin Shotliff
Consultant Physician and
Diabetologist
Beta Cell Diabetes Centre
Chelsea and Westminster Hospital
London, UK

Sara Suliman
Specialist Registrar in Diabetes,
Endocrinology and Metabolism,
and Diabetes UK Clinical Research
Fellow
Oxford Centre for Diabetes
Endocrinology and Metabolism
Churchill Hospital
Oxford, UK

Janet Sumner
Lead Diabetes Specialist Nurse
Churchill Hospital
Oxford, UK

Garry Tan
Consultant Diabetologist and
Endocrinologist
Derby Royal Infirmary, UK

Vivien Thornton-Jones
Lead Endocrine Specialist Nurse
Churchill Hospital
Oxford, UK

Helen E Turner
Consultant Endocrinologist
Department of Endocrinology
Churchill Hospital
Oxford, UK

John AH Wass
Professor of Endocrinology,
Department of Endocrinology
Churchill Hospital
Oxford, UK

John Wong
Consultant Chemical Pathologist
Kingston Hospital
Surrey, UK

Specialist readers

John S Bevan
Lead Consultant and Honorary
Reader in Endocrinology
Endocrine Unit
Aberdeen Royal Infirmary
Aberdeen
Scotland, UK

Polly Bingley
Professor of Diabetes
University of Bristol
Bristol, UK

Pierre Bouloux
Professor of Endocrinology
Royal Free and University College
Medical School
University College London, UK

John Connell
Professor of Endocrinology
BHF Glasgow Cardiovascular
Research Centre
University of Glasgow, UK

Sadaf Farooqi
Wellcome Trust Senior Clinical
Fellow and
Honorary Consultant Physician
Addenbrooke's Hospital
Cambridge, UK

Jayne A Franklyn
Professor of Medicine
Head of the School of Clinical and
Experimental Medicine
College of Medical and
Dental Sciences
University of Birmingham, UK

Neil Gittoes
Senior Lecturer in Endocrinology
University of Birmingham
Consultant and Lead Clinical
Endocrinologist
University Hospital Birmingham
Birmingham, UK

Mark Gurnell
University Lecturer in
Endocrinology and Honorary
Consultant Physician
University of Cambridge
Cambridge, UK

Linda Johnson
Consultant and Honorary
Senior Lecturer in Paediatric
Endocrinology Endocrine Centre
William Harvey Research Institute
Barts and the London Queen
Mary School of Medicine
London, UK

William Ledger
Professor of Obstetrics
Gynaecology and Head of Unit
Academic Unit of Reproductive
and Developmental Medicine
University of Sheffield
Sheffield Teaching Hospitals
NHS Trust,
Sheffield, UK

Hugh AW Neil
Professor of Clinical Epidemiology
University of Oxford and
Honorary Consultant Physician
Oxford Centre for Diabetes
Endocrinology and Metabolism
Churchill Hospital, Oxford, UK

Catherine Nelson-Piercy
Consultant Obstetric Physician
Guy's and St Thomas' Foundation
Trust and Queen Charlotte's and
Chelsea Hospital, Imperial College
Healthcare NHS Trust
London, UK

Anthony P Weetman
Professor of Medicine
University of Sheffield
Sheffield, UK

Symbols and abbreviations

📖	cross reference
↑	increased/ing
↓	decreased/ing
→	no change/normal
♂	male
♀	female
+ve	positive
−ve	negative
1°	primary
2°	secondary
5-FU	5-fluorouracil
ACE	angiotensin converting enzyme
ACEI	angiotensin converting enzyme inhibitor
AD	autosomal dominant
ADA	American Diabetes Association
ADH	antidiuretic hormone
ADHH	autosomal dominant hypocalcaemic hypercalciuria
AGE	advanced glycation end-products
AIH	amiodarone-induced hypothyroidism
AIT	amiodarone-induced thyrotoxicosis
ALT	alanine transaminase
ANP	atrial natriuretic peptide
APE	autoimmune polyglandular syndrome
APECED	autoimmune polyendocrinopthy, candidiasis and epidermal dystrophy
ART	assisted reproductive techniques
AST	aspartate transaminase
ATD	antithyroid drug
bd	*bis die* (twice a day)
BMD	bone mineral density
BP	blood pressure
CaE	calcium excretion
CAH	congenital adrenal hyperplasia
CBG	cortisol binding globulin
CHD	coronary heart disease

CMV	cytomegalovirus
CPA	cyproterone acetate
CRF	chronic renal failure
CRH	corticotrophin releasing hormone
CSF	cerebrospinal fluid
CSII	continuous subcutaneous insulin infusion
CSW	cerebral salt wasting syndrome
CT	computed tomography
CVP	central venous pressure
DCCT	Diabetes Control and Complications Trial
DCT	distal convolutued tubule
DDAVP	desamino-D-arginine vasopressin
DHEA	dihydroepiandrosterone
DHT	dihydrotestosterone
DI	diabetes insipidus
DIDMOAD	*d*iabetes *i*nsipidus, *DM*, optic *a*trophy + sensorineural *d*eafness (Wolfram's syndrome)
dL	decilitre
DVLA	Driver and Vehicle Licensing Agency
DVT	deep vein thrombosis
DXA	dual energy X-ray absorptiometry
EE2	ethinylestradiol
ESR	erythrocyte sedimentation rate
ESRF	end-stage renal failure
ETDRS	Early Treatment of Diabetic Retinopathy Study
FBC	full blood count
FCHL	familial combined hyperlipidaemia
FDB	familial defective apolipoprotein B-100
FFM	fat free mass
FH	familial hypercholesterolaemia
FHH	familial hypocalciuric hypercalcaemia
FIHP	familial isolated hyperparathyroidism
FMTC	familial medullary thyroid carcinoma
FNAC	fine needle aspiration cytology
FSH	follicle stimulating hormone
FTC	follicular carcinoma
g	gram
GAD	glutamic acid decarboxylase
GFR	glomerular filtation rate
GH	growth hormone
GHD	growth hormone deficiency

GI	gastrointestinal
GIFT	gamete intrafallopian transfer
GIP	gastric inhibitory peptide
GRTH	generalized resistance to thyroid hormone
h	hour/s
HAART	highly active antiretroviral therapy
HC	hydrocortisone
hCG	human chorionic gonadotrophin
HDL	high-density lipoprotein
HERS	Heart and Estrogen-Progestin Replacement Study
5HIAA	5-hydroxyindole acetic acid
HLA	human leukocyte antigens
HMG CoA	3-hydroxy-3-methylglutaryl coenzyme A
HNF	hepatic nuclear factor
HP	hypothalamus–pituitary
HPA	hypothalmic–pituitary–adrenal (axis)
HPT-JP	hyperparathyroidism-jaw tumour syndrome
HSG	hysterosalpingography
HZV	herpes zoster virus
ICSI	intracytoplasmic sperm injection
ID	intradermal
IDDM	insulin dependent diabetes mellitus (type 1)
IDL	intermediate-density lipoprotein
IFG	impaired fasting hyperglycaemia
IGF-I	insulin-like growth factor-1
IGT	impaired glucose tolerance
IHH	idiopathic hypogonadotrophic hypogonadism
IM	intramuscular
IPSS	inferior petrosal sinus sampling
IRMA	intraretinal microvascular abnormalities
ITT	insulin tolerance test
IU	international units
IUGR	intrauterine growth retardation
IUI	intrauterine insemination
IV	intravenous
IVF	*in vitro* fertilization
KS	Kaposi sarcoma
L	litre/s
LCAT	lecithin:cholesterol acyltransferase
LCCSCT	large cell calcifying Sertoli cell tumour

LDL	low-density lipoprotein
LFT	liver function test
LH	luteinizing hormone
MAI	*Mycobacterium avium intracellulare*
MC	mineralocorticoid
mcg	microgram
MDT	multi-disciplinary team
MEN	multiple endocrine neoplasia
MHC	major histocompatibility complex
MI	myocardial infarct
MIBG	[123]Iodine-metaiodobenzylguanidine
MIS	Müllerian inhibitory substance
mL	millilitre/s
od	*omni die* (once a day)
MODY	maturity onset diabetes of the young
MPH	mid-parental height
MRSA	methicillin-resistant *Staphylococcus aureus*
MTC	medullary thyroid cancer
NASH	non-alcoholic steatohepatitis
NF	neurofibromatosis
NFA	non-functioning pituitary adenoma
NG	nasogastric
NGF	nerve growth factor
NICH	non-islet cell hypoglycaemia
NIDDM	non-insulin dependent diabetes mellitus (type 2)
NVD	new vessels on the disc (diabetic retinopathy)
NVE	new vessels elsewhere (diabetic retinopathy)
OCP	oral contraceptive pill
OGTT	oral glucose tolerance test
25OHD	25-hydroxy vitamin D
17OHP	17-hydroxyprogesterone
OHSS	ovarian hyperstimulation syndrome
PAI	platelet activator inhibitor
PCOS	polycystic ovary syndrome
PCT	postcoital test
PET	positron emission spectrography
PID	pelvic inflammatory disease
PIH	pregnancy-induced hypertension
PO	*per os* (by mouth)
POMC	pro-opiomelanocortin

PMC	papillary microcarcinoma of the thyroid
PNMT	phenylethanolamine-*N*-methyl transferase
POEMS	progressive polyneuropathy, organomegaly, endocrinopathy, monoclonal gammopathy, and skin changes
POF	premature ovarian failure
POMC	pro-opiomelanocortin
PP	pancreatic polypeptide
PPAR	peroxisome proliferator activated receptor
PRH	post-prandial reactive hypoglycaemia
PPNAD	primary pigmented nodular adrenocortical disease
PPI	proton pump inhibitor
PRL	prolactin
PRTH	pituitary resistance to thyroid hormones
PSA	prostatic specific antigen
PTH	parathyroid hormone
PTHrP	parathyroid hormone related peptide
QALY	quality adjusted life year
QCT	quantitative computed tomography
QoL	quality of life
QUS	quantitative ultrasound
RCAD	renal cysts and diabetes
rhGH	recombinant human GH
RTH	thyroid hormone resistance
SC	subcutaneous
SD	standard deviation
SHBG	sex hormone binding globulin
$t^{1/2}$	half-life
T_3	tri-iodothyronine
T_4	thyroxine
TB	tuberculosis
TBG	T_4-binding globulin
TBPA	T_4-binding prealbumin
TBG	thyroid binding globulin
tds	three times a day
TFT	thyroid function test
TG	triglycerides
TGF	transforming growth factor
TNF	tumour necrosis factor
TPO	thyroid peroxidase

TRH	thyrotropin releasing hormone
TSAb	TSH stimulating antibodies
TSG	tumour suppressor genes
TSH	thyroid stimulating hormone
TSH-RAB	TSH receptor antibodies
TTR	transthyretin
U&Es	urea and electolytes
UFC	urinary free cortisol
UKPDS	Prospective Diabetes Study
US	ultrasound
VEGF	vascular endothelial growth factor
VHL	von Hippel–Lindau disease
VIP	vasoactive intestinal peptide
VLDL	very high-density lipoprotein
WDHA	watery diarrhoea, hypokalaemia, and achlorhydria
WHI	Women's Health Initiative
WHO	World Health Organization
ZE	Zollinger Ellison syndrome

Detailed contents

Part 2 **Pituitary**

Part 4 **Reproductive endocrinology**

Part 11 **Diabetes**

Part 1

Thyroid

Anatomy and physiology of the thyroid

Anatomy

The thyroid gland comprises
- A midline isthmus lying horizontally just below the cricoid cartilage.
- 2 lateral lobes that extend upward over the lower half of the thyroid cartilage.

The gland lies deep to the strap muscles of the neck, enclosed in the pre-tracheal fascia, which anchors it to the trachea, so that the thyroid moves up on swallowing.

Histology
- Fibrous septa divide the gland into pseudolobules.
- Pseudolobules are composed of vesicles called follicles or acini, surrounded by a capillary network.
- The follicle walls are lined by cuboidal epithelium.
- The lumen is filled with a proteinaceous colloid, which contains the unique protein thyroglobulin. The peptide sequences of T_4 and T_3 are synthesized and stored as a component of thyroglobulin.

Development
- Develops from the endoderm of the floor of the pharynx with some contribution from the lateral pharyngeal pouches.
- Descent of the midline thyroid anlage gives rise to the thyroglossal duct, which extends from the foramen caecum near the base of the tongue to the isthmus of the thyroid.
- During development the posterior aspect of the thyroid becomes associated with the parathyroid gland and the parafollicular C cells, derived from the ultimo-branchial body, which become incorporated into its substance.
- The C cells are the source of calcitonin and give rise to medullary thyroid carcinoma when they undergo malignant transformation.
- The fetal thyroid begins to concentrate and organify iodine at about 10–12 weeks' gestation.
- Maternal TRH readily crosses the placenta, maternal TSH and T_4 do not.
- T_4 from the fetal thyroid is the major thyroid hormone available to the fetus. The fetal pituitary–thyroid axis is a functional unit distinct from that of the mother—active at 18–20 weeks.

Thyroid examination

Inspection

- Look at the neck from the front. If a goitre (enlarged thyroid gland of whatever cause) is present, the patient should be asked to swallow a mouthful of water. The thyroid moves up with swallowing.
- Watch for appearance of any nodule not visible before swallowing, e.g. in an elderly patient with kyphosis the thyroid may be partially retrosternal.

Palpation

- Is the thyroid gland tender to touch?
- With index and middle finger feel below thyroid cartilage where the isthmus of the thyroid gland lies over the trachea.
- Palpate the 2 lobes of the thyroid, which extend laterally behind the sternomastoid muscle.
- Ask the patient to swallow again while you continue to palpate the thyroid.
- Assess *size*, whether it is *soft,* firm *or hard,* it is *nodular* or *diffusely* enlarged and whether it *moves* readily on swallowing.
- Palpate along the medial edge of the sternomastoid muscle on either side to look for a pyramidal lobe.
- Palpate for lymph nodes in the neck.

Percussion

Percuss upper mediastinum for retrosternal goitre.

Auscultation

- Auscultate to identify bruits, consistent with Graves' disease.
- Occasionally inspiratory stridor can be heard with a large or retrosternal goitre causing tracheal compression (□ see Pemberton's sign p.48).

Assess thyroid status

- Observe for signs of thyroid disease—exophthalmos, proptosis, thyroid acropachy, pretibial myxoedema, hyperactivity, restlessness, or whether immobile and uninterested.
- Take pulse; note presence or absence of tachycardia, bradycardia, or atrial fibrillation.
- Feel palms—whether warm and sweaty or cold.
- Look for tremor in outstretched hands.
- Examine eyes: exophthalmos (forward protrusion of the eyes—proptosis); lid retraction: sclera visible above cornea; lid lag; conjuctival injection or oedema (cheimosis); periorbital oedema; loss of full-range movement.

Physiology

- Thyroid hormone contains iodine. Iodine enters the thyroid in the form of inorganic or ionic iodide, which is organized by the thyroid peroxidase enzyme at the cell–colloid interface. Subsequent reactions result in the formation of iodothyronines.
- The thyroid is the only source of T_4.
- The thyroid secretes 20% of circulating T_3; the remainder is generated in extraglandular tissues by the conversion of T_4 to T_3 by deiodinases (largely in the liver and kidneys).

Synthesis of the thyroid hormones can be inhibited by a variety of agents termed *goitrogens*.
- Perchlorate and thiocyanate inhibit iodide transport.
- Thioureas and mercaptoimidazole inhibit the initial oxidation of iodide and coupling of iodothyronines.
- In large doses iodine itself blocks organic binding and coupling reactions.
- Lithium has several inhibitory effects on intrathyroidal iodine metabolism.

In the blood, T_4 and T_3 are almost entirely bound to plasma proteins. T_4 is bound in ↓ order of affinity to T_4 binding globulin (TBG), transthyretin (TTR), and albumin. T_3 is bound 10–20 times less avidly by TBG and not significantly bound by TTR. Only the free or unbound hormone is available to tissues. The metabolic state correlates more closely with the free than the total hormone concentration in the plasma. The relatively weak binding of T_3 accounts for its more rapid onset and offset of action. Table 1.1 summarizes those states associated with 1° alterations in the concentration of TBG. When there is primarily an alteration in the concentration of thyroid hormones, the concentration of TBG changes little (Table 1.2).

The concentration of free hormones does not necessarily vary directly with that of the total hormones; e.g. while the total T_4 level rises in pregnancy, the free T_4 level remains normal.

The levels of thyroid hormone in the blood are tightly controlled by feedback mechanisms involved in the hypothalamo–pituitary–thyroid axis (Fig. 1.1).
- TSH secreted by the pituitary stimulates the thyroid to secrete principally T_4 and also T_3. TRH stimulates the synthesis and secretion of TSH. T_4 and T_3 inhibit TSH synthesis and secretion directly.
- T_4 and T_3 are bound to TBG, TTR, and albumin. The remaining free hormones inhibit synthesis and release of TRH and TSH to influence growth and metabolism.
- T_4 is converted peripherally to the metabolically active T_3 or the inactive reverse T_3 (rT_3).
- T_4 and T_3 are metabolized in the liver by conjugation with glucuronate and sulphate. Enzyme inducers such as phenobarbital, carbamazepine, and phenytoin increase the metabolic clearance of the hormones without ↓ the proportion of free hormone in the blood.

Table 1.1 Disordered thyroid hormone–protein interactions

	Serum total T_4 and T_3	Free T_4 and T_3
Primary abnormality in TBG		
▲ Concentration	↑	Normal
▼ Concentration	↓	Normal
Primary disorder of thyroid function		
Hyperthyroidism	↑	↑
Hypothyroidism	↓	↓

Table 1.2 Circumstances associated with altered concentration of TBG

↑ TBG	↓ TBG
Pregnancy	Androgens
Newborn state	Large doses of glucocorticoids; Cushings' syndrome
OCP and other sources of oestrogens	Chronic liver disease
Tamoxifen	Severe systemic illness
Hepatitis A; chronic active hepatitis	Active acromegaly
Biliary cirrhosis	Nephrotic syndrome
Acute intermittent porphyria	Genetically determined
Genetically determined	Drugs, e.g. phenytoin

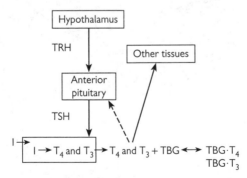

Fig. 1.1 Regulation of thyroid function. Solid arrows indicate stimulation, broken arrow indicates inhibitory influence. TRH, thyrotropin releasing hormone; TSH, thyroid stimulating hormone; T_4, thyroxine; T_3, tri-iodothyronine; I, iodine; TBG, thyroid binding globulin.

Molecular action of thyroid hormone

T_3 is the active form of thyroid hormone. It binds to thyroid hormone receptors (TRs), of which there are several isoforms and which are members of the nuclear hormone receptor superfamily. TR/T_3 complexes elicit action by binding to response elements in the DNA of gene promoters. Recruitment of co-activators alters the chromatin configuration allowing gene transcription to proceed, whilst co-repressors cause the opposite effect.

Abnormalities of development

- Remnants of the thyroglossal duct may be found in any position along the course of the tract of its descent:
  - In the tongue, it is referred to as '*lingual thyroid*'.
  - *Thyroglossal cysts* may be visible as midline swellings in the neck.
  - *Thyroglossal fistula* develops an opening in the middle of the neck.
  - Thyroglossal nodules *or*
  - The '*pyramidal lobe*', a structure contiguous with the thyroid isthmus which extends upwards.
- The gland can descend too far down to reach the anterior mediastinum.
- Congenital hypothyroidism results from failure of the thyroid to develop (agenesis). More commonly, however, congenital hypothyroidism reflects enzyme defects impairing hormone synthesis.

Thyroid investigations

Tests of hormone concentration

Highly specific and sensitive chemiluminescent and radioimmunoassays are used to measure serum T_4 and T_3 concentrations. Free hormone concentrations usually correlate better with the metabolic state than do total hormone concentrations because they are unaffected by changes in binding protein concentration or affinity.

Tests of homeostatic control

📖 See Table 2.1

- Serum TSH concentration is used as 1st line in the diagnosis of 1° hypothyroidism and hyperthyroidism. The test is misleading in patients with 2° thyroid dysfunction reflecting hypothalmic/pituitary disease.
- The TRH stimulation test, which can be used to assess the functional state of the TSH secretory mechanism, is now rarely used to diagnose 1° thyroid disease since it has been superseded by sensitive TSH assays. It is of limited use; its main use is in the differential diagnosis of elevated TSH in the setting of elevated thyroid hormone levels and in the differential diagnosis of resistance to thyroid hormone and a TSH-secreting pituitary adenoma (Table 2.3).

In interpreting results of TFTs, the effects of drugs that the patient might be on should be borne in mind. Table 2.2 lists the influence of drugs on TFTs. Table 2.3 sets out some examples of a typical thyroid function test.

Box 2.1 Thyroid hormone resistance (RTH)

- Syndrome characterized by reduced responsiveness to elevated circulating levels of free T_4 and free T_3, non-suppressed serum TSH and intact TSH responsiveness to TRH. Clinical features apart from goitre are usually absent but may include short stature, hyperactivity, attention deficits with mental deficiency or learning disability, and goitre.
- The cause is a mutation in the thyroid hormone receptor.
- Differential diagnosis includes TSH-secreting pituitary tumour.
- Most cases require no treatment. If needed it is usually B-adrenergic blockers to ameliorate some of the tissue effects of raised thyroid hormone levels.

Table 2.1 Thyroid hormone concentrations in various thyroid abnormalities

Condition	TSH	Free T_4	Free T_3
1° hyperthyroidism	Undetectable	↑↑	↑
T_3 toxicosis	Undetectable	Normal	↑↑
Subclinical hyperthyroidism	↓	Normal	Normal
2° hyperthyroidism (TSHoma)	↑ or normal	↑	↑
Thyroid hormone resistance	↑ or normal	↑	↑
1° hypothyroidism	↑	↓	↓ or normal
Subclinical hypothyroidism	↑	Normal	Normal
2° hypothyroidism	↓ or normal	↓	↓ or normal

Table 2.2 Influence of drugs on thyroid function tests

Metabolic process	↑	↓
TSH secretion	Amiodarone (transiently: becomes normal after 2–3 months) Sertraline St John's Wort	Glucocorticoids, dopamine agonists, phenytoin, dopamine
T_4 synthesis/release	Iodide	Iodide, lithium
Binding proteins	Oestrogen, clofibrate, heroin	Glucocorticoids, androgens, phenytoin, carbamazepine
T_4 metabolism	Anticonvulsants; rifampicin	
T_4/T_3 binding in serum		Salicylates, furosemide, mefenamic acid

Table 2.3 Atypical thyroid function tests

Test	Possible cause
Suppressed TSH and normal free T_4	T_3 toxicosis (approximately 5% of thyrotoxicosis)
Suppressed TSH and normal free T_4 and free T_3	Subclinical thyrotoxicosis Recovery from thyrotoxicosis Excess thyroxine replacement Sick euthyroidism
Detectable TSH and elevated free T_4 and free T_3	TSH secreting pituitary tumour Thyroid hormone resistance Heterophile antibodies leading to spurious measurements of free T_4 and free T_3
Elevated free T_4 and low normal free T_3, normal TSH	Amiodarone

Antibody screen

High titres of antithyroid peroxidase (anti-TPO) antibodies or antithyroglobulin antibodies are found in patients with autoimmune thyroid disease (Hashimoto's thyroiditis, Graves' disease, and sometimes euthyroid individuals). 📖 See Table 2.4.

Screening for thyroid disease[1]

The following categories of patients should be screened for thyroid disease:

- Patients with atrial fibrillation or hyperlipidaemia.
- Periodic (6-monthly) assessments in patients receiving amiodarone and lithium.
- Annual check of thyroid function in the annual review of diabetic patients.
- ♀ with type 1 diabetes in the 1st trimester of pregnancy and post delivery (because of the 3-fold increase in incidence of postpartum thyroid dysfunction in such patients).
- ♀ with past history of postpartum thyroiditis.
- Annual check of thyroid function in people with Down's syndrome, Turner's syndrome, and Addison's disease, in view of the high prevalence of hypothyroidism in such patients.
- ♀ with thyroid autoantibodies—8 × risk of developing hypothyroidism over 20 years compared to antibody −ve controls
- ♀ with thyroid autoantibodies and isolated elevated TSH—38× risk of developing hypothyroidism, with 4% annual risk of overt hypothyroidism.

1 Tunbridge WM and MP Vanderpump MP (2000). Population screening for autoimmune thyroid disease. *Endocrinol Metab Clin N Am* **29**(2), 239–53.

Table 2.4 Antithyroid antibodies and thyroid disease

Condition	Anti-TPO	Anti-thyroglobulin	TSH receptor antibody
Graves' disease	70–80%	30–50%	70–100% (stimulating)
Autoimmune hypothyroidism	95%	60%	10–20% (blocking)

Note: TSH receptor antibodies may be stimulatory or inhibitory. Heterophile antibodies present in patient sera may cause abnormal interference causing abnormally low or high values of free T_4 and free T_3, and can be removed with absorption tubes.

Scintiscanning

Permits localization of sites of accumulation of radioiodine or sodium pertechnetate [^{99m}Tc], which gives information about the activity of the iodine trap (Table 2.5). This is useful:

- To define areas of ↑ or ↓ function within the thyroid (Table 2.6) which occasionally helps in cases of uncertainty as to the cause of the thyrotoxicosis.
- To detect retrosternal goitre.
- To detect ectopic thyroid tissue.

The scan may be altered by:

- Agents which influence thyroid uptake, including intake of high-iodine foods and supplements, such as kelp (seaweed).
- Drugs containing iodine, such as amiodarone.
- Recent use of radiographic contrast dyes can potentially interfere with the interpretation of the scan.

Table 2.5 Radioisotope scans

	^{123}Iodine	^{99}Technitium pertechnetate
Half-life	Short	Short
Advantage	Low emission of radiation Have higher energy photons. Hence useful for imaging a toxic goitre with a substernal component	Maximum thyroid uptake within 30 min of administration. Can be used in breast-feeding women (discontinue feeding for 24h)
Disadvantage		Technetium is only trapped by the thyroid without being organified
Use	Functional assessment of the thyroid	Rapid scanning

Table 2.6 Radionuclide scanning (scintigram) in thyroid disease

Condition	Scan appearance
Graves' hyperthyroidism	Enlarged gland ↑ homogeneous radionucleotide uptake
Thyroiditis (e.g. de Quervain's)	Low or absent uptake
Toxic nodule	A solitary area of high uptake
Thyrotoxicosis factitia	Depressed thyroid uptake
Thyroid cancer	Successful ^{131}I uptake by tumour tissue requires an adequate level of TSH, achieved by stopping T_3 replacement 10 days before scanning or giving recombinant TSH injection

Ultrasound (US) scanning

Provides an accurate indication of thyroid size and is useful for differentiating cystic nodules from solid ones, but cannot be used to distinguish between benign and malignant disease.

- Microcalcification within nodules favours the diagnosis of malignancy; micro-calcifications <2mm in diameter are observed in ~60% of malignant nodules, but in <2% of benign lesions.
- Calcification is a prominent feature of medullary carcinoma of the thyroid.
- It can detect whether a nodule is solitary or part of a multinodular process.
- Sequential scanning can be employed to assess changes in size of thyroid over time.

Note neither scintigraphy or US is routinely indicated in a patient with goitre.

Fine needle aspiration (FNAC) cytology

- FNAC is now considered the most accurate test for diagnosis of thyroid nodules. It is performed in an outpatient setting. 1–2 aspirations are carried out at different sites for each nodule. Cytologic findings are *satisfactory* or *diagnostic* in approximately 85% of specimens and *non-diagnostic* in the remainder.
- In experienced hands FNAC is an excellent diagnostic technique, as shown in Table 2.7.
- Repeat FNAC after 3–6 months further reduces the proportion of false –ves.
- It is impossible to differentiate between benign and malignant follicular neoplasm using FNAC. Therefore surgical excision of a follicular neoplasm is always indicated.
- 📖 See Table 2.8 for diagnostic categories from FNAC.

Table 2.7 Diagnostic features of FNAC

Feature	Range (%)	Mean value (%)
Accuracy	85–100	95
Specificity	72–100	92
Sensitivity	65–98	83
False –ve	1–11	5

Table 2.8 Diagnostic categories from FNAC

Category		Action
Thy 1	Non-diagnostic Inadequate	Repeat sampling, using US if necessary
Thy 2	Non-neoplastic	Two samples 3–6 months apart showing benign appearances are indicated to exclude neoplasia. If rapid growth/pressure effects/high risk diagnostic lobectomy may be indicated.
Thy 3	(i) Follicular lesions	Lobectomy, with completion thyroidectomy if malignant
	(ii) Other suspicious findings	Discussion at thyroid cancer MDT
Thy 4	Suspicious of malignancy e.g. papillary, medullary, or anaplastic carcinoma/ lymphoma	Surgical excision for differentiated tumour
Thy 5	Diagnosis of malignancy	Surgical excision for differentiated thyroid cancer. Radiotherapy/ chemotherapy for anaplastic thyroid cancer, lymphoma/metastases

Computed tomography (CT)

- CT is useful in the evaluation of <u>retrosternal</u> and <u>retrotracheal</u> extension of an enlarged thyroid.
- Compression of the trachea and displacement of the major vessels can be identified with CT of the superior mediastinum.
- It can demonstrate the extent of intrathoracic extension of thyroid <u>malignancy and infiltration of a</u>djacent structures such as the carotid artery, internal jugular vein, trachea, oesophagus, and regional lymph nodes.

Additional laboratory investigations

Haematological tests

- Long-standing thyrotoxicosis may be associated with a *normochromic anaemia* and occasionally a *mild neutropaenia, lymphocytosis* and rarely a *thrombocytopaenia.*
- In hypothyroidism a macrocytosis is typical, although concurrent vitamin B12 deficiency should be considered.
- There may also be a *microcytic anaemia* due to menorrhagia and impaired iron utilization.

Biochemical tests

- *Alkaline phosphatase* may be elevated in thyrotoxicosis.
- Mild *hypercalcaemia* occasionally occurs in thyrotoxicosis and reflects ↑ bone resorption. *Hypercalciuria* is more common.
- In a hypothyroid patient, *hyponatraemia* may be due to reduced renal tubular water loss or less commonly due to co-existing cortisol deficiency.
- In hypothyroidism *creatinine* kinase is often raised and the lipid profile altered with ↑ LDL cholesterol.

Endocrine tests

- In untreated hypothyroidism there may be inadequate responses to provocative testing of the hypothalamo–pituitary–adrenal (HPA) axis.
- In hypothyroidism, serum prolactin may be elevated because ↑ TRH leads to ↑ prolactin secretion.
- In thyrotoxicosis there is an increase in *sex hormone binding globulin* (SHBG), and a complex interaction with sex steroid hormone metabolism, resulting in changes in the levels of androgens and oestrogens. The net physiological result is an increase in *oestrogenic* activity, with *gynaecomastia* and a decrease in libido in ♂ presenting with thyrotoxicosis.

Sick euthyroid syndrome (non-thyroidal illness syndrome)

- Biochemistry:
  - Low T_4 and T_3.
  - Inappropriately normal/suppressed TSH.
- Tissue thyroid hormone concentrations are very low.
- Context—starvation.
  - Severe illness e.g. ITU, severe infections, renal failure, cardiac failure, liver failure, end-stage malignancy.
- Thyroxine replacement is not indicated because there is no clear evidence that treatment provides benefit or is safe.

Atypical clinical situations

- *Thyrotoxicosis factitia:*
  - No thyroid enlargement.
  - Elevated free T_4 and suppressed TSH.
  - Depressed thyroid uptake on scintigraphy.
  - Low thyroglobulin differentiates from thyroiditis (which shows depressed uptake on scintigraphy but ↑ thyroglobulin) and all other causes of elevated thyroid hormones.
- *Struma ovarii* (ovarian teratoma containing hyperfunctioning thyroid tissue):
  - No thyroid enlargement.
  - Depressed thyroid uptake on scintigraphy.
  - Body scan after radioiodine confirms diagnosis.
- *Trophoblast tumours* hCG has structural homology with TSH and leads to thyroid gland stimulation, and usually mild thyrotoxicosis.
- *Hyperemesis gravidarum* Thyroid function tests may be abnormal with a suppressed TSH (see Chapter 3, p.34 and Chapter 70, p.431).
- *Choriocarcinoma of the testes* may be associated with gynaecomastia and thyrotoxicosis—measure hCG.

Thyrotoxicosis

Aetiology

Epidemiology

- 10 × more common in ♀ than in ♂ in the UK.
- Prevalence is approximately 2% of the ♀ population.
- Annual incidence is 3 cases per 1000 ♀.

Definition of thyrotoxicosis and hyperthyroidism

- The term *thyrotoxicosis* denotes the clinical, physiological, and biochemical findings that result when the tissues are exposed to excess thyroid hormone. It can arise in a variety of ways (Table 3.1).
It is essential to establish a specific diagnosis as this determines therapy choices and provides important information for the patient regarding prognosis.
- The term *hyperthyroidism* should be used to denote only those conditions in which hyperfunction of the thyroid leads to thyrotoxicosis.

Genetics of autoimmune thyroid disease (AITD)

- AITD consists of Graves' disease, Hashimoto's thyroiditis, atrophic autoimmune hypothyroidism, post-partum thyroiditis and thyroid associated ophthalmopathy, that appear to share a common genetic predisposition.
- There is a ♀ preponderance and sex steroids appear to play an important role.
- Twin studies show ↑ concordance for Graves' disease and autoimmune hypothyroidism, in monozygotic compared to dizygotic twins.
- It is estimated that genetic factors account for 79% of the susceptibility for Graves' disease.
- Sib studies indicate that sisters and children of ♀ with Graves' disease have a 5–8% risk of developing Graves' disease or autoimmune hypothyroidism.
- On the background of a genetic predisposition, environmental factors are thought to contribute to the development of disease.
- A number of interacting susceptibility genes are thought to play a role in the development of disease—a complex genetic trait.
- *CTLA-4* (cytotoxic T lymphocyte antigen 4) is associated with Graves' disease in Caucasian populations. In particular, the CT60 allele has a prevalence of 60% in the general population, but is also the allele most highly associated with Graves' disease. These data emphasise the complex nature of genetic susceptibility and the likely interplay of environmental factors.
- Association of major histocompatibility complex (MHC) loci with Graves' disease has been demonstrated in some populations, but not others. HLA-DR3 is associated with Graves' disease in whites. HLA-DQA1*0501 is associated in some populations, especially for men. However, the overall contribution of MHC genes to Graves' disease has been estimated to be only 10–20% of the inherited susceptibility.

Table 3.1 Classification of the aetiology of thyrotoxicosis

Associated with hyperthyroidism	
Excessive thyroid stimulation	Graves' disease, Hashitoxicosis
	Pituitary thyrotroph adenoma
	Pituitary thyroid hormone resistance syndrome (excess TSH)
	Trophoblastic tumours producing hCG with thyrotrophic activity
Thyroid nodules with autonomous function	Toxic solitary nodule, toxic multinodular goitre
	Very rarely, thyroid cancer
Not associated with hyperthyroidism	
Thyroid inflammation	Silent and postpartum thyroiditis, subacute (de Quervain's) thyroiditis
	Drug-induced thyroiditis (amiodarone)
Exogenous thyroid hormones	Overtreatment with thyroid hormone
	Thyrotoxicosis factitia (thyroxine use in non-thyroidal disease)
Ectopic thyroid tissue	Metastatic thyroid carcinoma
	Struma ovarii (teratoma containing functional thyroid tissue)

Manifestations of hyperthyroidism

Box 3.1 Manifestations of hyperthyroidism (all forms)

Symptoms
- Hyperactivity, irritability, altered mood, insomnia.
- Heat intolerance, ↑ sweating.
- Palpitation.
- Fatigue, weakness.
- Dyspnoea.
- Weight loss with ↑ appetite (weight gain in 10% of patients).
- Pruritus.
- ↑ stool frequency.
- Thirst and polyuria.
- Oligomenorrhoea or amenorrhoea, loss of libido.

Signs
- Sinus tachycardia, atrial fibrillation.
- Fine tremor, hyperkinesia, hyperreflexia.
- Warm, moist skin.
- Palmar erythema, onycholysis.
- Hair loss.
- Muscle weakness and wasting.
- Congestive (high output) heart failure, chorea, periodic paralysis (primarily in Asian ♂), psychosis (rare).

Investigation of thyrotoxicosis
- Thyroid function tests raised free T_4 and suppressed TSH (raised free T_3 in T_3 toxicosis).
- Thyroid antibodies—$\square$ see Table 2.4, p.11.
- Radionucleotide thyroid scan if diagnosis uncertain ($\square$ see p.12) but is seldom required.

Manifestations of Graves' disease (in addition to those in Box 3.1)
- Diffuse goitre.
- Ophthalmopathy ($\square$ see Graves' ophthalmopathy, p.42).
  - A feeling of grittiness and discomfort in the eye.
  - Retrobulbar pressure or pain, eyelid lag or retraction.
  - Periorbital oedema, chemosis*, scleral injection.*
  - Exophthalmos (proptosis).*
  - Extraocular muscle dysfunction.*
  - Exposure keratitis.*
  - Optic neuropathy.*
- Localized dermopathy (pretibial myxoedema, $\square$ see Graves' dermopathy, p.46).
- Lymphoid hyperplasia.
- Thyroid acropachy ($\square$ see Thyroid acropachy, p.46).

*Combination of these suggests congestive ophthalmopathy. Urgent action necessary if: corneal ulceration, congestive ophthalmopathy, or optic neuropathy ($\square$ see Graves' ophthalmopathy, p.42).

Conditions associated with Graves' disease

- Type 1 diabetes mellitus.
- Addison's disease.
- Vitiligo.
- Pernicious anaemia.
- Alopecia areata.
- Myasthenia gravis.
- Coeliac disease (4.5%).
- Other autoimmune disorders associated with the HLA-DR3 haplotype.

Treatment

Medical treatment

In general, the standard policy in Europe is to offer a course of antithyroid drugs (ATD) first. In the USA, radioiodine is more likely to be offered as first-line treatment.

Aims and principles of medical treatment

- To induce remission in Graves' disease.
- Monitor for relapse off treatment initially 6–8-weekly for 6 months, then 6-monthly for 2 years, and then annually thereafter or sooner if symptoms return.
- Use of a computerized thyroid follow-up register greatly facilitates monitoring and reduces the necessity for out-patient appointments.
- For relapse, consider definitive treatment such as radioiodine or surgery. A 2nd course of ATD almost never results in remission.

Choice of drugs—thionamides

- *Carbimazole*, which can be given as a single dose, is usually the drug of 1st choice in the UK. Carbimazole is converted to methimazole by cleavage of a carboxyl side chain on 1st liver passage. Methimazole and propylthiouracil are used widely in the USA and elsewhere in the world.
- During pregnancy and lactation *propylthiouracil* is the drug of choice because of its lower concentration in breast milk and the possible association of carbimazole with aplasia cutis.

Action of thionomides

- Thyroid hormone synthesis is inhibited by blockade of the action of thyroid peroxidase.
- Thionomides are especially actively accumulated in thyrotoxic tissue.
- Propylthiouracil also inhibits the deiodinase type 1 activity, and thus may have advantages when given at high doses in severe thyrotoxicosis.

Dose and effectiveness

- 5mg of carbimazole is roughly equivalent to 50mg of propylthiouracil. Propylthiouracil has a theoretical advantage of inhibiting the conversion of T_4 to T_3, and T_3 levels decline more rapidly after starting the drug.
- 30–40% of patients treated with an ATD remain euthyroid 10 years after discontinuation of therapy. If hyperthyroidism recurs after treatment with an ATD, there is little chance that a 2nd course of treatment will result in permanent remission. Young patients, smokers, those with large goitres, ophthalmopathy, or high serum concentrations of thyrotropin receptor antibody at the time of diagnosis are unlikely to have a permanent remission.
- *β-Adrenergic antagonists* Propranolol 20–80mg 3 × daily. Considerable relief from such symptoms as anxiety, tremor, and palpitations may be gained in the initial 4–8 weeks of treatment.

Atrial fibrillation

Should if present convert to sinus rhythm—otherwise cardiovert after 4 months euthyroid.

Side effects

- ATDs are generally well tolerated. Uncommonly, patients may complain of GI symptoms or an alteration in their sense of taste and smell.
- Agranulocytosis represents a potentially fatal but rare side effect of ATD occurring in 0.1–0.5% of patients. It is less frequent with carbimazole than with propylthiouracil and because cross reactivity of this reaction has been reported, one drug should never be substituted for the other after this reaction has been diagnosed. Agranulocytosis usually occurs within the first 3 months after initiation of therapy (97% within the first 6 months, especially on higher doses) but it is important to be aware of the documented cases, which have occurred (less frequently) a long time after starting treatment.
- As agranulocytosis occurs very suddenly and is potentially fatal, routine monitoring of FBC is thought to be of little use. Patients typically present with fever and evidence of infection, usually in the oropharynx, and *each patient should therefore receive written instructions to discontinue the medication and contact their doctor for a blood count should the situation arise.*
- Neutrophil dyscrasias occur more frequently in ♂, and are more often fatal in the elderly.
- Much more common are the allergic type reactions of rash, urticaria, and arthralgia, which occur in 1–5% of patients taking these drugs. These side effects are often mild and do not usually necessitate drug withdrawal, although one ATD may be substituted for another in the expectation that the second agent may be taken without side effects.
- Thionamides may cause cholestatic jaundice and elevated serum aminotransaminases have been reported, as has fulminant hepatic failure.
- All patients should be given written and verbal warnings about the potential side effects of thionamides.
- Rarely anti-neutrophil cytoplasmic antibody (ANCA) +ve vasculitis develops with propylthiouracil therapy. It may cause arthralgia, skin lesions, glomerulonephritis, fever, and alveolar haemorahge. Skin lesions include ulcers. Biopsy reveals vasculitis. Propylthiouracil should be stopped and steroids may be needed.

Treatment regimen

Two alternative regimens are practised for Graves' disease: dose titration and block and replace.

Dose titration regime

- The 1° aim is to achieve a euthyroid state with relatively high drug doses and then to maintain euthyroidism with a low stable dose. The dose of carbimazole or propylthiouracil is titrated according to the thyroid function tests performed every 4–8 weeks, aiming for a serum free T_4 in the normal range and a detectable TSH. High serum TSH indicates the need for a dose reduction. TSH may remain suppressed for weeks or months.
- The typical starting dose of carbimazole is 20–30mg/day. Higher doses (40–60mg) may be indicated in severe cases, with very high levels of JT4.

- The treatment is continued for 18 months, as this appears to represent the length of therapy which is generally optimal in producing the remission rate of up to 40% at 5 years after discontinuing therapy.
- Relapses are most likely to occur within the 1st year and may be more likely in the presence of a large goitre and high T_4 level at the time of diagnosis, or the presence of TSH-receptor antibodies at the end of treatment (📖 see p.22.)
- Patients with multinodular goitres and thyrotoxicosis always relapse on cessation of antithyroid medication, and definitive treatment with radioiodine or surgery is usually advised. Long-term thionomide therapy at low dose is also an option.

Block and replace regimen
- After achieving an euthyroid state on carbimazole alone, carbimazole at a dose of 40mg daily together with T_4 at a dose of 100mcg can be prescribed. This is usually continued for 6 months.
- The main advantages are fewer hospital visits for checks of thyroid function and shorter duration of treatment.
- Most patients achieve an euthyroid state within 4 – 6 weeks of carbimazole therapy.
- During treatment, FT_4 values are measured 4 weeks after starting thyroxine and the dose of thyroxine altered, if necessary, in 25mcg increments to maintain FT_4 in the normal range. Most patients do not require any dose adjustment.
- The originally reported higher remission rate was not confirmed in a large prospective multicentre European trial when combination treatment was compared to carbimazole alone but side effects were more common.[1]
- Relapses are most likely to occur within the 1st year.

1 Reinwein D, Benker G, Lazarus JH, et al. (1993). A prospective randomized trial of antithyroid drug dose in Graves' disease therapy. European Multicenter Study Group on Antithyroid Drug Treatment. *J Clin Endocrinol Metab* **76**, 1516–21.

Radioiodine treatment—radioiodine therapy

📖 See Table 3.2.

Indications
- Definitive treatment of multinodular goitre or adenoma.
- Relapsed Graves' disease.

Table 3.2 Recommended activity of radioiodine

Aetiology	Comments	Guide dose (MBq)
Graves' disease	First presentation; no significant eye disease	400–600
	Moderate goitre (40–50g)	
Toxic multinodular goitre in older person	Mild heart failure; atrial fibrillation or other concomitant disease, e.g. cancer	500–800
Toxic adenoma	Usually mild hyperthyroidism	500
Severe Graves' disease with thyroid eye disease	Postpone radioiodine till eye disease stable.	500–800
	Prednisolone 40mg to be administered at same time as radioiodine and for further 4–6 weeks (see below)	
Ablation therapy	Severe accompanying medical condition such as heart failure; atrial fibrillation or other concurrent medical disorders (e.g. psychosis)	500–800

Data taken from the use of radioiodine in benign thyroid disease. Royal College of Physicians, 2007.

Contra-indications
- Young children, because of the potential risk of thyroid carcinogenesis.
- Pregnant and lactating ♀.
- Situations where it is clear that the safety of other people cannot be guaranteed.
- *Graves' ophthalmopathy* There is some evidence that Graves' ophthalmopathy may worsen after the administration of radioactive iodine, especially in smokers. In cases of moderate-to-severe ophthalmopathy radioiodine may be avoided. Alternatively steroid cover in a dose of 40mg prednisolone should be administered on the day of administering radioiodine, 30mg daily for the next 2 weeks, 20mg daily for the following 2 weeks, reducing to zero over subsequent 3 weeks. It is essential that euthyroidism is closely maintained following radioiodine to avoid worsening of ophthalmopathy.

Caveats
- The control of disease may not occur for a period of weeks or a few months.
- >1 treatment may be needed in some patients, depending on the dose given; 15% require a 2nd dose and a few patients require a 3rd dose. The 2nd dose should be considered only at least 6 months after the 1st dose.
- Compounds that contain iodine, such as amiodarone, block iodine uptake for a period of several months following cessation of therapy; iodine uptake measurements may be helpful in this instance in determining the activity required and the timing of radioiodine therapy.
- ♀ of childbearing age should avoid pregnancy for a minimum of 6 months following radioactive iodine ablation.
- The prevalence of hypothyroidism is about 50% at 10 years, and continues to increase thereafter.

Side effects are rare
- Anterior neck pain caused by radiation-induced thyroiditis.
- Transient rise (72 hours) in thyroid hormone levels which may exacerbate heart failure if present.

Hypothyroidism after radioiodine
- After radioiodine administration, ATDs may be recommended. The ATDs should be withdrawn gradually guided by a 6–8-weekly thyroid function test. Early post-radioiodine hypothyroidism may be transient. TSH should be monitored initially, then annually after radioiodine to determine late hypothyroidism.
- In patients treated for autonomous toxic nodules the incidence of hypothyroidism is lower since the toxic nodule takes up the radioactive iodine while the surrounding tissue will recover normal function once the hyperthyroidism is controlled, though this is disputed by some experts.

Cancer risk after radioiodine therapy
In a recent large series, no overall excess risk of cancer was found. It is unclear whether the risk of death from thyroid cancer is slightly ↑.

Clinical guidelines
The recommendation is to administer enough radioiodine to achieve euthyroidism with the acceptance of a moderate rate of hypothyroidism, e.g. 15–20% at 2 years.

Instructions to patients before treatment
Discontinue ATDs 2–7 days before radioiodine administration since their effects last for 24h or more, though propylthiouracil has a prolonged radio-protective effect. ATDs may be recommended 3–7 days after radioiodine administration without significantly affecting the delivered radiation dose.

Administration of radioiodine (Table 3.2)
- Radioactive iodine-131 is administered orally as a capsule or a drink.
- There is no universal agreement regarding the optimal dose. Dosing according to size alone is not successful in 90% of cases.
- A dose of 400–800MBq should be sufficient to cure hyperthyroidism in 90%.
- Most patients are treated with 400–600MBq as the first dose, and 600–800MBq if thyrotoxicosis persists 6–12 months after the 1st dose.
- For precaution 🕮 see Table 3.3.

Outcomes of radioiodine treatment[1]
- In general 50–70% of patients have restored normal thyroid function within 6–8 weeks of receiving radioiodine. Shrinkage of goitre occurs but is slower.

---

1 Royal College of Physicians of London (2007). *The use of radioiodine in benign thyroid disease.*

Instructions to patients after treatment
Precautions for patients following treatment with radioiodine are summarized in Table 3.3.

Table 3.3 Number of days to apply caution after radioiodine

Precaution	Administered activity of 131-I MBq			
	≤200	≤400	≤600	≤800
Avoid journeys on public transport >1h	0	0	0	6
Avoid places of entertainment or close contact with other people (duration 3h)	1	5	8	11
Stay off work when travel alone by private transport and work does not involve close contact with other people	0	0	0	0
Stay off work which involves prolonged contact with other people at a distance of 1m, e.g. bank cashier	8	13	16	18
Stay off work which involves close contact with other people including pregnant ♀ or children, work of a radiosensitive nature, or commercial food production	11	17	20	22
Avoid non-essential close contact (<1m) with children, teenagers, pregnant women within the family	16*	22*	25*	27*
Avoid non-essential close contact and sleeping with another person	4	9	13	15

*These times need to be extended if the child concerned is young, fretful, and needs a lot of close contact

Note: These apply only in the UK, they are less stringent in the USA

Surgery

Total thyroidectomy is now considered the operation of choice because of the risk of relapse with partial thyroidectomy. All such patients go home on T4. 📖 See Box 3.2.

Box 3.2 Complications of thyroidectomy

Immediate

- Recurrent laryngeal nerve damage.
- Hypoparathyroidism.
- Thyroid crisis.
- Local haemorrhage, causing laryngeal oedema.
- Wound infection.

Late

- Hypothyroidism.
- Keloid formation.

Indications

- Documented suspicious or malignant thyroid nodule by FNAC.
- Pregnant mothers who are not adequately controlled by ATDs or in whom serious allergic reactions develop while being treated medically. Thyroidectomy is usually performed in the 2nd trimester.
- Patients:
  - Who reject or fear exposure to radiation.
  - With poor compliance to medical treatment.
  - In whom a rapid control of symptoms is desired.
  - With severe manifestations of Graves' ophthalmopathy, as total or near total thyroidectomy does not worsen eye manifestations.
  - With relapsed Graves' disease.
  - With local compressive symptoms which may not improve rapidly with radioiodine, whereas operation removes these symptoms in most patients.
  - With large thyroid glands and relatively low radioiodine uptake.

Preparation of patients for surgery

- ATDs should be used preoperatively to achieve euthyroidism.
- Propranolol may be added to achieve β-blockade especially in those patients where surgery must be performed sooner than achieving euthyroid state.
- Potassium iodide, 60mg 3 × daily can be used during the preoperative period to prevent an unwanted liberation of thyroid hormones during surgery. Preoperatively it should be given for 10 days. Operating later than this can be associated with exacerbation of thyrotoxicosis as the thyroid escapes from the inhibitory effect of the iodide. In practice it is rarely needed as good control of thyrotoxicosis can be achieved with ATDs in the majority of patients.
- In the patient who appears to be non-compliant with ATDs and remains thyrotoxic prior to surgery, it may be necessary to admit them as an inpatient for supervised administration of high dose ATDs, together with β-blockade, and measurement of FT_4 and FT_3 twice weekly. There is a risk of thyroid crisis, or storm if a patient undergoes operation when thyrotoxic. Most patients can be rendered euthyroid within 2–4 weeks and potassium iodide can be administered as above to coincide with the timing of surgery.
- Additional measures are as for thyroid storm.

Thyroid crisis (storm)

Thyroid crisis represents a rare but life-threatening exacerbation of the manifestations of thyrotoxicosis. It should be promptly recognized since the condition is associated with a significant mortality (30–50% depending on series), 📖 see Box 3.3. Thyroid crisis develops in hyperthyroid patients who:

• Have an acute infection.
• Undergo thyroidal or non thyroidal surgery or (rarely) radioiodine treatment.

Thyroid crisis should be considered in a very sick patient if there is:

• Recent history suggestive of thyrotoxicosis.
• Acute stressful precipitating factor such as surgery.
• History of previous thyroid treatment.

Box 3.3 Clinical signs suggestive of a thyroid storm

• Alteration in mental status.
• High fever.
• Tachycardia or tachyarrhythmias.
• Severe clinical hyperthyroid signs.
• Vomiting, jaundice, and diarrhoea.
• Multisystem decompensation: cardiac failure, respiratory distress, congestive hepatomegaly, dehydration, and prerenal failure.

Laboratory investigations

• Routine haematology may indicate a leukocytosis, which is well-recognized in thyrotoxicosis even in the absence of infection.
• The biochemical screen may reveal a raised alkaline phosphatase and mild hypercalcaemia.
• Thyroid function tests and thyroid antibodies should be requested although treatment should not be delayed while awaiting the results.
• The levels of thyroid hormones will be raised but may not be grossly elevated and are usually within the range of uncomplicated thyrotoxicosis.

Treatment
General supportive therapy

- The patient is best managed in an intensive care unit where close attention can be paid to the cardiorespiratory status, fluid balance, and cooling.
- Standard anti-arrhythmic drugs can be used, including digoxin (usually in higher than normal dose) after correction for hypokalaemia. If anticoagulation is indicated because of atrial fibrillation then it must be remembered that thyrotoxic patients are very sensitive to warfarin.
- Chlorpromazine (50–100mg IM) can be used to treat agitation and because of its effect in inhibiting central thermoregulation it may be useful in treating the hyperpyrexia.
- Broad-spectrum antibiotics should be given if infection is suspected.

Specific treatment

- Aim: to inhibit thyroid hormone synthesis completely.
  - Propylthiouracil 200–300mg 6-hourly via NG tube. Propylthiouracil is preferred because of its ability to block T_4 to T_3 conversion in peripheral tissues. There are no clinical data comparing propylthiouracil and carbimazole in this situation. ATDs should be commenced first.
- Potassium iodide 60mg via NG tube, 6-hourly, 6h *after* starting propylthiouracil will inhibit thyroid hormone release.
- B-adrenergic blocking agents are essential in the management to control tachycardia, tremor, and other adrenergic manifestations:
  - Propranolol 160–480mg/day in divided doses or as an infusion at a rate of 2–5mg/h.
- Calcium channel blockers can be tried in patients with known bronchospastic disease where β-blockade is contraindicated.
- High doses of glucocorticoids are capable of blocking T_4 to T_3 conversion: Prednisolone 60mg daily or hydrocortisone 40mg IM, 4 × daily.
- Plasmapheresis and peritoneal dialysis may be effective in cases resistant to the usual pharmacological measures.
- Colestyramine (3g tds) reduces the entero-hepatic circulation of thyroid hormones and may help improve thyrotoxicosis.

Subclinical hyperthyroidism

- Values of thyroid hormones should be repeated to exclude non thyroidal illness.
- Subclinical hyperthyroidism is defined as undetectable thyrotrophin (TSH) concentration in patients with normal levels of T_4 and T_3. Subtle symptoms and signs of thyrotoxicosis may be present.
- May be classified as endogenous in patients with thyroid hormone production associated with nodular thyroid disease or underlying Graves' disease; and as exogenous in those with undetectable serum thyrotropin concentrations as a result of treatment with levothyroxine.

The evidence that subclinical hyperthyroidism is a risk factor for the development of atrial fibrillation or osteoporosis is definitive[1].

- The ↑ risk of fracture reported in older ♀ taking thyroid hormone disappears when those with a history of hyperthyroidism are excluded.
- In many patients with endogeneous subclinical hyperthyroidism who do not have nodular thyroid disease or complications of excess thyroid hormone, treatment is unnecessary, but thyroid-function tests should be performed every 6 months. In older patients with atrial fibrillation or osteoporosis that could have been caused or exacerbated by the mild excess of thyroid hormone, ablative therapy with ^{131}I is the best initial option.
- In patients with exogenous subclinical hyperthyroidism, the dose of levothyroxine should be reduced, excluding those with prior thyroid cancer in whom thyrotropin suppression may be required. The dose of levothyroxine used for treating hypothyroidism may be reduced if the patient develops:
  - New atrial fibrillation, angina or cardiac failure.
  - Accelerated bone loss.
  - Borderline high serum triiodothyronine concentration.

1 Parle JV, Maisonneuve P, Sheppard MC, *et al.* (2001). Prediction of all-cause and cardiovascular mortality in elderly people from one low serum thyrotropin result: a 10-year cohort study. *Lancet* **358**(9285), 861–5.

Thyrotoxic hypokalaemic periodic paralysis

- More common in Asians (5–10% of all with thyrotoxicosis due to Graves' disease or multinodular goitre) (0.1–0.2% of non-Asian Europeans/North Americans).
- Aetiology is probably due to disordered function of ion channels in cell membranes.
- Most common form of acquired periodic paralysis.
- Usual age of onset 20–40 years, mostly ♂.
- Recurrent episodes of muscle weakness.
- Duration minutes to days.
- Flaccid paralysis, usually spreading from legs proximally.
- Clinical manifestations of thyrotoxicosis may be few and thus TSH should be checked in anyone presenting with periodic paralysis.
- Improves as thyrotoxicosis treated.
- Low serum potassium during attacks.
- CPK ↑ during recovery phase.
- Precipitated by carbohydrates, insulin, cold, vigorous exercise.
- Treatment with potassium replacement, usually by oral route, and treatment of thyrotoxicosis.
- Symptoms usually improve within 2–4 hours, full resolution in 24–48 hours.
- Non-selective β-blockers, such as propranolol (3mg/kg) help prevent attacks until a euthyroid state achieved.

Thyrotoxicosis in pregnancy

(📖 also see p.428.)

- Thyrotoxicosis occurs in about 0.2% of pregnancies.
- Graves' disease accounts for 90% of cases.
- Less common causes include toxic adenoma and multinodular goitre.
- Other causes are gestational hyperthyroidism (hyperemesis gravidarum) and trophoblastic neoplasia.
- Diagnosis of thyrotoxicosis during pregnancy may be difficult or delayed.
- Physiological changes of pregnancy are similar to those of hyperthyroidism.
- Total T_4 and T_3 are elevated in pregnancy because of an elevated level of TBG but, with free hormone assays available, this is no longer a problem.
- Physiological features of normal pregnancy include an increase in basal metabolic rate, cardiac stroke volume, palpitation, and heat intolerance.
- Serum free T_3 concentrations remain within the normal range in most pregnant ♀; serum TSH concentration decreases during the 1st trimester.

Symptoms

- Hyperemesis gravidarum is the classic presentation ($\frac{1}{3}$ are toxic). Tiredness, palpitations, insomnia, heat intolerance, proximal muscle weakness, shortness of breath, and irritability may be other presenting symptoms.
- Thyrotoxicosis may occasionally be diagnosed when the patient presents with pregnancy-induced hypertension or congestive heart failure.

Signs

- Failure to gain weight despite a good appetite.
- Persistent tachycardia with a pulse rate >90 beats/min at rest.
- Other signs of thyrotoxicosis as described previously.

Natural history of Graves' disease in pregnancy

There is aggravation of symptoms in the 1st half of the pregnancy; amelioration of symptoms in the 2nd half of the pregnancy, and often recurrence of symptoms in the postpartum period.

Transient hyperthyroidism of gestational hyperthyroidism (hyperemesis gravidarum)

- The likely mechanism is a raised β-hCG level.
- βhCG, LH, FSH, and TSH are glycoprotein hormones that contain a common α-subunit and a hormone-specific β-subunit. There is an inverse relationship between the serum levels of TSH and hCG, best seen in early pregnancy. There is also structural homology of the TSH and hCG receptors.
- Serum free T_4 concentration may be ↑ and the TSH levels suppressed in ♀ with hyperemesis gravidarum.
- Thyroid function tests recover after the resolution of hyperemesis.
- Pregnant ♀ with gestational hyperthyroidism (hyperemesis gravidarum), (which only accounts for 2/3 of hyperemesis) are not usually given ATD treatment but managed supportively with fluids, antiemetics, and nutritional support.
- There is no ↑ risk of thyrotoxicosis in subsequent pregnancies.
- Can be differentiated from Graves' disease by the absence of a goitre, antithyroid antibodies, or family history of Graves' disease, a history of other autoimmune phenomena and a previous history of ophthalmic Graves'.

Management of Graves' disease in the mother

- Aim of treatment is alleviation of thyroid symptoms and normalization of tests in the shortest time. Patients should be seen every 4–8 weeks and TFTs performed. Serum free T_4 is the best test to follow the response to ATDs. Block and replace regimen should not be used as this will result in fetal hypothyroidism.
- Both propylthiouracil (150mg bd.) and carbimazole (10–20mg once daily) are effective in controlling the disease in pregnancy. As propylthiouracil is more bound to plasma proteins, theoretically less of the drug would be transferred to the fetus. Most use propylthiouracil in pregnancy because this not associated with aplasia cutis which may be the case for carbimazole. A β-blocker (propranolol 20–40mg 6–8-hourly) is effective in controlling the hypermetabolic symptoms but should be used only for a few weeks until symptoms abate.
- The dosage of ATDs is frequently adjusted during the course of the pregnancy; therefore thyroid tests should be done at 2–4 week intervals, with the goal of keeping free thyroid hormone levels in the upper 1/3 of the reference range.
- Thyroid tests may normalize spontaneously with the progression of a normal pregnancy as a result of immunological changes.
- The use of iodides and radioiodine is contraindicated in pregnancy.
- Surgery is rarely performed in pregnancy. It is reserved for patients not responding to ATDs. It is preferable to perform surgery in the 2nd trimester.
- Breast-feeding mothers should be treated with the lowest possible dose of propylthiouracil.

Prepregnancy counselling

- Hyperthyroid ♀ who want to conceive should attain euthyroidism before conception, since uncontrolled hyperthyroidism is associated with an ↑ risk of congenital abnormalities (stillbirth and cranial synostosis are the most serious complications). 📖 See Box 3.4.
- There is no evidence that radioactive iodine treatment given to the mother 6 months or more before pregnancy has an adverse effect on the fetus or on an offspring in later life.
- Antithyroid medication requirements decrease during gestation; in about 50–60% of the dose may be discontinued in the last few weeks of gestation.
- The risk of recurrent hyperthyroidism should be discussed with the patient
- The rare occurrence of fetal and neonatal hyperthyroidism should be included during counselling sessions and the diagnosis of Graves' hyperthyroidism conveyed to the obstetrician and neonatologist.

Management of the fetus

- The hypothalamo–pituitary–thyroid axis is well developed at 12 weeks gestation but remains inactive until 18–20 weeks. Circulating TSH receptor antibodies (TSH-RAB) in the mother can cross the placenta. The risk of hyperthyroidism to the neonate can be assessed by measuring TSH-RAB in the maternal circulation at the beginning of the 3rd trimester. Antithyroglobulin antibody and thyroid peroxidase antibodies have no effect on the fetus.
- Long-term follow-up studies of children whose mothers received either carbimazole or propylthiouracil have not shown an ↑ incidence of any physical or psychological defects. The block and replace regimen using relatively high doses of carbimazole is contraindicated because the ATDs cross the placenta, but replacement T_4 does not, thus potentially rendering the fetus hypothyroid.
- Monitoring the fetal heart rate and growth rates are the standard means whereby fetal thyrotoxicosis may be detected. A rate >160 beats/min is suspicious of fetal thyrotoxicosis in the 3rd trimester. Fetal thyrotoxicosis may complicate the latter part of the pregnancy of ♀ with Graves' disease even if they have previously been treated with radioiodine or surgery since TSH receptor antibodies may persist. If there is evidence of fetal thyrotoxicosis, the dose of the ATD should be ↑. If this causes maternal hypothyroidism a small dose of T_4 can be added since, unlike carbimazole, T_4 crosses the placenta less. A paediatrician should be involved to monitor neonatal thyroid function and detect thyrotoxicosis.
- Hypothyroidism in the mother should be avoided because of the potential adverse effect on subsequent cognitive function of the neonate, 📖 see Box 3.4.
- If the mother has been treated with carbimazole, the post-delivery levels of T_4 may be low and neonatal levels of T_4 may only rise to the thyrotoxic range after a few days. In addition, TSH is usually absent in neonates who subsequently develop thyrotoxicosis. Clinical indicators of neonatal thyrotoxicosis include low birth weight, poor weight gain, tachycardia, and irritability. Carbimazole can be given at a dose of 0.5 mg/kg per day and withdrawn after a few weeks after the level of TSH-RAB declines.

Box 3.4 Potential maternal and fetal complications in uncontrolled hyperthyroidism in pregnancy

Maternal
- Pregnancy induced hypertension
- Preterm delivery
- Congestive heart failure
- Thyroid storm
- Miscarriage
- Abruptio placentae accidental haemorrhage

Fetal
- Hyperthyroidism
- Neonatal hyperthyroidism
- Intrauterine growth retardation
- Small-for-gestation age
- Prematurity
- Stillbirth
- Cranial synostosis

Postpartum thyroiditis

- Defined as a syndrome of postpartum thyrotoxicosis or hypothyroidism in ♀ who were euthyroid during pregnancy.
- Postpartum thyroid dysfunction, which occurs in ♀ with autoimmune thyroid disease, is characterized in a 1/3 by a thyrotoxic phase occurring in the first 3 months postpartum, followed by a hypothyroid phase that occurs 3–6 months after delivery, followed by spontaneous recovery. In the remaining 2/3, a single-phase pattern or the reverse occurs.
- 5–7% percent of ♀ develop biochemical evidence of thyroid dysfunction after delivery. An ↑ incidence is seen in patients with type I diabetes mellitus (25%), other autoimmune diseases, in the presence of anti-TPO antibodies and in the presence of a family history of thyroid disease.
- Hyperthyroidism due to Graves' disease accounts for 10–15% of all cases of postpartum thyrotoxicosis. In the majority of cases hyperthyroidism occurs later in the postpartum period (>3–6 months) and persists.
- Providing the patient is not breast-feeding, a radioiodine uptake scan can differentiate the 2 principal causes of autoimmune thyrotoxicosis by demonstrating ↑ uptake in Graves' disease and low uptake in postpartum thyroiditis.
- Graves' hyperthyroidism should be treated with ATDs. Propylthiouracil is preferable if the patient is breast-feeding. Thyrotoxic symptoms due to postpartum thyrotoxicosis are managed symptomatically using propranolol.
- 1/3 of affected ♀ with postpartum thyroiditis develop symptoms of hypothyroidism and may require T_4 for 6–12 months. There is a suggestion of an ↑ risk of postpartum depression in those with hypothyroidism.
- Histology of the thyroid in the case of postpartum thyroiditis shows lymphocytic infiltration with destructive thyroiditis and predominantly occurs at 16 weeks in ♀ with +ve antimicrosomal antibodies.
- There is an ↑ chance of subsequent permanent hypothyroidism in 25–30%. Patients with a history of postpartum thyroiditis should be followed up with annual TSH measurements.

Hyperthyroidism in children

Epidemiology

Thyrotoxicosis is rare before the age of 5 years. Although there is a progressive increase in incidence throughout childhood it is still rare and accounts for <5% of all cases of Graves' disease.

Clinical features

- Behavioural abnormalities, hyperactivity, declining school performance may bring the child to medical attention. Features of hyperthyroidism are as described previously.
- Acceleration of linear growth is common in patients increasing in height percentiles on the growth charts. The disease may be part of McCune–Albright syndrome and café-au-lait pigmentation, precocious puberty, and bony abnormalities should be considered during clinical examination.

Investigations

The cause of thyrotoxicosis in children is nearly always Graves' disease (with +ve antibodies to thyroglobulin, thyroid peroxidase, or both) although thyroiditis and toxic nodules have been described and a radioiodine scan may be useful if the diagnosis is not clear. Hereditary syndromes of thyroid hormone resistance often misdiagnosed as Graves' disease are now being increasingly recognized in children.

Treatment

ATDs represent the treatment of choice for thyrotoxic children. Therapy is generally started with propylthiouracil 2.5–5mg/kg (initial dose 75–150mg/day) or carbimazole 250mcg/kg (initial dose 10mg/day). Since relapse after withdrawal of ATDs is common, these drugs are often continued long term, until education is complete and definitive treatment with surgery or radioiodine can be offered.

Secondary hyperthyroidism

An elevated serum free T4 and non-suppressed serum TSH are characteristic of TSH secreting adenomas or resistance to thyroid hormone.
These conditions must be differentiated (Table 3.4).

TSH-secreting pituitary tumours

- <1% of all pituitary tumours.
- There are characteristically *elevated* serum free T_4 and T_3 concentrations and *non-suppressed* (inappropriately normal or frankly
  elevated) serum TSH levels.
- Among the 280 TSHomas reported in the literature (until 1998),
  72% secreted TSH alone; the remainder co-secreted growth hormone
  (16%), prolactin (11%), or rarely gonadotrophins. Approximately
  90% were macroadenomas (>1cm in diameter) and 71% exhibited
  suprasellar extension, invasion, or both into adjacent tissues
  (📖 see p.160).
- Patients with pure TSHomas present with typical symptoms and
  signs of thyrotoxicosis and the presence of a diffuse goitre. Patients
  may exhibit features of over secretion of the other pituitary
  hormones, e.g. prolactin or growth hormone. Headaches, visual field
  defects, menstrual irregularities, amenorrhoea, delayed puberty, and
  hypogonadotrophic hypogonadism have also been reported. Careful
  establishment of the diagnosis is the key to treatment. Inappropriate
  treatment of such patients with subtotal thyroidectomy or radioiodine
  administration not only fails to cure the underlying disorder but may be
  associated with subsequent pituitary tumour enlargement and an ↑ risk
  of invasiveness into adjacent tissues.
- Treatment options are:
  - Trans-phenoidal surgery.
  - Pituitary radiotherapy if surgical results are unsatisfactory, or
    surgery is contraindicated or not desired.
  - Medical therapy with somatostatin analogues such as octreotide
    or lanreotide may be useful preoperatively and suppresses TSH
    secretion in 80% of the cases.

Resistance to thyroid hormones

- Patients with generalized resistance to thyroid hormone (GRTH)
  may present with mild hyperthyroidism, deaf mutism, delayed bone
  maturation, raised circulating thyroid hormone concentrations,
  non-suppressed TSH, and failure of TSH to decrease normally upon
  administration of supraphysiological doses of thyroid hormones. Most
  patients present with goitre or incidentally found abnormal TFTs.
  Treatment is determined by thyroid status.
- In selective pituitary resistance to thyroid hormones (PRTH) the
  thyroid hormone resistance is more pronounced in the pituitary; thus
  the patient exhibits definite clinical manifestations of thyrotoxicosis.
- About 90% of thyroid hormone resistance syndromes result from
  mutations in the gene encoding TRβ. Mutant receptors have a reduced
  affinity for T_3 and are functionally deficient. It is usually inherited in

an autosomal dominant pattern with the affected individuals being heterozygous for the mutation.

- A subset of RTH receptors has been identified that are capable of inhibiting wild type receptor action. When co-expressed, the mutant proteins are able to inhibit the function of their wild type counterparts in a dominant −ve manner.
- Common features of patients with the thyroid hormones resistance syndromes include goitre (most commonly), and less so, tachycardia, hyperkinetic behaviour, emotional disturbances, ear, nose, and throat infections, language disabilities, auditory disorders, low body weight, cardiac abnormalities, and subnormal intelligence quotients.

Treatment options in RTH are not usually necessary. In PTR treatment may be needed but this is uncommon. Chronic suppression of TSH secretion with D T4, triiodo-thyroacetic acid, octreotide, or bromocriptine. If this is ineffective, thyroid ablation with radioiodine or surgery with subsequent close monitoring of thyroid hormone status and pituitary gland size.

Table 3.4 Tests useful in the differential diagnosis of TSHomas, PRTH, and GRTH

Test	TSHomas	PRTH	GRTH
Clinical thyrotoxicosis	Present	Present	Absent
Family history	Absent	Present	Present
TSH response to TRH	No change	Increase	Increase
TSH response to T$_3$ (100mcg/day + β-blockers)	No change	Decrease	Decrease
SHBG	Elevated–92%[a]	Normal[b]	Normal
α-subunit	Elevated–65%	2% elevated	
Pituitary MRI	Tumour–30% micoradenoma[c]	Normal	Normal
Fall in TSH on octreotide LAR 20mg/month for 2 months	95%	No change	No Change

[a] Not usually raised in mixed GH/TSH tumour.
[b] Peripheral markers of toxicosis sometimes affected (8% SHBG elevated).
[c] The best biochemical test is an elevated α-subunit

Further reading

Allahabadia A, Heward JM, Nithiyananthan R, et al. (2001). MHC class II region, CTLA4 gene, and ophthalmopathy in patients with Graves' disease. *Lancet* **358**(9286), 984–5.

Brent GP (2008). Grave's disease. *NEJM* **358**, 2594–605.

Brix TH, Kyvik KO, and Hegedus L (1998). What is the evidence of genetic factors in the etiology of Graves' disease? A brief review. *Thyroid* **8**, 727–34.

Franklyn JA, Maisonneuve P, Sheppard MC, et al. (1998). Mortality after the treatment of hyperthyroidism with radioactive iodine. *New Engl J Med* **338**, 712–8.

Franklyn JA, Maisonneuve P, Sheppard MC, et al. (1999). Cancer incidence and mortality after radioiodine treatment for hyperthyroidism: a population-based cohort study. *Lancet* **353**, 2111–15.

Gunji K, Kubota S, Swanson J, et al. (1998). Role of the eye muscles in thyroid eye disease: identification of the principal autoantigens. *Thyroid* **8**, 553–6 [Erratum *Thyroid* 1998, **8**, 1079].

Helfgott S and Smith RN (2002). Weekly clinicopathological exercises: Case 21-2002: A 21-year-old man with arthritis during treatment for hyperthyroidism. *New Engl J Med* **347**(2), 122–30.

Helfgott S and Smith RN (2002). Case records of the Massachusetts general hospital. Weekly clinicopathological exercises. Case 21-2002. A 21-year-old man with arthritis during treatment for hyperthyroidism. *New Engl J Med* **347**(2), 122–30.

Parle JV, Maisonneuve P, Sheppard MC, et al. (2001). Prediction of all-cause and cardiovascular mortality in elderly people from one low serum thyrotropin result: a 10-year cohort study. *Lancet* **358**(9285), 861–5.

Pearce SH (2004). Spontaneous reporting of adverse reactions to carbimazole and propylthiouracil in the UK. *Clin Endocrinol* **61**(5), 589–94.

Panzer C, Beazley R, Braverman L. (2004). Rapid preoperative preparation for severe hyperthyroid Graves' disease. *J Clin Endocrinol Metab* **89**(5), 2142–4.

Rivkees SA, Sklar C, and Freemark M (1998). The management of Graves's disease in children, with special emphasis on radioiodine treatment. *J Clin Endocrinol Metab* **83**, 3767–76.

Ron E, Doody MM, Becker DV et al. (1998). Cancer mortality following treatment for adult hyperthyroidism. Cooperative Thyrotoxicosis Therapy Follow-up Study Group. *JAMA* **280**, 347–55.

Toft AD (2001). Clinical practice. Subclinical hyperthyroidism *New Engl J Med* **345**(7), 512–16.

Weetman AP (2000). Graves's disease. *New Engl J Med* **343**(17), 1236–48.

Weetman AP, Pickerill AP, Watson P, et al. (1994). Treatment of Graves' disease with the block-replace regimen of antithyroid drugs: the effect of treatment duration and immunogenetic susceptibility on relapse. *QJM* **87**, 337–41.

Graves' ophthalmopathy, dermopathy, and acropachy

Graves' ophthalmopathy

(✍ see European Working Group on Graves' Ophthalmopathy www. EUGOGO.org)

- An organ-specific autoimmune disorder characterized by swelling of the extra-ocular muscles, lymphocytic infiltration, late fibrosis, muscle tethering, and proliferation of orbital fat and connective tissue.
- Clinically evident in ~30% of patients. Most have mild disease, but 5% have severe disease that threatens sight.
- Incidence higher in ♀ (except for severe disease where equal sex-incidence)
- Bimodal age distribution in ♀, with peak onsets between 40–44 years and 60–64 years. In ♂, a single peak incidence occurs at 65–69 years.
- There are 2 stages in the development of the disease, which can be recognized as an active inflammatory (dynamic) stage and a relatively quiescent static stage. 5% of patients with Graves' ophthalmopathy have hypothyroidism and 5% are euthyroid. 75% of patients develop Graves' disease within a year either side of Graves' ophthalmopathy developing. The lesions are due to localized accumulation of glycosaminoglycans.
- The appearance of eye disease follows a different time course to thyroid dysfunction and in a minority there is a lag period between the presentation of hyperthyroidism and the appearance of eye signs.
- Smoking and hypothyroidism moderately worsen Graves' ophthalmopathy.
- Current smokers (>20/day) are more likely to develop ophthalmopathy.
- The role of an endocrinologist during a routine review of Graves' patients is to record accurately the clinical features of Graves' eye disease and to identify ocular emergencies, such as corneal ulceration, congestive ophthalmopathy, and optic neuropathy, which should be referred urgently to an ophthalmologist.

Clinical features

- Retraction of eyelids is extremely common in thyroid eye disease. The margin of the upper eyelid normally rests about 2 mm below the limbus and retraction can be suspected if the lid margin is either level or above the superior limbus allowing the sclera to be visible. The lower lid normally rests at the inferior limbus and retraction is suspected when the sclera shows above the lid.
- Proptosis or exophthalmos can result in failure of lid closure, ↑ the likelihood of exposure keratitis and the common symptom of gritty eyes. This can be confirmed with a fluorescein or Rose Bengal stain. As papilloedema can occur, fundoscopy should be performed. Proptosis may result in periorbital oedema and chemosis because the displaced orbit results in less efficient orbital drainage.

- Persistent visual blurring may indicate an optic neuropathy and requires urgent treatment.
- Severe conjunctival pain may indicate corneal ulceration requiring urgent referral.
- Features are unilateral in approximately 15% of cases.

Investigation of proptosis

The 'NOSPECS' classification is not universally accepted, for detailed classification see ⚙ www.EUGOGO.org and The European Group on Graves' Orbitopathy[1].

- *Documentation using a Hertel exophthalmometer* The feet of the apparatus are placed against the lateral orbital margin as defined by the zygomatic bones. The marker on the body of the exophthalmometer is then superimposed on the reflection of the contralateral one by adjusting the scale. The position of each cornea can be read off against the reflections on a millimetre scale as seen on the mirror of the apparatus. A normal result is generally taken as being <20mm (<18mm in Asians, <22 in Afro-Carribeans). A reading of 21mm or more is abnormal and a difference of 2mm between the eyes is suspicious.
- *Soft tissue involvement* Soft tissue signs and symptoms include conjunctival hyperaemia, chemosis, and foreign body sensation. The soft tissue changes can be 2° to exposure but are often seen in the absence of these aetiological factors.
- *CT or MRI scan of the orbit* demonstrates enlargement of the extra-ocular muscles and this can be useful in cases of diagnostic difficulty. This is also more accurate for demonstration of proptosis.

Ophthalmoplegia

- Patients may complain of diplopia due to ocular muscle dysfunction caused by either oedema during the early active phase or fibrosis during the later phase. Assessment using a Hess chart may be helpful. Intra-optic pressure may increase on upgaze and result in compression of the globe by a fibrotic inferior rectus muscle. Ocular mobility may be restricted by oedema during the active inflammatory phase or by fibrosis during the fibrotic stage.
- The 2 most common findings are defective elevation caused by fibrotic contraction of the inferior rectus muscle and a convergence defect caused by fibrotic contraction of the medial rectus. Disorders of the medial rectus, superior rectus, and lateral rectus muscle produce typical signs of defective adduction, depression and abduction respectively.

1 The European Group on Graves' Orbitopathy (2006). Clinical assessment of patients with Graves' orbitopathy: recommendations to generalists, specialists and clinical researchers. *Eur J Endocrinol* **155**(3), 387–9.

Examining for possible optic neuropathy

- History of *poor vision*, a recent or *rapid change in vision*, or *poor colour vision* are reasons for prompt referral.
- A *visual acuity* of <6/18 warrants referral to an ophthalmologist. For *colour vision*, each eye should be evaluated by using a simple 15-plate Ishihara colour vision test. Colour vision is a subtle indicator of optic nerve function. Failure to identify >2 of the plates with either eye is an indication for referral. This is unhelpful in the 8% of ♂ who may be colour blind.
- *Marcus Gunn pupil* The 'swinging flashlight' test detects the presence of an *afferent pupillary defect*.

Medical treatment

📖 See Box 4.1.

Simple treatment for lid retraction

- Most patients do not require any treatment, since clinical signs usually improve with treatment of hyperthyroidism or spontaneously with time (40%).
- Sunglasses help with photophobia and excess tears.
- In patients with significant lid retraction and exposure keratopathy, topical lubricants improve symptoms (surgery to reduce the vertical lid fissures can be considered).
- Botulinum toxin injection may reduce upper lid retraction.
- Head elevation during sleep and diuretics may help congestion.

Acute treatment for active ophthalmopathy threatening sight

- Glucocorticoids at high dose (60–80mg/day) improve ophthalmopathy in 60–75% of cases.
- Effectiveness is more likely in those with diplopia at neutral gaze and an inflammatory component to ophthalmoplegia.
- Treatment should be given for 2 weeks and then tapered gradually.
- Urgent referral to ophthalmologist is indicated for any suspicion of optic neuropathy or corneal ulceration.

Orbital radiotherapy

- Indications for lens-sparing orbital radiotherapy are similar to those for high-dose glucocorticoids.
- Radiotherapy probably works by reducing the activity and number of activated lymphocytes in the retrobulbar tissues.
- 20 Gray delivered over 10 fractions is the standard regimen.
- Treatment with both radiotherapy and glucocorticoids is more effective than either alone.
- Effectiveness in 60% of cases <40 years.

Other medical therapies

- Other immunosuppressive regimens have no proven place in the general management of Graves' ophthalmopathy.
- Use of depot octreotide has been shown to be of no benefit in management.

Surgical treatment

📖 See Box 4.1.

Surgery for decompression

- Orbital decompression may be indicated for urgent treatment of optic neuropathy.
- Posteromedial wall of orbit usually removed.
- Complications include dysmotility of the eye, blindness, orbital cellulitis, CSF leak, cerebral haematoma, obstruction to nasolacrimal flow and anosmia.

Surgery for strabismus

- Should be performed after any necessary orbital decompression.
- Aims to allow correct binocular vision.
- Is performed when eyes are in a quiescent phase for at least 6 months after active disease.
- Involves alteration, loosening or tightening of eye muscles, often over several operations, to improve binocular vision.

Eye lid surgery

Is the final stage of any surgical approach and aims to adjust upper and lower eyelid position to improve comfort and appearance.

Box 4.1 Treatment of Graves' ophthalmopathy

General measures:

- Stop smoking
- Dark glasses, with eye protection
- Control thyroid function

Specific measures:

Problem	Treatment
Grittiness	Artificial tears and simple eye ointment
Eyelid retraction	Tape eyelids at night to avoid corneal damage. Surgery if risk of exposure keratopathy
Proptosis	Head elevation during sleep Diuretics Systemic steroids Radiotherapy Orbital decompression
Optic neuropathy	Systemic steroids Radiotherapy Orbital decompression
Ophthalmoplegia	Prisms in the acute phase Orbital decompression Orbital muscle surgery

Graves' dermopathy

- This is a rare complication of Graves' thyrotoxicosis (0.5%). It is usually pre-tibial in location (99%) and hence called *pre-tibial myxoedema*.
- Associated with ophthalmopathy (97%) and acropachy (18%)
- It typically appears as raised, discoloured, and indurated lesions on the front or back of the legs, or on the dorsum of the feet, and has occasionally been described in other areas, including the hands and the face.
- The lesions are due to localized accumulation of *glycosaminoglycans*. It is now recognized that there is a lymphocytic infiltrate. Lesions are characteristically asymptomatic but they can also be pruritic and tender. They can be very disfiguring.
- *Treatment* Usually not treated. Potent topical fluorinated steroids such as fluocinolone acetonide may be effective (4–8 weeks), not only in the treatment of localized pain and tenderness but also in some resolution of the visible skin signs. Surgery may worsen the condition.
- 25% remit completely; 50% are chronic on no therapy. topical steroids on remission rates is unproven.

Thyroid acropachy

- This is the rarest manifestation of Graves' disease.
- It presents as clubbing of the digits and sub-periosteal new bone formation. The soft tissue swelling is similar to that seen in localized myxoedema and consists of glycosaminoglycan accumulation.
- Patients almost inevitably have Graves' ophthalmopathy or pretibial myxoedema. If not, an alternative cause of clubbing should be looked for.
- It is typically painless and there is no effective treatment.

Further reading

Schwartz KM, Fatourechi V, Ahmed DD, et al. (1992). Dermopathy of Graves' disease (pretibial myxedema): long-term outcome. *J Clin Endocrinol Metab* **87**(2), 438–46

Tellez M, Cooper J, and Edmonds C (1992). Graves' ophthalmopathy in relation to cigarette smoking and ethnic origin. *Clin Endocrinol* **36**, 291–4.

The European Group on Graves' Orbitopathy (2006). Clinical assessment of patients with Graves' orbitopathy: recommendations to generalists, specialists and clinical researchers. *Eur J Endocrinol* **155**(3), 387–9.

Multinodular goitre and solitary adenomas

Background

Nodular thyroid disease denotes the presence of single or multiple palpable or non-palpable nodules within the thyroid gland.

- Prevalence rates range from 5–50% depending on population studied and sensitivity of detection methods. Prevalence increases linearly with age, exposure to ionizing radiation and iodine deficiency.
- Clinically apparent thyroid nodules are evident in ~10% of the UK population.
- Incidence of thyroid nodules is about 4 × more in ♀.
- Thyroid nodules always raise the concern of cancer, but <5% are cancerous.

Clinical evaluation

- An asymptomatic thyroid mass may be discovered either by a clinician on routine neck palpation or by the patient during self-examination.
- History should concentrate on:
  - An enlarging thyroid mass.
  - A previous history of radiation, especially childhood head and neck irradiation.
  - A family history of thyroid cancer.
  - The development of hoarseness or dysphagia.
- Nodules are more likely to be malignant in patients <20 or >60 years.
- Thyroid nodules are more common in ♀ but more likely to be malignant in ♂.
- Physical findings suggestive of malignancy include a firm or hard non-tender nodule; a recent history of enlargement, fixation to adjacent tissue, and the presence of regional lymphadenopathy.
- *Pemberton's sign* is facial erythema and jugular venous distension on raising the arms. It is a sign of superior venacaval obstruction caused by a sub-sternal mass.
- A hot nodule on a radioisotope scan makes malignancy less likely.
- 📖 See Box 5.1 for aetiology of thyroid nodules.

Box 5.1 Aetiology of thyroid nodules

Common causes
- Colloid nodule.
- Cyst.
- Lymphocytic thyroiditis.
- Benign neoplasms;
  - Hurthle cell.
  - Follicular.
- Malignancy:
  - Papillary.
  - Follicular.

Uncommon causes
- Granulomatous thyroiditis.
- Infections.
- Malignancy:
  - Medullary.
  - Anaplastic.
  - Metastatic.
  - Lymphoma.

Clinical features raising the suspicion of thyroid malignancy
- Age (childhood or elderly).
- Short history of enlarging nodule.
- Local symptoms including dysphagia, stridor, or hoarseness.
- Previous exposure to radiation.
- +ve family history of thyroid cancer or MEN syndrome.
- Gardner's syndrome (familial large intestinal polyposis).
- Familial polyposis coli.
- Cowden syndrome (autosomal dominantly inherited hamartoma syndrome).
- Lymphadenopathy.
- History of Hashimoto's disease (↑ incidence of lymphoma).

Investigations

- FNAC (🔲 see p.14).
- Serum TSH concentration.
- Respiratory flow loop especially for a large goitre possibly causing tracheal obstruction.
- CT scan or MRI if there are concerns about retrosternal goitre or tracheal compression.

Treatment

Toxic multinodular goitre or nodule

The patient should initially be rendered euthyroid with medical treatment.

ATDs

ATDs are effective in controlling the hyperthyroidism but are not curative. As the hot nodules are autonomous the condition will recur after stopping the drugs. Carbimazole is useful treatment to gain control of the disease in preparation for surgery or as long-term treatment in those patients unwilling to accept radioiodine or surgery.

Radioiodine

- This form of treatment is often considered as 1st choice for definitive treatment. ^{131}I is preferentially accumulated in hot nodules but not in normal thyroid tissue which, because of the thyrotoxic state, is non-functioning.
- Radioiodine treatment commonly induces a euthyroid state as the hot nodules are destroyed and the previously non-functioning follicles gradually resume normal function. A dose of 500–800MBq for small-to-medium and 600 or 800MBq for medium-to-large goitres is recommended

Surgery

- The aim of surgery is to remove as much of the nodular tissue as possible and if the goitre is large to relieve local symptoms. Postoperative follow-up should involve checks of thyroid function.
- Goitre recurrence, although rare, does occasionally occur.

Non-toxic multinodular goitre

Surgery

- Is the preferred treatment for patients with:
  - Local compression symptoms.
  - Cosmetic disfigurement.
- Solitary nodule with FNAC suspicious of malignancy.

Radioiodine

- Radioiodine may be particularly indicated in elderly patients in whom surgery is not appropriate. It may require admission. Up to 50% shrinkage of goitre mass has been reported in recent studies.
- Hypothyroidism following radioiodine is relatively low but is still recognized.

Medical treatment
Use of T_4 to suppress TSH is associated with risk of cardiac arrhythmias and bone loss. T_4 is useful only if TSH is detectable but is not generally indicated.

> **Box 5.2 Aetiology of goitre**
> - Autoimmune thyroid disease.
> - Sporadic.
> - Endemic (iodine deficiency, dietary origins).
> - Pregnancy.
> - Drug-induced (ATDs, lithium, amiodarone).
> - Thyroiditis syndromes.

Pathology

Thyroid nodules may be described as *adenomas* if the follicular cell differentiation is enclosed within a capsule; *adenomatous* when the lesions are circumscribed but not encapsulated.

Thyroid nodules in pregnant mothers

- Increase in size during gestation.
- Increase in number.
- Need FNA as higher risk of malignancy.
- Can be operated upon in 2nd trimester or post-partum.

Thyroiditis

Background

Inflammation of the thyroid gland often leads to a transient thyrotoxicosis followed by hypothyroidism. Overt hypothyroidism caused by autoimmunity has two main forms: *Hashimoto's (goitrous) thyroiditis* and *atrophic thyroiditis*.

Table 6.1 Causes and characteristics of thyroiditis

Cause	Characteristic features
Autoimmune thyroiditis (Hashimoto's)	Grossly lymphocytic and fibrotic thyrotoxicosis or hypothyroidism
Postpartum thyroiditis	Lymphocytic thyroditis, transient thyrotoxicosis or hypothyroidism
Drug induced	Particularly with amiodarone
Sub-acute (de Quervain)	Thought to be viral in origin, multinuclear giant cells
Riedel thyroiditis	Extensive fibrosis of the thyroid
Radiation thyroiditis	Radiation injury, transient thyrotoxicosis
Pyogenic (rare)	*Staph. aureus*, streptococci, *E. coli*, tuberculosis, fungal

Table 6.2 Clinical presentation of thyroiditis

Form of thyroiditis	Clinical presentation	Thyroid function
Suppurative (acute)	Painful, tender thyroid, fever	Usually normal
Subacute (de Quervain)	Painful anterior neck, arthralgia, antecedent upper respiratory tract infection; generalized malaise.	Early thyrotoxicosis, occasionally late hypothyroidism
Autoimmune	Hashimoto's : goitre Atrophic: no goitre	Usually hypothyroid Sometimes euthyroid Rarely early thyrotoxicosis
Riedel	Hard woody consistency of thyroid	Usually normal

Chronic autoimmune (atrophic or Hashimoto's) thyroiditis

📖 See Tables 6.1 and 6.2

- *Hashimoto's thyroiditis* Characterized by a painless, variably sized goitre with rubbery consistency and an irregular surface. The normal follicular structure of the gland is extensively replaced by lymphocytic and plasma cell infiltrates with formation of lymphoid germinal centres. The patient may have normal thyroid function, or subclinical, or overt hypothyroidism. Occasional patients present with thyrotoxicosis in association with a thyroid gland that is unusually firm and with high titres of circulating antithyroid antibodies.
- *Atrophic thyroiditis* Probably indicates end-stage thyroid disease. These patients do not have goitre and are antibody +ve. Biochemically, the picture is that of frank hypothyroidism.

Investigations

Investigations which are useful in establishing a diagnosis of Hashimoto's thyroiditis include:
- Testing of thyroid function.
- Thyroid antibodies (antithyroglobulin antibodies +ve in 20–25%, and antithyroperoxidase antibodies in >90%).
- Occasionally a thyroid biopsy to exclude malignancy in patients who present with a goitre and dominant nodule.

Prognosis

The long-term prognosis of patients with chronic thyroiditis is good because hypothyroidism can easily be corrected with T_4 and the goitre is not usually of sufficient size to cause local symptoms. In the atypical situation where Hashimoto's thyroiditis presents with rapidly enlarging goitre and pain a short course of prednisolone at a dose of 40mg daily may prove helpful.

Any unusual increase in size of the thyroid in patients known to suffer from Hashimoto's thyroiditis should be investigated with a FNA and possibly later a biopsy since there is an association between this condition and thyroid lymphoma (rare but risk ↑ by a factor of 70).

Other types of thyroiditis

Silent thyroiditis

Associated with transient thyrotoxicosis or hypothyroidism. A significant percentage of patients have a personal or family history of autoimmune thyroid disease. It may progress to permanent hypothyroidism.

Postpartum thyroiditis

📖 also see p.433. Thyroid dysfunction occurring within the first 6 months postpartum. Prevalence ranges from 5–7%. Postpartum thyroiditis develops in 30–52% of ♀ who have +ve thyroid peroxidase (TPO) antibodies. Most patients have a complete remission but some may progress to permanent hypothyroidism. It is thrice as common in patients with type I diabetes mellitus.

Chronic fibrosing (Riedel's) thyroiditis

A rare disorder characterized by intense fibrosis of the thyroid gland and surrounding structures leading to induration of the tissues of the neck. May be associated with mediastinal and retroperitoneal fibrosis, salivary gland fibrosis, sclerosing cholangitis, lachrymal gland fibrosis, and parathyroid gland fibrosis leading to hypoparathyroidism. Patients are usually euthyroid. Main differential diagnosis is thyroid neoplasia.

Management

Corticosteroids are usually ineffective. Surgery may be required to relieve obstruction and to exclude malignancy. Tamoxifen may be of benefit.

Pyogenic thyroiditis

- Rare. Usually anteceded by a pyogenic infection elsewhere.
  Characterized by tenderness and swelling of the thyroid gland, redness and warmth of the overlying skin, and constitutional signs of infection.
- Piriform sinus should be excluded. Excision of tract is preferable to incision and drainage.
- Treatment consists of antibiotic therapy and incision and drainage if a fluctuant area within the thyroid should occur.

Sub-acute thyroiditis (granulomatous, giant cell or de Quervain's thyroiditis)

- Viral in origin. Symptoms include pronounced asthenia, malaise, pain over the thyroid or pain referred to lower jaw, ear, or occiput. Less commonly the onset is acute with fever, pain over the thyroid, and symptoms of thyrotoxicosis. Characteristically signs include exquisite tenderness and nodularity of the thyroid gland. There is characteristically an elevated ESR and a depressed radionuclide (^{99m}Tc can be used) uptake. Biochemically, the patient may be initially thyrotoxic though later the patient may become hypothyroid (15%).

- In mild cases, non-steroidal anti-inflammatory agents offer symptom relief. In severe cases glucocorticoids (prednisolone 20–40mg/day) are effective. Propranolol can be used to control associated thyrotoxicosis. Treatment can be withdrawn when T_4 returns to normal. T_4 replacement is required if the patient becomes hypothyroid. Treatment with carbimazole or propylthiouracil is not indicated.

Drug-induced thyroiditis

Causes include:
- Amiodarone.
- Lithium.
- Interferon-α (15% develop thyroid peroxidase antibodies and or thyroid dysfunction).
- Interleukin 2.

Further reading

Lazarus JH, Hall R, Othman S, *et al.* (1996). The clinical spectrum of postpartum thyroid disease. *QJM* **89**, 429–35.

Muller AF, Drexhage HA, and Berghout A (2001). Postpartum thyroiditis and autoimmune thyroiditis in women of child bearing age: recent insights and consequences for antenatal and postnatal care. *Endocr Rev* **22**, 605–30.

Pearce EN, Farwell AP, Braverman LE (2003). Thyroiditis. *New Engl J Med* **348**(26), 2646–55.

Weetman AP (2000). Autoimmune thyroid disease. In *Endocrinology*, Vol. 2. DeGroot LJ and Jameson JL (eds.) WB Saunders & Co: Philadelphia.

Hypothyroidism

Background

Hypothyroidism results from a variety of abnormalities that cause insufficient secretion of thyroid hormones (Table 7.1). The commonest cause is autoimmune thyroid disease. *Myxoedema* is severe hypothyroidism in which there is accumulation of hydrophilic mucopolysaccharides in the ground substance of the dermis and other tissues leading to thickening of the facial features and doughy induration of the skin.

Epidemiology

- High TSH in 7.5% of ♀ and 2.5% of ♂ >65 years, 1.7% overt hypothyroidism, 13.7% subclinical hypothyroidism (Whickham Survey, UK).
- Incidence higher in whites than Hispanics or African-American populations.
- Incidence higher in areas of high iodine intake.
- An elevated TSH is associated with higher serum lipid concentrations, which may be an additional reason to initiate therapy.

Table 7.1 Classification of the causes of hypothyroidism

	TSH	Free T$_4$
Non-goitrous	↑	↓
Postablative (radioiodine, surgery)		
Congenital development defect		
Atrophic thyroiditis		
Postradiation (e.g. for lymphoma)		
Goitrous	↑	↓
Chronic thyroiditis (Hashimoto's thyroiditis)		
Iodine deficiency		
Drug elicited (amiodarone, aminosalicylic acid, iodides, phenylbutazone, lithium aminoglutethimide, interferon α, thalidomide, bexarotene, stavudine—antiretroviral)		
Heritable biosynthetic defects		
Maternally transmitted (antithyroid agents, iodides)		
Pituitary	↓	↓
Panhypopituitarism		
Isolated TSH deficiency		
Hypothalamic	↓	↓
Neoplasm		
Infiltrative (sarcoidosis)		
Congenital defects		
Infection (encephalitis)		
Self-limiting		
Following withdrawal of suppressive thyroid therapy		
Subacute thyroiditis and chronic thyroiditis with transient hypothyroidism		
Postpartum thyroiditis		

Clinical picture

Adult

- Insidious non-specific onset.
- Fatigue, lethargy, constipation, cold intolerance, muscle stiffness, cramps, carpal tunnel syndrome, menorrhagia, later oligo- or amenorrhoea.
- Slowing of intellectual and motor activities.
- ↓ appetite and weight gain.
- Dry skin; hair loss.
- Deep hoarse voice, ↓ visual acuity.
- Obstructive sleep apnoea.

Myxoedema

- Dull expressionless face, sparse hair, periorbital puffiness, macroglossia.
- Pale, cool skin that feels rough and doughy.
- Enlarged heart (dilation and pericardial effusion).
- Megacolon/ intestinal obstruction.
- Cerebellar ataxia.
- Prolonged relaxation phase of deep tendon reflexes.
- Peripheral neuropathy.
- Encephalopathy.
- Hyperlipidaemia.
- Hypercarotenaemia (also caused by hyperlipidaemia, diabetes mellitus, and porphyria).
- Psychiatric symptoms e.g. depression, psychosis.

Myxoedema coma

- Predisposed to by cold exposure, trauma, infection, administration of central nervous system depressants.
- Marked respiratory depression with ↑ arterial P_{CO2}
- Hyponatraemia from impaired water excretion and disordered regulation of vasopressin secretion.

Subclinical hypothyroidism

- This term is used to denote raised TSH levels in the presence of normal concentrations of free thyroid hormones.
- Treatment is indicated if the biochemistry is sustained in patients with a past history of radsioiodine treatment for thyrotoxicosis or +ve thyroid antibodies as in these situations progression to overt hypothyroidism is almost inevitable (at least 5% per year of those with +ve antithyroid peroxidase antibodies).
- 2 samples should be taken 2–3 months apart to distinguish from non-thyroidal illness.
- There is controversy over the advantages of T_4 treatment in patients with –ve thyroid antibodies and no previous radioiodine treatment.
- If treatment is not given, follow up with annual thyroid function tests is important.
- There is no generally accepted consensus of when patients should receive treatment. Some authorities suggest treatment when the serum TSH is >10U/L, because of ↑ rate of progression to overt hypothyroidism.
- Increased incidence of cardiac risk probably greater if < 65 years old.

Management

📖 See Fig. 7.1.

Treatment of hypothyroidism

- Normal metabolic state should be restored gradually as rapid increase in metabolic rate may precipitate cardiac arrhythmias
- The average replacement dose is 1.6mcg/kg/day, probably best at night.
- In the younger patients, start thyroxine at 50–100mcg. In the elderly, with a history of ischaemic heart disease, an initial dose of levothyroxine 25–50mcg can be ↑ by 25mcg increments at 4-week intervals until normal metabolic state is attained.
- Optimum dose determined by clinical criteria, the objective of treatment being to restore serum TSH to the normal range.
- TSH should be checked only 2 months after any dose change. Once stabilized TSH should be checked on an annual basis.
- In patients with 2° hypothyroidism, free T_4 is the most useful parameter to follow.
- Dose requirements can increase by 25–50% in pregnancy due to the increase in thyroid binding globulin (TBG). Recent data have shown that mild maternal hypothyroidism in the 1st trimester is associated with slightly impaired cognitive function in offspring. Thus, some now recommend routinely ↑ levothyroxine dose by 25mcg in any ♀ on replacement therapy when she learns she is pregnant.

Combined T_4 and T_3 replacement

Some studies have suggested that the additional replacement with T_3 and T_4 in combination improves well-being and cognitive function in patients in comparison to treatment with T_4 alone. A recent meta-analysis of double-blind cross-over studies showed no benefit of this therapy and is therefore not recommended.

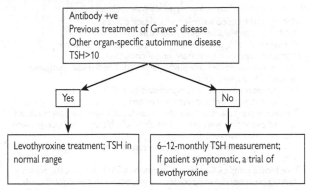

Fig. 7.1 Algorithm for management of subclinical hypothyroidism. Adapted from Lindsay and Toft (1997). Hypothyroidism. *Lancet* **349**, 413–17. Copyright 1997, with permission from Elsevier.

Management of myxoedema coma

- Identify and treat concurrent precipitating illness.
- Antibiotic therapy after blood cultures.
- Management of hypothermia by passive external rewarming.
- Manage in intensive treatment unit if comatose.
- Give warm humidified oxygen by facemask. Mechanical ventilation needed if hypoventilating.
- Aim for slow rise in core temperature (0.5°C/h).
- Cardiac monitor for supraventricular arrhythmias.
- Correct hyponatraemia (mild fluid restriction), hypotension (cautious volume expansion with crystalloid or whole blood), and hypoglycaemia (glucose administration).
- Monitor rectal temperature, oxygen saturation, BP, CVP, and urine output hourly.
- Take blood samples for thyroid hormones, TSH and cortisol before starting treatment. If hypocortisolaemic, administer glucocorticoids.
- Thyroid hormone replacement: no consensus has been reached. The following is an accepted regimen:
  - T_4 300–500mcg IV or by NG tube as a starting dose followed by 50–100mcg daily until oral medication can be taken
  - If no improvement within 24–48h, T_3 10mcg IV 8-hourly or 25mcg IV 8-hourly can be given in addition to above.
- Give hydrocortisone 50–100mg 6–8-hourly in case of cortisol deficiency.

Management of persistently elevated TSH despite thyroxine replacement

(📖 See Fig. 7.2).

- Elevated TSH despite thyroxine replacement is common, most usually due to lack of compliance.
- If TSH still elevated when levothyroxine dose at 1.6mcg/kg/day or higher careful questioning of compliance is needed.
- Consider malabsorption.
- Consider other drugs that may interfere with levothyroxine absorption (Box 7.1).

Box 7.1 Interference with absorption of thyroxine

- Coeliac disease.
- Drugs—colestyramine, aluminum hydroxide, sucralfate, omeprazole, rifampicin, phenytoin, iron, and calcium carbonate.
- Atrophic gastritis in *H. pylori* infection (↓ T4 by 30%)

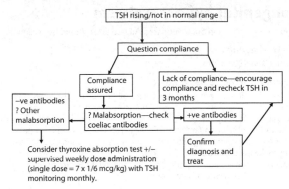

Fig. 7.2 Suggestions for investigations of elevated TSH despite thyroxine replacement therapy to >1.6mcg/kg/day

Congenital hypothyroidism

Incidence—about 1 in 5000 neonates. All neonates should be screened.

Thyroid agenesis

Occurs 1 in 1800 births.

Thyroid hormone dysgenesis

- Caused by inborn errors of thyroid metabolism. The disorders may be autosomal recessive, indicating single protein defects.
- Can be caused by inactivation of the TSH receptor, abnormalities of the thyroid transcription factors TTF1, TTF2, and PAX8, or due to defects in iodide transport, organification (peroxidase), coupling, deiodinase, or thyroglobulin synthesis.
- In a large proportion of patients with congenital hypothyroidism, the molecular background is unknown.

Pendred's syndrome

Characterized by overt or subclinical hypothyroidism, goitre, and moderate to severe sensorineural hearing impairment. The prevalence varies between 1 in 15 000 and 1 in 100 000. There is a partial iodide organification defect detected by ↑ perchlorate discharge. Thyroid hormone synthesis is only mildly impaired and so may not be detected by neonatal thyroid screening.

> **Box 7.2 Clinical features and congenital hypothyroidism**
> The following features are late sequelae of congenital hypothyroidism and, with routine screening now available, should never be seen nowadays.
> - Physiological jaundice.
> - Goitre.
> - Hoarse cry, feeding problems, constipation, somnolence.
> - Delay in reaching normal milestones of development; short stature.
> - Coarse features with protruding tongue, broad flat nose, widely-set eyes.
> - Sparse hair and dry skin, protuberant abdomen with umbilical hernia.
> - Impaired mental development, retarded bone age.
> - Epiphyseal dysgenesis, delayed dentition.

Laboratory tests

- Neonatal screening by measurement of serum TSH.
- Imaging procedure: ultrasonography or ^{123}I scintigraphy.
- Measurement of serum thyroglobulin and low molecular weight iodopeptides in urine to discriminate between the various types of defects.
- Measurement of neonatal and maternal autoantibodies as an indication of possible transient hypothyroidism.

Treatment

Irrespective of the cause of congenital hypothyroidism, early treatment is essential to prevent cerebral damage. Sufficient T_4 should be given to maintain the TSH in the normal range.

Further reading

Clyde PW, Harari AE, Getka EJ, et al. (2003). Combined levothyroxine plus liothyronine compared with levothyroxine alone in primary hypothyroidism: a randomized controlled trial. *JAMA* **290**(22), 2952–8.

de Vijlder JJM and Vulsma T (2000). In *Endocrinology*, Vol. 2, DeGroot LJ and Jameson JL (ed.). WB Saunders & Co: Philadelphia.

Escobar-Morreale HF, Botella-Carretero JI, Escobar del Rey F, et al. (2005). Treatment of hypothyroidism with combinations of levothyroxine plus liothyronine. *JCEM* **90**(8), 4949–54. Epub 2005 May 31.

Escobar-Morreale HF, Botella-Carretero JI, Gomez-Bueno M, et al. (2005). Thyroid hormone replacement therapy in primary hypothyroidism: a randomized trial comparing L-thyroxine plus liothyronine with L-thyroxine alone. *Ann Intern Med* **142**(6), 412–24.

Roberts CG, Ladenson PW (2004). Hypothyroidism. *Lancet* **363**(9411), 793–803.

Roberts CG and Ladenson PW (2004). Thyroxine adherence in primary hypothyroidism. *Lancet* **363** (9411), 793–803.

Amiodarone and thyroid function

Background

- Amiodarone has a high concentration of iodine (39% by weight). It is a benzofuranic derivative and its structural formula closely resembles that of thyroxine. On a dose of amiodarone between 200–600mg daily, 7–21mg iodine is made available each day. The optimal daily iodine intake is 150–200mcg. Amiodarone is distributed in several tissues from where it is slowly released. In one study terminal elimination half-life of amiodarone averaged 52.6 days with a standard deviation of 23.7 days.
- Abnormalities of thyroid function occur in up to 50% of patients (Table 8.1).
- In the UK and USA, 2% of patients on amiodarone develop thyrotoxicosis and about 13% develop hypothyroidism.
- Patients residing in areas with high iodine intake develop amiodarone induced hypothyroidism (AIH) more often than amiodarone induced thyrotoxicosis (AIT), but AIT occurs more frequently in regions with low iodine intake.
- AIT can present several months after discontinuing the drug because of its long half-life.
- Hypothyroidism is commoner in ♀ and in patients with thyroid autoantibodies.
- Thyroid function tests should be monitored initially and then every 6 months in patients taking amiodarone.

Pathogenesis

- The high iodine content of amiodarone may inhibit thyroid hormone synthesis and release causing AIH or leading to iodine-induced thyrotoxicosis (Jod-Basedow phenomenon).
- Thyrotoxicosis resulting from iodine excess and therefore ↑ hormone synthesis is referred to as *AIT type I*. Thyrotoxicosis due to a direct toxic effect of amiodarone is referred to as *AIT type II* (Table 8.2).
- Drug-induced destructive thyroiditis results in leakage of thyroid hormones from damaged follicles into the circulation and like subacute thyroiditis can be followed by a transient hypothyroid state before euthyroidism is restored.

Table 8.1 Thyroid function tests in clinically euthyroid patients after administration of amiodarone

Tests	1–3 months	>3 months
Free T$_3$	Decreased	Remains slightly decreased, but within normal range
TSH	Transient increase	Normal
Free T$_4$	Modest increase	Slightly increased compared to pretreatment values, may be in normal range or slightly increased.
Reverse T$_3$	Increased	Increased

Table 8.2 Characteristics of AIT (Some patients have a mixed form and classification is not always possible)

	AIT type I (10%)	AIT type II (90%)
Aetiology	Iodine toxicity	Thyroiditis
Signs of clinical thyroid disease	Yes	No
Goitre	Frequent	Infrequent
Thyroid antibodies	Positive	Negative
Radioiodine uptake	Normal	Decreased
Thyroglobulin	Normal or slightly elevated	Very elevated
Serum IL6 (research test)	Normal	Very elevated
Late hypothyroidism	No	Possible
Vascularity (Doppler)	Increased/normal	Reduced

Diagnosis and treatment

 See Table 8.3.

- After chronic administration of amiodarone, a steady state is achieved, typically reflected in mild elevation of free T_4 and reduction in free T_3. Thus in clinically euthyroid patients on amiodarone a slightly elevated T_4 is not indicative of hyperthyroidism, nor is a low T_3 indicative of hypothyroidism.
- Hyperthyroidism is indicated by significantly ↑ free T_4, together with elevated free T_3 and suppressed serum TSH.
- Hypothyroidism is indicated by elevation of TSH with low serum free T_4.
- Discontinuation of amiodarone does not always control the thyrotoxic state because of its long half-life (particularly in the obese) due to its very high volume of distribution and fat solubility.
- Numerous complex published algorithms exist for management, but since classification into type I and type II is often difficult (see Table 8.2), in practice most patients are treated with a ATDs ± glucocorticoids (see Table 8.4)
- The 1st line of treatment is ATDs (carbimazole or propylthiouracil).
- A combination of corticosteroids and ATDs may be effective in AIT type II. A high dose of prednisolone, 40–60mg daily, may be required for 8–12 weeks; studies where steroids have been discontinued after 2–3 weeks have been associated with a high relapse rate.
- Radioiodine is not usually effective because of reduced uptake by the thyroid gland reflecting the iodine load associated with the drug.
- Surgery remains a very successful form of treatment, with euthyroidism being restored within a matter of days. Achieving preoperative euthyroidism may be difficult, however.
- Cardiac function may be compromised by propranolol used in combination with amiodarone, since this may produce bradycardia and sinus arrest.
- Potassium perchlorate inhibits iodide uptake by the thyroid gland, reduces intrathyroidal iodine, and renders thionomides more effective. It can be given as a 1g daily dose together with carbimazole, a regimen shown to restore euthyroidism in a large percentage of patients with both type I and type II AIT. In small case studies a combination of potassium perchlorate and carbimazole has been effective while treatment with amiodarone was continued.

Box 8.1 Treatment of amiodarone induced hypothyroidism

Underlying thyroid abnormality (usually Hashimoto's thyroiditis):
- Amiodarone therapy can be continued.
- Add thyroxine replacement therapy.

Apparently normal thyroid:
- Discontinue amiodarone if possible and follow up for restoration of euthyrodism.
  - If amiodarone cannot be withdrawn, start thyroxine replacement therapy.

Table 8.3 Side effects and complications of amiodarone therapy

Side effect	Incidence (%)
Corneal microdeposits	100
Anorexia and nausea	80
Photosensitivity; blue/grey skin discolouration	55–75
Ataxia, tremors, peripheral neuropathy	48
Deranged liver function tests	25
Abnormal thyroid function tests	14–18
Interstitial pneumonitis	10–13
Cardiac arrhythmias	2–3

Table 8.4 Treatment of amiodarone induced thyrotoxicosis

	Type 1 AIT	Type 2 AIT
Step 1 Aim: Restore euthyroidism	Carbimazole up to 40mg/day or propylthiouracil 400mg/day in combination if necessary with potassium perchlorate 1g/day for 16–40 days. If possible discontinue amiodarone*	Discontinue amiodarone if possible* Prednisolone 40mg/day. In mixed forms add carbimazole or propylthiouracil as in type 1 AIT
Step 2: Definitive treatment	Radioiodine treatment or thyroidectomy	Follow up for possible spontaneous progression to hypothyroidism

*If amiodarone cannot be withdrawn and medical therapy is unsuccessful, consider total thyroidectomy.

Further reading

Bartalena L, Brogioni S, Grasso L, et al. (1996). Treatment of amiodarone-induced thyrotoxicosis, a difficult challenge: results of a prospective study. *J Clin Endocrinol Metab* **81**, 2930–33.

Martino E, Bartalena L, Bogazzi F, et al. (2001). The effects of amiodarone on the thyroid. *Endocr Rev* **22**(2), 240–54.

Newman CM, Price A, Davies DW, et al. (1998). Amiodarone and the thyroid. *Heart* **79**, 121–7.

Wiersinga WM (1997) Amiodarone and the thyroid. In *Pharmacotherapeutics of Thyroid Gland*, Weetman AP, Grossman A (ed.) Berlin: Springer-Verlag, pp.225–87.

Thyroid cancer

Epidemiology

- Clinically detectable thyroid cancer is rare. It accounts for <1% of all cancer and <0.5% of cancer deaths.
- Thyroid microcarcinoma (diameter <1cm) may be found in multinodular goitres.
- Thyroid cancers are commonest in adults aged 40–50, and rare in children and adolescents.
- ♀ are affected more frequently than ♂.

Table 9.1 Classification of thyroid cancer

Cell of origin	Tumour type	Frequency (%)
Papillary	Differentiated:	
	Papillary	>80
	Follicular	10
	Undifferentiated (anaplastic)	1–5
C-cells	Medullary	5–10
Lymphocytes	Lymphoma	1–5

Table 9.2 Comparison of papillary, follicular and anaplastic carcinomas of the thyroid

Characteristic	Papillary Ca	Follicular Ca	Anaplastic Ca
Age at presentation	30–50 (mean 44)	40–50	60–80
Spread	Lymphatic	Haematogenous	Haematogenous
Prognosis	Good	Good	Poor
Treatment	Initially: near total thyroidectomy Postoperative TSH suppression. High-risk patient: ^{131}I remnant ablation Postoperative total body radioiodine scan	Initially: near total thyroidectomy Postoperative TSH suppression ^{131}I remnant ablation Postoperative total body radioiodine scan	Total thyroidectomy with lymph node clearance Chemotherapy with doxorubicui and cisplatin External beam irradiation

Aetiology

Irradiation

- There does not appear to be a threshold dose of external irradiation for thyroid carcinogenesis; doses of 200–500cGy seem to produce thyroid cancer at a rate of about 0.5%/year.
- There is no evidence that therapeutic or diagnostic ^{131}I administration can induce thyroid cancer, although there is a small increase in death rates from thyroid cancer after ^{131}I. At present it is unclear whether this is due to an effect of ^{131}I or part of the natural history of the underlying thyroid disease.
- External irradiation at an age <20 years is associated with an ↑ risk of thyroid nodule development and thyroid cancer (most commonly papillary). The radioactive fallout from the Chernobyl nuclear explosion in 1986, resulted in a 4.7-fold increase in thyroid cancer in the regions of Belarus from 1985 to 1993, including a 34-fold increase in children. Most of these were papillary carcinomas.
- The risk is greater for ♀ and when irradiation occurs at an younger age.
- There is a latency of at least 5 years with maximum risk at 20 years following exposure, though this was not seen following the Chernobyl disaster.

Other environmental factors

Most investigators agree that iodine supplementation has resulted in a decrease in the incidence of follicular carcinoma.

Genetic syndromes and oncogenes

- *RET/PTC1* proto-oncogene abnormalities in the long arm of chromosome 10 are associated with some papillary tumours (5–30%), especially after irradiation (60–80%). It is similar to the abnormality associated with medullary thyroid carcinoma in MEN2A.
- 2 new proto-oncogenes have been have been identified: *RET/PTC2* and *RET/PTC3* TRK (less common).
- The tumour suppressor gene *p53* has been found to be mutated in some de-differentiated cancers.
- Overexpression of the *ras* and *PTTG* oncogenes is found in papillary thyroid cancers and were found to be markers for adverse prognosis.
- c-*myc* mRNA expression has been correlated with histologic markers of papillary cancer aggression.

Papillary microcarcinoma of the thyroid (PMC)

- PMC is defined by WHO as a tumour focus of 1.0cm or less in diameter. It is detected coincidentally on histopathological examination of the thyroid following resection of multinodular goitre or any thyroid resected
- Autopsy studies show:
  - Prevalence ranges from 1–35.6%.
  - No significant difference in the prevalence rates of papillary micro-carcinoma has been demonstrated between the sexes.
  - PMC rarely progresses to clinically apparent thyroid cancer with advancing age.

- PMC can be multifocal.
- Cervical lymph node metastasis from PMC ranges from 4.3–18.2%.
- Lymph node metastasis was most often associated with multifocal tumours.
- Although exposure to irradiation increases the likelihood of developing papillary thyroid cancer, the tumours will usually be >1.0cm in diameter and thus not PMC.
- Follow-up studies suggest that PMC is a slow growing lesion which rarely spreads to distant sites and which carries a good prognosis.
- The recommendations for treatment of PMC vary widely:
  - The low morbidity and long survival mean that collection of randomized prospective data has never been performed and comparisons of therapies are based on retrospective studies.
  - The treatment of PMC should not cause more morbidity than the disease process itself.
  - Surgical treatment recommendations range from simple excision to ipsilateral lobectomy.
  - With adjuvant therapy the consensus is routine use of T_4, but not the use of radioiodine as there is no difference in the recurrence rate. There is some evidence to keep TSH below the reference range but robust data are not available.

Papillary thyroid carcinoma

- Constitutes almost >80% of all thyroid cancers.
- Commoner in ♀ (3:1).
- Rare in childhood, peaks occur in 2nd and 3rd decades and again in later life (bimodal frequency).
- Incidence: 3–5 per 100 000 population.

Pathology

- Slow growing, usually non-encapsulated, may spread through the thyroid capsule to structures in the surrounding neck, especially regional lymph nodes. Multifocal in 30% of cases.
- Recognized variants are follicular, papillary, dorsal, columnar cell, tall cell, and diffuse sclerosing.
- *Histology* the tumour contains complex branching papillae that have a fibrovascular core covered by a single layer of tumour cells.
- Nuclear features include:
  - Large size with pale staining, 'ground-glass' appearance (*orphan Annie-eye nucleus*).
  - Deep nuclear grooves.
- The characteristic and pathognomonic cytoplasmic feature is the 'psammoma body' which is a calcified, laminated, basophilic, stromal structure.
- It is confined to the neck in over 95% of cases, although 15–20% have local extra thyroidal invasion. Metastases (1–2% of patients) occur via lymphatics to local lymph nodes and more distantly to lungs.
- Several prognostic scoring systems are in use, none of which permits definitive decisions to be made for individual patients.
- Low risk—JNM stage I (under 45, no metastases)

Management

Primary treatment: surgery

- Should be performed by an experienced thyroid surgeon at a centre with adequate case load to maintain surgical skills.
- In general, as near total thyroidectomy as possible should be performed.
- Clinically evident cervical lymph node metastasis is best treated with radical modified neck dissection with preservation of sternocleido-mastoid muscle, spinal accessory nerve, and internal jugular vein.

Adjuvant therapy—radioiodine therapy

- Postoperative radioiodine therapy is advised in the high-risk patient with differentiated thyroid cancer. After surgery in a low risk group, some thyroidologists argue that ^{131}I is not required. A dose of 3.1GBq is used for thyroid ablation. A whole body scan done 4–6 months after administration of 150MBq ^{131}I helps determine the presence of any residual disease. In the presence of metastasis a dose of approximately 5.5–7.4GBq radioiodine is used. Liothyronine should be administered for 4–6 weeks in place of thyroxine. It is then omitted for 10 days prior to the scan, allowing TSH to rise. A low-iodine diet for 2 weeks increases the effective specific activity of the administered iodine.

- The patient should be isolated until residual dose meter readings indicate <30 MBq.
- Chronic suppression of serum TSH levels to <0.10mU/L is standard practice in patients with differentiated thyroid carcinoma. Inhibition of TSH secretion reduces recurrence rate as TSH stimulates growth of the majority of thyroid cancer cells.

Patients are followed up with thyroglobulin levels. After effective treatment thyroglobulin levels are undetectable. A trend of ↑ thyroglobulin values should be investigated with a radioiodine uptake scan. Liothyronine (T_3) is substituted for T_4 4–6 weeks before the scan, and omitted for 10 days immediately beforehand.

Thyroglobulin

- A very sensitive marker of recurrence of thyroid cancer.
- Secreted by the thyroid tissue.
- After total thyroidectomy and radioactive iodine ablation, the levels of thyroglobulin should be <2ng/L.
- Measurement of thyroglobulin levels could be made difficult in the presence of antithyroglobulin antibodies, which should be checked.
- There is controversy over whether the patient should come off T_4 or T_3 or be started on recombinant TSH before checking the thyroglobulin levels. Coming off thyroid hormones or giving TSH increases the sentivity of thyroglobulin to detect recurrence, but this may not affect survival rates.

Recurrent disease/distant metastases

- In the case of recurrence, treatment employs all methods used in 1° and adjuvant therapy.
- Surgery for local metastases.
- External radiotherapy is indicated in tumours that do not take up ^{131}I.
- Bony and pulmonary metastases (usually osteolytic) may be treated with ^{131}I.
- Unfortunately only 50% of metastases concentrate ^{131}I and bony metastases are often very difficult to irradiate.
- Some advocate use of external beam radiation.
- Response to chemotherapy is usually poor.

Recombinant TSH

- Avoids morbidity of hypothyroidism during T_4 withdrawal.
- Useful for patients with TSH deficiency (hypopituitarism).
- Comparable thyroglobulin rise but reduced ^{131}I scan sensitivity compared to T_4 withdrawal.
- Give 0.9mg of recombinant TSH on day 1 and 2 and measure thyroglobulin on day 5.

Follicular carcinoma (FTC)

- Constitutes 15% of all thyroid cancers.
- Mean patient age in most studies is 50 years.
- Commoner in ♀ (2:1).
- Relatively more common in endemic goitre areas.

Pathology

- Follicular carcinoma is a neoplasm of the thyroid epithelium that exhibits follicular differentiation and shows capsular or vascular invasion.
- Differentiation of benign follicular adenoma from encapsulated low-grade or minimally invasive tumours can be impossible to diagnose, particularly for the cytopathologist, and surgery is usually necessary for a follicular adenoma.
- FTC may be minimally invasive or widely invasive.
- Metastases (15–20% cases) are more likely to be spread by haematogenesis to the lung and bones and less likely to local lymph nodes.
- Hurthle cell carcinoma is an aggressive type of follicular tumour with a poor prognosis because it fails to concentrate ^{131}I.

Treatment

as for Papillary thyroid carcinoma, pp.74–75.

Follow-up of papillary and FTC

- Follow-up usually involves an annual clinical review, with clinical examination for presence of suspicious lymph nodes and measurements of serum TSH (to ensure adequate TSH suppression to <0.1mU/L) and thyroglobulin.
- Serum thyroglobulin should be undetectable in patients with total thyroid ablation. However, detectable levels may be seen for up to 6 months after thyroid ablation. A trend of ↑ thyroglobulin level requires investigations with ^{131}I uptake scan (off thyroid hormones or with TSH stimulation) and other imaging modalities, such as u/s of the neck, CT scan of the lungs, or bone scans. Thyroglobulin antibodies must be checked, as there may be interactions with the thyroglobulin assays.
- Radioiodine scans are done annually for the first 3 years and if –ve, not repeated unless there are clinical indications, like an ↑ thyroglobulin level.
- Isolated lymph node metastases can occasionally be associated with normal thyroglobulin. Stopping thyroid hormone replacement, or using recombinant TSH, before the measurement of thyroglobulin can increase sensitivity of detecting persistent recurrent disease.
- Detectable thyroglobulin and absent uptake on radioiodine uptake scan may be due to dedifferentiation of the tumour and failure to take up iodine. A PET scan may be useful in this situation. If a PET scan is not available, an iodine uptake scan following 150 MBq ^{131}I can be useful.

Box 9.1 Thyroid cancer in children

- Uncommon, with an incidence of 0.2–5 per million per year.
- >85% are papillary, but with more aggressive behaviour than in adults (local invasion and distant metastases are commoner).
- Recently an ↑ incidence in children in Belarus and Ukraine has been reported following the Chernobyl nuclear accident in 1986. RET oncogene rearrangements are common in these tumours.
- Management is similar to adults, with a similar controversy as to the extent of initial surgery.
- Various studies report an overall recurrence rate of 0–39%; disease-free survival of 80–93%, and disease-specific mortality of 0–10%.
- Evidence is currently lacking on the independent risks or benefits of radioactive iodine or extensive surgery.
- Many investigators recommend lifelong follow-up with a combination of thyroglobulin and radionuclide scanning.

Thyroid cancer and pregnancy
- The natural course of thyroid cancer developing during pregnancy may be different from that in non-pregnant ♀.
- Any ♀ presenting with a thyroid nodule in pregnancy appears to have an ↑ risk for thyroid cancer.
- Evaluation should be undertaken with FNAC. Radioiodine scan is contraindicated.
- Lesions <2cm diameter or any lesion appearing after 24 weeks' gestation should be treated with TSH suppression and further evaluations carried out postpartum.
- If FNAC is suspicious or diagnostic, operation should be performed at the earliest safe opportunity—generally the 2nd trimester or immediately postpartum.
- ^{131}I ablation should be scheduled for the postpartum period and the mother advised to stop breast-feeding.
- Avoid pregnancy for 6 months after any ^{131}I ablation.

Medullary thyroid carcinoma (MTC)

📖 also see Chapter 100, MEN type 2, p.622.

- Accounts for 5–10% of all thyroid cancers.
- Should be managed by a dedicated regional service.

Presentation

- Lump in neck.
- Systemic effects of calcitonin-flushing/diarrhea.

Diagnosis

- FNAC
- Unsuspected at surgery.
- Comprehensive family history and screening in search for features of MEN-2 is needed.
- Pathology specimens show immunostaining for calcitonin and staining for amyloid.

Management

- Baseline plasma calcitonin.
- Baseline biochemical investigations for phaeochromocytoma and hyperparathyroidism.
- Genetic screening.
- Staging with thoraco-abdominal CT/MRI.
- MIBG and pentavalent ^{99m}Tc DMSA scintography may also be used.

Treatment

- Total thyroidectomy and central node dissection is the 1° treatment modality.
- Germline RET mutation carriers should ideally undergo thyroidectomy before 5 years of age.

Adjuvant therapy

- Radioiodine and TSH suppression does not play a role.
- External radiotherapy and systemic chemotherapy has not been shown to be benefit.
- Therapeutic MIBG may help in some cases.

Follow-up

All patients should have lifelong follow-up at the dedicated regional service.

Anaplastic (undifferentiated) thyroid cancer

- Rare.
- Peak incidence: 7th decade. $♀:♂$ = 1:1.5.
- Characterized by rapid growth of a firm/hard fixed tumour.
- Often infiltrates local tissue such as larynx and great vessels and so does not move on swallowing. Stridor and obstructive respiratory symptoms are common.
- Aggressive, with poor long-term prognosis—7% 5-year survival rate and a mean survival of 6 months from diagnosis.
- Optimal results occur following total thyroidectomy. This is usually not possible and external irradiation is used, sometimes in association with chemotherapy.

Lymphoma

- Uncommon.
- Almost always associated with autoimmune thyroid disease (Hashimoto's thyroiditis). Occurs more commonly in ♀ and in patients aged >40 years.
- Characterized by rapid enlargement of the thyroid gland.
- May be limited to thyroid gland or part of a more extensive systemic lymphoma (usually non-Hodgkin's lymphoma). Trucut biopsy may be required.
- Treatment with radiotherapy alone or chemotherapy if more extensive often produces good results.

Further reading

British Thyroid Association (2007). *Guidelines for the management of thyroid cancer*, 2nd edn. Royal College of Physicians: London.

Hay I and Wass JAH (2008). *Clinical Endocrine Oncology*, 2nd edn. Blackwell-Wiley. pp.109–71.

Mazzaferri EL, Robbins RJ, Spencer CA, et al. (2003). A consensus report of the role of serum thryoglobulin as a monitoring method for low-risk patients with papillary thyroid carcinoma. *JCEM* **88**(4), 1433–41.

Sherman SI (2003). Thyroid carcinoma. *Lancet* **361**(9356), 501–11

Wartofsky L, Sherman SI, Gopal J, et al. (1998). The use of radioactive iodine in patients with papillary and follicular thyroid cancer. *J Clin Endocrinol Metab* **83**, 4195–203.

www.british-thyroid-association.org/guidelines.htm

Anatomy and physiology of anterior pituitary gland

Anatomy

The pituitary gland is situated in the pituitary fossa (Fig. 10.1). Below is the sphenoid air sinus, on either side the internal carotid artery and cavernous sinus, and above the posterior pituitary is continuous with the pituitary stalk of the basal hypothalamus, which with the pituitary portal vessels passes down through the dura mater which roofs the pituitary fossa.

The posterior pituitary gland is supplied by the inferior hypophyseal branches of the internal carotid artery, and the anterior pituitary gland by the hypothalamohypophyseal portal veins.

Physiology

Prolactin (PRL) secretion[*]

Single chain polypeptide. Pulsatile secretion in a circadian rhythm with around 14 pulses/24h, and a superimposed bimodal 24h pattern of secretion, with a nocturnal peak during sleep and a lesser peak in the evening.

Growth hormone (GH) secretion[*]

Single chain polypeptide. Pulsatile—GH is usually undetectable in the serum apart from 5–6 90min pulses/24h that occur more commonly at night.

LH/FSH secretion

Glycoprotein hormone, with α chain common to LH, FSH (also TSH and hCG), but β chain specific for each hormone. Pulsatile secretion.

Thyroid stimulating hormone (TSH) secretion

Pulsatile, with 9 ± 3 pulses/24h, and ↑ amplitude of pulses at night.

Adrenocorticotrophic hormone (ACTH)[*]

- Single-chain polypeptide cleaved from pro-opiomelanocortin (POMC).
- Circadian rhythm of secretion, beginning to rise from 3 a.m. to a peak before waking in the morning, and falling thereafter.

Posterior pituitary—📖 see p.196.

---

[*]Concentrations ↑ with stress: NB venepuncture.

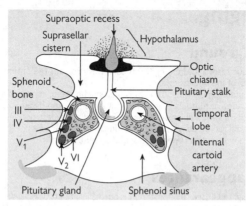

Fig. 10.1 Reproduced with permission from by Weatherall DJ, Ledingham JGG, and Warrell DA (eds) (1996). *Oxford Textbook of Medicine*, 3rd edn. Oxford University Press: Oxford.

Imaging

Background

- Magnetic resonance imaging (MRI) currently provides the optimal imaging of the pituitary gland.
- Computed tomography (CT) scans may still be useful in demonstrating calcification in tumours (e.g. craniopharyngiomas) and hyperostosis in association with meningiomas, or evidence of bone destruction.
- Plain skull radiography may show evidence of pituitary fossa enlargement but has been superseded by MRI.

MRI appearances

- T1-weighted images demonstrate cerebrospinal fluid (CSF) as dark grey, and brain as much whiter. This imaging is useful for demonstrating anatomy clearly. The normal posterior pituitary gland appears bright white (due to neurosecretory granules and phospholipids) on T1-weighted images, in contrast to the anterior gland which is of the same signal as white matter. The bony landmarks have low signal intensity on MRI, and air in the sphenoid sinus below the fossa shows no signal. Fat in the dorsum sellae may shine white. T2-weighted images may sometimes be used to characterize haemisoderin and fluid contents of a cyst.
- IV gadolinium compounds are used for contrast enhancement. Because the pituitary and pituitary stalk have no blood–brain barrier, in contrast to the rest of the brain, the normal pituitary gland enhances brightly following gadolinium injection. Particular uses are the demonstration of cavernous sinus involvement and microadenomas. (e.g. Cushing's disease)
- The normal pituitary gland has a flat or slightly concave upper surface. In adolescence or pregnancy, the surface may become slightly convex.

Pituitary adenomas

On T1-weighted images, pituitary adenomas are of lower signal intensity than the remainder of the normal gland. The size and extent of the pituitary adenomas are noted in addition to the involvement of other structures such as invasion of the cavernous sinus, erosion of the fossa, and relations to the optic chiasm. Larger tumours may show low intensity areas compatible with necrosis or cystic change, or higher intensity signal due to haemorrhage. The presence of microadenomas may be difficult to demonstrate. Contrast enhancement may assist, as may asymmetry of the gland or stalk position.

Neuroradiological classification

📖 See p.167

Craniopharyngiomas

These appear as suprasellar (occasionally intrasellar) masses with cystic and/or calcified portions.

Further reading

Naidich MJ and Russell EJ (1999). Current approaches to imaging of the sellar region and pituitary. *Endocrinol Metab Clin N Am* **28**, 45.

Pituitary function—dynamic tests

Insulin tolerance test (ITT)

Indications
- Assessment of ACTH reserve.
- Assessment of GH reserve.

Physiology
IV insulin is used to induce hypoglycaemia (glucose <2.2mmol/L with signs of glycopenia) which produces a standard stress causing ACTH and GH secretion.

Contraindications
- Basal cortisol <100nmol/L.
- Untreated hypothyroidism.
- Abnormal ECG.
- Ischaemic heart disease.
- Seizures.

NB Patients should discontinue oral estrogen replacement for 6 weeks before the test as ↑ CBG will make the cortisol results difficult to interpret. Progesterone and transdermal estrogen may be continued.

Box 12.1 Procedure

- Continued medical surveillance is essential throughout.
- Patient is fasted overnight. Weight is checked.
- Insert cannula. Check basal (time 0) glucose, cortisol, and GH.
- Administer IV soluble insulin 0.15U/kg (occasionally 0.3U/kg needed in untreated Cushing's syndrome and acromegaly because of ↑ insulin resistance).
- Measure glucose, GH, and cortisol at 30, 45, 60, 90, and 120min. Repeat insulin dose if a bedside stick test for glucose does not show hypoglycaemia at 45min.
- Test is terminated if prolonged hypoglycaemia—may need to administer 25mL of 25% glucose and IV 100mg hydrocortisone after sampling for cortisol and GH.
- Ensure patient eats lunch and has normal glucose before discharge.

Response
- The normal response is for glucose to fall to <2.2mmol/L, and for cortisol to rise to >580nmol/L and GH to >20mU/L.
- In the presence of inadequate hypoglycaemia, the test cannot be interpreted.
- A normal cortisol response demonstrates ability to withstand stress (including major surgery) without requiring glucocorticoid cover.

- A subnormal response in an asymptomatic patient (e.g. peak cortisol 450–580nmol/L) may be managed by administration of glucocorticoids at time of stress only.
- Other patients with subnormal responses require glucocorticoid replacement treatment (📖 see Glucocorticoids, p.106).
- A GH response <10mU/L is indicative of severe GH deficiency and in the appropriate clinical situation (📖 see p.108) GH replacement therapy may be recommended. Values between 10 and 20 are borderline.

Glucagon test

Indications
- Assessment of ACTH reserve.
- Assessment of GH reserve.

Physiology
Glucagon leads to release of insulin which then leads to GH and ACTH release. The response may be 2° to the drop in glucose seen after the initial rise following glucagon injection, or may relate to the nausea induced by glucagon.

Contraindications
- Often unreliable in patients with diabetes mellitus.
- NB Patients should discontinue oral oestrogen replacement for 6 weeks before the test as ↑ CBG will make the cortisol results difficult to interpret.

Box 12.2 Procedure

The test is performed at 9 a.m. following an overnight fast. Basal GH and cortisol are measured then 1mg (1.5mg if patient weighs >90kg) glucagon is administered SC. Samples for GH, cortisol, and glucose are checked from 90min every 30min until 240min.

Response
- The normal response is a rise in glucose to a maximum at 90min. Cortisol rises to >580nmol/L and GH rises to >20mU/L.
- This is a less reliable test than the ITT as 20% normal individuals may fail to respond.

ACTH stimulation test

Short Synacthen® test (tetracosactide test).

Indication
- Assessment of adrenal cortical function.
- Assessment of ACTH reserve.

Physiology
Low cortisol that does not rise following administration of ACTH demonstrates adrenal cortical disease. Prolonged ACTH administration will lead to cortisol secretion in ACTH deficiency but not in 1° adrenal disease. It *can* be used to assess ACTH reserve, as in ACTH deficiency the adrenal cortex is unable to respond to a stimulatory signal within 30min.

Box 12.3 Procedure
- The test can be done at any time of the day; the response is not time dependent.
- Synacthen® is administered 250mcg IM, and cortisol measured at 0, 30, and 60min. When this test is used to measure ACTH reserve, only the 0 and 30min values are required. The dose may also be given IV with identical results.
- NB Patients should discontinue oestrogen replacement for 6 weeks before the test as ↑ CBG will make the cortisol results difficult to interpret.

Response
The post-stimulation cortisol should rise to >580nmol/L at 30min. This is an unreliable test of ACTH reserve within 6 weeks of an insult e.g. surgery to the pituitary.

Arginine test

Indication
2nd line test for assessment of GH reserve.

Physiology
Arginine leads to GH release.

Contraindications
None.

Box 12.4 Procedure

- Fast from midnight, and administer 0.5g/kg (max 30g) arginine IV in 100mL normal saline over 30min from time 0 (9 a.m.).
- Sample glucose and GH at 0, 30, 60, 90, and 120min.

Response
A normal response is a rise in GH to >15–20mU/L.

Clomifene test

Indications

Assessment of gonadotrophin deficiency (e.g. Kallmann's syndrome).

Physiology

Clomifene has mixed oestrogen and antioestrogenic effects. The basis of the test is competitive inhibition of oestrogen binding at the hypothalamus and pituitary gland, leading to ↑ LH and FSH after 3 days.

Contraindications

- Avoid in those with liver disease.
- May transiently worsen depression.

Box 12.5 Procedure

- Advise patient of possible side-effects—visual disturbance (peripheral flickering of vision), and also of possible ovulation in ♀ (contraceptive advice).
- Measure LH and FSH on days 0, 4, 7, and 10. In ♀ measure day 21 progesterone to detect whether ovulation has occurred.
- Administer clomifene 3mg/kg (max 200mg/day) in divided doses for 7 days.

Response

- The normal response is a doubling of gonadotrophins by day 10, usually rising beyond the normal range.
- In hypothalamic disease no gonadotropin rise is seen. Pre-pubertal patients may show a fall in gonadotrophins.
- Ovulation is presumed if day 21 progesterone is >30nmol/L.

hCG test

Indications

To examine Leydig cell function, 📖 see Clinical assessment, p.374–5.

GnRH test

Indication
Assessment of LH/FSH reserve.

Physiology
Synthetic GnRH leads to pituitary gland release of FSH and LH.

Contraindications
None.

Box 12.6 Procedure
- Because of variations through the menstrual cycle, this is usuavlly performed in ♀ during the follicular phase if patients are cycling.
- Sample LH and FSH 0, 20, and 60min after administration of GnRH.

Response
- LH levels rise quickly to peak at 20min whereas FSH levels are maximal at 60min.
- This test does not diagnose gonadotrophin deficiency, as subnormal, normal, or exaggerated responses may be seen. It demonstrates the amount of pituitary reserve of LH/FSH secretion. It is now rarely used.
- Occasional patients with acromegaly have a GH response.

TRH test

This is rarely required with currently available sensitive TSH assays.

Indications

- Differentiation of pituitary TSH and hypothalamic TRH deficiency.
- Differentiation of TSH-secreting tumour from thyroid hormone resistance (📖 see Table 3.4, p.40).
- Diagnosis of hyperthyroidism (largely superseded by sensitive TSH assay).

Box 12.7 Procedure

- Administer TRH 200mcg IV to supine patient.
- Measure T_4 and TSH at time 0, and TSH at 20 and 60min.
- Note occasional reports of pituitary tumour haemorrhage. TRH induces a rise in blood pressure.

Response

- Normal response is rise in TSH by more than 2mU/L to >3.4mU/L, with a maximum at 20min and lower values at 60min.
- A delayed peak (60min rather than 20min) is typically found in hypothalamic disease.
- In hyperthyroidism there is no TSH response to TRH.
- The TRH test is also used rarely in investigation of hyperprolactinaemia and acromegaly (📖 see p.116; p.124).

Hypopituitarism

Definition

Hypopituitarism refers to either partial or complete deficiency of anterior and/or posterior pituitary hormones, and may be due to 1° pituitary disease or to hypothalamic pathology which interferes with the hypothalamic control of the pituitary.

Causes

- Pituitary tumours.
- Parapituitary tumours—craniopharyngiomas, meningiomas, secondary deposits (breast, lung), chordomas, gliomas.
- Radiotherapy—pituitary, cranial, nasopharyngeal.
- Pituitary infarction (apoplexy), Sheehan's syndrome.
- Infiltration of the pituitary gland—sarcoidosis, lymphocytic hypophysitis, haemochromatosis, Langerhans' cell histiocytosis, Erdheim-Chester disease.
- Empty sella.
- Infection—tuberculosis, pituitary abscess.
- Trauma.
- Isolated hypothalamic releasing hormone deficiency—e.g. Kallmann syndrome due to GnRH deficiency.
- Russell viper snake bite.

Features

- The clinical features depend on the severity of pituitary hormone deficiency and the rate of development, in addition to whether there is intercurrent illness. In the majority of cases, the development of hypopituitarism follows a characteristic order, with secretion of GH, then gonadotrophins being affected first followed by TSH and ACTH secretion at a later stage. PRL deficiency is rare, except in Sheehan's syndrome associated with failure of lactation. ADH deficiency is virtually unheard of with pituitary adenomas, but may be seen rarely with infiltrative disorders and trauma.
- The majority of the clinical features are similar to those occurring when there is target gland insufficiency. There are important differences e.g. lack of pigmentation and normokalaemia in ACTH deficiency in contrast to ↑ pigmentation and hyperkalaemia (due to aldosterone deficiency) in Addison's disease.
- NB *Houssay phenomenon* amelioration of diabetes mellitus in patients with hypopituitarism due to reduction in counter-regulatory hormones.

Apoplexy

Apoplexy refers to infarction of the pituitary gland due to either haemorrhage or ischaemia. It occurs most commonly in patients with pituitary adenomas, usually macroadenomas, but other predisposing conditions include postpartum (Sheehan's syndrome), radiation therapy, diabetes mellitus, anticoagulant treatment, disseminated intravascular coagulopathy, reduction in intracranial pressure.

It may present with a syndrome which is difficult to differentiate from any other intracranial haemorrhage with sudden onset headache, vomiting, meningism, and visual disturbance and cranial nerve palsy. The diagnosis is based on the clinical features and pituitary imaging which shows high signal on T1- and T2-weighted images (📖 see p.88). It has been suggested that early surgery (within 8 days) provides the optimal chance for neurological recovery. However, some patients may be managed conservatively if the patient has no significant visual or other neurological loss.

Empty sella syndrome

An enlarged pituitary fossa, which may be 1° (due to arachnoid herniation through a congenital diaphragmatic defect) or 2° to surgery, radiotherapy, or pituitary infarction. The majority of patients have normal pituitary function. Hypopituitarism (and or hyperprolactinaemia) is found in <10%. A radiologically empty sella may rarely be associated with a functioning pituitary tumour.

Sheehan's syndrome

Haemorrhagic infarction of the enlarged postpartum pituitary gland causing hypopituitarism, following severe hypotension usually due to blood loss, e.g. postpartum haemorrhage. It can be fatal and survivors require life replacement therapy. Improvement in obstetric care has made this a rare occurrence in the developed world.

Investigations

The aims of investigation of hypopituitarism are to biochemically assess the extent of pituitary hormone deficiency and also to elucidate the cause.

Basal hormone levels

Basal concentrations of the anterior pituitary hormone as well as the target organ hormone should be measured, as the pituitary hormones may remain within the normal range despite low levels of target hormone. Measurement of the pituitary hormone alone does not demonstrate that the level is inappropriately low, and the diagnosis may be missed.

- LH and FSH, and testosterone (9 a.m.) or oestradiol.
- TSH and thyroxine.
- 9 a.m. cortisol.
- PRL.
- IGF-1 (NB May be normal in up to half of GHD depending on age).

Box 13.1 Dynamic tests

- Dynamic tests, such as the ITT (📖 Insulin tolerance test p.90) or glucagon test (📖 Glucagon test, p.92) if the ITT is contraindicated, are used to assess cortisol and GH reserve.
- Some centres use the short Synacthen® test to assess ACTH reserve using the 0 and 30min values of cortisol (📖 ACTH stimulation test, p.93). There are few false –ves using this investigation, and it is simpler to perform than the former tests but gives no measure of GH reserve. It is important to note that falsely normal results occur when hypopituitarism is of recent onset because the test relies on the fact that ACTH deficiency causes atrophy of the adrenal cortex and therefore a delayed response to Synacthen®. Less than 6 weeks of ACTH deficiency may allow a 'normal' adrenal response.

Posterior pituitary function

- It is important to assess and replace corticotroph function before assessing posterior pituitary hormone production because ACTH deficiency leads to reduced GFR and the inability to excrete a water load, which may therefore mask diabetes insipidus (DI).
- Plasma and urine osmolality are often adequate as baseline measures. However, in patients suspected to have DI, a formal water deprivation test should usually be performed (📖 see Box 33.2, p.200).

Investigation of the cause

- Pituitary imaging—MRI ± contrast.
- Investigation of hormonal hypersecretion if a pituitary tumour is demonstrated.
- Investigation of infiltrative disorders as discussed in Chapter 27 (📖 see Parasellar inflammatory conditions, pp.176–77), e.g. serum and CSF ACE, ferritin, hCG.
- Occasionally biopsy of the lesion is required.

Table 13.1 Summary of clinical features of hypopituitarism

Hormone deficiency	Clinical features
GH	Adult GHD (📖 see p. 108)
	Reduced exercise capacity, reduced lean body mass, impaired psychological well-being, ↑ cardiovascular risk
LH/FSH	Anovulatory cycles, oligo/amenorrhoea, dyspareunia in ♀
	Erectile dysfunction and testicular atrophy in ♂
	Reduced libido, infertility and loss of 2° sexual hair (often after many years) in both sexes
ACTH	As in Addison's disease, except lack of hyperpigmentation, absence of hyperkalaemia (📖 p. 252)
TSH	As in 1° hypothyroidism (📖 see p. 56)
PRL	Failure of lactation
ADH	Polyuria and polydipsia

Treatment

Treatment involves adequate and appropriate hormone replacement (□ see p.104, p.108, and p.198), and management of the underlying cause.

Isolated defects of pituitary hormone secretion

Rarely, patients have isolated insufficiency of only 1 anterior pituitary hormone. The aetiology of these disorders is largely unknown, although loss of hypothalamic control may play a role; an autoimmune pathology has been suggested in some and genetic mutations in others

- GnRH deficiency (Kallman syndrome—congenital GnRH deficiency ± anosmia).
- Isolated ACTH deficiency.
- *Pit1* gene mutation (leads to isolated GH, PRL, and TSH deficiency).
- *Prop1* gene mutation (leads to isolated GH, PRL, TSH and gonadotrophin deficiency).

Anterior pituitary hormone replacement

Background

Anterior pituitary hormone replacement therapy is usually performed by replacing the target hormone rather than the pituitary or hypothalamic hormone that is actually deficient. The exceptions to this are GH replacement (☐ see Growth hormone replacement therapy in adults, p.108) and when fertility is desired (☐ see Management, p.410).

Table 14.1 Usual doses of hormone replacement therapy

Hydrocortisone	10mg on waking, 5mg at lunch time, and 5mg early evening or twice daily regimen with a total dose of 15–30mg/d
or	
Prednisolone	3mg on waking and 2mg early evening (total dose 5–7.5mg/d)
Levothyroxine	100–150mcg/d
GH	0.2–0.6mg/d (0.4–1.5IU)
Oestrogens/testosterone	Depends on formulation

Thyroid hormone replacement

This is discussed in the section on 1° hypothyroidism (📖 p.56).

Monitoring of therapy

In contrast to replacement in 1° hypothyroidism, the measurement of TSH cannot be used to assess adequacy of replacement in TSH deficiency due to hypothalamopituitary disease. Therefore, monitoring of treatment in order to avoid under- and over-replacement should be via both clinical assessment and by measuring free thyroid hormone concentrations.

Sex hormone replacement

📖 See Hormone replacement therapy in women, p.332; Androgen replacement therapy, p.378.

Oestrogen/testosterone administration is the usual method of replacement, but gonadotrophin therapy is required if fertility is desired (📖 see Ovulation induction in males, p.410).

Glucocorticoids

Replacement therapy

Patients with ACTH deficiency usually need glucocorticoid replacement only and do not require mineralocorticoids, in contrast to patients with Addison's disease.

The normal production rate of cortisol is 9.9 ± 2.7mg/day. The glucocorticoid most commonly used for replacement therapy is *hydrocortisone*. It is rapidly absorbed with a short half-life (90–120min). *Prednisolone* and *dexamethasone* can occasionally be used for glucocorticoid replacement. The longer half-lives of these 2 drugs makes them useful where sustained ACTH suppression is required in, for example, congenital adrenal hyperplasia (CAH). Dexamethasone is useful when monitoring endogenous production as it is not detected in most cortisol assays. Cortisol acetate was previously used for glucocorticoid replacement therapy but requires hepatic conversion to active cortisol.

Monitoring of replacement

This is important to avoid over-replacement which is associated with ↑ BP, elevated glucose and insulin, and reduced bone mineral density (BMD). Under-replacement leads to the nonspecific symptoms as seen in Addison's disease (📖 see p.252). A clinical assessment is important but biochemical monitoring using plasma and urine cortisol (UFC) measurements are used by most endocrinologists. The aim is to keep the UFC within the reference range (<220nmol/24h). Many centres use plasma cortisol measurements on a hydrocortisone day curve. The aim is to keep the plasma cortisol between 150–300nmol/L, avoiding nadirs of <50nmol/L pre-doses. Conventional replacement (20mg hydrocortisone/24h) may overtreat patients with partial ACTH deficiency.

Safety

Patients should be encouraged to wear a MedicAlert indicating that they are cortisol deficient, to carry a steroid card, and to keep a vial of parenteral hydrocortisone at home to be administered in emergency situations.

Equivalent oral glucocorticoid doses

Prednisolone 5mg is approximately equivalent to:
• Hydrocortisone 20mg.
• Dexamethasone 750mcg.
• Methylprednisolone 4mg.

Acute/severe intercurrent illness

- *Mild disease without fever* No change in glucocorticoid replacement.
- *Pyrexial illness* Double replacement dose (e.g. hydrocortisone 20, 10, 10mg) for duration of fever.
- *Vomiting or diarrhoea* Parenteral therapy 100mg IM (from GP/trained relative; useful for patient to have vial of hydrocortisone at home with instruction sheet for emergency administration by suitable trained personnel).
- *Severe illness/operation* Parenteral therapy with IM hydrocortisone 50–100mg 6-hourly (e.g. 72h for major surgery, 24h for minor surgery). An alternative is a continual IV infusion of 1–3mg/h hydrocortisone.

Box 14.1 Hydrocortisone day curve

There are various protocols for this test ranging from a 3-point curve to detect under-replacement (used with 24h UFC to detect over-replacement)—serum cortisol checked at 9. a.m., 12.30 p.m. (before the lunch time dose), and 5 p.m. (pre evening dose), to more frequent sampling to detect over and under-replacement. This involves serum cortisol at time 0, then administration of the morning dose of hydrocortisone. Plasma cortisol is then checked at 30min, 1, 2, 3, and 5h (prelunchtime dose specimen), and 7 and 9h (pre evening dose) followed by samples at 10 and 11h.

- Oral oestrogen therapy should be stopped 6 weeks before the test as ↑ CBG leading to higher cortisol values will make the test uninterpretable.
- This test is only valid for hydrocortisone replacement. Prednisolone or dexamethasone replacement can only be monitored clinically.

Growth hormone (GH) replacement therapy in adults

Background

There is now a considerable amount of evidence that there are significant and specific consequences of GH deficiency (GHD) in adults, and that many of these features improve with GH replacement therapy. GH replacement for adults has now been approved in many countries.

Definition

It is important to differentiate between adult and childhood onset GHD.
- Although *childhood onset* GHD occurs 2° to structural lesions such as craniopharyngiomas and germinomas, and following treatment such as cranial irradiation, the commonest cause in childhood is an isolated variable deficiency of GH releasing hormone (GHRH) which may resolve in adult life because of maturation of the hypothalamo-somatotroph axis. It is therefore important to retest patients with childhood onset GHD when linear growth is completed (50% recovery of this group).
- *Adult onset* GHD usually occurs 2° to a structural pituitary or parapituitary condition or due to the effects of surgical treatment or radiotherapy.

Prevalence

- Adult onset GHD 1/10 000.
- Adult GHD due to adult and childhood onset GHD 3/10 000.

Benefits of GH replacement

- Improved QoL and psychological well-being.
- Improved exercise capacity.
- ↑ lean body mass and reduced fat mass.
- Prolonged GH replacement therapy (more than 12–24 months) has been shown to increase BMD, which would be expected to reduce fracture rate.
- There are as yet no outcome studies in terms of cardiovascular mortality. However, GH replacement does lead to a reduction (approximately 15%) in cholesterol. GH replacement also leads to improved ventricular function and ↑ left ventricular mass.

NICE guidelines for GH replacement

Adult criteria

- Severe GHD—GH <9mU/L.
- Impaired QoL (AGHDA Q.L. score >/=11).
- Treatment for other pituitary hormone deficiencies.

Reassessment of treatment after 9 months treatment (3 month dose titration followed by 6 month therapeutic trial)—GH discontinued if improvement in AGHDA <7.

Young adults (up to 25 years)

- GH discontinued for 3 months at completion of linear growth (<2cm/ year) and GH status reassessed.
- If severe GH deficiency confirmed, GH continued at adult dose till age 25 years (peak bone mass).
- Age 25 and above—adult criteria apply.

Diagnosis

The diagnosis of GHD depends on appropriate biochemical testing in the presence of an appropriate clinical context. The latter is important, because distinguishing 'partial GHD' from physiological causes of reduced GH secretion such as obesity or ageing and pathological causes, e.g. hypercortisolaemia in Cushing's syndrome, can be problematic. In these situations GHD can be diagnosed when there is supportive evidence such as pituitary disease and other anterior pituitary hormone deficiencies.

Who should be tested?

As the features of GHD may be non-specific, and biochemical tests can be misleading in certain clinical situations such as obesity, investigation of GHD should only be performed in the following groups of patients:

- Patients with hypothalamo–pituitary disease (GHD occurs early in hypopituitarism, and is almost invariable in patients with other anterior pituitary hormone deficiencies).
- Patients who had childhood onset GHD.
- Patients who have received cranial irradiation.

Investigation of GH deficiency

Dynamic tests of GH secretion

- ITT most widely used test. Peak GH <10mU/L (3mcg/L) are diagnostic of GHD. GH values of 10–20mU/L indicate partial GHD.
- Alternative tests if the ITT is contraindicated include a combination of GHRH (1mcg/kg) and arginine (0.5g/kg) IV over 30min or GH releasing peptide-6 (GHRP-6). The GH peak should be >30mU/L (10mcg/L). Another alternative is pyridostigmine (120mg) at 60min, following GHRH (1mcg/kg) at 0min. The clonidine test, although useful in paediatric practice, is not helpful in the diagnosis of adult GHD. The recently described natural ligand for the GHRH receptor GHrelin may prove useful in the future. Further validation of these newer tests and determination of cut-off values is required.
- A 2nd confirmatory dynamic biochemical test is recommended, particularly in patients who have suspected isolated GH deficiency. A single GH dynamic test is sufficient to diagnose GHD in patients with 2 or 3 pituitary hormonal defects.

IGF-1

IGF-1 concentrations may remain within the age-matched reference range despite severe GHD in up to 50% of patients, and therefore do not exclude the diagnosis, and reduced IGF-1 is seen in a number of conditions.

For causes of lowered IGF-1 levels 📖 see Box 15.1.

Box 15.1 Causes of lowered IGF-1 levels

- GHD.
- Malnutrition.
- Poorly controlled diabetes mellitus.
- Hepatic disease.
- Renal disease.
- Severe intercurrent illness.

Abnormalities in adult GH deficiency

- Stimulated GH <10mU/L (3mcg/L).
- Low or low–normal IGF-1 (IGF-1 may be normal in up to 50%, depending on age).
- ↓ BMD.
- ↑ insulin resistance.
- Hyperlipidaemia (↑ LDL).
- Impaired cardiac function.

Clinical features of GH deficiency

- Impaired well-being.
- Reduced energy and vitality (depressed mood, ↑ social isolation, ↑ anxiety).
- Reduced muscle mass and impaired exercise capacity.
- ↑ central adiposity (↑ waist:hip ratio) and ↑ total body fat.
- ↓ sweating and impaired thermogenesis.
- ↑ cardiovascular risk.
- ↑ fracture risk (osteoporosis).

Treatment of GH deficiency

All patients with GHD should be considered for GH replacement therapy. In particular, patients with impaired QoL, reduced mineral density, an adverse cardiovascular risk profile, and reduced exercise capacity should be considered for treatment.

Dose

- Unlike paediatric practice, where GH doses are determined by body weight and surface area, most adult endocrinologists use dose titration using serial IGF-1 measurements to increase the dose of GH until the IGF-1 approaches the middle to upper end of the age-matched IGF-1 reference range. This reduces the likelihood of side-effects, mainly related to fluid retention, which were frequently observed in the early studies of GH replacement in adults when doses equivalent to those used in paediatric practice were used.
- The normal production of GH is 200–500mcg/day in an adult. Current recommendations are a starting dose of 150–300mcg/day. The maintenance dose is usually 200–600mcg/day. The dose in ♀ is often higher than for age-matched ♂.

Monitoring of treatment

- A clinical examination, looking for reduction in overall body weight (a good response is loss of 3–5kg in 12 months), and reduced waist to hip ratio. BP may fall in hypertensive patients because of reduction in peripheral systemic vascular resistance.
- IGF-1 is monitored to avoid over-replacement, aiming to keep values within the age-matched reference range. During dose titration, IGF-1 should be measured every 1–2 months. Once a stable dose is reached, IGF-1 should be checked at least once a year.
- The adverse effects experienced with GH replacement usually resolve with dose reduction, and tend to be less frequent with the lower starting doses used in current practice.
- GH treatment may be associated with impairment of insulin sensitivity, and therefore markers of glycaemia should be monitored.
- Lipids should be monitored annually. Bone mineral density should be monitored every 2 years, particularly in those with ↓ BMD.
- It may be helpful to monitor quality of life using a questionnaire such as the AGHDA (adult GHD assessment) questionnaire.
- As the long-term safety and efficacy of GH replacement in adults is as yet unknown, it is recommended that patients receiving GH therapy should remain under the care of an endocrinologist. There are large databases of patients receiving GH in order to monitor and determine these questions regarding long-term benefits and safety, particularly with regard to cardiovascular risk.

GH therapy in special situations

- *Pregnancy* There are currently no data on GH replacement in pregnancy. There are occasional reports of continued GH replacement throughout pregnancy with no adverse effect.

- *Critical illness* There is no good evidence for a beneficial effect of GH replacement during critical illness. Patients should continue GH replacement during non-severe illness, but many endocrinologists would suggest that GH should be discontinued in patients who are severely ill: for example, receiving major surgery or on ITU.
- *Cardiac failure* GH treatment has recently been suggested as a potential therapy in dilated cardiomyopathy. Longer term data are required in this group of patients.

Adverse effects of GH replacement

- Sodium and water retention:
  - Weight gain.
  - Carpal tunnel syndrome.
- Hyperinsulinaemia.
- Arthralgia (possibly due to intra-articular cartilage swelling).
- Myalgia.
- Benign intracranial hypertension (resolves on stopping treatment).
- No data suggest that GH therapy affects tumour development. (No evidence from long-term studies in children of ↑ risk of recurrence with GH treatment. Insufficient long-term data in adults.) No evidence of ↑ risk of tumour recurrence in adolescents and adults following childhood malignancy.

Box 15.2 Contraindications to GH replacement

- Active malignancy.
- Benign intracranial hypertension.
- Pre-proliferative/proliferative retinopathy in diabetes mellitus.

Further reading

Carroll PV, Christ ER, Bengtsson BA *et al.* (1998). GH deficiency in adulthood and the effects of GH replacement: a review. *J Clin Endocrinol Metab* **83**, 382–95.

Consensus Guidelines for the Diagnosis and Treatment of Adults with GH deficiency (1998). Summary Statement of the GH Research Society Workshop on adult GH deficiency. *J Clin Endocrinol Metab* **83**, 379–81.

Pituitary tumours

Pathogenesis

The mechanism of pituitary tumourigenesis remains largely unclear. Pituitary adenomas are monoclonal, supporting the theory that there are intrinsic molecular events leading to pituitary tumourogenesis. However, the mutations (e.g. p53) found in other tumour types are only rarely found. A role for hormonal factors and in particular the hypothalamic hormones in tumour progression is likely.

Table 16.1 Approximate relative frequencies of pituitary tumours

Tumour type	Prevalence	Annual incidence
Incidental pituitary microadenomas	0.1%	
Clinically overt pituitary adenomas		1–2/100 000
Acromegaly	0.1%	4 cases/million
Cushing's syndrome		2 cases/million
Non-functioning adenoma		6 cases/million
Prolactinomas	0.5%	10 cases/million (if hyperprolactinaemia is considered, then higher incidence)

NB Good epidemiological data are lacking except in acromegaly. Many of these figures derive from the pre-MRI era.

Molecular mechanisms of pituitary tumour pathogenesis

Activation of oncogenes

- *Gsα mutation* found in up to 40% GH-secreting tumours (less in non-Caucasians), and also described in a minority of NFAs and ACTH-secreting tumours.
- *Ras mutation* found in aggressive tumours and mainly pituitary carcinomas. ?role in malignant transformation.
- *Pituitary tumour transforming gene (PTTG)* has recently been described and found to be over-expressed in pituitary tumours. Its role in tumour pathogenesis is as yet uncertain.

Inactivation of tumour suppressor genes (TSG)

- *MEN-1 gene* loss of heterozygosity (LOH) at 11q13 had been previously demonstrated in up to 20% sporadic pituitary tumours; however, the expression of the *MEN-1* gene product, menin, is not down-regulated in the majority of sporadic pituitary tumours.
- *Retinoblastoma gene* Mutations in mice lead to intermediate lobe corticotroph adenomas; however, no mutations have been demonstrated in human pituitary adenomas.

Cyclins and modulators of cyclin activity

- Mutations of the cyclin-dependent kinases p27 and p18 are rare in human pituitary tumours (unlike tumours in mice). p27 may be translationally down-regulated and p16 may be transcriptionally silenced by methylation of its gene. Cyclin D1 over-expression may be an early step in pituitary tumourogenesis as it is commonly found in different tumour types.
- Mutations are rare in pituitary tumours.

Alterations in receptor and growth factor expression (e.g. TGF, activin, bFGF)

No consistent patterns have emerged.

Further reading

Asa SL, Ezzat S (1998). The cytogenesis and pathogenesis of pituitary adenomas. *Endocr Rev* **19**, 798–827.

Prolactinomas

Epidemiology

- Prolactinomas are the commonest functioning pituitary tumour.
- Postmortem studies show microadenomas in 10% the population.
- During life, microprolactinomas are commoner than macroprolactinomas, and there is a ♀ preponderance of microprolactinomas.

Pathogenesis

Unknown. Occur in 20% of patients with MEN-1. (Prolactinomas are commonest pituitary tumour in MEN-1 and may be more aggressive than sporadic prolactinomas.) Malignant prolactinomas are very rare and may harbour *ras* mutations.

Clinical features

Hyperprolactinaemia (microadenomas and macroadenomas)

- Galactorrhoea (up to 90% ♀, <10% ♂).
- Disturbed gonadal function in ♀ presents with menstrual disturbance (up to 95%)—amenorrhoea, oligomenorrhoea, or with infertility, and reduced libido.
- Disturbed gonadal function in ♂ presents with loss of libido and/or erectile dysfunction. Presentation with reduced fertility and oligospermia or gynaecomastia is unusual.
- Hyperprolactinaemia is associated with a long-term risk of ↓ BMD.
- Hyperprolactinaemia inhibits GnRH release, leading to ↓ LH secretion. There may be a direct action of PRL on the ovary to interfere with LH and FSH signalling which inhibits oestradiol and progesterone secretion and also follicle maturation.

Mass effects (macroadenomas only)

- Headaches and visual field defects (uni- or bitemporal field defects).
- Hypopituitarism.
- Invasion of the cavernous sinus may lead to cranial nerve palsies.
- Occasionally very invasive tumours may erode bone and present with a CSF leak or 2° meningitis.

📖 See Box 17.1 for causes of hyperprolactinaemia.

Box 17.1 Causes of hyperprolactinaemia

- *Physiological:*
  - Pregnancy.
  - Sexual intercourse.
  - Nipple stimulation/suckling.
  - Neonatal.
  - Stress.
- *Pituitary tumour:*
  - Prolactinomas.
  - Mixed GH/PRL secreting tumour.
  - Macroadenoma compressing stalk.
  - Empty sella.
- *Hypothalamic disease*—mass compressing stalk (craniopharyngioma, meningioma, neurofibromatosis).
- *Infiltration*—sarcoidosis, Langerhans' cell histiocytosis.
- *Stalk section*—head injury, surgery.
- *Cranial irradiation.*
- *Drug treatment:*
  - Dopamine receptor antagonists (metoclopramide, domperidone).
  - Neuroleptics* (perphenazine, thioridazine, chlorpromazine, trifluoperazine, haloperidol, sulpiride, risperidone, fluphenazine, flupenthixol).
  - Antidepressants (tricyclics, selective serotonin reuptake inhibitors, monoamine oxidase inhibitors, sulpiride, amisulpiride, imipramine, clomipramine, amitriptyline, pargyline, clorgyline).
  - Cardiovascular drugs—verapamil, methyldopa, reserpine.
  - Opiates.
  - Cocaine.
  - Protease inhibitors—e.g. ritonavir, indinavir, zidovudine.
  - Oestrogens.
  - Others—bezafibrate, omeprazole, H_2 antagonists.
- *Metabolic:*
  - Hypothyroidism—TRH increases PRL.
  - Chronic renal failure—reduced PRL clearance.
  - Severe liver disease—disordered hypothalamic regulation.
- *Other:*
  - PCOS—can make differential diagnosis of menstrual problems difficult.
  - Chest wall lesions—zoster, burns, trauma (stimulation of suckling reflex).
- *No cause found:*
  - 'Idiopathic' hyperprolactinaemia.

*clozapine, quetiapine and olanzapine are antipsychotics with little or no effect on prolactin.

Investigations

Serum PRL

- The differential diagnosis of elevated PRL is shown in Box 17.1, p.117. Note that the stress of venepuncture may cause mild hyperprolactinaemia, so 2–3 levels should be checked, preferably through an indwelling cannula after 30min.
- Serum PRL <2000mU/L is suggestive of a tumour—either a microprolactinoma or a non-functioning macroadenoma compressing the pituitary stalk with loss of dopamine inhibitory tone to the lactotroph and subsequent hyperprolactinaemia.
- Serum PRL >4000mU/L is diagnostic of a macroprolactinoma.
- *Hook effect* This occurs where the assay utilizes antibodies recognizing 2 ends of the molecule. 1 is used to capture the molecule, and 1 to label it. If PRL levels are very high, it may be bound by 1 antibody but not by the other. Thus above a certain concentration, the signal will reduce rather than increase and very high PRL levels will be spuriously reported as normal or only slightly raised.

Thyroid function and renal function

Hypothyroidism and chronic renal failure are causes of hyperprolactinaemia.

Imaging

- *MRI* Microadenomas usually appear as hypointense lesions within the pituitary on T1-weighted images. Negative imaging is an indication for contrast enhancement with gadolinium. Stalk deviation or gland asymmetry may also suggest microadenoma.
- Macroadenomas are space-occupying tumours often associated with bony erosion and/or cavernous sinus invasion

Macroprolactin ('Big' PRL)

Occasionally, aggregate forms (150–170 kDa) of PRL are detected in the circulation. Although these are measurable in the prolactin assay, they do not interfere with reproductive function but may be found in 10% patients referred. Typically there is hyperprolactinaemia with regular ovulatory menstrual cycles. Assays for macroprolactin are available using PEG (polyethylene glycol) precipitation where low recovery of PRL demonstrates presence of macroprolactin, or gel filtration chromatography (gold standard).

Hyperprolactinaemia and drugs

(📖 See p.117)

Antipsychotic agents are the most likely psychotropic agents to cause hyperprolactinaemia. If dose reduction is not possible or not effective, then an MRI to exclude a prolactinoma, and treatment of hypogonadism may be indicated. Where dopamine antagonism is the mechanism of action of the drug, then dopamine agonists may reduce efficacy. Drug-induced increases in PRL are usually <3000mU/L.

'Idiopathic' hyperprolactinaemia

When no cause is found following evaluation as above, the hyperprolactinaemia is designated idiopathic, but in many cases is likely to be due to a tiny microprolactinoma which is not demonstrable on current imaging techniques. In other cases it may be due to alterations in hypothalamic regulation. Follow-up of these patients shows that in $1/3$, PRL levels return to normal, in 10–15% there is a further increase in PRL, and in the remainder PRL levels remain stable.

Treatment

Aims of therapy

- *Microprolactinomas* restoration of gonadal function.
- *Macroprolactinomas*
  - Reduction in tumour size and prevention of tumour expansion.
  - Restoration of gonadal function.
- Although microprolactinomas may expand in size without treatment, the majority do not (<93%). Therefore although restoration of gonadal function is usually achieved by lowering PRL levels, ensuring adequate sex hormone replacement is an alternative if the tumour is monitored in size.
- Macroprolactinomas, however, will continue to expand and lead to pressure effects. Definitive treatment of the tumour is therefore necessary.

Drug therapy—dopamine agonists

- Dopamine agonist treatment (☐ see Dopamine agonists, p.192) leads to suppression of PRL in most patients, with 2° effects of normalization of gonadal function and termination of galactorrhoea. Tumour shrinkage occurs at a variable rate (from 24h to 6–12 months) and extent, and must be carefully monitored. Continued shrinkage may occur for years. Slow chiasmal decompression will correct visual field defect in the majority of patients and immediate surgical decompression is not necessary. Lack of improvement of visual fields despite tumour shrinkage makes improvement with surgery unlikely. Restoration of other hormonal axes may occur with tumour shrinkage.
- *Cabergoline* is more effective in normalization of PRL in microprolactinoma (83% compared with 59% on bromocriptine) with fewer side-effects than *bromocriptine*.
- Dopamine agonist resistance (☐ see Box 17.2) may occur when there are reduced numbers of D2 receptors.
- Tumour enlargement following initial shrinkage on treatment is usually due to non-compliance. A rare possibility however is carcinoma.

Drug therapy—oestrogens

Oestrogen replacement rather than dopamine agonist therapy may be appropriate in ♀ with idiopathic hyperprolactinaemia or microprolactin-momas where fertility and galactorrhoea are not issues. Small short-term series suggest no evidence of tumour enlargement. However individual cases where tumour enlargement has occurred make monitoring of PRL important.

> **Box 17.2 Dopamine agonist resistance**
> - *Definition*: failure to normalize prolactin. Failure to decrease tumour size to <50%.
> - Occurs with 24% treated with bromocriptine, 13% with pergolide, and 11% with cabergoline.
> - D2 receptors are reduced in number but not efficacy.
> - Treatment options include switch dopamine agonist, increase dose of dopamine agonist, surgery, fertility treatment, or oestrogen replacement (± DXR for macroprolactinomas).

Surgery

📖 see Trans-sphenoidal surgery, p.182.

- Since the introduction of dopamine agonist treatment, trans-sphenoidal surgery is indicated only for patients who are resistant to or intolerant of dopamine agonist treatment. The cure rate for macroprolactinomas treated with surgery is poor (30%), and therefore drug treatment is 1st-line in tumours of all size. Occasionally surgery may be required for patients with CSF leak 2° to an invasive macroprolactinoma. Cure rates for microprolactinomas treated with surgery are >80%, but the risk of hypopituitarism (GH deficient in 25%) and recurrence (4% at 5 years) makes this a 2nd-line option.
- The surgical management of a CSF leak can be very difficult in patients with very invasive tumours. Tumour shrinkage with dopamine agonists will either precipitate or worsen the leak, with the subsequent risk of meningitis. There is no evidence for the long-term use of prophylactic antibiotics in this group, but patients at risk should be informed of the warning symptoms and advised to seek expert medical attention urgently.

Radiotherapy

📖 see technique, p.188.

- Standard pituitary irradiation leads to slow reduction (over years) of PRL in the majority of patients. While waiting for radiotherapy to be effective, dopamine agonist therapy is continued, but should be withdrawn on a biannual basis at least to assess if it is still required.
- Radiotherapy is not indicated in the management of patients with microprolactinomas. It is useful in the treatment of macroprolactinomas once the tumour has been shrunk away from the chiasm, only if the tumour is resistant.

Prognosis

- The natural history of microprolactinomas is difficult to assess. However, they are a common post-mortem incidental finding, and <7% show any increase in tumour size. It has been demonstrated that hyperprolactinaemia in approximately $\frac{1}{3}$ of ♀ will resolve particularly after the menopause or pregnancy. This shows that patients receiving dopamine agonist treatment for microprolactinoma should have treatment withdrawn intermittently to assess the continued requirement for it, and certainly the dose may be titrated downwards over time.

- There are few data on dopamine agonist withdrawal in macroprolactinomas in the absence of definitive treatment (radiotherapy or surgery). There are data suggesting that cautious attempts at dose reduction could be considered after 2–5 years, if PRL normal and MRI shows no tumour. These patients would need close monitoring and scans.

Management of prolactinomas in pregnancy

📖 see Prolactinoma in pregnancy, p.438.

Further reading

Bevan JS, Webster J, Burke CW, et al. (1992). Dopamine agonists and pituitary tumour shrinkage. *Endocrinol Rev* **13**, 220–40.

Casaneuva FF, Molitch ME, Schlechte JA, et al. (2006). Guidelines of the Pituitary Society for the diagnosis and management of prolactinomas. *Clin Endocrinol* **65**(2), 265–73.

Colao A, Di Sarno A, Capabianca P, et al. (2003). Withdrawal of long-term cabergoline therapy for tumoural ad nontumoural hyperprolactinaemia *New Engl J Med* **349**, 2023–33.

Karavitaki N, Thanabalasinggham G, Shore HC (2006). Do the limits of serum prolactin in disconnection hyperprolactinaemia need re-definition? A study of 226 patients with histologically verified non-functioning pituitary macroadenoma. *Clin endocrinol* **65**(4), 524–9.

Molitch ME (1985). Pregnancy and the hyperprolactinaemic woman. *New Engl J Med* **312**, 1364–70.

Molitch ME (1992). Pathologic hyperprolactinaemia. *Endocrinol Metabo Clin N Am* **21**, 877–910.

Molitch ME (2002). Medical management of prolactinomas. *Pituitary* **5**, 55–65.

Molitch ME (2003). Dopamine resistance of prolactinomas. *Pituitary* **6**(1), 19–27.

Molitch ME (2008). Drugs and prolactin. *Pituitary* **11**, 209–218.

Suliman SG, Gurlek A, Byrne JV (2007). Non-surgical cerebrospinal fluid rhinorrhoea in invasive macroprolactinoma: incidence, radiological and clinicopathological features. *J Clin Endocrinol Metab* **92**, 3829–3835 PMID: 17623759.

Acromegaly

Definition

Acromegaly is the clinical condition resulting from prolonged excessive GH and hence, IGF-1 secretion in adults. GH secretion is characterized by blunting of pulsatile secretion and failure of GH to become undetectable during the 24-h day, unlike normal controls.

Epidemiology

- Rare. Equal sex distribution.
- Prevalence 40–60 cases/million population. Annual incidence of new cases in the UK is 4/million population.
- Onset is insidious, and there is therefore often a considerable delay between onset of clinical features and diagnosis. Most cases are diagnosed at 40–60 years. Typically acromegaly occurring in an older patient is a milder disease with lower GH levels and a smaller tumour.

Pituitary gigantism

The clinical syndrome resulting from excess GH secretion in children prior to fusion of the epiphyses.

- Rare.
- ↑ growth velocity without premature pubertal manifestations should arouse suspicion of pituitary gigantism.
- *Differential diagnosis* Marfan syndrome, neurofibromatosis, precocious pubertal disorders, cerebral gigantism (large at birth with accelerated linear growth, and disproportionately large extremities—associated normal IGF-1 and GH).
- Arm span >standing height is compatible with eunochoid features, and suggests onset of disease before epiphyseal fusion (pituitary gigantism).

Causes

- *Pituitary adenoma* (>99% of cases) Macroadenomas >microadenomas. Local invasion is common, but frank carcinomas are very rare.
- *GHRH secretion*
  - Hypothalamic secretion.
  - Ectopic GHRH e.g. carcinoid tumour (pancreas, lung) or other neuroendocrine tumours
- *Ectopic GH secretion* Very rare. One report of a pancreatic islet cell tumour secreting GH and one of a lymphoreticulosis.
- There has been some progress on the molecular pathogenesis of the GH secreting pituitary adenomas—as mutations of the Gsα are found in up to 40% of tumours. This leads to an abnormality of the G protein that usually inhibits GTPase activity in the somatotroph.

Associations

- *MEN-1* less common than prolactinomas (see MEN type 1, p.616).
- *Carney complex* AD, spotty cutaneous pigmentation, cardiac and other myxomas, and endocrine overactivity, particularly Cushing's syndrome due to nodular adrenal cortical hyperplasia and GH secreting pituitary tumours in less than 10% of cases. Mainly due to activating mutations of protein kinase A (see p.610).
- *Isolated familial somatotrophinomas* existence of 2 or more cases of acromegaly or gigantism in a family that does not exhibit MEN-1 or Carney complex. (Possibly linked to chromosome 11q13.)

Clinical features

The clinical features arise from the effects of excess GH/IGF-1, excess PRL in some (as there is co-secretion of PRL in a minority (30%) of tumours, or rarely stalk compression), and the tumour mass.

Symptoms

- ↑ sweating—>80% of patients.
- Headaches—independent of tumour effect.
- Tiredness and lethargy.
- Joint pains.
- Change in ring or shoe size.

Signs

- *Facial appearance* Coarse features, oily skin, frontal bossing, enlarged nose, deep nasolabial furrows, prognathism and ↑ interdental separation.
- *Deep voice*—laryngeal thickening (Table 18.1).
- *Tongue enlargement*—macroglossia.
- *Musculoskeletal changes* enlargement of hands and feet, degenerative changes in joints lead to osteoarthritis. Generalized myopathy.
- *Soft tissue swelling* may lead to entrapment neuropathies such as carpal tunnel syndrome (40% of patients).
- *Goitre and other organomegaly*—liver, heart, kidney.

NB Fabry disease causes thickening of the lips

Complications

- Hypertension (40%).
- Insulin resistance and impaired glucose tolerance (40%)/diabetes mellitus (20%).
- Obstructive sleep apnoea—due to soft tissue swelling in nasopharyngeal region.
- ↑ risk of colonic polyps and colonic carcinoma—extent currently considered controversial.
- Ischaemic heart disease and cerebrovascular disease.
- Congestive cardiac failure, and possible ↑ prevalence of regurgitant valvular heart disease.

Effects of tumour

- Visual field defects.
- Hypopituitarism.

Table 18.1 Macroglossia—causes

- Acromegaly
- Hypothyroidism
- Beckwith–Widemann Syndrome (macrosomia, visceromegaly)—associated with hypoglycaemia and malignancies
- Simpson Golah Behmel Syndrome (macrosomnia, and renal skeletal abnormalities)
- Tongue amyloidoses (primary, or secondary to myeloma)
- Mucopolysaccharidoses/lysosomal storage disease
- Focal tongue lesions, eg haemorrhage
- Down's Syndrome

Investigations

Oral glucose tolerance test (OGTT)

- In acromegaly, there is failure to suppress GH to <1mU/L in response to a 75g oral glucose load. In contrast, the normal response is GH suppression to undetectable levels. Note reports of occasional patients with mild acromegaly with elevated IGF-1 but basal and glucose suppressed GH <2mU/L.
- *False +ves*—chronic renal and liver failure, malnutrition, diabetes mellitus, heroin addiction, adolescence (due to high pubertal GH surges).

Random GH

Not useful in the diagnosis of acromegaly as although normal healthy subjects have undetectable GH levels throughout the day, there are pulses of GH which are impossible to differentiate from the levels seen in acromegaly. However, in untreated patients, a random GH <1mU/L excludes the diagnosis.

IGF-1

Useful in addition to the OGTT in differentiating patients with acromegaly from normals, as it is almost invariably elevated in acromegaly except in severe intercurrent illness. It has a long half-life as it is bound to binding proteins, and reflects the effect of GH on tissues. However, abnormalities of GH secretion may remain while IGF-1 is normal.

IGFBP3

IGFBP3 concentrations correlate with IGF-1, and the use of this assay in both the diagnosis and monitoring of acromegaly has been advocated. It does not give such clear differentiation in the diagnosis as IGF-1.

TRH test

📖 also see TRH test, p.97. The normal GH response at 20 and 60min following 200g TRH IV is GH suppression; however, 80% of patients with acromegaly show an increase (by 50% of basal). This test is usually not required as the OGTT and IGF-1 usually provide the diagnosis. It may be helpful in patients with equivocal results.

MRI

MRI usually demonstrates the tumour (98%), and whether there is extrasellar extension either suprasellar or into the cavernous sinus.

Pituitary function testing

📖 also see Insulin tolerance test (ITT), p.90. Serum PRL should be measured as some tumours co-secrete both GH and PRL.

Serum calcium

Some patients are hypercalciuric due to ↑ 1,25-DHCC as GH stimulates renal 1α-hydroxylase. There may be an ↑ likelihood of renal stones due to hypercalcaemia as well as hypercalciuria (which occurs in 80%). Rarely hypercalcaemia may be due to associated MEN-1 and hyperparathyroidism.

GHRH

Occasionally it is not possible to demonstrate a pituitary tumour, or pituitary reveals global enlargement and histology reveals hyperplasia. A serum GHRH in addition to radiology of the chest and abdomen may then be indicated to identify the cause, usually a GHRH-secreting carcinoid of lung or pancreas.

GH day curve (GHDC)

- GH taken at 4–5 time points during the day.
- This is used to assess response to treatment following surgery or radiotherapy, and also to assess GH suppression on somatostatin analogues, in order to determine whether an increase in dose is required.
- It does not have a role in the diagnosis of acromegaly, but in acromegaly GH is detectable in all samples in contrast to normal. The degree of elevation of GH is relevant to the response to all forms of treatment; the higher the GH the less frequent is treatment by surgery, drugs, or radiotherapy effective.

Box 18.1 Differential diagnosis of elevated GH

- Pain.
- Pregnancy.
- Puberty.
- Adolescence if tall.
- Stress.
- Chronic renal failure.
- Chronic liver failure.
- Heart failure.
- Diabetes mellitus.
- Malnutrition.
- Prolonged fast.
- Severe illness.
- Heroin addiction.

Note on units for GH assay

- GH concentrations may be measured in mU/L or μg/L. The equivalent ratio of mU/L to mcg/L was previously considered to be 2 and now 3.
- To improve standardization, it is recommended that the GH reference preparation should be a recombinant 22 kDa hGH; presently 88/624.
- There is currently no acceptable IGF-1 reference preparation.

Management

The management strategy depends on the individual patient, and also on the tumour size. A tumour causing compressive effects requires definitive management, whereas microadenomas do not necessarily need tumour removal. Lowering of GH is essential in all situations.

Trans-sphenoidal surgery

📖 also see Trans-sphenoidal surgery, p.182.

- This is usually the 1st line for treatment in most centres.
- Reported cure rates vary: 40–91% for microadenomas and 10–48% for macroadenomas, depending on surgical expertise.
- A GHDC should be performed following surgery to assess whether 'safe' levels of GH and IGF-1 have been attained. If the mean GH is <5mU/L then the patient can be followed up with annual IGF-1 and/or GH assessment. If safe levels of GH have not been achieved, then medical treatment and/or radiotherapy is indicated.

Role of preoperative octreotide Lanreotide treatment

This leads to some tumour shrinkage in at least 40% of cases, and it has been suggested that it may lead to reduced operative morbidity, and possibly improve surgical results.

Tumour recurrence following surgery

This is defined as tumour regrowth and increase in GH levels leading to active acromegaly following postoperative normalization of GH levels. Using the definition of postoperative cure as mean GH <5mU/L, the reported recurrence rate is low (6% at 5 years).

Radiotherapy

📖 also see Technique, p.188.

- This is usually reserved for patients following unsuccessful trans-sphenoidal surgery, only occasionally is it used as 1° therapy. The largest fall in GH occurs during the first 2 years, but GH continues to fall after this. However, normalization of mean GH may take several years and during this time adjunctive medical treatment (usually with somatostatin analogues) is required. With a starting mean GH >50mU/L, it takes on average 6 years to achieve mean GH <5mU/L compared with 4 years with starting mean GH <50mU/L.
- After radiotherapy, somatostatin analogues should be withdrawn on an annual basis to perform a GHDC to assess progress and identify when mean GH <5mU/L and therefore radiotherapy has been effective and somatostatin analogue treatment is no longer required.

Definition of cure

- Epidemiological data suggest that a mean GH <5mU/L should be the aim of treatment, as this is associated with reduction of the ↑ mortality associated with acromegaly to that of the normal population. More recently normalization of IGF-1 has also been shown in 1 study to be associated with reduction of ↑ mortality to normal.
- For this reason, patients are monitored during treatment using a GH aiming for a mean of <5mU/L. Others use suppression to <1mU/L on an OGTT as this has been shown to correlate well with mean GH. These values may be too high if more sensitive and modern assays are used. It is likely that normalization of IGF-1 may also be used, but there are limited epidemiological data on this approach. Possible ↑ risk of recurrence if abnormal nadir GH despite normal IGF-1.

Colonic polyps and acromegaly

- ↑ incidence of *colonic polyps and colonic carcinoma* has been reported by many groups. Both retrospective and prospective studies have demonstrated that 9–39% of acromegalic patients studied have colonic polyps and 0–5% have been shown to have colonic carcinoma.
- *Mechanism* IGF-1 and/or GH are implicated as both may stimulate colonic mucosal turnover. However, some studies have failed to demonstrate a direct relationship between serum levels and polyps/carcinoma.
- *Importance* Patients with acromegaly are probably at slightly ↑ risk and therefore need screening for polyps. All patients aged >40 years should have routine colonoscopy, and those with polyps should receive 3–5 years repeat colonoscopy. Agreement has not been reached, though on the frequency of follow up colonoscopy.

Drug treatment

Somatostatin analogues (📖 also see Somatostatin analogues, p.194)

- Somatostatin analogues lead to suppression of GH secretion in 60% of patients with acromegaly. At least 40% of patients are complete responders and somatostatin analogues will lead to normalization of GH (<5mU/L) and IGF-1. However, some patients are partial responders and although somatostatin analogues will lead to lowering of mean GH, they do not suppress to normal despite dose escalation.
- Acute response to these drugs is assessed by measuring GH at hourly intervals for 6h following the injection of 50–100mcg octreotide SC. This predicts long-term response.
- Depot preparations lanreotide SR, Lanreotide Autogel®, and octreotide LAR® are available. Octreotide LAR® 20mg IM is administered every 4 weeks, with dose alterations either down or up to 10–30mg every 3 months. Lanreotide Autogel® 90mg (deep SC) is administered every 4 weeks with dose alteration either down to 60mg or up to 120mg every 3 months. Patients can be taught to self administer lanreotide.
- These drugs may be used as 1° therapy where the tumour does not cause mass effects, or in patients who have received surgery and or radiotherapy who have elevated mean GH.

Dopamine agonists (📖 also see Dopamine agonists, p.192)
These drugs do lead to lowering of GH levels, but very rarely lead to normalization of GH or IGF-1 (<10%). They may be helpful particularly if there is coexistent secretion of PRL, and in these cases there may be significant tumour shrinkage. Cabergoline has recently been shown to be more effective than bromocriptine and may lead to IGF-1 normalization in up to 30%.

GH receptor antagonists (pegvisomant)
Normalization of IGF-1 in >90% of patients is reported. More data on the effect on tumour size are required as GH rises during treatment. GH levels cannot therefore be used to guide treatment and IGF-1 is used to monitor therapy. Monitoring of liver biochemistry is necessary for safety. It is indicated for somastatin non-responders. Liver function tests should be monitored 6-weekly for 6 months. MRI of the pituitary is indicated 6-monthly in case of pituitary enlargement. Therapy may be continued with octreotide or lanreotide to decrease the frequency of pegvisomant injections.

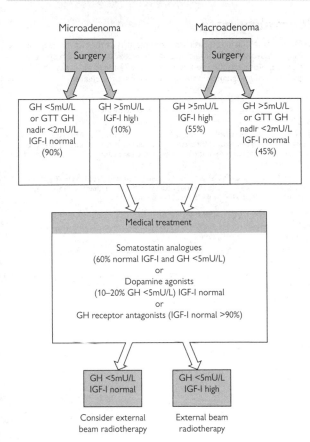

Fig. 18.1 Treatment paradigms in acromegaly. Reproduced with permission from from Wass J, (2001) *Handbook of Acromegaly*, p.81. BioScientifica Ltd.

Mortality data

- Mortality in untreated patients is double that of the normal population.
- Major causes include cardiovascular, cerebrovascular, and respiratory disease. More effective treatment has now ↑ life expectancy and the true risk of malignancy in this group will become clearer.

Further reading

Bates AS, Van't Hoff W, Jones JM, *et al.* (1993). An audit of outcome of treatment in acromegaly. *QJM* **86**, 293–99.

Bevan JS, Atkin SL, Atkinson AB, *et al.* (2002). Primary medical therapy for acromegaly: an open, prospective, multicenter study of the effects of subcutaneous and intramuscular slow-release ocreotide on growth hormone, insulin-like growth factor-I, and tumor size. *J Clin Endocrinol Metab* **87**(10), 4554–63.

Jenkins PJ, Bates P, Carson MN, *et al.* (2006). Conventional pituitary irradiation is effective in lowering serum growth hormone and insulin-like growth factor-I in patients with acromegaly. *J Clin Endocrinol Metab* **91**(4), 1239–45. Epub 2006 Jan 10.

Melmed S (2006). Medical progress: Acromegaly. *New Engl J Med* **55**(24), 2558–73.

Melmed S, Casanueva FF, Cavagnini F, *et al.* (2002). Guidelines for acromegaly management. J Clin Endocrinol Metab **87**(9), 4054–8.

Orme SM, McNally RJQ, Cartwright RA, *et al.* (1998). Mortality and Cancer Incidence in Acromegaly: A retrospective cohort study *JCEM* **83**, 2730–4.

Trainer PJ, Drake WM, Katznelso L, *et al.* (2000). Treatment of acromegaly with the growth hormone-receptor antagonist pegvisomant. *New Engl J Med* **342**(16), 1171–7.

Wass JAH (ed.) (2001). *Handbook of Acromegaly.* BioScientifica: Bristol.

Cushing's disease

Definition

Cushing's syndrome is an illness resulting from excess cortisol secretion which has a high mortality if left untreated. There are several causes of hypercortisolaemia which must be differentiated, and the commonest cause is iatrogenic (oral, inhaled, or topical steroids). It is important to decide whether the patient has true Cushing's syndrome rather than pseudo-Cushing's associated with depression or alcoholism. Secondly, ACTH-dependent Cushing's must be differentiated from ACTH-independent disease (usually due to an adrenal adenoma or rarely carcinoma—📖 see p.238). Once a diagnosis of ACTH-dependent disease has been established, it is important to differentiate between pituitary dependent (Cushing's disease) and ectopic secretion.

Epidemiology

- Rare, annual incidence approximately 2/million.
- Commoner in ♀ (3–15:1, ♀:♂).
- Age—most commonly 20–40 years.

Pathophysiology

- The vast majority of Cushing's syndrome is due to a pituitary ACTH-secreting corticotroph microadenoma. The underlying aetiology is ill-understood.
- Occasionally corticotroph adenomas reach larger sizes (macroadenomas) and rarely become invasive or malignant. The tumours typically maintain some responsiveness to the usual feedback control factors that influence the normal corticotoph (e.g. high doses of glucocorticoids, and CRH). However, this may be lost and the tumours become fully autonomous, particularly in Nelson's syndrome.
- NB Crooke's hyaline change is a fibrillary appearance seen in the non-tumorous corticotroph associated with elevated cortisol levels from any cause.

For Causes of Cushing's syndrome 📖 see Box 19.1.

Box 19.1 Causes of Cushing's syndrome

- Pseudo-Cushing's syndrome:
  - Alcoholism <1%
  - Severe depression 1%
- ACTH-dependent:
  - Pituitary adenoma 68% (Cushing's disease)
  - Ectopic ACTH syndrome 12%
  - Ectopic CRH secretion <1%
- ACTH-independent:
  - Adrenal adenoma 10%
  - Adrenal carcinoma 8%
  - Nodular (macro or micro) hyperplasia 1%
  - Carney complex (📖see p.610)
- Exogenous steroids including skin creams e.g. clobetasol.

Clinical features

The features of Cushing's syndrome are progressive and may be present for several years prior to diagnosis. A particular difficulty may occur in a patient with cyclical Cushing's, where the features and biochemical manifestations appear and disappear with a variable periodicity. Features may not always be florid and clinical suspicion should be high.

- *Facial appearance*—round plethoric complexion, acne and hirsutism, thinning of scalp hair
- *Weight gain*—truncal obesity, buffalo hump, supraclavicular fat pads.
- *Skin* thin and fragile due to loss of SC tissue, purple striae on abdomen, breasts, thighs, axillae (in contrast to silver healed postpartum striae), easy bruising, tinea versicolor, occasionally pigmentation due to ACTH.
- Proximal *muscle weakness*.
- *Mood disturbance*—labile, depression, insomnia, psychosis.
- *Menstrual disturbance*.
- *Low libido and impotence*.
- *Growth arrest* in children.

Associated features

- Hypertension (>50%) due to mineralocorticoid effects of cortisol. (cortisol overwhelms the renal 11β-hydroxysteroid dehydrogenase enzyme protecting the mineralocorticoid receptor from cortisol). Cortisol may also increase angiotensinogen levels.
- Impaired glucose tolerance/diabetes mellitus (30%).
- Osteopenia and osteoporosis (leading to fractures of spine and ribs).
- Vascular disease due to metabolic syndrome.
- Susceptibility to infections.

Investigations

Does the patient have Cushing's syndrome?

Outpatient tests

- *2–3 × 24h urinary free cortisol* This test can be useful for outpatient screening—however the false −ve rate of 5–10% means that it should not be used alone. (Fenofibrate, carbamazepine and digoxin may lead to false +ves depending on assay and reduced GFR <30 mL/min may lead to false −ves). In children: correct for body surface area. Mild elevation occurs in pseudo-Cushing's and normal pregnancy.
- *Overnight dexamethasone suppression test* Administration of 1mg dexamethasone at midnight is followed by a serum cortisol measurement at 9 a.m. Cortisol <50nmol/L makes Cushing's unlikely. (NB False +ves with poor dexamethasone absorption or hepatic enzyme induction). The false −ve value is 2% of normal individuals but rises to <20% in obese or hospitalized patients.
- If both the above tests are normal, Cushing's syndrome is unlikely.

Inpatient tests

- *Midnight cortisol* Loss of circadian rhythm of cortisol secretion is seen in Cushing's syndrome and this is demonstrated by measuring a serum cortisol at midnight (patient must be asleep for this test to be valid and ideally after 48h as an in-patient). In normal subjects the cortisol at this time is at a nadir (<50nmol/L), but in patients with Cushing's syndrome it is elevated. Late-night salivary cortisol may be promising particularly in those with possible cyclical Cushing's.
- *Low dose dexamethasone suppression test* Administration of 0.5mg dexamethasone 6-hourly (30mcg/hg/day) for 48h at 9 a.m., 3 p.m., 9 p.m., and 3 a.m. should lead to complete suppression of cortisol to <50nmol/L in normal subjects. Serum cortisol is measured at time 0 and 48h (day 2).
- Interfering conditions should be considered with all dexamethasone testing: ↓ dexamethasone absorption, hepatic enzyme inducers (e.g. phenytoin, carbamazepine, and rifampicin), and ↑ CBG.

Pseudo-Cushing's

- Patients with pseudo-Cushing's syndrome will also show loss of diurnal rhythm and lack of low dose suppressibility. However, alcoholics return to normal cortisol secretory dynamics after a few days' abstinence in hospital. Severe depression can be more difficult to differentiate, particularly since this may be a feature of Cushing's syndrome itself.
- Typically patients with pseudo-Cushing's show a normal cortisol rise with hypoglycaemia (tested using ITT), whereas patients with true Cushing's syndrome show a blunted rise. However, this is not 100% reliable, as up to 20% of patients with Cushing's syndrome (especially those with cyclical disease) show a normal cortisol rise with hypoglycaemia.

- The combined dexamethasone suppression test-CRH test (0.5mg dexamethasone 6-hourly for 48h starting at 12 p.m., followed by ovine CRH 1mcg/kg IV at 8 a.m. (2h after last dose dexamethasone) may be helpful as patients with pseudo-Cushing's are thought to be under chronic CRH stimulation thus showing a blunted response to CRH after dexamethasone suppression (Cortisol 15min after CRH >38nmol/L in Cushing's and <38nmol/Lin pseudo-Cushing's).
- IV desmopressin 10mcg increases ACTH in 80–90% with Cushing's but rarely in patients with pseudo-Cushing's.
- No screening tests are fully capable of distinguishing all case of Cushing's syndrome from normal individuals/pseudo-Cushing's.

Box 19.2 Cyclical Cushing's

A small group of patients with Cushing's syndrome have alternating normal and abnormal cortisol levels on an irregular basis. All causes of Cushing's syndrome may be associated with cyclical secretion of cortisol. Clearly the results of dynamic testing can only be interpreted when the disease is shown to be active (elevated urinary cortisol secretion and loss of normal circadian rhythm and suppressability on dexamethasone).

Table 19.1 Screening tests for Cushing's syndrome

Test	False +ves	False −ves	Sensitivity
24h urinary free cortisol	1%	5–10%	95%
Overnight 1mg dexamethasone suppression test	2% normal 13% obese 23% hospital Inpatients	2%	
Midnight cortisol	?	0	100%
Low-dose dexamethasone suppression test	<2%	2%	98%

What is the underlying cause?
ACTH
- Once the presence of Cushing's syndrome has been confirmed, a serum basal ACTH should be measured to differentiate between ACTH dependent and ACTH independent aetiologies (Fig. 19.1). ACTH may not be fully suppressed in some adrenal causes of Cushing's; however ACTH >4pmol/L are suggestive of ACTH dependent aetiology.
- The basal ACTH is, however, of very little value in differentiating between pituitary-dependent Cushing's syndrome and ectopic Cushing's syndrome as there is considerable overlap between the 2 groups although patients with ectopic disease tend to have higher ACTH levels (Fig. 19.1).

Serum potassium
A rapidly spun potassium is a useful discriminatory test as hypokalaemia <3.2mmol/L is found in almost 100% of patients with ectopic secretion of ACTH but <10% of patients with pituitary dependent disease.

High dose dexamethasone suppression test
The high dose dexamethasone suppression test is performed in an identical way to the low dose test but with 2mg doses of dexamethasone (120mcg/kg/day). In Cushing's disease the cortisol falls by >50% of the basal value. In ectopic disease, there is no suppression. However, approximately 10% of cases of ectopic disease, particularly those due to carcinoid tumours, show >50% suppression, and 10% of patients with Cushing's disease do not suppress.

Corticotrophin releasing hormone test (Fig. 19.2)
- The administration of 100mcg of CRH IV (SE transient flushing, very rare apoplexy reported) leads to an exaggerated rise in cortisol (14–20%) and ACTH (35–50%) in 95% of patients with pituitary-dependent Cushing's syndrome. There are occasional reports of patients with ectopic disease who show a similar response.

Inferior petrosal sinus sampling (Fig. 19.3)
- Bilateral simultaneous inferior petrosal sinus sampling with measurement of ACTH centrally and in the periphery in the basal state and following stimulation with IV CRH (100mcg) allows differentiation between pituitary dependent and ectopic disease. A central to peripheral ratio of >2 prior to CRH is very suggestive of pituitary dependent disease, and >3 following CRH gives a diagnostic accuracy of approaching 90–95% for pituitary-dependent disease. The test should be performed when cortisol levels are elevated.
- The accurate lateralization of a tumour using the results from inferior petrosal sinus sampling (IPSS) is difficult as differences in blood flow and catheter placement, etc. will affect the results.

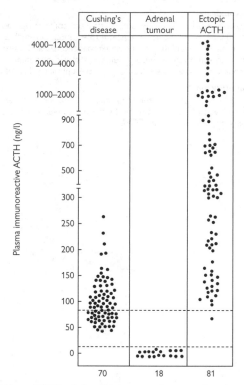

Fig. 19.1 Plasma ACTH levels (9 a.m.) in patients with pituitary-dependent Cushing's disease, adrenal tumours and ectopic ACTH secretion. From Besser M and Thorner GM (1994). *Clinical Endocrinology 2nd edn.* Mosby.

Table 19.2 Investigation of ACTH-dependent Cushing's syndrome

Test	Pituitary dependent disease (% with this finding)	Ectopic disease (% with this finding)
Serum potassium <3.2mmol/L	10	100
Suppression of basal cortisol to over 50% on high dose dexamethasone suppression test	90	10
Exaggerated rise in cortisol on CRH test	95	<1

Reproduced from Besser M and Thorner GM (1994). Clinical Endocrinology 2nd edn, Mosby, Copyright Elsevier, with permission.

Pituituary imaging

MRI following gadolinium enhancement localizes corticotroph adenomas in up to 80% of cases. However, it should be remembered that at least 10% of the normal population harbour microadenomas and therefore the biochemical investigation of these patients is essential as a patient with an ectopic source to Cushing's syndrome may have a pituitary 'incidentaloma'.

Other pituitary function

Hypercortisolism suppresses the thyroidal, gonadal, and GH axes leading to lowered levels of TSH and thyroid hormones as well as reduced gonadotrophins, gonadal steroids and GH.

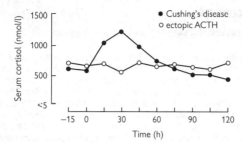

Fig. 19.2 CRH test in pituitary-dependent and ectopic disease. In the patient with pituitary-dependent disease, the characteristic marked plasma cortisol rise after an IV bolus of 100mcg of CRH is seen. Serum cortisol levels are unaltered in the patient with ectopic ACTH secretion. Reproduced from Besser M and Thorner GM (1994). *Clinical Endocrinology, 2nd edn.* Mosby. Copyright Elsevier, with permission.

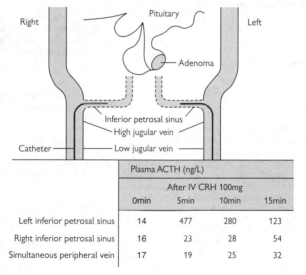

	Plasma ACTH (ng/L)			
	After IV CRH 100mg			
	0min	5min	10min	15min
Left inferior petrosal sinus	14	477	280	123
Right inferior petrosal sinus	16	23	28	54
Simultaneous peripheral vein	17	19	25	32

Fig. 19.3 Simultaneous bilateral inferior petrosal sinus and peripheral vein sampling for ACTH. The ratio of >3 between the left central and peripheral vein confirm a diagnosis of Cushing's disease. Reproduced from Besser M and Thorner GM (1994). *Clinical Endocrinology, 2nd edn.* Mosby. Copyright Elsevier, with permission.

Treatment

Trans-sphenoidal surgery (📖 also see Trans-sphenoidal surgery, p.182)

- This is the 1st-line option in most cases. Selective adenomectomy gives the greatest chance of cure with a reported remission rate of up to 90%. However, strict criteria of a postoperative cortisol of <50nmol/L lead to lower cure rates, but much lower recurrence rates (<10% compared with up to 50% in those with detectable postoperative cortisols). This should be the current definition of successful surgery as the long-term outcome is significantly better in this group of patients.
- Complications of surgery may be higher in these patients as their preoperative general status and the condition of the tissues is poorer than other patients who are referred for surgery. It is often useful to administer medical treatment for at least 6 weeks prior to surgery to allow improvement in wound healing and reduce anaesthetic risk in those with severe metabolic problems.
- Risk of relapse lasts for at least 10 years.

Pituitary radiotherapy (📖 also see p.188)

This is usually administered as 2nd-line treatment following unsuccessful trans-sphenoidal surgery. As control of cortisol levels may take months to years, medical treatment to control cortisol levels while waiting for cortisol levels to fall is essential. A more rapid response to radiotherapy is seen in childhood.

Adrenalectomy

- This used to be the favoured form of treatment. It successfully controls cortisol hypersecretion in the majority of patients. Occasionally a remnant is left and leads to recurrent hypercortisolaemia.
- Nelson's syndrome may occur in up to 30% of patients. The administration of prophylactic radiotherapy ↓ the likelihood of this complication. Careful follow-up of these patients is therefore essential to allow prompt treatment of the tumour. These tumours are associated with marked increase in ACTH, and associated pigmentation is common. Loss of normal responsiveness to glucocorticoids is characteristic and therefore biochemical monitoring should be performed at least 6 months first and then annually by measuring a basal ACTH and re-checking it 1 and 2h after the morning dose of glucocorticoid (ACTH curve).
- Bilateral adrenalectomy may still be indicated when pituitary surgery, radiotherapy, and medical treatment have failed to control the disease. It is also helpful in Cushing's syndrome due to ectopic disease, when the ectopic source remains elusive or inoperable. Laparoscopic surgery minimizes morbidity and complications.

Peri- and postoperative management following trans-sphenoidal surgery for Cushing's disease

- Perioperative hydrocortisone replacement is given in the standard way as it is assumed that the patient will become cortisol deficient after successful removal of the tumour.
- After 3–4 days, the evening steroid replacement is omitted and 9 a.m. cortisol and ACTH checked the following day, and 24h later after withholding steroids. Undetectable cortisol (<50nmol/L) is suggestive of cure and glucocorticoid replacement is commenced. Cortisol 50–300nmol/L is compatible with resolution of symptoms and a day curve should be performed. Patients with levels >300nmol/L should be considered for re-exploration and/or radiotherapy.
- Ante-thrombotic prophylaxis should be considered as Cushing's is associated with a thrombophilic state.

Box 19.3 Nelson's syndrome

- Occurs in patients with Cushing's disease following adrenalectomy.
- Hyperpigmentation and an enlarging (often invasive) pituitary tumour associated with markedly elevated ACTH levels.
- Usually within 2 years of adrenalectomy.
- Overall incidence is 50% at 10 years. However if pituitary adenoma visible at time of adrenalectomy, incidence is 80% at 3 years. MRI and ACTH monitoring is important for at least 6 years post-adrenalectomy, and should be initiated 6 months after adrenalectomy.

Medical treatment

- This is indicated during the preoperative preparation of patients, or while awaiting radiotherapy to be effective or if surgery or radiotherapy are contra-indicated.
- Inhibitors of steroidogenesis: *metyrapone* is usually used 1st line, but *ketoconazole* should be used as 1st line in children as it is unassociated with ↑ adrenal metabolites. There is also a suggestion that ketoconazole may have a direct action on the corticotroph as well as lowering cortisol secretion.
- Disadvantages of these agents inhibiting steroidogenesis are the need to increase the dose to maintain control as ACTH secretion will increase as cortisol concentrations decrease.
- Steroidogenesis inhibitors may be used in a *complete* inhibition and glucocorticoid replacement regimen, or with an aim for *partial* inhibition of cortisol production.
- The dose of these drugs needs to be titrated against the cortisol results from a day curve (cortisol taken at 9 a.m., 12 noon, 3 p.m., 6 p.m.) aiming for a mean cortisol of 150–300nmol/L as this approximates the normal production rate.
- Response rates for drugs that reduce ACTH/CRH synthesis/release e.g. somatostatin agonists, bromocriptine, valproate and cyproheptadine are poor but there are no large-scale published studies.
- Successful treatment (surgery or radiotherapy) of Cushing's disease leads to cortisol deficiency, and therefore glucocorticoid replacement therapy is essential. In addition patients who have undergone bilateral adrenalectomy require fludrocortisone. These patients should all receive instructions for intercurrent illness and carry a MedicAlert bracelet and steroid card.

Table 19.3 Drug treatment of Cushing's syndrome

Drug	Dose	Action	Side effects
Metyrapone	1–4g/d (usually given in 4 divided doses)	11β-hydroxylase inhibitor	Nausea ↑ androgenic and mineralocorticoid precursors lead to hirsutism and hypertension
Ketoconazole	200–400mg tds 1st line in children NB Avoid if taking H2 antagonists as acid required to metabolize active compound.	Direct inhibitor of P450 enzymes at several different sites	Abnormalities of liver function (usually reversible) Gynaecomastia
Mitotane (o-p- DDD)	4–12g/d (begin at 0.5–1g/d and gradually increase dose)	Inhibits steroidogenesis at the side-chain cleavage, 11 and 18-hydroxylase and 3β-hydroxysteroid dehydrogenase Adrenolytic	Nausea and vomiting Cerebellar disturbance Somnolence Hypercholesterolaemia NB May increase clearance of steroids— replacement dosage may need to be ↑ NB May be teratogenic. Avoid if fertility desired.
Etomidate	Useful when parenteral treatment is required.	Inhibits side-chain cleavage and 11β-hydroxylase.	

Follow-up

Successful treatment for Cushing's disease leads to a cortisol that is undetectable (<50nmol/L) following surgery. (This is due to the total suppression of cortisol production from the normal corticotrophs in Cushing's disease). An undetectable postoperative cortisol leads to a significantly higher chance of long-term cure compared to the patients who had postoperative cortisols between 50—300nmol/L.

- The aim of follow-up is
  - To detect recurrent Cushing's, and also
  - To recognize when recovery of the pituitary adrenal axis occurs which may take several years (80% recovered by 2 years).
- Therefore patients need to have regular assessment of cortisol production off glucocorticoid replacement. When cortisol is detectable following surgery, recurrent disease must be excluded (UFC and low dose dexamethasone suppression). If recurrence is excluded, it is then important to document the adequacy of the stress response once weaned off glucocorticoid replacement (ITT).

Prognosis

- Untreated disease leads to an approximately 30–50% mortality at 5 years owing to vascular disease and ↑ susceptibility to infections.
- Treated Cushing's syndrome has a good prognosis. Patients who have an undetectable postoperative cortisol are very unlikely to recur (0–20%), whereas 50–75% recur if the postoperative cortisol is detectable.
- Although the physical features and severe psychological disorders associated with Cushing's improve or resolve within weeks or months of successful treatment, more subtle mood disturbance may persist for longer. Adults also have impaired cognitive function. In addition, it is likely that there is an ↑ cardiovascular risk.
- Osteoporosis will usually resolve in children, but may not improve significantly in older patients. Bone mineral density therefore requires monitoring and may need specific treatment. *Alendronic acid* has been shown to be effective therapy leading to improved bone mineral density in patients with Cushing's syndrome and osteoporosis.
- Hypertension has been shown to resolve in 80% and diabetes mellitus in up to 70%.

Cushing's syndrome in children

In a series of 59 patients aged 4–20 years the following factors were found:

Causes

- Pituitary dependent disease 85%.
- Adrenal disease 10%.
- Ectopic ACTH secretion 5%.

Initial presentation

- Excessive weight gain 90%.
- Growth retardation 83%.

Below the age of 5 years, adrenal causes are common. In neonates and young children the McCune–Albright syndrome should be considered, whereas in late childhood and early adolescence, ACTH independence may suggest Carney complex (🕮 also see Carney complex, p.610).

Treatment

- Trans-sphenoidal surgery is used as 1st-line therapy in pituitary-dependent Cushing's in children as in adults and is usually successful.
- Radiotherapy cures up to 85% children and this may be considered 1st-line in some patients. Ketoconazole is the preferred medical therapy in this age group as it is not associated with ↑ adrenal androgens.
- The long-term management of children with Cushing's syndrome requires careful attention to growth as growth failure is a very common presentation of this condition. Postoperatively or after radiotherapy, GH therapy may restore growth and final height to normal.

Further reading

Arnaldi G, Angeli A, Atkinson AB, et al. (2003). Diagnosis and complications of Cushing's syndrome: a consensus statement. *J Clin Endocrinol Metab* **88**, 5593–602.

Assié G, Bahurel H, Coste J, et al. (2007). Corticotroph tumor progression after adrenalectomy in Cushing's disease: A reappraisal of Nelson's syndrome. *J Clin Endocrinol Metab* **92**(1), 172–9.

Isidori AM, Kaltsas GA, Pozza C, et al. (2006). The ectopic adrenocorticotropin syndrome: clinical features, diagnosis, management, and long-term follow-up. *J Clin Endocrinol Metab* **91**(2), 371–7. Epub 2005 Nov 22.

Magiakou MA, Mastorakos G, Oldfield EH, et al. (1994). Cushing's syndrome in children and adolescents. *New Engl J Med* **331**, 629–36.

Newell-Price J, Morris DG, Drake WM, et al. (2002). Optimal response criteria for the human CRH test in the differential diagnosis of ACTH-dependent Cushing's Syndrome. *J Clin Endocrinol Metab* **87**(4), 1640–5.

Newell-Price J, Trainer P, Besser M, et al. (1998). The diagnosis and differential diagnosis of Cushing's syndrome and pseudo-Cushing's states. *Endocrinol Rev* **19**(5), 647–72.

Nieman LH (2002). Medical management of Cushing's disease *Pituitary* **5**, 77–82.

Nieman CH et al. (2008). The Diagnosis of Cushing's Syndrome. An Endocrine Society Clinical Practice Guideline. *JCEM* **93**, 1526–40.

Non-functioning pituitary tumours

Background

These pituitary tumours are unassociated with clinical syndromes of anterior pituitary hormone excess.

Epidemiology

- Non-functioning pituitary tumours (NFA) are the commonest pituitary macroadenoma. They represent 25% of all pituitary tumours.
- There is an equal sex distribution and the majority of cases present in patients aged >50 years.
- 50% enlarge if left untreated, at 5 years.

Pathology

- Despite the fact that NFAs are unassociated with hormone production, they may immunostain for:
  - Glycoprotein hormones (most commonly gonadotrophins)—LH, FSH, the α or β subunits or TSH.
  - ACTH (silent corticotroph adenomas), or
  - Be −ve on immunostaining—either null cell tumours or oncocytomas (characteristically contain multiple mitochondria on electron microscopy).
- Tumour behaviour is variable, with some tumours behaving in a very indolent slow-growing manner and others invading the sphenoid and cavernous sinus.

Clinical features

Mass effects

- Visual field defects (uni- or bitemporal quadrantanopia or hemianopia).
- Headache.
- Ophthalmoplegia (III, IV, and VI cranial nerves—rarely).
- Optic atrophy (rarely, following long-term optic nerve compression).
- Apoplexy (rarely).

Hypopituitarism

📖 also see Hypopituitarism, p.98.
  At diagnosis, approximately 50% are gonadotrophin deficient.

Incidental finding

A NFA may be detected on the basis of imaging performed for other reasons.

Investigations

- *Pituitary imaging* MRI/CT demonstrates the tumour and/or invasion into the cavernous sinus or supraoptic recess.
- *Visual fields assessment* Abnormal in up to $^2/_3$ of cases.
- *PRL* Essential to exclude a PRL secreting macroadenoma (📖 see p.118).
  - Mild elevation (<3000mU/Usually 2,000mU/c) may occur secondary to stalk compression
- *Pituitary function* Assessment for hypopituitarism (📖 see Pituitary function—dynamic tests, p.90, 100).

Management

Surgery

- The initial definitive management in virtually every case is surgical. This removes mass effects and may lead to some recovery of pituitary function in around 10%. The majority of patients can be operated on successfully via the trans-sphenoidal route.
- Close follow-up is necessary after surgery as tumour regrowth can only be detected using pituitary imaging and visual field assessment.

Radiotherapy

- The use of postoperative radiotherapy remains controversial. Some centres advocate its use for every patient following surgery; others reserve its use for those patients who have had particularly invasive or aggressive tumours removed or those with a significant amount of residual tumour remaining (e.g. in the cavernous sinus).
- The regrowth rate at 10 years without radiotherapy approaches 45% and there are no good predictive factors for determining which tumours will regrow. However, administration of postoperative radiotherapy reduces this regrowth rate to less than 10%. 📖 as discussed in Complications, p.190, however, there are sequelae to radiotherapy—with a significant long-term risk of hypopituitarism and a possible ↑ risk of visual deterioration and malignancy in the field of radiation p.188

Medical treatment

- Unlike the case for GH and PRL-secreting tumours, medical therapy for NFAs is usually unhelpful, although there have been reports of the somatostatin agonist octreotide leading to tumour shrinkage and/or visual field improvement in some cases.
- Hormone replacement therapy is required to treat any hypopituitarism (📖 see p.104).
- Visual field defects at diagnosis may improve following surgery in the majority and improvement may continue for a year following tumour debulking.

Prediction of regrowth of NFAs?

No markers that provide certainty. However the following have been suggested as useful markers to raise suspicion of aggressive behaviour:

- Younger age.
- Preoperative cavernous sinus invasion and postoperative suprasellar extension.
- Atypical features on histology (elevated mitotic index, MIB-1 labelling index >3% and macronucleoli).

Biochemical markers for NFAs?
- The majority of patients lack a hormone marker—despite approximately half immunostain positively for gonadotrophins and contain secretory granules at the EM level.
- A minority of patients have elevated circulating FSH/LH levels, see section on gonadotrophinomas (see p.158).
- The use of the response of α subunit or LH/FSH as a tumour marker has been suggested. Small series have shown that up to 70% of patients with functionless tumours show a 50% rise in serum gonadotrophin/ subunit after 200mcg IV TRH. As this response disappears after tumour resection it may be a useful tumour marker, although this is not widely practised.

Follow-up

- Patients who have not received postoperative irradiation require careful long-term follow-up with serial pituitary imaging and visual field assessment. The optimal protocol is still not known but an accepted practice is to image in the first 3 months following surgery and then re-image annually for 5 years and then biannually thereafter. Tumour recurrence has been reported at up to 15 years following surgery and therefore follow-up needs to be long-term.
- In patients who have received postoperative radiotherapy, follow-up with annual visual field assessment and imaging only if a deterioration is noted.
- Dopamine agonists may decrease recurrences but this needs a proper prospective study.

Prognosis

Patients with NFAs have a good prognosis once the diagnosis and appropriate treatment including replacement of hormone deficiency is performed. The main concern is the risk of tumour regrowth with subsequent visual failure. As mentioned earlier, the administration of radiotherapy, although not without potential complications itself significantly reduces this risk. Unirradiated patients require very close follow-up in order to detect regrowth and perform repeat surgery or administer radiotherapy.

Further reading

Karavitaki N, Thanabalasingham G, Shore HC, Trifanescu R, Ansorge O, Meston N, Turner HE, Wass JA (2006). Do the limits of serum prolactin in disconnection hperprolactinaemia need re-definition? A study of 226 patients with histologically verified non-functioning pituitary macroadenoma *Clin Endocrinol* (Oxf). **65**(4), 524–9.

Gonadotrophinomas

Background

These are tumours that arise from the gonadotroph cells of the pituitary gland and produce FSH, LH, or the α subunit. They are often indistinguishable from other non-functioning pituitary adenomas as they are usually silent and unassociated with excess detectable secretion of LH and FSH, although studies demonstrate gonado-trophin/α subunit secretion *in vitro*. Occasionally however, these tumours do produce detectable excess hormone *in vivo*.

Clinical features

- Gonadotrophinomas present in the same manner as other non-functioning pituitary tumours with mass effects and hypopituitarism (📖 see p.152).
- The rare FSH-secreting gonadotrophinomas may lead to macroorchidism in ♂.
- May cause ovarian hyperstimulation in premenopausal females.

Investigations

The secretion of FSH and LH from these tumours is usually undetectable in the plasma. Occasionally elevated FSH, and more rarely LH, is measured. This finding is often ignored, particularly in postmenopausal ♀, although elevated gonadotrophins together with ACTH and/or TSH deficiency in the presence of a macroadenomas should raise the suspicion of a functioning gonadotrophinoma.

Management

These tumours are managed as non-functioning tumours. The potential advantage of FSH/LH secretion from a functioning gonadotrophinoma is that it provides a biochemical marker of presence of tumour for follow-up.

Thyrotrophinomas

Epidemiology

These are rare tumours comprising approximately 1% of all pituitary tumours. The diagnosis may be delayed, because the significance of an unsuppressed TSH in the presence of elevated free thyroid hormone concentrations may be missed. Approximately $1/3$ of cases in the literature have received treatment directed at the thyroid in the form of radioiodine treatment or surgery, before diagnosis.

Unlike 1° hyperthyroidism, thyrotrophinomas are equally common in ♂ and ♀. 5% associated with MEN1.

Tumour biology and behaviour

- The majority are macroadenomas (90%) and secrete only TSH often with α-subunit in addition, but some co-secrete GH (55%), and/or PRL (15%).
- The pathogenesis of thyrotoxicosis in the presence of normal TSH levels is poorly understood, but there are reports of secretion of TSH with ↑ bioactivity possibly due to changes in posttranslational hormone glycosylation.
- The observation that prior thyroid ablation is associated with deleterious effects on the size of the tumour suggests some feedback control, and is similar to the aggressive tumours seen in Nelson's syndrome after bilateral adrenalectomy has been performed for Cushing's disease. Thyrotropin-secreting pituitary carcinoma has been very rarely reported.
- 5% are associated with MEN1.

Clinical features

(📖 see p.20)

- Clinical features of *hyperthyroidism* are usually present, but often milder than expected given the level of thyroid hormones. In mixed tumours, hyperthyroidism may be overshadowed by features of *acromegaly*.
- *Mass effects* visual field defects and hypopituitarism.

Investigations

($\square$ see also p.40)

- *TSH is inappropriately normal or elevated* The range of TSH that has been described is <1–568 mU/L, and $^1/_3$ untreated patients had TSH in the normal range. There is no correlation between TSH and T_4.
- *Free thyroid hormones* elevated 65% patients.
- *α-subunit (raised in 65%)* Typically patients have an ↑ α-subunit: TSH molar ratio(>1)(81%).
- *Other anterior pituitary hormone levels* PRL and/or GH may be elevated in mixed tumours (an OGTT may be indicated to exclude acromegaly).
- *SHBG* elevated into the hyperthyroid range.
- *TRH test* absent TSH response to stimulation with TRH (useful to differentiate TSH-secreting tumours from thyroid hormone resistance where the TSH response is normal or exaggerated).
- *T_3 suppresion test* (Lack of suppression of TSH following 100mcg/day for 10 days).
- *Thyroid antibodies* In contrast to Graves' disease, the incidence of thyroid antibodies is similar to that in the general population.
- *Pituitary imaging* MRI scan will demonstrate a pituitary tumour (macroadenoma) in the majority of cases (90%).

Causes of an elevated FT_4 in the presence of an inappropriately unsuppressed TSH

($\square$ see p.40)

- TSH-secreting tumour.
- Thyroid hormone resistance.
- Amiodarone therapy.
- Inherited abnormalities of thyroid-binding proteins.

Management

Surgery

- Surgery leads to cure in approximately $1/3$ of patients as judged by apparent complete removal of tumour mass and normalization of thyroid hormone levels, with another $1/3$ improved with normal thyroid hormone levels but incomplete removal of the adenoma.
- Microadenomas are cured in higher proportions.

Radiotherapy

Radiotherapy is useful following unsuccessful surgery, and leads to gradual (over years) reduction in TSH.

Medical treatment

Somatostatin analogues

- Medical treatment with the somatostatin agonists octreotide and lanreotide is successful in the majority of patients in suppressing TSH secretion and leading to tumour shrinkage. In 1 study, octreotide reduced TSH secretion in almost all patients treated, and normalized thyroid hormone levels in 73% of patients. There was partial tumour shrinkage in 40%.
- Drug therapy is useful in the preoperative preparation of these patients to ensure that they are fit for general anaesthetic and also while waiting for radiotherapy to be effective.

Anti-thyroid medication

Treatment with antithyroid drugs has been associated with ↑ TSH in approximately 60% of patients reported. It should be avoided if possible and the more appropriate somatostatin agonist therapy utilized.

Further reading

Beck-Peccoz P, Brucker-Davis F Persani L, et al. (1996). Thyrotropin-secreting pituitary tumours. Endocr Rev **17**, 610–38.

Chanson P, Weintraub BD, and Harris AG (1993). Octreotide therapy for thyroid stimulating hormone-secreting pituitary adenomas. Ann Intern Med **119**, 236–40.

Pituitary incidentalomas

Definition

The term incidentaloma refers to an incidentally detected lesion that is unassociated with hormonal hyper- or hyposecretion and has a benign natural history.

The increasingly frequent detection of these lesions with technological improvements and more widespread use of sophisticated imaging has led to a management challenge—which, if any lesions need investigation and/or treatment, and what is the optimal follow-up strategy (if required at all)?

Epidemiology

- Autopsy studies have shown that 10–20% of pituitary glands unsuspected of having pituitary disease harbour pituitary adenomas. Approximately half the tumours stain for PRL and the remainder are –ve on immunostaining.
- Imaging studies using MRI demonstrate pituitary microadenomas in approximately 10% of normal volunteers.
- Incidentally detected macroadenomas have been reported when imaging has been performed for other reasons. However, these are not true incidentalomas as they are often associated with visual field defects, and/or hypopituitarism.

Natural history

Incidentally detected microadenomas are very unlikely to increase in size (<10%) whereas larger incidentally detected meso- and macroadenomas are more likely to enlarge (40–50%). Thus conservative management in selected patients may be appropriate for microadenomas which are incidentally detected as long as careful follow-up imaging is in place and patients are truly asymptomatic. Macroadenomas should be treated if possible.

Clinical features

By definition, a patient with an incidentaloma should be asymptomatic. Any patient who has an incidentally detected tumour should have visual field assessment and a clinical review to ensure that this is not the initial presentation of Cushing's syndrome acromegaly as a prolactinoma.

Investigations

- Aims:
  - Exclude any hormone hypersecretion from the tumour.
  - Detect hypopituitarism.
- Investigation of hypersecretion of hormones should include measurement of PRL, IGF-1, and an OGTT if acromegaly is suspected, 24h urinary free cortisol and overnight dexamethasone suppression test and thyroid function tests (unsuppressed TSH in the presence of elevated T_4).
- Others suggest that this approach is unnecessary, but with limited data most endocrinologists would perform investigations as above.

Management

- All extra-sellar macroadenomas (incidentally detected but by definition not true incidentalomas) require definitive treatment.
- Tumours with excess hormone secretion require definitive treatment.
- Mass <1cm repeat MRI at 1, 2, and 5 years.
- Mass >1cm diameter—repeat MRI at 6 months, 1, 2, and 5 years.

Further reading

Turner HE, Moore NR, Byrne JV, et al. (1998). Pituitary, adrenal and thyroid incidentalomas. *Endocr-rel Cancer* **5**, 131–50.

Karavitaki N, Collison K, Halliday J, Byrne JV, Price P, Cudlip S, Wass JA (2007). What is the natural history of nonoperated nonfunctioning pituitary adenomas? Clin Endocrinol (Oxf). **67**(6), 938–43. (PMID: 17692109)

Pituitary carcinoma

Definition

Pituitary carcinoma is defined as a 1° adenohypophyseal neoplasm with craniospinal and/or distant systemic metastases.

Epidemiology

These are extremely rare tumours, and only approximately 60 cases have been reported in the world literature.

Pathology and pathogenesis

- The initial tumours and subsequent carcinomas show higher proliferation indices than the majority of pituitary adenomas. They are also likely to demonstrate p53 positivity and have an ↑ mitotic index. However, histology is unable to reliably distinguish between benign invasive pituitary adenomas and carcinomas.
- The aetiology of these tumours is unknown, but the adenoma–carcinoma sequence is followed in ACTH-secreting tumours: pituitary adenoma causing Cushing's disease, followed by locally invasive adenoma (Nelson's syndrome) leading to pituitary carcinoma.
- Metastatic spread outside the CNS is via lymphatic and vascular routes, while intra-CNS spread is local invasion and tumour seeding.

Features

Virtually all pituitary carcinomas initially present as invasive pituitary macroadenomas. After a variable interval of time (mean 6.5 years) the majority present with local recurrence. There is a tendency to systemic (liver, lymph nodes, lungs, and bones) rather than craniospinal metastases but metastases do not usually predominate in the clinical picture.

Table 24.1 Types of pituitary carcinoma

Type	Proportion of reported cases
PRL	30%
ACTH	28%
GH	2%
Non-functioning	30%

NB Many 'non-functioning' carcinomas were reported prior to routine measurement of PRL or routine immunostaining, and therefore the true incidence of PRL-producing carcinomas may be higher.

Invasive adenomas

Invasive pituitary adenomas behave more aggressively than other benign pituitary adenomas, however they are not frankly malignant.

Approximately 10% pituitary adenomas may be defined as invasive according to neuroradiological criteria and up to 40% according to intra-operative inspection.

Neuroradiological classification of pituitary adenomas (modified Hardy criteria)

- Grade 1—microadenoma.
- Grade 2—macroadenoma with or without suprasellar extension.
- Grade 3—locally invasive tumour with boney destruction and tumour in the cavernous or sphenoid sinus.
- Grade 4—spread within the CNS or extracranial dissemination.

Grades 3 and 4 are termed 'invasive'.

Treatment

Treatment involves surgery, radiotherapy, and medical treatment. As mass effects often predominate, initial debulking surgery may provide relief. It may need to be repeated to maintain local control. Some advocate a trans-sphenoidal route as less likely to disseminate tumour.

Radiotherapy or medical treatment provide palliation only. Radiotherapy has been reported to be successful in some cases in controlling growth and occasionally leading to regression. Stereotactic radiosurgery may play a role. Medical treatment with dopamine agonists for malignant prolactinomas and acromegaly has been reported with varying results. Many pituitary carcinoma are dedifferentiated and therefore escape from control. Various chemotherapy regimes have been reported with occasional success (e.g. CCNU, 5FU and folinic acid or cisplatinum, procarbazine, lomustine and vincristine).

Prognosis

Most patients die within a year of diagnosis.

Further reading

Kaltsas GA and Grossman AB (1998). Malignant pituitary tumours. *Pituitary* **1**(1), 69–81.

Pernicone PJ, Scheithauer BW, and Sebo TJ, et al. (1997). Pituitary carcinoma. *Cancer* **79**, 804–12.

Pituitary metastases

Incidence
0.1–28% autopsy series, <1% trans-sphenoidal surgery.

Epidemiology
Equal sex distribution. Age >60 (occasionally younger).

Features
Diabetes insipidus in almost 100%. Symptomatic pituitary failure and cranial nerve defects less common. Often difficult to differentiate neuroradiologically from other pituitary mass lesions (adenoma, cyst, or inflammatory pituitary mass). Many do not have symptoms as features of end-stage malignancy predominate. Disconnection hyperprolactinaemia may be a feature, and very rare cases of endocrine hyperfunction related to metastasis within a primary adenoma have been reported. 📖 See Box 24.1.

Box 24.1 Primary tumours associated with pituitary metastases

Breast ⎤
Lung ⎥ account for $^2/_3$
GI.   ⎦
Prostate.
Kidney.

Diagnosis
Histology is required to confirm.

Treatment
- Of 1° tumour where possible.
- Management of endocrine symptoms.
- Decompression may be indicated for visual field defects.

Prognosis
Mean survival 6–7 months.

Craniopharyngiomas and perisellar cysts

Prevalence

0.065/1000.

Epidemiology

Any age, only 50% present in childhood (<16 years).

Pathology

- Tumour arising from squamous epithelial remnants of Rathke's pouch.
- Histology may be either adamantinous epithelial, with cyst formation and calcification, or squamous papillary (generally associated with a better prognosis).
- Cyst formation and calcification is common.
- Benign tumour, although infiltrates surrounding structures. hCG is present in cyst fluid.

Features

- Raised intracranial pressure.
- Visual disturbance.
- Hypothalamopituitary disturbance.
- Growth failure in children.
- Precocious puberty and tall stature are less common.
- Anterior and posterior pituitary failure, including DI.
- Weight gain.

Other perisellar cysts

- Arachnoid.
- Epidermoid.
- Dermoid.

Investigations

- MRI/CT (CT may be helpful to evaluate boney erosion).
- Visual field assessment.
- Anterior and posterior pituitary assessment (see p.100 and 200).

Box 25.1 Rathke's cleft cysts

Pathology

Derived from the remnants of Rathke's pouch, lined by epithelial cells (ciliated cuboidal/columnar epithelium, compared with squamous for craniopharyngiomas) and filled with fluid.

Features

Usually asymptomatic, although may present with headache and amenorrhoea, and rarely hypopituitarism and hydrocephalus.

Investigation

CT/MRI—variable enhancement.

Management

- Decompression if symptomatic.
- Recurrence is rare.

Management

- Gross total removal is the aim of treatment as this is associated with a significantly lower recurrence rate. This may be via a transfrontal or trans-sphenoidal route. If total removal cannot be safely achieved, adjuvant radiotherapy is beneficial in reducing recurrence.
- Restoration of pituitary hormone deficiencies is extremely unlikely following surgery.
- Cystic lesions may be treated with aspiration alone, although radiotherapy reduces the likelihood of reaccumulation.

Prognosis

- Craniopharyngiomas are associated with ↓ survival (up to 5 × the mortality of the general population).
- Recurrence following initial treatment may present early or several decades following initial treatment. Childhood and adult-onset lesions behave similarly.

Further reading

Karivitaki N, Cudlip S, Adams CB, *et al.* (2006). Craniopharyngiomas. *Endocr Rev* **27**(4), 371–93.

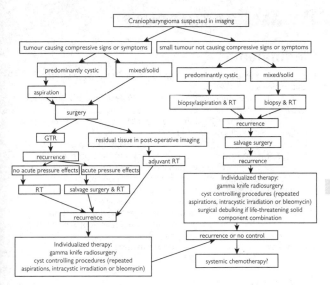

Fig. 25.1 Treatment algorithm for craniopharyngiomas. Reproduced with permission from Karavitaki N, Cudlip S, Adams CB, Wass JA (2006). Craniopharyngiomas. *Endocr Rev* **27** (4), pp.371–97. Epub 2006 Mar 16, copyright 2006, The Endocrine Society.

Parasellar tumours

Meningiomas

- Suprasellar meningiomas arise from the tuberculum sellae or the chiasmal sulcus.
- Usually present with a chiasmal syndrome where loss of visual acuity occurs in 1 eye followed by reduced acuity in the other eye.
- Differentiation from a 1° pituitary tumour can be difficult where there is downward extension into the sella.
- MRI is the imaging of choice. T1-weighted images demonstrate meningiomas as isodense with grey matter and hypointense with respect to pituitary tissue, with marked enhancement after gadolinium.
- Cerebral angiography also demonstrates a tumour blush.
- Management is surgical and may also be complicated by haemorrhage as these are often very vascular tumours. They are relatively radioresistant but inoperable or partially removed tumours may respond. As they are slow-growing, a conservative approach with regular imaging may be appropriate.
- Associations include type 2 neurofibromatosis.

Clivus chordomas

- Rare. Arise from embryonic crest cells of the notochord.
- May present with cranial nerve palsies (III, VI, IX, X) or pyramidal tract dysfunction.
- Anterior and posterior pituitary hypofunction is reported.
- Often invasive and relentlessly progressive.
- Treatment is surgical followed by radiotherapy in some cases, although they are relatively radioresistant. Data on radiosurgery are not yet available, but this may be considered.

Hamartomas

- Non-neoplastic overgrowth of neurones and glial cells.
- Rare. May present with seizures—typically gelastic (laughing).
- May release GnRH leading to precocious puberty or very rarely GHRH leading to disorders of growth or acromegaly.
- Appear as homogeneous isointense with grey matter, pedunculated or sessile non-enhancing tumours on T1-weighted MRI scans.

Management

Tumours do not enlarge, and therefore treatment is of endocrine consequences—most commonly precocious puberty.

Ependymomas

- Intracranial ependymomas typically affect children and adolescents.
- Pituitary insufficiency may follow craniospinal irradiation.
- Occasionally 3rd ventricle tumours may interfere with hypothalamic function

Further reading

Whittle IR, Smith C, Navoo P, et al. (2004). Meningiomas. *Lancet* **363**(9420), 1535–43.

Parasellar inflammatory conditions

Neurosarcoidosis

Pituitary and hypothalamus may be affected by meningeal disease. Most patients with hypothalamic sarcoidosis also have involvement outside the CNS.

Features

Hypopituitarism and DI, in addition to hypothalamic syndrome of absent thirst, somnolescence, and hyperphagia.

Investigations

- Serum and CSF ACE may be raised.
- CSF examination may reveal a pleocytosis, oligoclonal bands, and low glucose.
- MRI may demonstrate additional enhancement, e.g. meningeal.
- Gallium scan may reveal ↑ uptake in lacrimal and salivary glands.

Management

- High doses of glucocorticoids (60–80mg prednisolone) for initial treatment. Subsequent treatment with 40mg/day is often required for several months. Pulsed methylprednisolone may also be useful. Steroid sparing agents such as azathioprine may be helpful.
- Management of hormonal deficiency can be very difficult particularly in the context of absent thirst and poor memory.

Langerhans' cell histiocytosis

- >50% of cases occur in children.
- Most frequent endocrine abnormalities are DI and growth retardation due to hypothalamic infiltration by Langerhans' cells or involvement of the meninges adjacent to the pituitary. Rarely hyperprolactinaemia and panhypopituitarism develop. In adults, DI may precede the bone and soft tissue abnormalities making diagnosis difficult.

Management

The role of radiotherapy is controversial, with some workers reporting improvement, and others questioning the efficacy. If radiotherapy is used, rapid institution of treatment appears to be important (within 10 days of diagnosis). High dose glucocorticoids can lead to transient improvement, but chemotherapy does not alter the course of DI although it may lead to temporary regression of lesions.

Tuberculosis

TB may present as a tuberculoma which may compromise hypotha-lamic or pituitary function. DI is common. Most patients have signs of TB elsewhere, but not invariably so. Trans-sphenoidal biopsy is therefore sometimes required. An alternative strategy is antituberculous treatment with empirical glucocorticoid treatment.

Further reading

Freda PU and Post KD (1999). Differential diagnosis of sellar masses. *Endocrinol Metabol Clin N Am* **28**, 81.

Lymphocytic hypophysitis

Background

This is a rare inflammatory condition of the pituitary.

Epidemiology

Lymphocytic hypophysitis occurs more commonly in ♀, and usually presents during late pregnancy or the 1st year thereafter.

Pathogenesis

Ill-understood—probably autoimmune. Approximately 25% of cases of lymphocytic hypophysitis have been associated with other autoimmune conditions—Hashimoto's thyroiditis in the majority, but also pernicious anaemia.

Pathology

- Somatotroph and gonadotroph function are more likely to be preserved than corticotroph or thyrotroph function, unlike the findings in hypopituitarism due to a pituitary tumour. The posterior pituitary is characteristically spared so that DI is not part of the picture, but there are occasional reports of coexistent or isolated DI, presumably because of different antigens.
- Lymphocytic hypophysitis has occasionally involved the cavernous sinus and extra-ocular muscles.
- Light microscopy typically reveals a lymphoplasmacytic infiltrate, occasionally forming lymphoid follicles, with variable destruction of parenchyma and fibrosis.

Clinical features

- Mass effects leading to headache and visual field defects.
- Often a temporal association with pregnancy.
- Hypopituitarism (ACTH and TSH deficiency, less commonly gonadotrophin and GH deficiency).
- Posterior pituitary involvement and cavernous sinus involvement occur less commonly.

Investigations

- Investigation of hypopituitarism is essential, and may not be thought of because gonadotrophin secretion often remains intact, leaving the potentially life-threatening ACTH deficiency unsuspected.
- MRI shows an enhancing mass, with variably loss of hyperintense bright spot of neurohypophysis, thickening of pituitary stalk, enlargement of the neurohypophysis. Suprasellar extension often appears tongue-like along the pituitary stalk. There may be central necrosis but no calcification.
- Biopsy of the lesion is often required, but may be avoided in the presence of typical features.
- The presence of antipituitary antibodies has been investigated by some groups and shown to be variably present. This is, however, a research tool and an unreliable marker.

Box 28.1 Classification of hypophysitis

- Acute:
  - Bacterial infections.
- Chronic:
  - Lymphocytic hypophysitis
  - Xanthomatous—characterized by lipid-laden macrophages.
- Granulomatous:
  - Tuberculosis.
  - Sarcoidosis.
  - Syphilis.
  - Giant cell—?variant of lymphocytic hypophysitis.

Treatment

- Treatment of hypopituitarism.
- Most often, no specific treatment is necessary. There is anecdotal evidence only of the effectiveness of immunosupressive doses of glucocorticoids—for example prednisolone 60mg/day for 3 months and progressive reduction for 6 months. This has been reported to be associated with reduction in the mass and gradual recovery of pituitary function. However, relapse after discontinuing therapy is also reported.
- Spontaneous recovery may also occur.
- Surgery has also been used to improve visual field abnormalities

Natural history

Variable—some progress rapidly to life-threatening hypopituitarism, while others spontaneously regress.

Relationship to other conditions

Lymphocytic hypophysitis remains an ill-understood condition but has been suggested to be the underlying cause of other conditions such as isolated ACTH deficiency and the empty sella syndrome.

Further reading

Thodou E, Asa SL, Kontogeorgos G, et al. (1995). Clinical case seminar: lymphocytic hypophysitis: clinicopathological findings. *J Clin Endocrinol Metab* **80**, 2302–311.

Caturegli P, Newschaffer C, Olivi A, et al (2005). Autoimmune hypophysitis. *Endocr Rev* **26**(5), 599–614. Epub 2005 Jan 5.

Surgical treatment of pituitary tumours

Trans-sphenoidal surgery

This is now the favoured technique for pituitary surgery, and is 1st-line for virtually every case. It is preferred to the previously used technique of craniotomy because there is minimal associated morbidity as a result of the fact that the cranial fossa is not opened and there are therefore no immediate sequelae due to direct cerebral damage (particularly frontal lobe) and no long-term risk of epilepsy. There is reduced duration of hospital stay and improved cure rates as there is better visualization of small tumours. Unfortunately the technique may be inadequate to deal with very large tumours with extensive suprasellar extension. In these situations craniotomy is required if adequate debulking is not possible following the trans-sphenoidal approach. 📖 See Box 29.1 for indications for surgery.

Preparation for trans-sphenoidal surgery

Pretreatment before surgery

- Pretreatment with *metyrapone* or *ketoconazole* to improve the condition of patients with Cushing's syndrome is often given for at least 6 weeks. This allows some improvement in healing and also improves the general state of the patient.
- Patients with macroprolactinomas will in the majority of cases have received treatment with dopamine agonists in any case, and surgery is usually indicated for resistance or intolerance. There is a risk of tumour fibrosis, with long-term (>6 months) dopamine agonist therapy.

Immediately preoperative

- Immediate preoperative treatment requires appropriate anterior pituitary hormone replacement. In particular, a decision as to whether perioperative glucocorticoid treatment is required. The majority of microprolactinomas will not require perioperative hydrocortisone, but patients with Cushing's syndrome will require peri-and postoperative glucocorticoid treatment (📖 see trans-sphenoidal surgery/craniotomy, p.146). Patients with macroadenomas and an intact preoperative pituitary–adrenal axis do not usually require perioperative steroids, but those who are deficient or whose reserve has not been tested need to be given perioperative glucocorticoids. TSH deficiency should be corrected with levothyroxine. Ensure the patient is not taking aspirin.
- Prophylactic antibiotics are started in some centres the night before surgery to reduce the chances of meningitis.

Complications

📖 See also Box 29.2 and Table 29.1.

- Patients should be counselled about the possible complications of trans-sphenoidal surgery prior to consent. The commonest complications are DI which may be transient or permanent (5% and 0.1% respectively; often higher in Cushing's disease and prolactinoma) and the development of new anterior pituitary hormonal deficiencies (uncommon with microadenomas, approximately 10% of TSA for macroadenomas).

- The risk of meningitis can be reduced by preoperative and peri-operative prophylactic antibiotic administration. In Oxford our practice is to give 5 days of oral antibiotics (*amoxicillin* and *flucloxacillin*, or *clorithromycin* if penicillin allergic) starting the night before surgery. Other complications include CSF leak, visual deterioration, haemorrhage (rare), and transient hyponatraemia usually 7 days postoperatively.

Cerebral salt wasting

A rare but important complication of trans-sphenoidal surgery, more commonly seen after subarachnoid haemorrhage is cerebral salt wasting syndrome (CSW). This typically oc-curs at day 5–10 postoperatively and is associated with often massive urinary salt loss, and hypovolaemia. It needs to be differentiated from SIADH which may also occur at this stage (often using central venous pressure measurement to demonstrate hypovolaemia in CSW compared with euvolaemia in SIADH). The management of CSW involves administration of saline, whereas fluid restriction is indicated for SIADH.

Box 29.1 Indications for surgery

- Non-functioning pituitary adenoma.
- GH-secreting adenoma.
- ACTH secreting tumour.
- Nelson's syndrome.
- Prolactinoma—if patient dopamine agonist resistant or intolerant.
- Recurrent pituitary tumour.

Less common

- Gonadotrophin-secreting tumours.
- TSH-secreting adenoma.
- Craniopharyngioma.
- Pituitary biopsy to define diagnosis e.g. hypophysitis, pituitary metastases.
- Chordoma.
- Rathke's cleft cyst.
- Arachnoid cyst.

Box 29.2 Post-operative disorders of fluid balance

- Acute post-operative transient DI.
- SIADH.
- Triphasic response: initial DI due to axon shock (hours–days) followed by antidiuretic phase due to uncontrolled release of ADH from damaged posterior pituitary (2–14 days) followed by DI due to depletion of ADH.
- Transient hyponatraemia (isolated second phase) at 5–10 days post-operative, usually mild and self-limiting.

Table 29.1 Complications of trans-sphenoidal surgery

Complications of any surgical procedure	Anaesthetic related
	Venous thrombosis and pulmonary embolism
Immediate	Haemorrhage
	Hypothalamic damage
	Meningitis
Permanent	Visual deterioration or loss
	Cranial nerve damage (e.g. oculomotor nerve palsies)
	Hypopituitarism
	DI
	SIADH
Transient	DI
	CSF rhinorrhoea
	Visual deterioration
	Cerebral salt wasting

Trans-frontal craniotomy

Indications

- Pituitary tumours with major suprasellar and lateral invasion where trans-sphenoidal surgery is unlikely to remove a significant proportion of the tumour.
- Craniopharyngiomas.
- Parasellar tumours, e.g. meningioma.

Complications

- In addition to the complications of trans-sphenoidal surgery, brain retraction leads to cerebral oedema or haemorrhage.
- Manipulation of the optic chiasm may lead to visual deterioration.
- Vascular damage.
- Damage to the olfactory nerve.

Perioperative management

Similar to that for patients undergoing trans-sphenoidal surgery (📖 see Trans-sphenoidal surgery, p.182).

Postoperative management

- Recovery is typically slower than after trans-sphenoidal surgery.
- Prophylactic anticonvulsants are administered for up to 1 year.
- The DVLC must be advised of surgery, and driving is allowed following adequate visual recovery, but drivers of group 2 vehicles (HGV) cannot drive for 6 months.

Further reading

Laws ER and Thapar K (1999). Pituitary surgery. *Endocrinol Metab Clin N Am* **28**, 119.

Pituitary radiotherapy

Indications

> See Box 30.1.

- Pituitary radiotherapy is an effective treatment used to reduce the likelihood of tumour regrowth, to further shrink a tumour, and to treat persistent hormone hypersecretion following surgical resection.
- Occasionally it is used as a 1° therapeutic option, but its usual role is following non-curative surgery or following macroprolactinoma shrinkage with dopamine agonists.
- Pituitary radiotherapy is usually only administrable once in a lifetime.

Technique

- Conventional external beam 3-field radiotherapy is able to deliver a beam of ionizing irradiation accurately to the pituitary fossa.
- Accurate targeting requires head fixation in a moulded plastic shell to keep the head immobilized. The fields of irradiation are based on simulation using MRI or CT scanning and the volume is usually the tumour margins plus 0.5cm in all planes. The preoperative tumour volume is used for planning, whereas the post-drug (dopamine agonist) shrinkage films are used for prolactinomas. There are 3 portals, 2 temporal and 1 anterior.
- The standard dose is 4500cGy in 25 fractions over 35 days, but 5000 cGy may be used for relatively 'radioresistant' tumours such as craniopharyngiomas.

Efficacy

Radiotherapy is effective in reducing the chances of pituitary tumour regrowth. For example, in a large series of 400 patients who received pituitary radiotherapy over a period of 20 years, the progression-free survival rate was 97% at 10 years and 92% at 20 years. Comparison of functionless tumour recurrence following surgery and radiotherapy compared with surgery alone, shows that radiotherapy is effective in reducing the likelihood of regrowth (Fig. 30.1)

Box 30.1 Indications for pituitary radiotherapy

Tumour	Aim of treatment
Non-functioning pituitary adenoma	To shrink residual mass or reduce liklihood of regrowth
GH/PRL/ACTH secreting tumour	To reduce persistent hormonal hypersecretion and shrink residual mass
Craniopharyngioma	To reduce likelihood of regrowth
Recurrent tumour	

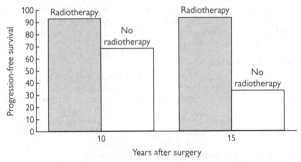

Fig. 30.1 Recurrence rates following radiotherapy. Modified from Gittoes NJL, Bates AS, Tse W, *et al.* (1998). Radiotherapy for non-functioning pituitary tumours. *Clin Endocrinol* **48**, 331–7. With permission from Wiley Blackwell.

Complications

Short term
- Nausea.
- Headache.
- Temporary hair loss at radiotherapy portals of entry.

Hypopituitarism
- Anterior pituitary hormone deficiency occurs due to the effect of irradiation on the hypothalamus leading to reduced hypothalamic releasing hormone secretion. The total dose of irradiation determines the speed, incidence and extent of hypopituitarism. In addition the presence of pre-existing hormonal deficiency increases the chances of post-radiotherapy hypopituitarism (Table 30.1).
- The onset of hypopituitarism is gradual, and the order of development of deficiency is as for any other cause of developing hypopituitarism—namely GH first followed by gonadotrophin and ACTH followed finally by TSH. Posterior pituitary deficiencies are very rare, but 2° temporary mild hyperprolactinaemia may be seen after about 2 years which gradually returns to normal.

Visual impairment
- The optic chiasm is particularly radioresistant, but may undergo damage thought to be due to vascular damage to the blood supply. Visual deterioration typically occurs within 3 years of irradiation, and is progressive.
- The literature suggest that the risk is greatest with high total and daily doses. A standard total dose of 4500 cGy and daily dose of 180 cGy appears to pose very little, if any, risk to the chiasm.
- Our practice is to avoid administration of radiotherapy where possible when the chiasm is under pressure from residual tumour.

Radiation oncogenesis
- There is controversy as to whether pituitary irradiation leads to the development of 2nd tumours. There have been reports of sarcomas, gliomas and meningiomas developing in the field of irradiation after 10–20 years. However, there are also reports of gliomas and meningioma occurring in unirradiated patients with pituitary adenomas. A retrospective review of a large series of patients given pituitary irradiation suggested a risk of 2nd tumour of 1.9% by 20 years after irradiation when compared to the normal population (but not patients with pituitary tumours).
- More subtle changes in neurocognition have been suggested.

Table 30.1 Development of new hypopituitarism at 10 years following pituitary radiotherapy

	No previous surgery	Surgery
Gonadotrophin deficiency	47%	70%
ACTH deficiency	30%	54%
Thyrotrophin deficiency	16%	38%

Box 30.2 Focal forms of radiotherapy

Stereotactic radiosurgery uses focused radiation to deliver a precise dose of radiation:

• Gamma knife 'radiosurgery'—ionizing radiation from a cobalt 60 source delivered by convergent collimated beams.
• Linear accelerator focal radiotherapy—photons focused on a stationary point from a moving gantry
• Potential advantages are that a single high dose of irradiation is given which can be sharply focused on the tumour with minimal surrounding tissue damage.
• Long-term data are required to demonstrate endocrine efficacy, but it may have a particular role in recurrent or persistent tumours which are well-demarcated and surgically inaccessible e.g. in the cavernous sinus.
• Potential limitations include proximity to the optic chiasm.

Further reading

Brada M, Ford D, Ashley S et al. (1992). Risk of second brain tumour after conservative surgery and radiotherapy for pituitary adenoma. *BMJ* **304**, 1343–6.

Jackson IMD and Noren G (1999). Role of gamma knife therapy in the management of pituitary tumours. *Endocrinol Metab Clin N Am* **28**, 133.

Jones A (1991). Radiation oncogenesis in relation to treatment of pituitary tumours. *Clin Endocrinol* **35**, 379

Plowman PN (1999). Pituitary adenoma radiotherapy. *Clin Endocrinol* **51**, 265–71.

Drug treatment of pituitary tumours

Dopamine agonists

Types

- *Bromocriptine*—the 1st ergot alkaloid to be used, short acting, taken daily. Usually administered orally, although vaginal and IM formulations can be used and may reduce GI intolerance.
- *Quinagolide*—non-ergot, longer acting, taken daily.
- *Cabergoline*—ergot derivative. Long acting—taken once or twice a week.
- *Less commonly used*—pergolide and lisuride.

Mechanism of action

Activation of D2 receptors.

Side-effects

Commonly at initiation of treatment

- Nausea.
- Postural hypotension.

Less common

- Headache, fatigue, nasal stuffiness, constipation, abdominal cramps, and a Raynaud-like phenomenon in hands.
- Very rarely patients have developed hallucinations and psychosis (usually at higher doses).
- Side-effects may be minimized by slow initiation of therapy (e.g. 1.25mg bromocriptine or 250mcg cabergoline), taking medication before going to bed, and taking the tablets with food.

Box 31.1 Uses of dopamine agonists

Hyperprolactinaemia (📖 see p.120)

- D2 receptor stimulation leads to inhibition of PRL secretion and reduction in cell size leading to tumour shrinkage. The PRL often falls before significant tumour shrinkage is seen.
- Problems may arise when patients are either intolerant of the medication or resistant. Cabergoline appears to be better tolerated than bromocriptine and it is often worth trying an alternative in the case of intolerance, although true intolerance is probably a class effect. Dopamine agonist resistance macro>micro adenomas, (10–25% patients) may be due to differences in receptor subtype (e.g. loss of D2 receptors) or possibly altered intracellular signalling.

GH-secreting tumours

- Although administration of L-dopa to normal individuals leads to acute increase in GH due to hypothalamic dopamine and noradrenaline synthesis and inhibition of somatostatin secretion, >50% of patients with GH-secreting tumours given dopamine agonists have a fall in GH. Dopamine acts directly on somatotroph tumours to inhibit GH release.
- Patients with acromegaly often need larger doses of dopamine agonist than patients with prolactinomas. Tumour shrinkage is most likely if there is concomitant secretion of PRL from the tumour. Dopamine agonists are currently usually reserved for 2nd-line drug therapy in patients who are somatostatin agonist resistant or as a co-prescription with somatostatin agonists in patients with mixed GH-and PRL-secreting tumours.

Pregnancy

Bromocriptine is licensed for use in pregnancy, but cabergoline is not licensed in the UK, although it has not thus far been associated with any ↑ teratogenicity.

Somatostatin analogues

Mechanism of action

- Since the half-life of somatostatin is very short, a longer acting analogue were synthesized—octreotide and lanreotide. These have a half-life of 110min in the circulation, inhibits GH secretion 45 × more actively than native somatostatin, with none of the rebound hypersecretion that occurs with somatostatin.
- The somatostatin analogues act predominantly on the somatostatin receptors 2 and 5. Unlike dopamine agonists, somatostatin analogues do not lead to dramatic tumour sh rinkage, but some shrinkage is still seen in the majority of tumours.

Types

- Octreotide LAR® (10–30mg IM) administered every 4–6 weeks.
- Lanreotide Autogel® (60–120mg IM) administered every 4 weeks.
- SC octreotide (50–200mcg) administered 3 × daily.
- Lanreotide SR (30mg IM) administered every 7–14 days.

Side effects

- Gallstones at least 20–30% of patients develop gallstones or sludge on octreotide (thought by most to antedate stone formation), but only 1%/year develop symptoms. The incidence is unknown on octreotide LAR® or lanreotide. Symptoms may particularly occur if SMS analogue therapy is withdrawn.
- GI due to inhibition of motor activity and secretion leading to nausea, abdominal cramps, and mild steatorrhoea. These usually settle with time.
- Injection site pain Obviated by allowing vial to warm to room temperature before injecting.
- Hair loss (<10%).

Box 31.2 Uses of somatostatin analogues

- Acromegaly.
- Carcinoid tumours.
- Pancreatic neuroendocrine tumours.
- TSH-secreting pituitary tumours.

Growth hormone receptor antagonist

Pegvisomant—newly developed novel treatment for acromegaly.

Mechanism of action

- Binds to GH receptor and induces internalization but blocks receptor signalling leading to reduction in IGF-1 (but not GH) production.
- Studies sugest that it is the most potent available medical therapy. Normalization of IGF-1 in >90% treated patients.

Usage

- May be used with somatostatin analogues to decrease frequency of injections.

Problems

- High cost.
- Further data required on the effects on pituitary tumour growth.
- Occasional deterioration in liver biochemistry.
- IGF-1 used to monitor effectiveness of treatment.

Further reading

Feenstra J, de Herder WW, ten Have SM, van den Beld et al. (2005). Combined therapy with somatostatin analogues and weekly pegvisomant in active acromegaly. Lancet 7–13:365 (9471), 1644–6.

Karivitaki N and Wass JAH (2004). Pegvisamant: a new treatment modality for acromegaly. Hormones **3**, 27–36.

Paisley AN, Roberts ME, and Trainer PJ (2007). Withdrawal of somastatin analogue therapy in patients with acromegaly is associated with an ↑ risk of acute biliary problems. Clin Endocrinol **66**(5), 723–6. Epub 2007 Mar 27.

Trainer PJ, Drake WM, Katznelson L et al. (2000). Treatment of acromegaly with the growth hormone receptor antagonist pegvisomant New Engl J Med **342**, 1171–7.

Van der Lely AJ, Hutson R, Trainer PJ et al. (2001). Long-term treatment of acromegaly with pegvisomant, a growth hormone receptor antagonist Lancet **358**, 1754–9.

Posterior pituitary

Physiology and pathology

The posterior lobe of the pituitary gland arises from the forebrain, and comprises up to 25% of the normal adult pituitary gland. It produces arginine vasopressin and oxytocin. Both hormones are synthesized in the hypothalamic neurons of the supra-optic and paraventricular nuclei and migrate as neurosecretory granules to the posterior pituitary before release into the circulation. The hormones are unbound in the circulation and their half-life is short.

Oxytocin

- Oxytocin has no known role in ♂. It may aid contraction of the seminal vesicles.
- In ♀, oxytocin contracts the pregnant uterus and also causes breast duct smooth muscle contraction leading to breast-milk ejection during breastfeeding. Oxytocin is released in response to suckling and also to cervical dilatation during parturition. However, oxytocin deficiency has no known adverse effect on parturition or breast-feeding.
- There are several as yet ill-understood features of oxytocin physiology. For example, osmotic stimulation may also lead to oxytocin secretion. Oxytocin may play a role in the ovary and testis, as ovarian luteal cells and testicular cells have both been shown to synthesize it, although its subsequent role is not known.

Vasopressin and neurophysin

- Arginine vasopressin is the major determinant of renal water excretion and therefore fluid balance. Its main action is to reduce free water clearance.
- Vasopressin is a nonapeptide, and derives from a large precursor with a signal peptide, and a neurophysin. The vasopressin gene is located on chromosome 20, and is closely linked to the oxytocin gene. Vasopressin travels to the posterior pituitary and undergoes cleavage as it travels. Neurophysin is released with vasopressin but has no further role after acting as a carrier protein in the neurons.
- Release of vasopressin occurs in response to changes in osmolality detected by osmoreceptors in the hypothalamus. Large changes in blood volume (5–10%) also influence vasopressin secretion. Many substances modulate vasopressin secretion including the catecholamines and opioids.
- The main site of action of vasopressin is in the collecting duct and the thick ascending loop of Henle where it increases water permeability so that solute-free water may pass along an osmotic gradient to the interstitial medulla. Vasopressin in higher concentrations has a pressor effect. It also acts as an ACTH secretagogue synergistically with CRH.

Diabetes insipidus (DI)

Definition

DI is defined as the passage of large volumes (>3L/24h) of dilute urine (osmolality <300mOsmol/kg).

Classification

Cranial

Due to deficiency of circulating arginine vasopressin (anti-diuretic hormone).

Nephrogenic

Due to renal resistance to vasopressin.

Primary polydipsia

- Polyuria due to excessive drinking.
- In addition to suppressed levels of vasopressin due to low plasma osmolality, there may be impaired renal effectiveness because of wash out of solute and therefore reduced urine-concentrating ability.

Features

- *Adults*—polyuria, nocturia, and thirst.
- *Children*—polyuria, enuresis, and failure to thrive.
- NB Clinical syndrome of cranial DI may be masked by cortisol deficiency as this results in failure to excrete a water load.
- Syndrome may worsen in pregnancy due to placental breakdown (vasopressinase) of circulating vasopressin.

📖 See Box 33.1 for causes of DI.

Box 33.1 Causes of DI

Cranial
10% vasopressin cells should be sufficient to keep the urine volume <4L/day.

Familial
- Autosomal dominant (vasopressin gene).
- DIDMOAD syndrome (DI, diabetes mellitus, optic atrophy, deafness).

Acquired
- Trauma—head injury, neurosurgery.
- Tumours—craniopharyngiomas, pituitary infiltration by metastases.
- Inflammatory conditions—sarcoidosis, tuberculosis, Langerhans' cell histiocytosis, lymphocytic hypophysitis.
- Infections—meningitis, encephalitis.
- Vascular—Sheehan's syndrome, sickle cell disease.
- Idiopathic.

Nephrogenic
Familial
- X-linked recessive—vasopressin receptor gene.
- Autosomal recessive—aquaporin-2 gene.

Acquired
- Drugs—lithium, demeclocycline.
- Metabolic—hypercalcaemia, hypokalaemia, hyperglycaemia.
- Chronic renal disease.
- Post-obstructive uropathy.

Primary polydipsia
- Psychological.

Investigations

Diagnosis of type of DI

- Confirm large urine output (> 3000mL/day).
- Exclude diabetes mellitus and renal failure (osmotic diuresis).
- Check electrolytes. Hypokalaemia and hypercalcaemia (nephrogenic DI).
- Fluid deprivation test (□ see Box 33.2) and assessment of response to vasopressin.
- Occasionally further investigations are required, particularly when only partial forms of the condition are present;
- Measurement of plasma vasopressin, osmolality, and thirst threshold:
  - In response to infusion of 0.05mL/kg per min 5% hypertonic saline for 2h for cranial DI (no ↑ vasopressin).
  - In response to fluid deprivation for nephrogenic DI (vasopressin levels rise with no ↑ urine osmolality).
- An alternative is a therapeutic trial of desmopressin with monitoring of sodium and osmolality.

Investigation of the cause

- MRI head:
  - Looking for tumours—hypothalamic, pineal, or infiltration.
  - Often demonstrates loss of bright spot of posterior pituitary gland.
- Serum ACE (sarcoidosis) and tumour markers, e.g. βHCG (pineal germinoma).

Box 33.2 Fluid deprivation test

1. Patient is allowed fluids overnight. If psychogenic polydipsia suspected, consider overnight fluid deprivation to avoid morning overhydration.
2. Patient is then deprived of fluids for 8h or until 5% loss of body weight if earlier. Weigh patient hourly.
3. Plasma osmolality is measured 4-hourly and urine volume and osmolality every 2h.
4. The patient is then given 2mcg IM desmopressin with urine volume, and urine and serum osmolality measured over the next 4h.

Results

If serum osmolality >305mOsm/kg: patient has DI and test is stopped.

Urine osmolality (mOsm/kg)

Diagnosis	After fluid deprivation	After desmopressin
Cranial DI	<300	>800
Nephrogenic DI	<300	<300
1° polydipsia	>800	>800
Partial DI or polydipsia	300–800	<800

Treatment

Maintenance of adequate fluid input

In patients with partial DI, and an intact thirst mechanism, then drug therapy may not be necessary if the polyuria is mild (<4L/24h).

Drug therapy

Desmopressin

- Vasopressin analogue, acting predominantly on the V2 receptors in the kidney, with little action on the V1 receptors of blood vessels. It thus has reduced pressor activity and ↑ antidiuretic efficacy, in addition to a longer half-life than the native hormone.
- Drug may be administered in divided doses, orally (100–1000mcg/day), intranasally (10–40mcg/day) or parenterally (SC, IV, IM) (0.1–2mcg/day) or bucally. There is wide variation in the dose required by an individual patient.
- Monitoring of serum sodium and osmolality is essential as hyponatraemia or hypo-osmolality may develop.

Lysine vasopressin

- The antidiuretic hormone of the pig family.
- Not used very often as its effects are short lived (1–3h) and it may retain pressor activity. Intranasal administration. Dose 5–20U/day.

Chlorpropamide (100–500mg/day) and carbamazepine enhance the action of vasopressin on the collecting duct.

Nephrogenic DI

- Correction of underlying cause (metabolic or drugs).
- High doses of desmopressin (e.g. up to 5mcg IM) can be effective.
- Maintenance of adequate fluid input.
- Thiazide diuretics and prostaglandin synthase inhibitors (decrease the action of prostaglandins which locally inhibit the action of vasopressin in the kidney), e.g. indomethacin, can be helpful.

Polydipsic polyuria

Management is difficult. Treatment of any underlying psychiatric disorder is important.

Hyponatraemia

📖 See Table 34.1.

Incidence

- 1–6% hospital admissions Na <130mmol/L.
- 15–22% hospital admissions Na <135mmol/L.

Causes

Box 34.1 Causes of hyponatraemia

Excess water (dilutional)
- Excess water intake.
- ↑ water reabsorption (cirrhosis, congestive cardiac failure, nephrotic syndrome).
- Reduced renal excretion of a water load (SIADH, glucocorticoid deficiency).

Salt deficiency
- Renal loss (salt wasting nephropathy —tubulointerstitial nephritis, polycystic kidney disease, analgesic nephropathy, recovery phase of acute tubular necrosis, relief of bilateral ureteric obstruction).
- Non-renal loss (skin, GI tract [bowel sequestration, high fistulae]).
- Renal sodium conservation of sodium is efficient and therefore low salt intake alone never causes sodium deficiency.

Pseudohyponatraemia
- Lipids, proteins (e.g. paraproteinaemia).
- Sodium only in aqueous phase of plasma, therefore, depending on assay, total sodium concentration may be spuriously low if concentrations of lipid or protein are high.

Solute
- Glucose, mannitol, ethanol.
- Addition of solute confined to the ECF causes water to shift from the ICF lowering ECF sodium concentration.

Sick cell syndrome
- Symptomless hyponatraemia at 120–130mmol/L.
- True clinically apparent hyponatraemia is associated with either excess water or salt deficiency. The other causes can usually be easily excluded.

Table 34.1 Hyponatraemia investigations

Hypovolaemic		Euvolaemic		Hypervolaemic	
NaU <20mmol/L	NaU >20mmol/L	NaU <20mmol/L	NaU >20mmol/L Serum osmolality <270mOsm/kg Urine osmolality >100mOsm/kg	NaU <20mmol/L	NaU >20mmol/L Serum osmolality <270mOsm/kg Urine osmolality >100mOsm/kg
Non-renal sodium loss	Renal sodium loss	Depletional ECF loss with inappropriate fluid replacement	Distal dilution	Excess water	
?GIT loss	?Salt losing nephropathy		SIADH	Cirrhosis	SIADH
?Skin loss	?Mineralocorticoid deficiency		GC deficiency	Nephrotic syndrome	
				CCF	

GC = glucocorticoid

Features

- Depend on the underlying cause and also on the rate of development of hyponatraemia. May develop once the sodium reaches 115mmol/L or earlier if the fall is rapid. 100mmol/L or less are life threatening.
- Features of excess water are mainly neurological because of brain injury, and depend on the age of the patient and rate of development. They include confusion and headache, progressing to seizures and coma. In hypervolaemic forms of excess water (where the fluid is confined to the ECF e.g. cardiac failure, nephrotic syndrome, and cirrhosis) oedema and fluid overload are apparent. In contrast, in the syndromes of excess water associated with SIADH the fluid is distributed throughout the ECF and ICF and there is no apparent fluid overload. Salt deficiency presents with features of hypovolaemia with tachycardia and postural hypotension.

Investigations

(Table 34.1)
- Urinary sodium is very helpful in differentiating the underlying cause.
- Assess volume status.
- Other investigations as indicated e.g. serum and urine osmolality, cortisol, thyroid function, liver biochemistry.

Treatment

Salt deficiency (renal or non-renal)

- Increase dietary salt.
- May need IV normal saline if dehydrated.

Excess water (cirrhosis, nephrotic syndrome, CCF)

- Fluid restriction to 500–750mL/24h.
- Occasionally hypertonic (3%) saline (513mmol/L) may be required in patients with acute symptomatic hyponatraemia. The appropriate infusion rate can be calculated from the formula:

  Rate of sodium replacement (mmol/h) = total body water (60% of body weight) × desired correction rate (0.5–1mmol/h).

  E.g. for a 70 kg ♂:

  $$Na^+ = 60\% \times 70 \text{ kg} \times 1 \text{ mmol/h} = 42\text{mmol/h}$$

  $$= 42 \times \frac{1000}{513} \qquad\qquad = 82\text{mL/h of 3\% saline}$$

- Rapid normalization (faster than 0.5mmol/h) of sodium may be associated with central pontine myelinolysis.

SIADH

📕 See Syndrome of inappropriate ADH (SIADH), p.206 and p.684.

Neurosugical hyponatraemia

- Injudicious fluids.
- Diuretics.
- Drugs e.g. carbamazepine, opiates.
- SIADH.
- Glucocorticoid deficiency.
- Cerebral salt wasting.

Unexplained hyponatraemia

- Common in elderly (↑ ADH release in response to ↑ osmolality and less effective suppression of ADH).
- ↑ risk of hyponatraemia with SSRIs.

Syndrome of inappropriate ADH (SIADH)

Definition

SIADH is a common cause of hyponatraemia. It is clinically normovolaemic hyponatraemia, since the ↑ water is distributed through all compartments. (NB The elderly are more prone to SIADH as they are unable to suppress ADH as efficiently, and therefore investigation is probably only necessary if Na <130mmol/L in this group).

Criteria for diagnosis

- Hyponatraemia and hypotonic plasma (osmolality <270mOsm/kg).
- Hyper proteinaemia and hyperlipidaemia may cause hyponatraemia but not hypotonic plasma.
- Inappropriate urine osmolality >100mOsm/kg.
- Excessive renal sodium loss (>30mmol/L, often >50mmol/L).
- Absence of clinical evidence of hypovolaemia or of volume overload.
- Normal renal, adrenal, and thyroid function (all must be excluded).
- NB Fluid restriction may reduce sodium loss.
- Differentiate from cerebral salt wasting (📖 see Trans-sphenoidal surgery, p.183).

📖 See Box 35.1 for causes of SIADH.

Types of SIADH

- Type 1—erratic excess ADH secretion, unrelated to plasma osmolality commonest (40%) associated (not exclusively) with tumours.
- Type 2—'reset osmostat': patients autoregulate around a lower serum osmolality.
- Chest and CNS disease.
- Type 3—'leaky osmostat' normal osmoregulation until plasma hypotonicity develops when vasopressin secretion continues.
- Type 4—normal osmoregulated vasopressin secretion, possible receptor defect or alternative antidiuretic hormone.

Investigation of aetiology of SIADH

- Plasma and serum osmolalities and biochemistry.
- Thyroid function tests.
- Synacthen® test.
- Chest x-ray.
- Optional or if not explained—MRI head, CT chest, HIV serology, bronchoscopy, lumbar puncture.

Box 35.1 Causes of SIADH

- Tumours
  - Small cell lung carcinoma, thymoma, lymphoma, leukaemia, sarcoma, mesothelioma
- Chest disease
  - Infections (pneumonia, tuberculosis, empyema)
  - Pneumothorax
  - Asthma
  - Positive pressure ventilation
- CNS disorders
  - Pituitary, macroadenomsa
  - Infections (meningitis, encephalitis, abscess)
  - Head injury
  - Guillain Barré
  - Vascular disorders (subarachnoid haemorrhage, cerebral thrombosis)
  - Psychosis
- Drugs
  - Chemotherapy (vincristine, vinblastine, cyclophosphamide)
  - Psychiatric drugs (phenothiazines, MAOI)
  - Carbamazepine
  - Clofibrate
  - Chlorpropamide
- Metabolic
  - Hypothyroidism
  - Glucocorticoid deficiency
  - Acute intermittent porphyria
- Idiopathic

Treatment

- Treatment of the underlying cause.
- Fluid restriction to 500–750mL/24h.
- If the problem is not temporary and fluid restriction long-term can be difficult for the patient, drug treatment may be tried. *Demeclocycline* may be effective by inducing partial nephrogenic DI. New specific vasopressin antagonists are under trial. (e.g. tolvaptan)
- In an emergency, saline infusion may be required—great care is required as rapid overcorrection of hyponatraemia may cause central pontine myelinolysis (demyelination). This can be avoided if the rate of correction does not exceed 0.5 mmol/L per hour.

Hypothalamus

Pathophysiology

- The hypothalamus releases hormones that act as releasing hormones at the anterior pituitary gland. It also produces dopamine that inhibits PRL release from the anterior pituitary gland. It also synthesizes arginine vasopressin and oxytocin (📖 see p. 196).
- The commonest syndrome to be associated with the hypothalamus is abnormal GnRH secretion leading to reduced gonadotrophin secretion and hypogonadism. Common causes are stress, weight loss, and excessive exercise. Management involves treatment of the cause if possible. Administration of pulsatile GnRH is usually effective at reversing the abnormality but rarely undertaken.

Hypothalamic syndrome

Uncommon but may occur due to a large tumour, following surgery for a craniopharyngioma, or due to infiltration from e.g. Langerhans' cell histiocytosis. The typical features are hyperphagia and weight gain, loss of thirst sensation, DI, somnolence, and behaviour change. Management can be challenging e.g. DI with the loss of thirst sensation may require the prescription of regular fluid in addition to desmopressin, and monitoring with daily weights and fluid balance as a routine.

> **Box 36.1 Metabolic effects of hypothalamic mass lesions**
>
> - Appetite:
>   - Hyperphagia and obesity.
>   - Anorexia.
> - Thirst:
>   - Adipsia.
>   - Compulsive drinking.
> - Temperature:
>   - Hyperthermia.
>   - Hypothermia.
> - Somnolence and coma.

Eating disorders

Anorexia nervosa

Features

- Typical presentation is a ♀ aged <25 with weight loss, amenorrhoea, and behavioural changes.
- There is a long-term risk of severe osteoporosis associated with >6 months of amenorrhoea. There is loss of bone mineral content and bone density with little or no recovery after resolution of the amenorrhoea. Bone loss occurs at 2.5% per annum.

Endocrine abnormalities

- Deficiency of GnRH, low LH and FSH, normal PRL, and low oestrogen in ♀ or testosterone in ♂.
- Elevated circulating cortisol (usually non-suppressible with dexamethasone).
- Low normal thyroxine, reduced T_3, and normal TSH.
- Elevated resting GH levels.
- In addition, it is common to find various metabolic abnormalities such as reduced magnesium, zinc, phosphorus, and calcium levels in addition to hyponatraemia, hypoglycaemia, and hypokalaemia.
- Weight gain leads to a reversion of the prepubertal LH secretory pattern to the adult-like secretion. Administration of GnRH in a pulsatile pattern leads to normalization of the pituitary–gonadal axis, demonstrating that the 1° abnormality is hypothalamic.

Management

- The long-term treatment of these patients involves treatment of the underlying condition and then management of osteoporosis, although many patients will refuse oestrogen replacement.
- Resumption of menstrual function is important for recovery of spine bone mineral density (BMD). Weight gain is important for hip BMD recovery. Oral contraceptives do not help BMD recovery.

Bulimia

Features

- Typically occurs in ♀ who are slightly older than the group with anorexia nervosa. Weight may be normal and patients often deny the abnormal eating behaviour. Patients gorge themselves, using artificial means of avoiding excessive weight gain (laxatives, diuretic abuse, vomiting). This may be a cause of 'occult' hypokalaemia.
- These patients may or may not have menstrual irregularity. If menstrual irregularity is present, this is often associated with inadequate oestrogen secretion and anovulation.

Further reading

Miller KK, Lee EE, Lawson EA, et al. (2006). Determinants of skeletal loss and recovery in anorexia nervosa. *J Clin Endocrinol Metab* **91**(8), 2931–7. Epub 2006 May 30.

Pineal gland

Physiology

- The pineal gland lies behind the 3rd ventricle, is highly vascular, and produces melatonin and other peptides.
- During daylight, light-induced hyperpolarization of the retinal photoreceptors inhibits signalling and the pineal gland is quiescent.
- Darkness stimulates the gland, and there is synthesis and release of melatonin.
- Melatonin levels are usually low during the day, rise during the evening, peak at midnight and then decline independent of sleep.
- Exposure to darkness during the day does not increase melatonin secretion.

Jet lag

- It is claimed that pharmacological doses of melatonin can reset the body clock.
- Studies have suggested that melatonin may reduce the severity or duration of jet lag. There are few safety data, and currently melatonin does not have a product licence in the UK.

Pineal and intracranial germ cell tumours

- *Incidence* 0.5%–3% intracranial neoplasms.
- *Epidemiology* ♂>♀. All ages. 2/3 present between age 10 and 21 years.
- Germ cell tumours are now classified as germinomas or nongerminomatous germ cell tumours (choriocarcinoma, teratoma). The latter term includes the tumours previously called 'true' pinealomas.

Features

- Raised intracranial pressure (compression of cerebral aqueduct), headache, and lethargy.
- Visual disturbance (pressure on quadrigeminal plate).
- Parinaud's syndrome (paralysis of upward gaze, convergent nystagmus, Argyll–Robertson pupils).
- Ataxia.
- Pyramidal signs.
- Hypopituitarism.
- DI.
- Sexual precocity in boys (excess hCG secretion mimics LH leading to Leydig cell testosterone secretion, or related to space-occupying mass).

Investigations

- Imaging of craniospinal axis MRI/CT (may detect 2nd tumour/ metastases).
- CSF examination.
- Tumour markers (hCG, α-fetoprotein).
- Cytology.
- Biopsy if tumour markers unhelpful.
- Pituitary function assessment.

Management

- External beam radiotherapy—standard therapy is to irradiate the whole craniospinal axis.
- Germinomas are exquisitely radiosensitive.
- Chemotherapy may be indicated, e.g. vincristine, etopside, carboplatin.
- Cranio spinal irradiation cures the majority of patients (90%).

Prognosis

Excellent for germinomas (70–85% 5-year survival), but nongerminomatous germ cell tumours have a worse prognosis (15–40% 5-year survival).

Adrenals

Anatomy and physiology

Anatomy

The normal adrenal glands weigh 4–5g. The cortex represents 90% of the normal gland and surrounds the medulla. The arterial blood supply arises from the renal arteries, aorta, and inferior phrenic artery. Venous drainage occurs via the central vein into the inferior vena cava on the right, and into the left renal vein on the left.

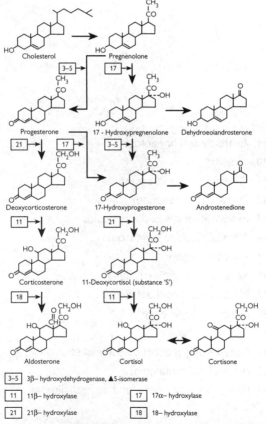

Fig. 39.1 Pathways and enzymes involved in synthesis of glucocorticoids, mineralocorticoids, and adrenal androgens from a cholesterol precursor. Reproduced from Besser M and Thorner GM (1994). *Clinical Endocrinology*, Mosby: St Louis. With permission from Elsevier.

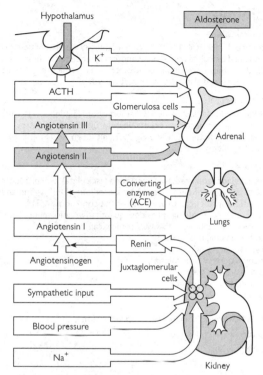

Fig. 39.2 Physiological mechanisms governing the production and secretion of aldosterone. Reproduced from Besser M and Thorner GM (1994). *Clinical Endocrinology*, Mosby: St Louis. With permission from Elsevier.

Physiology

Glucocorticoids

Glucocorticoid (cortisol 10–20mg/day) (Table 39.1) production occurs from the zona fasciculata and adrenal androgens arise form the zona reticularis. Both of these are under control of ACTH, which regulates both steroid synthesis, and also adrenocortical growth.

Mineralocorticoids

Mineralocorticoid (aldosterone 100–150mcg/d) (Table 39.1) synthesis occurs in zona glomerulosa predominantly under the control of the renin–angiotensin system (🕮 see Fig 39.2), although ACTH also contributes to its regulation.

Androgens

The adrenal gland (zona reticularis and zona fasciculata) also produces sex steroids, in the form of dehydroepiandrostenedione (DHEA) and androstenedione. The synthetic pathway is under the control of ACTH.

Urinary steroid profiling provides quantitative information on the biosynthetic and catabolic pathways. Profiling can be useful in:
- Mineralocorticoid hypertension.
- Polycystic ovary syndrome.
- Congenital adrenal hyperplasia.
- Steroid producing tumours.
- Precocious puberty/virilization.
- Hirsutism.

Table 39.1 Adrenal cortex steroid production

Adrenal cortex	Cortisol	Aldosterone	DHEA	DHEAS
Production rate/24h	10	100mcg	10mg	25mg
t½	80min	20min	20min	9h
Control	ACTH	Renin	ACTH	ACTH

Further reading

Taylor, NF (2006). Urinary steroid profiling. *Method Mol Biol* **324**, 159–75.

Imaging

Computed tomography (CT) scanning

CT is the most widely used modality for imaging the adrenal glands. It is able to detect masses >5mm in diameter. It can be useful in differentiating between different adrenal cortical pathologies.

Magnetic resonance imaging (MRI)

MRI can also reliably detect adrenal masses >5–10mm in diameter, and in some circumstances provides additional information to CT, e.g. differentiation of cortical from medullary tumours.

Ultrasound (US) imaging

US detects masses >20mm in diameter, but normal adrenal glands are not usually visible except in children. Body morphology and bowel gas can provide technical difficulties.

Normal adrenal

Normal adrenal cortex is assessed by measuring limb thickness, and is considered enlarged at >5mm approximately the thickness of the diaphragmatic crus nearby.

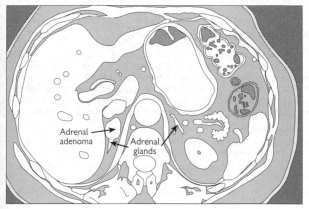

Fig. 40.1 Typical appearance of adrenal adenoma on CT scan.

Radionucleotide imaging

- *123Iodine-metaiodobenzylguanidine* (MIBG) is a guanethidine analogue, concentrated in some phaeochromocytomas, paragangliomas, carcinoid tumours, and neuroblastomas, and is useful diagnostically. A different isotope, *131I-MIBG*, may be used therapeutically, e.g. in malignant phaeochromocytomas when the diagnostic imaging shows uptake.
- *75Se 6β-selenomethyl-19-norcholesterol* This isotope is concentrated in functioning steroid synthesizing tissue, and is used to image the adrenal cortex. It can be used in determining whether a nodule is functioning or not and can be helpful in localizing residual adrenal tissue following failed bilateral adrenalectomy. However, high resolution CT and MRI have largely replaced it in localizing functional adrenal adenomas.

Positron emission tomography (PET)

PET can be useful in locating tumours and metastases. Radiopharmaceuticals for specific endocrine tumours are being developed e.g. [11C] metahy-droxyephedrine for phaeochromocytoma: combined with CT (PET-CT) it may offer particular value in localizing occult neuroendocrine tumours.

Venous sampling

Adrenal vein sampling can be useful to lateralize an adenoma, or to differentiate an adenoma from bilateral hyperplasia. It is technically difficult—particularly catheterizing the right adrenal vein because of its drainage into the IVC. It may also be used to confirm the diagnosis of bilateral phaeochromocytoma. It is of particular value in lateralising small aldosterone producing adenomas that cannot easily be visualised on CT or MRI.

Further reading

Pacak K, Eisenhofer G, Goldstein DS (2004). Functional imaging of endocrine tumors: role of positron emission tomography. *Endocr Rev* **25**(4), 568–80.

Peppercorn PD, Grossman AB, et al. (1998). Imaging of incidentally discovered adrenal masses. *Clin Endocrinol* **48**, 379–88.

Reznek RH and Armstrong P (1994). The adrenal gland. *Clinical Endocrinology* **40**, 561–76.

Mineralocorticoid excess

Definitions

The majority of cases of mineralocorticoid excess are due to excess aldosterone production which may be 1° or 2° and are typically associated with hypertension and hypokalaemia.

- *Primary hyperaldosteronism* is a disorder of autonomous aldosterone hypersecretion with suppressed renin levels.
- *Secondary hyperaldosteronism* occurs when aldosterone hypersecretion occurs 2° to elevated circulating renin levels. This is typical of heart failure, cirrhosis, or nephrotic syndrome, but can also be due to renal artery stenosis and, occasionally a very rare renin-producing tumour (reninoma).
- Other mineralocorticoids may occasionally be the cause of this syndrome (☐ see Box 41.1).

Box 41.1 Causes of mineralocorticoid excess

Primary hyperaldosteronism
- Conn's syndrome (aldosterone-producing adrenal adenoma) 35%.
- Bilateral adrenal hyperplasia 60%.
- Glucocorticoid remedial aldosteronism (GRA) <1%.
- Aldosterone-producing adrenal carcinoma.

Secondary hyperaldosteronism
- Renal artery stenosis.
- Renal hypoperfusion.
- Cirrhosis.
- Congestive cardiac failure.
- Nephrotic syndrome.
- Renin-secreting tumour.

Other mineralocorticoid excess syndromes
- Apparent mineralocorticoid excess (🕮 p.234).
- Liquorice ingestion (p.236) (inhibits II β HSOH) ↓ aldosterone,
  ↓ renin, ↓ K^+ found in sweets, chewing tobacco, cough mixtures,
  herbal medicines.
- Deoxycorticosterone and corticosterone (🕮 p.236).
- Ectopic ACTH secretion (🕮 p.142).
- Congenital adrenal hyperplasia (🕮 p.302).
- Exogenous mineralocorticoids.

'Pseudoaldosteronism' due to abnormal renal tubular transport
- 🕮 Bartter's syndrome (p.245)
- 🕮 Gitelman's syndrome (p.246)
- 🕮 Liddle's syndrome (p.244)

Primary aldosteronism

Epidemiology

Primary hyperaldosteronism is present in around 10% of hypertensive patients. The most common cause is bilateral adrenal hyperplasia (see Table 42.1).

Pathophysiology

Aldosterone causes renal sodium retention and potassium loss. This results in expansion of body sodium content, leading to suppression of renal renin synthesis. The direct action of aldosterone on the distal nephron causes sodium retention and loss of hydrogen and potassium ions, resulting in a hypokalaemic alkalosis, although serum potassium may not be significantly reduced and may be normal in up to 50% of cases.

Aldosterone has pathophysiological effects on a range of other tissues, causing cardiac fibrosis, vascular endothelial dysfunction and nephrosclerosis.

Clinical features

- Moderately severe hypertension, which is often resistant to conventional therapy. There may be disproportionate left ventricular hypertrophy.
- Hypokalaemia is usually asymptomatic. Occasionally patients may present with tetany, myopathy, polyuria and nocturia (hypokalaemic nephrogenic diabetes insipidus) due to severe hypokalaemia.

Table 42.1 Causes of 1° hyperaldosteronism

Condition	Relative frequency	Age	Sex	Pathology
Aldosteronoma (Conn's adenoma)	30%	3rd–6th decade	Predominant in ♀	Benign, adenoma, <2.5cm diameter, yellow because of high cholesterol content
Idiopathic aldosteronism/ adrenal hyperplasia	50%	Older than Conn's	No sex difference	Macronodular or micronodular hyperplasia
Adrenal carcinoma	Rare	5th–7th decade (occasionally young)	More common in ♀	Tumour >4cm in diameter – often larger, may be evidence of local invasion
Glucocorticoid suppressible hyperaldosteronism	Rare	Childhood	No sex difference	Bilateral hyperplasia of zona glomerulosa

Conn's syndrome— aldosterone-producing adenoma

Very high levels of the enzyme aldosterone synthase are expressed in tumour tissue. Although aldosterone production is autonomous, ACTH has a greater stimulatory effect than angiotensin II (aldosterone often displays a diurnal variation that mirrors that of cortisol), although a subtype that remain more responsive to angiotensin II has been described. Very rarely, Conn's adenomas may be part of the MEN1 syndrome.

Bilateral adrenal hyperplasia (bilateral idiopathic hyperaldosteronism)

This is the most common form of 1° hyperaldosteronism in adults. Hyperplasia is more commonly bilateral than unilateral, and may be associated with micronodular or macronodular hyperplasia. Note however that CT demonstrable nodules have a prevalence of 2% in the general population, including hypertensive patients without excess aldosterone production. The pathophysiology is not known although aldosterone secretion is very sensitive to circulating angiotensin II. The pathophysiology of bilateral adrenal hyperplasia is not understood, and it is possible that it represents an extreme end of the spectrum of low renin essential hypertension.

Glucocorticoid-remedial aldosteronism (GRA)

This is a rare autosomal dominantly inherited condition due to the presence of a chimeric gene (8q22) containing the 5′ sequence which determines regulation of the 11β-hydroxylase gene (*CYP11B1*) coding for the enzyme catalysing the last step in cortisol synthesis, and the 3′ sequence from the aldosterone synthase gene (*CYP11B2*) coding for the enzyme catalysing the last step in aldosterone synthesis. This results in expression of aldosterone synthase in the zona fasiculata as well as the zona glomerulosa and aldosterone secretion becomes under ACTH control. Glucocorticoids lead to suppression of ACTH and suppression of aldosterone production.
• Early hypertension and family history.
• Hybrid steroids (18OHcortisol and 18oxocortisol) elevated.

Aldosterone-producing carcinoma

Rare, and usually associated with excessive secretion of other corticosteroids (cortisol, androgen, oestrogen). Hypokalaemia may be profound, and aldosterone levels very high.

Screening

Indications

- Patients resistant to conventional antihypertensive medication (i.e. not controlled on 3 agents).
- Hypertension associated with hypokalaemia (potassium < 3.7mmol/L, irrespective of thiazide use).
- Hypertension developing before age of 40 years.
- Adrenal incidentaloma.

Method

False −ves and false +ves can occur if the test is not performed under controlled circumstances

- Give oral supplements of potassium to control hypokalaemia.
- Stop medication that can interfere with the test using appropriate washout period (Table 42.2).
- BP can be controlled using doxazosin or verapamil (rather than other calcium antagonists).
- *Measure aldosterone: renin ratio*
  - A high ratio is suggestive of 1° hyperaldosteronism (aldosterone [pmol/L]/plasma renin activity [ng/mlLh] >750 or aldosterone [ng/dL]/plasma renin activity [ng/mL/h] >30–50). Note that newer assays that measure renin mass (rather than activity) will require development of different cut-offs.
  - The greater the ratio, the more likely the diagnosis of 1° aldosteronism.
  - A false −ve can occur in patients with chronic renal failure due to an inappropriately high plasma renin activity.

Table 42.2 Effect of medication on renin and aldosterone measurement

Drug	Washout	Magnitude of effect	Effect on screening test
Methyl-dopa			False +ves
Clonidine	–	–	False +ves
Beta blockers e.g. atenolol	2	62% (± 82)	False +ves
Alpha blockers e.g. doxazosin	na	−5% (± 26)	Little effect
ACE inhibitors e.g. fosinopril	2	−30% (± 24)	False −ves
ARB e.g. irbesartan	2	−43% (± 24)	False −ves
Ca Antagonists e.g. amlodipine	2	−17% (± 32)	False −ves
Diuretics	6	–	False −ves

NSAIDS give false +ves

Confirmation of diagnosis

Confirmation of autonomous aldosterone production is made by demonstrating failure to suppress aldosterone in face of sodium/volume loading. This can be achieved by a number of mechanisms after optimizing test conditions as described.

- Dietary sodium loading: patients can be given instruction to take a diet with a high sodium content (sufficient to raise the sodium intake to 200mmol per day for 3 days. If necessary, this can be achieved by adding supplemental sodium chloride tablets (slow sodium). It is important to ensure that potassium is maintained during this period and potassium supplementation may also be required. Failure to suppress 24 urinary aldosterone secretion at the end of this period is diagnostic of primary aldosteronism.
- *Fludrocortisone suppression test:*
  - Give fludrocortisone 100mcg 6-hourly for 4 days.
  - Measure plasma aldosterone basally and on last day.
  - Aldosterone fails to suppress in 1° aldosteronism.
- *Saline infusion test:*
  - Administer 2L normal saline over 4h.
  - Measure plasma aldosterone at 0, 2, 3, and 4h.
  - Aldosterone fails to suppresses to <140pmol/L, (140–280 equivocal) in 80–90% of 1° aldosteronism.
- Other tests such as the captopril suppression test are described but are of lesser value in this circumstance, lacking appropriate sensitivity or specificity in the diagnosis of 1° aldosteronism.
- A number of tests have been described that are said to differentiate between the various subtypes of 1° aldosteronism (solitary Conn's adenoma; bilateral adrenal hyperplasia; GRA). However, none of these are sufficiently specific to influence management decisions and more specific investigations (imaging and adrenal vein sampling) are necessary if there is doubt. Additional tests such as postural response of aldosterone and the measurement of urinary 18-hydroxycortisol have been largely superseded because of this. Diagnosis of GRA is best made using a specific genetic test rather than on the ability of dexamethasone (0.5mg 6-hourly for 3 days) to suppress aldosterone.

Other dynamic tests

If these tests are non-diagnostic then it is usual to proceed to venous sampling rather than dynamic testing however such tests can sometimes be helpful.

Captopril suppression test

- Plasma aldosterone is measured in the sitting position, basally and 60min after captopril 25mg.
- Inhibition of angiotensin II leads to a fall in aldosterone in patients with idiopathic hyperaldosteronism but not in Conn's syndrome.

Fludrocortisone suppression test

- Give fludrocortisone 100mcg 6-hourly for 4 days.
- Measure aldosterone basally and on last day.
- Aldosterone suppressed in hyperplasia but unchanged in adenomas.

Saline infusion test
- Administer 2L normal saline over 4h.
- Measure aldosterone at 0, 2, 3, and 4h.
- Aldosterone fails to suppresses to 140pmol/L in 80–90% of adenomas.
- Also suppressed in 60% of normokalaemic hyperaldosteronism.

Table 42.3 Differential diagnosis of 1° hyperaldosteronism.

Test		Upright posture and time	ACE inhibitor	Dexamethasone suppression
Normal	PRA	↑	↑	→
	Aldosterone	↑	↓	→
Aldosterone-producing adenoma	PRA	→	→	→
	Aldosterone	↓	→	→
Angiotensin-responsive adenoma (?~20% adenomas)	PRA	↑	↑	→
	Aldosterone	↑	↓	→
Idiopathic adrenal hyperplasia	PRA	↑	↑	→
	Aldosterone	↑	↓	→
Glucocorticoid-suppressible hyperaldosteronism	PRA	→	→	↑
	Aldosterone	↓	→	↓

Localization and confirmation of differential diagnosis

CT/MRI scan

CT and MRI scanning are of value in identifying adrenal adenomas. It should be noted, however, that the frequency of adrenal incidentalomas rises with age and, for this reason, it is prudent to consider adrenal vein sampling in older patients (age >50) with 1° aldosteronism who have an apparent solitary adenoma on scanning.

- Identifies most adenomas >5mm diameter. Bilateral abnormalities or tumours <1cm in diameter require further localization procedures.
- In bilateral adrenal hyperplasia both glands can appear enlarged or normal in size.
- Macronodular hyperplasia may result in identifiable nodules on imaging.
- A mass >4cm in size is suspicious of carcinoma but is unusual in Conn's syndrome.
- NB In essential hypertension nodules are described.

Adrenal vein sampling

Aldosterone measurements from both adrenal veins allow a gradient between the 2 sides to be identified in the case of unilateral disease. It is the gold standard for differentiation between uni- and bilateral aldosterone production, but cannulating the right adrenal vein is technically difficult as it drains directly into the inferior vena cava. Cortisol measurements must also be taken concomitantly with aldosterone, to confirm successful positioning within the adrenal veins and should be more than thrice a peripheral sample (central\peripheral ratio >3). The aldosterone/cortisol ratio with an adenoma is >4.1.

Radiolabelled iodocholesterol scanning

This test has low sensitivity specificity and offers no advantage over a high resolution CT or MRI with, where necessary, adrenal vein sampling.

Treatment

Surgery

- Laparascopic adrenalectomy is the treatment of choice for aldosterone secreting adenomas and is associated with lower morbidity than open adrenalectomy.
- Surgery is not indicated in patients with idiopathic hyperaldosteronism as even bilateral adrenalectomy may not cure the hypertension.
- Presurgical spironolactone treatment may be used to correct potassium stores before surgery.
- The BP response to treatment with spironolactone (50–400mg/day) before surgery can be used to predict the response to surgery of patients with adenomas.
- Hypertension is cured in about 70%.

- If it persists (more likely in those with long-standing hypertension and increased age) it is more amenable to medical treatment.
- Overall 50% become normotensive in 1 month and 70% within 1 year.

Medical treatment

Medical therapy remains an option for patients with a solitary adrenaladenoma who are unlikely to be cured by surgery, who are unfit for operation or who express a preference for medical management.

- The aldosterone antagonist *spironolactone* (50–400mg/day) has been used successfully for many years to treat the hypertension and hypokalaemia associated with bilateral adrenal hyperplasia and idiopathic hyperaldosteronism.
- There may be a delay in response of hypertension of 4–8 weeks. However, combination with other antihypertensive agents (ACEI and calcium channel blockers) is usually required.
- Side-effects are common—particularly gynaecomastia and impotence in ♂, menstrual irregularities in ♀, and GI effects.
- *Eplerenone* (50–100mg/day) is a mineralocorticoid antagonist without antiandrogen effects and greater selectivity than spironolactone.
- Alternative drugs include the potassium-sparing diuretics *amiloride* and *triamterene*. Amiloride may need to be given in high dose (up to 40mg/day) in 1° aldosteronism, and monitoring of serum potassium is essential. Calcium channel antagonists may also be helpful.
- Glucocorticoid-remedial aldosteronism can be treated with low dose *dexamethasone* (0.5mg on going to bed). Side effects often limit therapy, and spironolactone or amiloride treatment is often preferred.
- Adrenal carcinoma Surgery and postoperative adrenolytic therapy with *mitotane* is usually required, but the prognosis is usually poor (📖 see Treatment, p.240).

Further reading

Allolio, B., S. Hahner, Weismann D, et al. (2004). Management of adrenocortical carcinoma. *Clin Endocrinol* **60**, 273–28.

Espiner, E. A., D. G. Ross, Yandle, TG, et al. (2003). Predicting surgically remedial primary aldosteronism: role of adrenal scanning, posture testing, and adrenal vein sampling *J Clin Endocrinol Metab* **88**(8), 3637–44.

Funder JW et al. (2008). Case detection, diagnosis, and treatment of patients with primary aldosteronism: an Endocrine Society clinical practice guideline.

Ganguly A (1998). Primary aldosteronism. *New Engl J Med* **339**, 1828–33.

Young, WF (2007). Primary aldosteronism—renaissance of a syndrome. *Clin Endocrinol* **66**, 607–18.

Excess other mineralocorticoids

Epidemiology

Occasionally, the clinical syndrome of hyperaldosteronism is not associated with excess aldosterone, and a process due to another mineralocorticoid is suspected. This can either be due to an increase in an alternative mineralcorticoid or due to ↑ mineralocorticoid effect of cortisol.

These conditions are rare.

Apparent mineralocorticoid excess

- The aldosterone receptor has an equal affinity for cortisol and aldosterone, but there is a 100-fold excess of circulating cortisol over aldosterone.
- The receptor is usually protected from the effects of stimulation by cortisol by the 11β-hydroxysteroid type 2 dehydrogenase enzyme which converts cortisol to cortisone.
- In this syndrome there is a deficiency of the 11β-hydroxysteroid dehydrogenase (HSD) enzyme type 2 encoded on chromosome 16q22.
- Congenital absence (autosomal recessive) of the enzyme or inhibition of its activity allows cortisol to stimulate the receptor and leads to severe hypertension.

Type 1 is seen predominantly in children, presenting with failure to thrive, thirst, polyuria, and severe hypertension. Patients are not cushingoid as there is intact −ve feedback, and circulating cortisol levels are not raised. The urinary terahydrocortisol and allo-tetrahydro-cortisol to terahydrocortisone ratio is raised to 10 × normal.

Type 2 is a milder form that may be a cause of hypertension in adolescence\early adulthood. The urinary terahydrocortisol and allo-tetrahydrocortisol to terahydrocortisone ratio is normal.

However multiple mutations have been found in the 11β-HSD2 gene for both types and some authors believe there is a spectrum of disease: mild forms may present with salt sensitive hypertension.

Biochemistry

- Suppression of renin and aldosterone.
- Hypokalemic alkalosis.
- Urinary free cortisol/cortisone ratio ↑.
- Ratio of urinary tetrahydrocortisol and *allo*-tetrahydro-cortisol to tetrahydrocortisone is raised (>10 ×) in type 1 but is normal in type 2.
- Confirm with genetic testing.

Treatment

- *Dexamethasone* leads to suppression of ACTH secretion, reduced cortisol concentrations, and lowered BP in 60%. It has a much lower affinity for the mineralocorticoid receptor.
- Other antihypertensive agents are often required.
- One patient with hypertensive renal failure was cured with a renal transplant.

Liquorice ingestion

- Liquorice contains glycyrrhetinic acid which is used as a sweetener.
- It inhibits the action of 11β-HSD making the aldosterone receptor more sensitive to cortisol.
- It is found in candies, chewing tobacco, cough mixtures, and some herbal medicines.

Ectopic ACTH syndrome

(see p.138)

In the syndrome of ectopic ACTH, the 11β-HSD protection is overcome because of high cortisol secretion rates, which saturate the enzyme, leading to impaired conversion of cortisol to cortisone, and thus hypokalaemia and hypertension.

Deoxycorticosterone (DOC) excess

2 forms of congenital adrenal hyperplasia (see Part 4 p.302) are associated with excess production of deoxycorticosterone which acts as an agonist at the mineralocorticoid receptor, resulting in hypertension with suppression of renin.

- 17α-hydroxylase deficiency.
- 11β-hydroxylase deficiency.

Glucocorticoid replacement to inhibit ACTH is effective treatment for these conditions.

Adrenal tumours rarely secrete excessive amounts of deoxycorticosterone. Usually this is concomitant with excessive aldosterone production, but occasionally it may occur in an isolated fashion.

Adrenal Cushing's syndrome

Definition and epidemiology

- Cushing's syndrome results from chronic excess cortisol, and is described in Chapter 19 (📖 Cushing's disease, p.136).
- The causes may be classified as ACTH dependent and ACTH independent. This section describes ACTH-independent Cushing's syndrome, which is due to adrenal tumours (benign and malignant), and is responsible for 10–20% cases of Cushing's syndrome.
- Adrenal tumours causing Cushing's syndrome are commoner in ♀. The peak incidence is in the 4th and 5th decade.
- Causes and relative frequencies of adrenal Cushing's syndrome in adults:
  - Adrenal adenoma   10%.
  - Adrenal carcinoma   8%.
  - Bilateral micronodular adrenal hyperplasia   1%.
  - Bilateral macronodular hyperplasia   1%.

Pathophysiology

- Benign adenomas are usually encapsulated, and <6cm in diameter. They are usually associated with pure glucocorticoid excess.
- Adrenal carcinomas are usually >6cm in diameter, although they may be smaller, and are often associated with local invasion and metastases at the time of diagnosis. They may be associated with secretion of excess androgen production in addition to cortisol. Occasionally they may be associated with mineralocorticoid or oestrogen secretion.
- *Carney complex* (📖 see Carney complex, p.610) is an autosomal dominant condition characterized by atrial myxomas, spotty skin pigmentation, peripheral nerve tumours, and endocrine disorders e.g. Cushing's syndrome due to pigmented adrenal nodular hyperplasia.
- Adrenal hyperplasia may be micronodular (<1cm diameter) or macronodular (>1cm).

Bilateral macronodular adrenal hyperplasia

- The majority of cases of bilateral macronodular hyperplasia do not have an identifiable cause.
- Abnormal gastric inhibitory peptide (GIP), vasopressin, β agonist, human chorionic gonadotrophin\luteinizing hormone and serotonin receptors have been described.
- Several 'food-dependant' Cushing's syndrome cases have been described due to GIP receptor expression.

Clinical features

- The clinical features of ACTH-independent Cushing's syndrome are as described in 🕮 Clinical features, p.138 in Chapter 19, Cushing's disease.
- It is important to note that in patients with adrenal carcinoma, there may also be features related to excessive androgen production in ♀, and also a relatively more rapid time course of development of the syndrome.

Investigations

- Once the presence of Cushing's syndrome is confirmed (🕮 see Clinical features, p.138) subsequent investigation of the cause depends on whether ACTH is suppressed (ACTH independent) or measurable/elevated (ACTH dependent).
- Patients with ACTH-independent Cushing's syndrome do not suppress cortisol to <50% basal on high dose dexamethasone testing, and fail to show a rise in cortisol and ACTH following administration of CRH. (The latter test is often important when patients have borderline/low ACTH to differentiate pituitary dependent disease from adrenal.)
- ACTH-independent causes are adrenal in origin, and the mainstay of further investigation is adrenal imaging.
- CT scan allows excellent visualization of the adrenal glands and their anatomy.
- Adenomas are usually small and homogeneous, and usually associated with contralateral gland atrophy.
- Adrenal carcinomas are usually >6cm in diameter, heterogeneous with calcification and necrosis, and evidence of local invasion.

Bilateral macronodular adrenal hyperplasia

- Monitor ACTH and cortisol response to a mixed meal, LHRH, and posture.
- ACTH independent.
- Medical treatment may be possible e.g. octreotide for GIP dependent disease.

Treatment

(📖 see Treatment, p. 149)

Adrenal adenoma

- Unilateral adrenalectomy (normally laparoscopic) is curative.
- Postoperative temporary adrenal insufficiency ensues because of long-term suppression of ACTH and the contralateral adrenal gland, requiring glucocorticoid replacement for up to 2 years.

Adrenal carcinoma

- Surgery is useful to debulk tumour mass, and occasionally adrenalectomy and local clearance leads to cure. However, most patients have distant metastases at the time of diagnosis.
- Postoperative drug treatment with the adrenolytic agent *mitotane* (*ortho-para* DDD) 3–12g daily may prolong survival. This may lead to adrenal insufficiency and glucocorticoid replacement may be required. Side-effects may limit therapy—nausea and vomiting, dizziness, and diarrhoea. Monitoring of drug levels can be helpful to ensure concentrations within the therapeutic range (14–20mcg/mL), and so limit unwanted side effects.
- Other drugs may be required to control cortisol hypersecretion (e.g. *metyrapone*).
- Newer treatments such as *suramin*, *5-fluorouracil*, and *gossypol* have also been tried without evidence of benefit.

Bilateral adrenal hyperplasia

- Bilateral adrenalectomy is curative. Lifelong glucocorticoid and mineralocorticoid treatment is required.
- Medical treatment may be possible for cases with aberrant receptors e.g. octreotide for GIP dependant disease.

Prognosis

- Adrenal adenomas, which are successfully treated with surgery, have a good prognosis, and recurrence is unlikely. The prognosis depends on the long-term effects of excess cortisol before treatment—in particular atherosclerosis and osteoporosis.
- The prognosis for adrenal carcinoma is very poor, despite surgery. Reports suggest a 5-year survival of 22%, and median survival time of 14 months. Age >40 years and distant metastases are associated with a worse prognosis.

Subclinical Cushing's syndrome

- Describes a subset of 5–10% of patients with an adrenal incidentaloma with autonomous glucocorticoid production which is insufficient to produce overt Cushing's syndrome.
- Urinary free cortisol measurement may be within the normal range but there is a failure to suppress with low dose dexamethasone.
- An associated ↑ risk of diabetes mellitus, osteoporosis, and hypertension has been reported.
- Data are insufficient to indicate the superiority of a surgical or nonsurgical approach to management.
- Hypoadrenalism post adrenalectomy has been reported due to suppression of the contralateral adrenal gland. Perioperative steroid cover is therefore required with re-evaluation postoperatively.

Further reading

Allolin B and Fassnacht M (2006). Clinical review: Adrenocortical carcinoma: clinical update. *J Clin Endocrinol Metab* **91**(6), 2027–37. Epub Mar 21 2006.

Lacroix A, N'Diaye N, Tremblay J, *et al.* (2001). Ectopic and abnormal hormone receptors in adrenal Cushing's syndrome. *Endocr Rev* **22**(1), 75–110.

Terzolo M, Angeli A, Fasscacht M, *et al.* (2007). Adjuvant mitotane treatment for adrenocortical carcinoma. *New Engl J Med* **356**(23), 2372–80.

Adrenal surgery

Adrenalectomy

Open adrenalectomy may still be necessary for large and complex pathology. However, laparoscopic adrenalectomy (first performed in 1992) has become the procedure of choice for removal of most adrenal tumours. Retrospective comparisons with open approaches suggest reduced hospital stay and analgesic requirements and lower postoperative morbidity. However, there are few long-term outcome data on this technique. It is most useful in the management of small (<6cm) benign adenomas. Laparoscopic bilateral adrenalectomy, although technically demanding, offers a useful approach to patients with macronodular hyperplasia and in selected patients with ACTH-dependent Cushing's syndrome where alternative therapeutic options are not appropriate.

Further reading

Dudley NE and Harrison BJ (1999). Comparison of open posterior versus transperitoneal laparoscopic adrenalectomy. *Br J Surg* **86**, 656–60.

McCallum R and Connell JMC (2001). Laparoscopic adrenalectomy. *Clin Endocrinol* **55**, 435–6.

Wells SA, Merke DP, Cutler GB, *et al.* (1998). The role of laparoscopic surgery in adrenal disease. *J Clin Endocrinol Metab* **83**, 3041–9.

Preoperative preparation of patients

- Cushing's—metyrapone or ketoconazole (🕮 see p.148)
- Phaeochromocytoma—α- and β-blockade (🕮 see p.280).

Perioperative management

🕮 see Box 45.1.

Box 45.1 Perioperative management of patients undergoing adrenalectomy

Adrenal cortical tumours (benign and malignant)/bilateral adrenalectomy for Cushing's syndrome.

- Perioperative glucocorticoid cover is required, as even 'silent' adenomas may be associated with subclinical excess cortisol secretion and hence suppression of the contralateral adrenal gland.
- Hydrocortisone is given as for pituitary surgery – 100mg IM with the premedication, and then continued every 6h for 24–48h, until the patient can take oral medication and is eating and drinking.
- This is changed to oral hydrocortisone at double replacement dose—20mg on waking, 10mg at lunchtime and 10mg at 5 p.m., and mineralocorticoid replacement commenced if bilateral adrenalectomy has been performed (100mcg fludrocortisone daily). Electrolytes and BP guide adequacy of treatment. Normal replacement hydrocortisone (10, 5, 5mg) can be commenced when the patient is recovered and may be omitted altogether if the patient did not have preoperative evidence of Cushing's syndrome/suppression of the contralateral gland/bilateral adrenalectomy. Mineralocorticoid replacement is only required in patients who have had bilateral adrenalectomy.
- A short Synacthen® test (off hydrocortisone for at least 24h) is performed after at least 2 weeks to demonstrate adequate function of the contralateral adrenal. However, in patients with ACTH-independent Cushing's syndrome, it may take up to 2 years for full recovery of the contralateral adrenal gland to recover.
- The exception is patients undergoing adrenalectomy for mineralocorticoid-secreting tumours. These patients do not usually require peroperative glucocorticoid replacement, but preoperative amiloride or spironolactone allows recovery of potassium stores and control of hypertension prior to surgery.

Renal tubular abnormalities

Background

Bartter's syndrome and Gitelman's syndrome are both associated with hypokalaemic alkalosis and activation of the renin–angiotensin system, but without hypertension—in contrast, BP tends to be low in these conditions. Liddle's syndrome is associated with hypokalaemic alkalosis and hypertension but low renin and aldosterone levels.

Liddle's syndrome

A rare autosomal dominant (AD) condition with variable penetrance. Mutations have been localized to genes on chromosome 16.

Cause

A mutation in the gene encoding the β or γ subunit of the highly selective epithelial sodium channel in the distal nephron. This leads to constitutive activation of sodium transport independent of circulating mineralocorticoid; 2° activation of the sodium/potassium exchange occurs.

Features

Hypokalaemia and hypertension.

Investigation

- Hypokalaemic alkalosis.
- Suppressed renin and aldosterone levels.
- 📖 See Table 46.1.

Treatment

Hypertension responds to amiloride (doses up to 40mg/day) but not spironolactone, because amiloride acts on the sodium channel directly whereas spironolactone acts on the mineralocorticoid receptor.

Bartter's syndrome

Cause

Loss of function of the bumetanide-sensitive Na–K–2Cl co-transporter in the thick ascending limb of the loop of Henle. Mutations in 3 genes have been reported to account for the phenotype—these encode regulatory ion channels (*NKCC2; ROMK; CLCNKB*). Inactivation of the co-transporter leads to salt wasting, activation of the renin–angiotensin system, and ↑ aldosterone which leads to ↑ sodium reabsorption at the distal nephron and causes hypokalaemic alkalosis. Reabsorption of calcium also occurs in the thick ascending loop and thus inactivation leads to hypercalciuria. The lack of associated hypertension is thought to be due to ↑ prostaglandin production from the renal medullary interstitial tissue in response to hypokalaemia.

- Rare (~1/million) autosomal recessive hypokalaemic metabolic alkalosis associated with salt wasting and normal or reduced BP.
- Usually present at an early age (<5 years).

Features

- Intravascular volume depletion.
- Seizures.
- Tetany.
- Muscle weakness.

There is also an antenatal variant which is a life-threatening disorder of renal tubular hypokalaemic alkalosis and hypercalciuria.

Investigations

- Hypokalaemic alkalosis.
- ↑ PRA and aldosterone.
- Hypercalciuria.

Treatment

Potassium replacement Potassium sparing diuretics may be helpful. However, they are usually inadequate in correcting hypokalaemia. Prostaglandin synthase inhibitors (NSAIDS) e.g. indometacin 2–5mg/kg per day or ibuprofen may be required.

Gitelman's syndrome

Cause

- Loss of function in the thiazide-sensitive Na–Cl transporter of the distal convoluted tubule (DCT) due to mutations in the *SCL12A3* gene that encodes it (located on chromosome 16q13). This leads to salt wasting, hypovolaemia, and metabolic alkalosis.
- Hypovolaemia leads to activation of the renin–angiotensin system, and ↑ aldosterone levels.
- Hypokalaemic alkalosis in conjunction with hypocalciuria and hypomagnaesaemia.
- Present at older ages without overt hypovolaemia (essentially a less severe phenotype of Bartter's syndrome).

Investigations

- Hypokalaemic alkalosis, in association with ↑ renin and aldosterone.
- Hypomagnaesaemia.
- Hypocalciuria.

Treatment

- Potassium and magnesium replacement.
- Potassium sparing diuretics may be required.
- 📖 See Table 46.1.

Further reading

Amirlak I and Dawson KP (2000). Bartter's syndrome. *QJM* **93**, 207–15.

Furuhashi, M., K. Kitamura, Adachi, M et al. (2005). Liddle's syndrome caused by a novel mutation in the proline-rich PY motif of the epithelial sodium channel β-subunit. *J Clin Endocrinol Metab* **90**(1), 340–4.

Table 46.1 Summary of features of renal tubular abnormalities

Syndrome*	BP	Renin	Aldosterone	Urinary calcium	Other
Bartter's	N	↑	↑	↑	
Gitelman's	N	↑	↑	↓	↓ Mg
Liddle's	↑	↓	↓	N	

*All 3 conditions have hypokalaemic alkalosis

Mineralocorticoid deficiency

Epidemiology

Rare, apart from the hyporeninaemic hypoaldosteronism associated with diabetes mellitus.

Causes

Congenital

- *Adrenal hypoplasia*–X-linked failure of development of the adrenal gland. Presents in infancy with salt losing state. Differentiated from CAH by normal external genitalia and steroid levels.
- *CAH*—certain types, most commonly 21-hydroxylase deficiency, are associated with MC deficiency; 📖 see p.302.
- Rare *inherited disorders* of aldosterone biosynthesis.
- *Adrenoleukodystrophy*–X-linked affecting 1/20 000 ♂, where very long chain fatty acids cannot be oxidized in peroxisomes and accumulate in tissues. CNS symptoms may be absent but progressive demyelination can lead to hypertonic tetraparesis, dementia, epilepsy, coma or death.
- *Pseudohypoaldosteronism*—inherited resistance to the action of aldosterone, 📖 see p.707. Autosomal dominant and recessive forms are described. Usually presents in infancy. Treated with sodium chloride.

Acquired

- Adrenal insufficiency—📖 see p.250.
- *Drugs*—heparin(heparin for >5 days, may cause severe hyperkalaemia due to a toxic effect on the zona glomerulosa); ciclosporin.
- *Hyporeninaemic hypoaldosteronism*—interference with the renin– angiotensin system leads to mineralocorticoid deficiency and hyperkalaemic acidosis (type IV renal tubular acidosis) e.g. diabetic nephropathy. Treatment is fludrocortisone and potassium restriction. ACEI may produce a similar biochemical picture, but here the PRA will be elevated as there is no angiotensin II feedback on renin.

Treatment

Fludrocortisone.

Adrenal insufficiency

Definition

Adrenal insufficiency results from inadequate adrenocortical function, and may be due to destruction of the adrenal cortex (1° or Addison's disease), or due to disordered pitutary and hypothalamic function (2°).

Epidemiology

- The prevalence of Addison's disease is approximately 93–140/million adults. Incidence 4.7–6.2 per million in white population.
- 2° adrenal insufficiency is most commonly due to suppression of pituitary–hypothalamic function by exogenous glucocorticoid administration.

Causes of secondary adrenal insufficiency

Lesions of the hypothalamus and/or pituitary gland
- Tumours—pituitary tumour, metastases, craniopharyngioma,
- Infection—tuberculosis,
- Inflammation—sarcoidosis, histiocytosis X, haemochromatosis, lymphocytic hypophysitis,
- Iatrogenic—surgery, radiotherapy,
- Other—isolated ACTH deficiency, trauma.

Suppression of the hypothalamo–pituitary–adrenal axis
- Glucocorticoid administration.
- Cushing's disease (after pituitary tumour removal).

Features of secondary adrenal insufficiency

As 1° (◻ see Clinical features, p.98), except:
- Absence of pigmentation—skin is pale.
- Absence of mineralocoticoid deficiency.
- Associated features of underlying cause, e.g. visual field defects if pituitary tumour.
- Other endocrine deficiencies may manifest due to pituitary failure (◻ see p.98).
- Acute onset may occur due to pituitary apoplexy.

Isolated ACTH deficiency

- Rare.
- Pathogenesis unclear—may be autoimmune (associated with other autoimmune conditions, and antipituitary antibodies described in some patients).
- Absent ACTH response to CRH.
- POMC mutations and POMC processing abnormalities (e.g. proconvertase PC1).

Pathophysiology

Primary

- Adrenal gland destruction or dysfunction occurs due to a disease process which usually involves all 3 zones of the adrenal cortex, resulting in inadequate glucocorticoid, mineralocorticoid, and androgen secretion. The manifestations of insufficiency do not usually appear until at least 90% of the gland has been destroyed, and are usually gradual in onset, with partial adrenal insufficiency leading to an impaired cortisol response to stress, and the features of complete insufficiency occurring later. Acute adrenal insufficiency may occur in the context of acute septicaemia (e.g. meningococcal or haemorrhage).
- Mineralocortcoid deficiency leads to reduced sodium retention and hypotension with ↓ intravascular volume, in addition to hyperkalaemia due to ↓ renal potassium and hydrogen ion excretion.
- Androgen deficiency presents in ♀ with reduced axillary and pubic hair and reduced libido. (Testicular production of androgens is more important in ♂.)
- Lack of cortisol −ve feedback increases CRH and ACTH secretion. An increase in other POMC-related peptides leads to skin pigmentation and other mucous membranes.

Secondary

- Inadequate ACTH results in deficient cortisol production (and ↓ androgens in ♀).
- There is no pigmentation because ACTH and POMC secretion is reduced. Mineralocorticoid secretion remains normal as it is mainly regulated by the renin–angiotensin system.
- The onset is usually gradual with partial ACTH deficiency resulting in reduced response to stress. Prolonged ACTH deficiency leads to atrophy of the zona fasiculata and reduced ability to respond acutely to ACTH.

Investigations

📖 see p.100 for pituitary/hypothalamic disease and p.266 for long-term endogenous or exogenous glucocorticoids.

Addison's disease

Causes of primary adrenal insufficiency

- Autoimmune—commonest cause in developed world (approximately 70% cases).
- Autoimmune polyglandular deficiency—type 1 or 2 (□ see p.254).
- *Malignancy:*
  - Metastatic (lung, breast, kidney—adrenal metastases found in ~50% of patients, but symptomatic adrenal insufficiency much less common).
  - Lymphoma.
- *Infiltration:*
  - Amyloid.
  - Haemochromatosis.
- *Infection:*
  - Tuberculosis (medulla more frequently destroyed than cortex).
  - Fungal e.g. histoplasmosis, cryptococcosis.
  - Opportunistic infections in e.g. AIDS—CMV, mycobacterium intracellulare, cryptococcus (up to 5% patients with AIDS develop 1° adrenal insufficiency in the late stages).
- *Vascular haemorrhage:*
  - Anticoagulants.
  - Waterhouse–Friedrichson syndrome in meningococcal septicaemia.
- *Infarction*—e.g. 2° to thrombosis in antiphospholipid syndrome.
- *Adrenoleucodystrophy:*
  - Inherited disorder of fatty acid metabolism.
  - Diagnosed by measuring very long chain fatty acids.
  - Presents in childhood.
  - Progresses to quadraparesis and dementia in association with adrenal failure).
  - Treat with Lorenzo's oil.
- *Congenital adrenal hyperplasia*—□ see p.302.
- *Congenital adrenal hypoplasia*—rare familial failure of adrenal cortical development due to mutations/deletion of *DAX 1* gene.
- *Iatrogenic:*
  - Adrenalectomy.
  - Drugs: ketoconazole and fluconazole (inhibit cortisol synthesis), phenytoin, rifampicin (increases cortisol metabolism), etomidate, aminoglutethamide (usually do not cause hypoadrenalism unless reduced adrenal or pituitary reserve).

Autoimmune adrenalitis

- Mediated by humoral and cell-mediated immune mechanisms. Autoimmune insufficiency associated with polyglandular autoimmune syndrome is more common in ♀ (70%).
- Adrenal cortex antibodies are present in the majority of patients at diagnosis, and although titres decline and eventually disappear, they are still found in approximately 70% of patients 10 years later. Up to 20% patients/year with +ve adrenal antibodies develop adrenal insufficiency. Antibodies to 21-hydroxylase are commonly found, although the exact nature of other antibodies that block the effect of ACTH for example are yet to be elucidated.
- Antiadrenal antibodies are found in <2% of patients with other autoimmune endocrine disease (Hashimoto's thyroiditis, diabetes mellitus, autoimmune hypothyroidism, hypoparathyroidism, pernicious anaemia). In addition, antibodies to other endocrine glands are commonly found in patients with autoimmune adrenal insufficiency (thyroid microsomal in 50%, gastric parietal cell, parathyroid, and ovary and testis).
- Polyglandular autoimmune conditions (📖 see Autoimmune polyglandular syndrome (APS) type 1, p.254; APS types 2–4, p.255). The presence of 17-hydroxylase antibodies in association with 21-hydroxylase antibodies is a good marker of patients at risk of developing premature ovarian failure in association with 1° adrenal failure.
- Patients with type 1 diabetes mellitus and autoimmune thyroid disease only rarely develop autoimmune adrenal insufficiency. Approximately 50% of patients with Addison's disease have other autoimmune or endocrine disorders.

Clinical features

Chronic

- Anorexia and weight loss (>90%).
- Tiredness.
- Weakness—generalized, no particular muscle groups.
- Pigmentation—generalized, but most common in light exposed areas, and areas exposed to pressure (elbows and knees, and under bras and belts), mucosae and scars acquired after onset of adrenal insufficiency. Look at palmar creases in Caucasians.
- Dizziness and postural hypotension.
- GI symptoms—nausea and vomiting, abdominal pain, diarrhoea.
- Arthralgia and myalgia.
- Symptomatic hypoglycaemia—rare in adults.
- ↓ axillary and pubic hair and reduced libido in ♀.
- Pyrexia of unknown origin—rarely.

Associated conditions

- Vitiligo.
- Features of other autoimmune endocrinopathies.

Laboratory investigations

- Hyponatraemia.
- Hyperkalaemia.
- Elevated urea.
- Anaemia (normocytic normochromic).
- Elevated ESR.
- Eosinophilia.
- Mild hypercalcaemia—↓ absorption, ↓ renal absorption of calcium.

Autoimmune polyglandular syndrome (APS) type 1

- Also known as autoimmune polyendocrinopthy, candidiasis and epidermal dystrophy (APECED).
- Autosomal recessive with childhood onset.
- Chronic mucocutaneous candidiasis.
- Hypoparathyroidism (90%),1° adrenal insufficiency (60%).
- 1° gonadal failure.
- 1° hypothyroidism.
- Rarely hypopituitarism, diabetes insipidus, type 1 diabetes mellitus.
- Associated chronic active hepatitis (20%),malabsorption (15%), alopecia (40%), pernicious anaemia, vitiligo.
- Mutations in the AIRE (autoimmune regulator) gene located on chromosome 21p22.3.

APS types 2–4

- Autosomal recessive, autosomal dominant, polygenic.
- Adult onset.
- Adrenal insufficiency (100%).
- 1° hypothyroidism (69%).
- Type 1 diabetes mellitus. (52%)
- 1° gonadal failure (4-10%).
- Rarely diabetes insipidus (<0.1%).
- Associated vitiligo, myasthenia gravis, alopecia, pernicious anaemia, immune thrombocytopenic purpura.
- APS3—thyroid disease without adrenal insufficiency.
- APS4—adrenal insufficiency without thyroid disease.

Eponymous syndromes

- Schmidt syndrome:
  - Addison's disease *and*
  - Autoimmune hypothyroidism.
- Carpenter syndrome:
  - Addison's disease *and*
  - Autoimmune hypothyroidism *and/or*
  - Type 1 diabetes mellitus.

Screening recommendations

- 2.4% of patients with a monoglandular autoimmune endocrinopathy have APS2 on subsequent follow up
- Functional screening is recommended every 3 years until the age of 75 years
  - Serum Na^+, K^+, Ca^{2+}, blood cell count.
  - TSH, free T_4.
  - FSH, LH, testosterone, or oestradiol.
  - Fasting morning cortisol and glucose.
  - Optional: ACTH stimulation test.
- If a 2nd endocrinopathy is diagnosed then measure organ-specific autoantibodies and consider functional screening in 1st degree relatives
  - Islet cells, GAD, IA2.
  - TPO, TSH receptor.
  - Cytochrome P450 enzymes.
  - H^+-K^+-ATPase of the parietal cells, intrinsic factor.
  - Transglutaminase, gliadin.

Further reading

Dittmar M and Kahaly GJ (2003). Polyglandular autoimmune syndromes: immunogenetics and long-term follow-up. *J Clin Endocrinol Metab* **88**(7), 2983–92.

Investigation of primary adrenal insufficiency

Electrolytes
- Hyponatraemia is present in 90% and hyperkalaemia in 65%.
- Elevated urea.

Serum cortisol and ACTH
- Undetectable serum cortisol is diagnostic of adrenal insufficiency, but the basal cortisol is usually in the normal range. A cortisol >580nmol/L precludes the diagnosis. At times of acute stress, an inappropriately low cortisol is very suggestive of the diagnosis.
- Simultaneous 9 a.m. cortisol and ACTH will show an elevated ACTH for the level of cortisol. This is a very sensitive means of detecting Addison's disease.
- NB drugs causing ↑ cortisol-binding globulin (e.g. oestrogens) will result in higher total cortisol concentration measurements.

Response to ACTH
Short Synacthen® test
- Following basal cortisol measurement, 250mcg Synacthen® is administered IM and serum cortisol checked at 30 and 60min.
- Serum cortisol should rise to a peak of 580nmol/L (note that this cutoff may depend on local assay conditions).
- Failure to respond suggests adrenal failure.
- A long Synacthen® test may be required to confirm 2° adrenal failure if ACTH is equivocal.
- Recent onset 2° adrenal failure (2 weeks) may produce a normal response to a short Synacthen® test.

Long Synacthen® test
- Following basal cortisol level, depot Synacthen® 1mg IM is administered, and serum cortisol measured at 30, 60, 120min, 4, 8, 12 and 24h. A normal response is an elevation in serum cortisol to >1000nmol/L.
- Differentiation of 2° from 1° adrenal failure can be made more reliably following 3 days IM ACTH 1mg. This is because the test relies on the ability of the atrophic adrenal glands to respond to ACTH in 2° adrenocortical failure, whereas in 1° adrenal failure the diseased gland is already maximally stimulated by elevated endogenous levels of ACTH and therefore unable to respond to further stimulation.
- Serum cortisol responses within the first 60min are superimposable with the short Synacthen® test.
- There is a progressive rise in cortisol secretion in 2° adrenal insufficiency, but little or no response on 1° adrenal insufficiency.

Increased plasma renin activity (assessment of mineralocorticoid sufficiency)
This is one of the earliest abnormalities in developing 1° adrenal insufficiency.

Thyroid function tests

Reduced thyroid hormone levels and elevated TSH may be due to a direct effect of glucocorticoid deficiency (cortisol inhibits TRH) or due to associated autoimmune hypothyroidism. Re-evaluation is therefore required after adrenal insufficiency has been rectified.

Establish cause of adrenal insufficiency

- *Adrenal autoantibodies* (detect antibodies to adrenal cortex, and more recently specific antibodies to 21-hydroxylase, side-chain-cleavage enzyme, and 17-hydroxylase). 21-hydroxylase antibodies are the major component of adrenal cortex antibodies and are present in 80% of recent onset autoimmune adrenalitis. Adrenal cortex antibodies (present in 80% patients of recent onset autoimmune adrenalitis) are not detectable in non-autoimmune 1° adrenal failure.
- *Imaging:*
  - Adrenal enlargement with or without calcification may be seen on CT of the abdomen, suggesting tuberculosis, infiltration or metastatic disease. The adrenals are small and atrophic in autoimmune adrenalitis.
  - Percutaneous CT guided adrenal biopsy is occasionally required.
- *Specific tests*—e.g. serological, or microbiological investigations directed at particular infections, very long chain fatty acids (adrenoleucodystrophy) in ♂ and ♀ with antibody –ve isolated 1° adrenal insufficiency.

Acute adrenal insufficiency

Clinical features

- Shock.
- Hypotension (often not responding to measures such as inotropic support).
- Abdominal pain (may present as 'acute abdomen').
- Unexplained fever.
- Often precipitated by major stress such as severe bacterial infection, major surgery, unabsorbed glucocorticoid medication due to vomiting.
- Occasionally occurs due to bilateral adrenal infarction.

Investigations

- As chronic.
- In the acute situation if the diagnosis is suspected, an inappropriately low cortisol (i.e. <600nmol/L) is often sufficient to make the diagnosis.

📖 See Box 48.1 for Emergency management.

Box 49.1 Emergency management of acute adrenal insufficiency

- This is a life-threatening emergency, and should be treated if there is strong clinical suspicion rather than waiting for confirmatory test results.
- Blood should be taken for urgent analysis of electrolytes and glucose, in addition to cortisol and ACTH.

Fluids

Large volumes of 0.9% saline may be required to reverse the volume depletion and sodium deficiency. Several litres may be required in the first 24–48h, but caution should be exercised where there has been chronic hyponatremia; in this circumstance rapid correction of the deficit exposes the patient to risk of central pontine myelinolysis. If plasma sodium is <120mmol/L at presentation, aim to correct by no more than 10mmol/L in the 1st 24h.

Hydrocortisone

- A bolus dose of 100mg hydrocortisone is administered intravenously. Hydrocortisone 100mg IM is then continued 6-hourly for 24–48h, or until the patient can take oral therapy. Double replacement dose hydrocortisone (20, 10, and 10mg orally) can then be instituted until well.
- This traditional regimen causes supraphysiological replacement and some authors suggest lower doses e.g. 150mg IV/24h.
- Specific mineralocorticoid replacement is not required as the high dose glucocorticoid has sufficient mineralocorticoid effects (40mg hydrocortisone ~ 100mcg fludrocortisone). Once the dose of glucocorticoid is reduced after a couple of days, and the patient is taking food and fluids by mouth, fludrocortisone 100mcg/day can be commenced.

Glucose supplementation

Occasionally required because of risk of hypoglycaemia (low glycogen stores in the liver as a result of glucocorticoid deficiency).

Investigate and treat precipitant

This is often infection.

Monitoring treatment

Electrolytes, glucose, and urea.

Treatment

Maintenance therapy

Glucocorticoid replacement

- Hydrocortisone is the treatment of choice for replacement therapy, as it is reliably and predictably absorbed and allows biochemical monitoring of levels.
- It is administered 3 × daily 10mg on waking, 5mg at midday, and 5mg at 6 p.m. Some patients can be managed adequately with twice daily administration of hydrocortisone.
- An alternative is prednisolone 3mg on waking and 1–2mg at 6 p.m. This has the disadvantage that levels cannot be biochemically monitored, but its longer t½ may lead to better suppression of ACTH if pigmentation and markedly elevated morning ACTH levels are a problem. Occasionally dexamethasone is required for this purpose.

Mineralocorticoid replacement

- Fludrocortisone (9-flurohydrocortisone) is given at a dose of 100mcg daily. Aim to avoid significant postural fall in BP (>10mmHg).
- Occasionally lower (0.05mg) or higher (0.2mg) doses are required.
- 40mg hydrocortisone has the equivalent mineralocortisone effects as 100mcg fludrocortisone.
- Renin activity can help guide adequacy of therapy.

DHEA replacement

- Dihydroepiandrosterone (DHEA) is also deficient in hypoadrenalism.
- DHEA replacement (25–50mg/day) may improve mood and well-being.
- DHEA is not available on prescription but is available from the USA as a dietary supplement.

Monitoring of therapy

Clinical

- For signs of glucocorticoid excess e.g ↑ weight.
- BP (including postural change).
- Hypertension and oedema suggest excessive mineralocorticoid replacement, whereas postural hypotension and salt craving suggest insufficient treatment.

Biochemical

- Serum electrolytes.
- Plasma renin activity (elevated if insufficient fludrocortisone replacement). Very dependant on when the last dose was taken.
- Cortisol day curve to assess adequacy of treatment (📖 see p.107).
- ACTH levels prior to and following morning glucocorticoids replacement if patient develops ↑ pigmentation. If elevated or rising with little suppression following glucocorticoid, MRI scan to exclude rare possibility of pituitary hyperplasia or very rarely the development of a corticotroph adenoma.

Intercurrent illness

- Cortisol requirements increase during severe illness or surgery.
- For moderate elective procedures or investigations, e.g. endoscopy or angiography, patients should receive a single dose of 100mg hydrocortisone before the procedure.
- For major surgery, patients should take 20mg hydrocortisone orally or 100mg intramuscularly with the premedication, and receive:
  - 50–100mg IM hydrocortisone 6-hourly for the first 3 days or
  - 100–150mg per 24h IV in 5% dextrose before reverting rapidly to a maintenance dose.
- To cover severe illness, e.g. pneumonia, patients should receive 50–100mg IM hydrocortisone 6-hourly until resolution of the illness.

Box 49.2 Pregnancy

📖 Also see Normal changes during pregnancy, p.433.
- During normal pregnancy:
  - Cortisol-binding globulin gradually increases.
  - Free cortisol increases in the 3rd trimester.
  - Progesterone increases exerting an antimineralocorticoid effect.
  - Renin levels increases.
- In Addison's disease therefore:
  - The usual glucocorticoid and mineralocorticoid replacement is continued initially.
  - Increase the hydrocortisone 50% in the 3rd trimester.
  - Adjust mineralocorticoids to BP and serum potassium (not renin).
- Severe hyperemesis gravidarum during the 1st trimester may require temporary parenteral therapy and patients should be warned about this to avoid precipitation of a crisis.
- During labour and for 24–48h.
  - Parenteral glucocorticoid therapy is administered (100mg IM every 6h).
  - Or hydrocortisone 100mg IV in 5% dextrose per 24h.
  - Fluid replacement with IV 0.9% saline may be required.

Drug interactions

- Rifampicin:
  - Increases the clearance of cortisol.
  - Double usual dose of hydrocortisone.
- Mitotane:
  - Increases cortisol binding globulin.
  - Double usual dose of hydrocortisone.

Education of the patient

- Patient education is the key to successful management. Patients must be taught never to miss a dose. They should be encouraged to wear a MedicAlert/SOS bracelet or necklace and always to carry a steroid card.
- Every patient should know how to double the dose of glucocorticoid during febrile illness, and to get medical attention if unable to take the tablets because of vomiting. They should have a vial of 100mg hydrocortisone with syringe, diluent, and needle for times when parenteral treatment may be required.

Further reading

Arlt W and Allolio B (2003). Adrenal insufficiency. *Lancet* **361**, 1881–93.

Hunt PJ, Gurnell EM, Huppert FA, *et al.* (2000). Improvement in mood and fatigue after dehydroepiandrosterone replacement in addison's disease in a randomized, double blind trial. *J Clin Endocrinol Metab* **85**(12), 4650–6.

Kong MF, Lawden M, Howlett T (2008). The Addison's disease dilemma—autoimmune or ALD? *Lancet* **371**, 1970.

Oelkers W (1996). Adrenal insufficiency. *New Engl J Med* **335**, 1206–12.

Long-term glucocorticoid administration

Both exogenous glucocorticoid administration and endogenous excess glucocorticoids (Cushing's syndrome) lead to a −ve feedback effect on the hypothalamo–pituitary axis (HPA), leading to suppression of both CRH and ACTH secretion and atrophy of the zonae fasiculata and reticularis of the adrenal cortex.

Short-term steroids

- Any patient who has received glucocorticoid treatment for <3 weeks is unlikely to have clinically significant adrenal suppression, and if the medical condition allows it, glucocorticoid treatment can be stopped acutely. A major stress within a week of stopping steroids should, however, be covered with glucocorticoids.
- Exceptions to this are patients who have other possible reasons for adrenocortical insufficiency, who have received more than 40mg prednisolone (or equivalent), where a short course has been prescribed within 1 year of cessation of long-term therapy, or evening doses (↑ HPA axis suppression).

Steroid cover

While receiving glucocorticoid treatment and within 1 year of steroid withdrawal, patients should receive standard steroid supplementation at times of stress, e.g. major trauma, surgery and infection (📖 p.261).

Box 50.1 Steroid equivalents

- 1mg Hydrocortisone.
- 1.25mg cortisone acetate.
- 0.25mg prednisolone.
- 37.5mcg dexamethasone.

4mg prednisolone ≡ 20mg hydrocortisone ≡ 75mcg dexamethasone.

Box 50.2 Dehydroepiandrosterone
- DHEA is an abundant circulating adrenal androgen, with a production rate of 25–50mg/day. Its levels undergo a progressive decline with ↑ age, and there has been interest in its physiological role.
- Epidemiological data suggest a link between changes in DHEA and age-related changes including an inverse relationship between DHEA and cardiovascular disease, Alzheimer disease, and malignancy.
- Although animal studies have suggested potential therapeutic benefit of DHEA therapy, small studies in humans have so far failed to demonstrate convincing benefit otherwise and apart from short-term improvement in well-being.
- Recent evidence suggests that DHEA replacement in patients with Addison's disease may have beneficial effects on well-being.

Long-term steroids

- When patients are receiving supraphysiological doses (>5.0mg prednisolone, or equivalent) of glucocorticoid, dose reduction depends on disease activity.
- Once a daily equivalent of 5.0mg prednisolone is reached, the rate of reduction should be slower to allow recovery of the HPA axis.
- If concerned about disease resolution, then the rate of reduction of glucocorticoids is determined by the disease process until 6.0mg equivalent is reached.
- If the disease has resolved, the dose can be rapidly reduced to 6.0mg prednisolone by a reduction of 2.5mg every 3–5 days.
- Once the patient is established on 6.0mg prednisolone, consider changing to hydrocortisone (20mg in the morning), as this has a shorter t½ and will therefore lead to less prolonged suppression of ACTH.
- Daily hydrocortisone dose should be reduced by 2.5mg every 1–2 weeks, or as tolerated until a dose of 10mg is reached. After 2–3 months a 9 a.m. cortisol is checked 24h after last dose of hydrocortisone. If it is >300nmol/L, then hydrocortisone can be stopped and a short Synacthen® test performed. If the 9 a.m. cortisol is <300nmol/L, then continue hydrocortisone 10mg for another 2–3 months and repeat the 9 a.m. cortisol. When basal cortisol is >400nmol/L, stop regular hydrocortisone and administer in emergency only. Once a short Synacthen® test demonstrates a normal response, it is helpful to perform an ITT to confirm full recovery of the HPA axis. Supplemental steroids during intercurrent illness are not required.

Cushing's syndrome

Patients with Cushing's syndrome on metyrapone or with recently treated disease, whatever the cause, may also have HPA axis suppression and may therefore need steroid replacement at times of stress.

Further reading

Baulieu E (1996). DHEA: A fountain of youth? *J Clin Endocrinol Metab* **81**, 3147–51.

Nippoldt TB and Nair KS (1998). Is there a case for DHEA replacement? *Ballière Clin Endocrinol Metab* **12**, 507–20.

Adrenal incidentalomas

Definition and epidemiology

- A true incidentaloma is an incidentally detected lesion with no pathophysiological significance, and needs to be differentiated from incidentally detected but clinically relevant masses.
- The incidental detection of an adrenal mass is becoming more common, as ↑ numbers of imaging procedures are performed, and with technological improvements in imaging.
- Autopsy studies suggest an incidence of adrenal adenomas of 1–6%.
- Imaging studies suggest an incidence of approximately 3.5%.

Importance

It is important to determine whether the incidentally discovered adrenal mass is:
- Malignant.
- Functioning and associated with excess hormonal secretion.

Differential diagnosis of an incidentally detected adrenal nodule

- Cortisol-secreting adrenal adenoma causing Cushing's syndrome or subclinical Cushing's syndrome (5.2%).
- Mineralocorticoid-secreting adrenal adenoma.
- Androgen-secreting adenoma.
- CAH.
- Adrenal carcinoma (12%).
- Metastasis (2%).
- Phaeochromocytoma (11%).
- Adrenal cysts (5%).
- Lipoma.
- Myelolipoma (8%).
- Haematoma.
- Ganglioneuroma (4%).

Investigations

- Clinical assessment for symptoms and signs of excess hormone secretion and signs of extra-adrenal carcinoma.
- Urinary free cortisol and overnight dexamethasone suppression test.
- Urinary free catecholamines/ metadrenalines.
- Plasma free metanephrines if available (☐ see p.274).
- Aldosterone/renin ratio if hypertensive or hypokalaemic.
- A homogeneous mass with a low attenuation value (<10 HU) on CT scan is likely to be a benign adenoma.
- Additional tests if adrenal carcinoma suspected:
  - 24h urinary excretion of corticosteroid metabolites.
  - DHEA, 17α OH progesterone.
  - 17α oestradiol (in ♂ only).
  - Testosterone, androstendione (in virilizing tumours).

Management

- Up to 20% of patients may develop hormonal excess during follow up.
- Unlikely if tumour <3cm.
- Cortisol is the commonest excess hormone.
- Surgery if there is/are:
  - Evidence of a syndrome of hormonal excess attributable to the tumour.
  - Biochemical evidence of Phaeochromocytoma.
  - Mass diameter >4cm (↑ likelihood of malignancy and definitely if >6cm in diameter).
  - Imaging features suggestive of malignancy (e.g. lack of clearly circumscribed margin, vascular invasion).
- Non-surgical management:
  - Repeat MRI at 6 and 12 months.
  - Repeat biochemical screening annually.
  - In patients with tumours that remain stable on 2 imaging studies carried out at least 6 months apart and do not exhibit hormonal hypersecretion over 4 years, further follow up may not be warranted.

Further reading

Chidiak RM and Aron DC (1997). Incidentalomas. Endocrinol Metab Clin N Am 26, 233–53.

Kloos RT, Gross MD, Francis IR, et al. (1995). Incidentally discovered adrenal masses. Endocr Rev 16, 460–84.

Mansmann G, Lau J, Balk E, et al. (2004). The clinically inapparent adrenal mass: update in diagnosis and management. Endocr Rev 25(2), 309–40.

Newell-Price J and Grossman A (1996). Adrenal incidentaloma. Postgrad Med J 72, 207–10.

Turner HE, Moore NR, Byrne JV, et al. (1998). Pituitary, adrenal and thyroid incidentalomas. Endocr Rel Cancer 5, 131–50.

Young WF Jr (2007). Clinical practice. The incidentally discovered adrenal mass. New England J Med 356(6), 601–10.

Phaeochromocytomas and paragangliomas

Definition

- *Phaeochromocytomas* are adrenomedullary catecholamine-secreting tumours.
- *Paragangliomas* are tumours arising from extra-adrenal medullary neural crest derivatives, e.g. organ of Zuckerkandl (sympathetic) or carotid body, aorticopulmonary, intravagal, or jugulotympanic (parasympathetic). They are usually in the head and neck and only 25% are secretory.
- *Glomus jugulare tumours*.

Incidence

Rare tumours, accounting for <0.1% of causes of hypertension. However, it is a very important diagnosis due to:

- The development of potentially fatal hypertensive crises.
- The reversibility of all its manifestations after surgical removal of the tumour.
- The lack of long-term efficacy of medical treatment.
- The appreciable incidence of malignancy.

Epidemiology

- Equal sex distribution, and most commonly present in the 3rd and 4th decades. Up to 50% may be diagnosed postmortem.
- Tumours may be bilateral, particularly where part of an inherited syndrome (Table 52.1).

Table 52.1 Syndromes associated with phaeochromocytomas

Familial phaeochromocytomas	Isolated autosomal dominant trait
MEN-IIa and b 📖 see p.622	Mutation in RET proto-oncogene (chromosome 10)
	Hyperparathyroidism and medullary thyroid carcinoma associated with phaeochromocytoma
	MEN IIb also associated with marfanoid phenotype 📖 see p.622
Von Hippel–Lindau syndrome 📖 see p.606	Mutation of VHL tumour suppressor gene (chromosome 3)
	Renal cell carcinoma, cerebellar haemangioblastoma, retinal angioma, renal and pancreatic cysts
	Phaeochromocytomas in 25%
Neurofibromatosis 📖 see p.604	Autosomal dominant condition caused by mutations of NF1 gene on chromosome 17
	Phaechromocytomas in 0.5–1.0%
Familial carotid body tumour	Dominantly inhyerited disorder characterized by vascular tumors in the head and the neck, most frequently at the carotid and bifurcation
	Succinate dehydrogenase gene (subunit D)
Familial paraganglionoma	Succinate dehydrogenase (subunits B,C,D)

Pathophysiology

Sporadic tumours are usually unilateral, and <10cm in diameter. Tumours associated with familial syndromes are more likely to be bilateral, and associated with pre-existing medullary hyperplasia.

Malignancy

- Approximately 15–20% are malignant and these are characterized by local invasion or distant metastasis rather than capsular invasion.
- Differentiating benign and malignant tumours is difficult and mainly based on presence of metastases although chromosomal ploidy may be useful.
- Paragangliomas are more likely to be malignant, and to recur.
- Typical sites for metastases are retroperitoneum, lymph nodes, bone, liver, and mediastinum.

Secretory products

- Catecholamine secretion is usually adrenaline or noradrenaline and may be constant or episodic.
- Phenylethanolamine-*N*-methyl transferase (PNMT) is necessary for methylation of noradrenaline to adrenaline, and is cortisol dependent.
- Paragangliomas (exception—organ of Zuckerkandl) secrete noradrenaline only, as they lack PNMT.
- Small adrenal tumours tend to produce more adrenaline, whereas larger adrenal tumours produce more noradrenaline as a proportion of their blood supply is direct rather than corticomedullary, and therefore lower in cortisol concentrations.
- Pure dopamine secretion is rare, and may be associated with hypotension. These tumours are more likely to be malignant.
- Other non-catecholamine secretory products may also be produced, including VIP, neuropeptide Y, ACTH (associated with Cushing's syndrome), PTH, and PTHrP.

Clinical features

- Sustained or episodic *hypertension* often resistant to conventional therapy.
- *General:*
  - Sweating and heat intolerance >80%.
  - Pallor or flushing.
  - Feeling of apprehension.
  - Pyrexia.
- *Neurological*—headache (throbbing or constant) (65%), paraesthesiae, visual disturbance, seizures.
- *Cardiovascular*—palpitations (65%), chest pain, dyspnoea, postural hypotension.
- *GI*—abdominal pain, constipation, nausea.

Complications

- *Cardiovascular*—left ventricular failure, dilated cardiomyopathy (reversible), dysrhythmias.
- *Respiratory*—pulmonary oedema.
- *Metabolic*—carbohydrate intolerance, hypercalcaemia.
- *Neurological*—cerebrovascular, hypertensive encephalopathy.

Box 52.1 Who should be screened for the presence of a phaeochromocytoma?

- Patients with a family history of MEN, VHL, neurofibromatosis, SDH gene mutations.
- Patients with paroxysmal symptoms.
- Young patients with hypertension.
- Patient developing hypertensive crisis during general anaesthesia/ surgery.
- Patients with unexplained heart failure.
- Patients with an adrenal incidentaloma

Factors precipitating a crisis

- Straining.
- Exercise.
- Pressure on abdomen—tumour palpation, bending over.
- Surgery.
- Drugs:
    - Anaesthetics.
    - Unopposed β-blockade.
    - IV contrast agents.
    - Opiates.
    - Tricyclic antidepressants.
    - Phenothiazines.
    - Metoclopramide.
    - Glucagon.

Investigations

Demonstrate catecholamine hypersecretion

24h urine collection is the standard test for screening for a phaeochromocytoma. In a patient with suggestive symptoms this is usually sufficient to confirm or exclude the diagnosis. False –ves are more common when patients are asymptomatic and early in the disease. Particular care is needed in familial cases, incidentalomas and in those in whom a general anaesthetic has precipitated a hypertensive episode. Metadrenalines (either urine or plasma) offer more specific diagnostic tools than measurement of unmetabolized catecholamines and provide the best biochemical tests for diagnosing phaeochromocytoma.

24h urine collection for catecholamines/metadrenalines (see Table 52.2)

- Urine is collected into bottles containing acid (warn patient).
- Because of the episodic nature of catecholamine secretion, at least 2 × 24h collections should be performed. It is useful to perform a collection while a patient is having symptoms, if episodic secretion is suspected.
- The sensitivity of urinary VMAs is less than free catecholamines or metadrenalines, and also influenced by dietary intake and should not be used.
- NB tricyclic antidepressants and labetalol interfere with adrenaline measurements and should be stopped for 4 days.

Plasma catecholamine measurement

- Intermittent secretion, and the short t½ of catecholamines, makes this test of limited use in screening.
- Plasma metadrenalines may be more useful as their t½ is longer and offer high specificity.
- Normal levels drawn during an episode are strongly against the diagnosis.
- Routine measurement requires controlled conditions—supine and cannulated for 30min, 10mL blood drawn into a lithium heparin tube and cold spun.
- Plasma catecholamines are elevated by renal failure, caffeine, nicotine, exercise, and some drugs.
- Plasma catecholamines 3 × the upper limit of normal are suspicious of a phaeochromocytoma in symptomatic individuals.
- Catecholamine levels in asymptomatic individuals investigated for an adrenal incidentaloma or due to a familial condition are often diagnosed at an earlier stage and may therefore have lower catecholamines.

Suppression tests (see Box 52.3, p.275)

These tests may be used to differentiate patients who have borderline catecholamine levels, but may offer little advantage over the screening tests already described.

- Pentolinium 2.5mg IV—elevated plasma catecholamines at 10min are seen in phaeochromocytomas, whereas the normal response is suppression into the normal range.

- *Clonidine 300mcg orally*—failure of suppression of plasma
  catecholamines into the normal range at 120 and 180min is suggestive
  of a tumour.

Provocative tests

These are not used routinely as they do not enhance diagnostic accuracy
and are potentially dangerous.

Table 52.2 Substances interfering with urinary catecholamine levels

Increased catecholamines	Decreased catecholamines	Variable effect
α-Blockers	Mono-amine oxidase inhibitors	Levodopa
β-Blockers	Clonidine	Tricyclic antidepressants
Levodopa	Guanethidine and other adrenergic neurone blockers	Phenothiazines
Drugs containing catecholamines, e.g. decongestants		Calcium channel inhibitors
Metoclopramide		ACE inhibitors
Domperidone		Bromocriptine
Hydralazine		
Diazoxide		
Glyceryltrinitrate		
Sodium nitroprusside		
Nicotine		
Theophylline		
Caffeine		
Amphetamine		

Table 52.3 Sensitivity and specificity of tests

Test	Sensitivity	Specificity
2 × 24 h urinary free catecholamines	100%	95%
Urinary metanephrines	80%	86%
Urinary VMA	65%	88%
Clonidine suppression test	97%	
MRI	98%	70%
CT	93%	70%
MIBG	80%	95%

Localization of tumour

Imaging

- These are large tumours, in contrast to Conn's syndrome, and not easily missed with good quality imaging to the bifurcation of the aorta. Approximately 98% will be detected in the abdomen.
- <2% are in the chest and 0.02% are in the head.
- Adrenal imaging with non-ionic contrast should be performed initially, then body imaging (ideally MRI) if tumour not localized in adrenal.
- *MRI* bright hyperintense image on T2.
- *CT* less sensitive and specific—less good at distinguishing between different types of adrenal tumours.

^{123}I-MIBG scan (📖 see Box 52.2, p.278)

- *Meta*-Iodobenzylguanidine is a chromaffin-seeking analogue. Imaging using MIBG is +ve in 60–80% phaeochromocytomas, and may locate tumours not visualized on MRI e.g. multiple and extra-adrenal tumours.
- Specificity is nearly 100%.
- Performed preoperatively to exclude multiple tumours.
- NB phenoxybenzamine may lead to false –ve MIBG imaging, so these scans should be preformed before commencing this drug.
- 18F fluorodopamine PET scanning is superior to MBG in localizing metastatic disease. No K^+ iodide is necessary to block thyroid uptake.

Positron emission tomography

- [18F]fluorodeoxyglucose (FDG) and the norepinephrine analogue [11C]metahydroxyephedrine (mHED) have both been used as radionucleotides.
- Current data are insufficient to determine which radionucleotide has the greatest sensitivity and specificity.
- Sensitivity is better than MIBG and approaches 100% but specificity is worse with false +ves being reported.

Venous sampling

- Used to localize a phaeochromocytoma/paraganglioma if imaging is unhelpful.
- Caution: α- and β-blockade should be administered before the procedure.
- Reversal of the ratio of noradrenaline:adrenaline ratio (N <1) in the adrenal vein is suggestive of a phaeochromocytoma.

Screening for associated conditions

Up to 24% of patients with apparently sporadic phaeochromocytomas may have a familial disorder and high-risk patients should therefore be screened for the presence of associated conditions, even if asymptomatic. Screening can either be performed by looking for associated clinical manifestations or by genetic testing.

Genetic testing in nonsyndromic phaeochromocytoma has shown a hereditary predisposition in 24% of which 45% had germ-line mutations in VHL, 20% had mutations in RET, 18% mutations in SDHD, and 17% mutations in SDHB.

MEN (p.622)
- Serum calcium.
- Serum calcitonin (phaeochromocytomas precede medullary thyroid carcinoma in 10%).

VHL (p.606)
- Opthalmoscopy—retinal angiomas are usually the 1st manifestation.
- MRI posterior fossa and spinal cord.
- US of kidneys—if not adequately imaged on MRI of adrenals.

NF1 (☐ see p.604)
Clinical examination for café au Lait spots and cutaneous neuromas.

Succinate dehydrogenase (subunits B, C, D)

- Reports of renal carcinomas: ensure adequate imaging of kidneys.
- The SDH enzyme consists of 4 subunits (A, B, C and D). SHDC and SDHD anchor the 2 other components which form the catalytic core, to the inner-mitochondrial membrane. The enzyme is a component of Kreb's cycle, and also regulates the downregulation of the transcription factor HIF1α.
- The succinate dehydrogenase D subunit gene is located at chromosome 11q21–23 and the B subunit on chromosome 1p35–6.
- Mutations in SDHB, SDHC, and SDHD may cause hereditary paraganglioma and glomus tumours.
- Mutations in SDHD have been associated with familial carotid body tumours.
- Germline SDHA mutations are associated with juvenile encephalopathy.
- SHD mutations show maternal imprinting so that only carriers who inherit the mutation paternally are at risk of developing a tumour.
- Rates of penetrance and malignancy vary: SDHB mutation may be associated with a more malignant phenotype.

Indications for screening for genetic conditions as a cause for a phaeochromocytoma

- Bilateral tumours
- Extra-adrenal tumour including head and neck
- Age of onset (< 50 years 45% +ve, > 40 years 7% +ve, > 50 years 1% +ve)
- Malignancy.

Box 52.2 Drugs interfering with MIBG uptake in phaeochromocytoma*

- Opioids.
- Cocaine.
- Tramadol.
- Tricyclic antidepressants:
  - Amitriptyline.
  - Imipramine.
- Sympathomimetics:
  - Phenylpropanolamine, pseudoephedrine, amphetamine, dopamine, salbutamol.
- Antihypertensives/cardiovascular agents:
  - Labetalol, metoprolol, amiodarone, reserpine, guanethidine, calcium channel blockers nifedipine and amlodipine, ACE inhibitors captopril and enalapril.

*should be discontinued 7–14 days prior to scan.

Box 52.3 Test procedures

Clonidine suppression test
- Patient supine and cannulated for 30min.
- Clonidine 300 mcg orally.
- Plasma catecholamines measured at time 0, 120, and 180min.
- Failure to suppress into the normal range is suggestive of a tumour.
- 1.5% false +ve rate in patients with essential hypertension.

Management

Medical

- It is essential that any patient is fully prepared with α- and β-blockade before receiving IV contrast, or undergoing a procedure such as venous sampling, or surgery.
- α-blockade must be commenced before β-blockade to avoid precipitating a hypertensive crisis due to unopposed α-adrenergic stimulation.
- *α-blockade*—commence phenoxybenzamine, as soon as diagnosis made. Start at 10mg 2 × day by mouth, and increase up to 20mg 4 × day.
- *β-blockade*—use a beta-blocker such as propranolol 20-80mg 8-hourly by mouth 48–72h after starting phenoxybenzamine and with evidence of adequate α-blockade blockade (generally noted by a postural fall in BP).
- Treatment is commenced in hospital. Monitor BP, pulse, and haematocrit. The goal is a BP of 130/80 or less sitting and 100mg systolic standing, pulse 60–70 sitting and 70–80 standing. Reversal of α-mediated vasoconstriction may lead to haemodilution (check Hb preoperatively).
- To ensure complete blockade before surgery, IV *phenoxybenzamine* (1mg/kg over 4h in 100mL 5% dextrose) is administered on the 3 days before surgery. There is less experience with competetive α-adrenergic blockade such as prazosin.

Surgical

- Surgical resection is curative in the majority of patients, leading to normotension in at least 75%.
- Mortality from elective surgery is <2%. It is essential that the anaesthetic and surgical teams have expertise of management of phaechromocytomas perioperatively.
- Surgery may be laparoscopic if the tumour is small and apparently benign. Careful perioperative anaesthetic management is essential as tumour handling may lead to major changes in BP and also occasionally cardiac arrythmias. *Phentolamine, nitroprusside or IV nicardipine* are useful to treat perioperative hypertension, and e*smolol or propranolol* for perioperative arrythmias. Hypotension (e.g. after tumour devascularization) usually responds to volume replacement, but occasionally requires inotropic support.

Follow-up

- Cure is assessed by 24h urine free catecholamine measurement, but since catecholamines may remain elevated for up to 10 days following surgery, these should not be performed until 2 weeks postoperatively.
- Lifelong follow-up is essential to detect recurrence of a benign tumour, or metastasis from a malignant tumour, as it is impossible to exclude malignancy on a histological specimen.
- Chromogranin A is also a useful marker (falsely elevated with proton pump therapy, steroids, and renal failure).

Malignancy

- Malignant tumours require long-term α- and β-blockade. The tyrosine kinase inhibitor α-*methylparatyrosine* may help control symptoms.
- High dose ^{131}I MIBG can be used to treat metastatic disease.
- Chemotherapy using *cyclophosphamide*, *vincristine*, *adriamycin*, and *dacarbazine* has been associated with symptomatic improvement.
- Radiotherapy can be useful palliation in patients with bony metastases.

Prognosis

- Hypertension may persist in 25% patients who have undergone successful tumour removal.
- 5-year survival for 'benign' tumours is 96%, and the recurrence rate is <10%.
- 5-year survival for malignant tumours is 44%.
- SHB gene mutation patients are associated with a shorter survival.

Further reading

Astuti D, Latif F, Dallol A, et al. (2001). Gene mutations in the succinate dehydrogenase subunit SDHB cause susceptibility to familial pheochromocytoma and to familial paraganglioma. *A J Hum Genet* **69**, 49–54.

Erickson D, Kudva YC, Ebersold MJ, et al. (2001). Benign paragangliomas: clinical presentation and treatment outcomes in 236 patients. *J Clin Endocrinol Metab* **86**(11), 5210–16.

Gimm O, Armanios M, Dziema H, et al. (2000). Somatic and occult germ-line mutations in SDHD, a mitochondrial complex II gene, in nonfamilial pheochromocytoma. *Cancer Res* **60**(24), 6822–5.

Ilias I, Yu J, Carrasquillo JA, et al. (2003). Superiority of 6-[18F]-fluorodopamine positron emission tomography versus [131I]-metaiodobenzylguanidine scintigraphy in the localization of metastatic pheochromocytoma. *J Clin Endocrinol Metab* **88**(9), 4083–7.

Kudva YC, Sawka AM, Young WF Jr. (2003). The laboratory diagnosis of adrenal pheochromocytoma: the Mayo Clinic experience. *J Clin Endocrinol Metab* **88**(10), 4533–9.

Neumann HP, Bausch B, McWhinney SR, et al. (2002). Germ-line mutations in nonsyndromic pheochromocytoma. *New Engl J Med* **346**(19), 1459–66.

Reproductive endocrinology

Hirsutism

Definition

Hirsutism (not a diagnosis in itself) is the presence of excess hair growth in ♀ as a result of ↑ androgen production and ↑ skin sensitivity to androgens. 📖 See Table 53.1 for causes.

Physiology of hair growth

Before puberty the body is covered by fine unpigmented hairs, or vellus hairs. During adolescence, androgens convert vellus hairs into coarse, pigmented terminal hairs in androgen-dependent areas. The extent of terminal hair growth depends on the concentration and duration of androgen exposure as well as on the sensitivity of the individual hair follicle. The reason different body regions respond differently to the same androgen concentration is unknown but may be related to the number of androgen receptors in the hair follicle. Genetic factors play an important role in the individual susceptibility to circulating androgens, as evidenced by racial differences in hair growth.

Androgen production in women

In ♀, testosterone is secreted primarily by the ovaries and adrenal glands although a significant amount is produced by the peripheral conversion of androstenedione and DHEA. Ovarian androgen production is regulated by lutenizing hormone, whereas adrenal production is ACTH dependent. The predominant androgens produced by the ovaries are testosterone and androstenedione, and the adrenal glands are the main source of DHEA. Circulating testosterone is mainly bound to sex hormone binding globulin (SHBG) and it is the free testosterone which is biologically active. Testosterone is converted to dihydrotestosterone in the skin by the enzyme 5α-reductase. Androstenedione and DHEA are not significantly protein-bound. 📖 See Fig. 53.1.

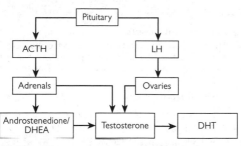

Fig. 53.1 Regulation of androgen production in ♀.

Box 53.1 Signs of virilization

- Frontal balding.
- Deepening of voice.
- ↑muscle size.
- Clitoromegaly.

Table 53.1 Causes of hirsutism

Ovarian	PCOS	95%
	Androgen-secreting tumours	<1%
Adrenal	Congenital adrenal hyperplasia	1%
	Cushing's syndrome	<1%
	Androgen-secreting tumours	<1%
	Acromegaly	<1%
	Severe insulin resistance	<1%

Evaluation

Androgen-dependent hirsutism

Normally develops following puberty. Hairs are coarse and pigmented and typically grow in ♂ pattern. It is often accompanied by other evidence of androgen excess such as acne, oily skin and hair, and ♂-pattern alopecia.

Box 53.2 Androgen-independent hair growth

Excess vellus hairs over face and trunk including forehead. It does not respond to anti-androgen treatment.

Causes of androgen-independent hair growth
- Drugs, e.g. phenytoin, ciclosporin, glucocorticoids.
- Anorexia nervosa.
- Hypothyroidism.
- Familial

History

- *Age and rate of onset of hirsutism* Slowly progressive hirsutism following puberty suggests a benign cause, whereas rapidly progressive hirsutism of recent onset requires further immediate investigation to rule out an androgen-secreting neoplasm.
- *Menstrual history* ?oligomenorrhoeic.
- Presence of other evidence of *hyperandrogenism*, e.g. acne or bitemporal hair recession.
- *Drug history* Some progestins used in oral contraceptive preparations may be androgenic (e.g. norethisterone).

Physical examination

- Distinguish beween *androgen-dependent* and *androgen-independent* hair growth.
- Assess the *extent* and *severity* of hirsutism. The Ferriman–Gallwey score (🕮 see Table 53.2) assesses the degree of hair growth in 11 regions of the body. This provides a semi-objective method of monitoring disease progression and treatment outcome.
- *Virilization* should be looked for, as this indicates severe hyperandrogenism and should be further investigated (Box 53.1 p. 285).
- *Acanthosis nigricans* is indicative of insulin resistance and probable PCOS.
- *Rare causes* of hyperandrogenism such as Cushing's syndrome and acromegaly should be ruled out.

Laboratory investigation

Serum testosterone should be measured in all ♀ presenting with hirsutism. If this is <5 nmol/L then the risk of a sinister cause for her hirsutism is low. Further investigations and management of the individual disorders will be discussed in the following chapters.

Further reading

Martin KA, Chang JR, Ehrmann DA, *et al* (2008). Evaluation and treatment of Hirsutism in pre-menopausal woman: an endocrine society clinical practice guideline. *JCEM* **93**, 1105–20.

Table 53.2 Assessment of hirsuitism—the Ferriman–Gallway score[1]

Site	Grade	Definition
Upper lip	1	A few hairs at outer margin
	2	A small moustache at outer margin
	3	A moustache extending halfway from outer margin
	4	A moustache extending to midline
Chin	1	A few scattered hairs
	2	Scattered hairs with small concentrations
	3	Complete cover, light
	4	Complete cover, heavy
Chest	1	Circumareolar hairs
	2	With midline hair
	3	Fusion of these areas
	4	Complete cover
Upper back	1	A few scattered hairs
	2	More, but still scattered
	3	Complete cover, light
	4	Complete cover, heavy
Lower back	1	Sacral tuft of hair
	2	Some lateral extension
	3	Three-quarter cover
	4	Complete cover
Upper abdomen	1	A few midline hairs
	2	Rather more, still midline
	3	Half cover
	4	Full cover
Lower abdomen	1	A few midline hairs
	2	A midline streak of hair
	3	A midline band of hair
	4	An inverted V-shaped growth
Arm	1	Sparse growth affecting not more than a quarter of the limb surface
	2	More than this, cover still incomplete
	3	Complete cover, light
	4	Complete cover, heavy
Forearm	1,2,3,4	Complete cover of dorsal surface, 2 grades of light and 2 grades of heavy growth
Thigh	1,2,3,4	As for arm
Leg	1,2,3,4	As for arm
Total score		

[1] Reproduced with permission from Ferriman-Gallwey (1961). Clinical assessment of body hair growth in women. *J Clin Endocrinol and Metab* **21**(11), 1440–7.

Polycystic ovary syndrome (PCOS)

Definition

- A heterogeneous genetic clinical syndrome characterized by hyperandrogenism (both ovarian and adrenal), ovulatory dysfunction, and hyperinsulinaemia in which other causes of androgen excess have been excluded (see Box 53.3).
- The diagnosis is further supported by the presence of characteristic ovarian morphology on US.

> **Box 53.3 2003 Joint European Society of Human Reproduction and Embryology and American Society of Reproductive Medicine Consensus on the diagnosis criteria for PCOS (Rotterdam criteria)**
>
> At least 2 out of 3 of the following:
> - Oligo/amenorrhoea.
> - Hyperandrogenism (clinical or biochemical).
> - Polycystic ovaries on US.
>   and exclusion of other disorders.

Epidemiology

- PCOS is the most common endocrinopathy in ♀ of reproductive age. 95% of ♀ presenting to outpatients with hirsutism have PCOS.
- The estimated prevalence of PCOS ranges from 5–10% on clinical criteria. Polycystic ovaries on US alone are present in 20–25% of ♀ of reproductive age.

Secondary causes of PCOS

- Congenital adrenal hyperplasia.
- Acromegaly.
- Cushing's syndrome.
- Testosterone secreting tumours.

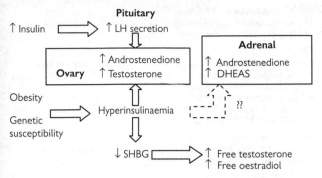

Fig. 54.1 Abnormalities of hormone secretion in PCOS.

Pathogenesis (Box 54.1 p. 289)

The fundamental pathophysiological defect is unknown but both genetic and environmental factors are thought to play a role.

Genetic

- Familial aggregation of PCOS in 50% of ♀. A family history of type 2 diabetes mellitus is also more common in ♀ with PCOS.
- PCOS is probably an oligogenic or polygenic disorder.
- Insulin synthesis genes, steroid enzyme biosynthesis genes and genes involved in reproduction and metabolism are likely candidates, e.g. *INS*, *VNTR*, and *CYP11* genes; also FTO gene.

Hyperandrogenism

- The main source of hyperandrogenaemia is the ovaries although there may also be adrenal androgen hypersecretion in approximately 25% of ♀.
- The biochemical basis of ovarian dysfunction is unclear. Studies suggest an abnormality of cytochrome P-450c17 α activity but this is unlikely to be the 1° event but rather an index of ↑ steroidogenesis by ovarian theca cells.
- There is also an increase in the frequency and amplitude of GnRH pulses, resulting in the increase in LH concentration which is characteristic of the syndrome. This is probably 2° to anovulation and low progesterone levels.

Hyperinsulinaemia

- Approximately 70% of ♀ with PCOS are insulin resistant. The defect in insulin sensitivity appears to be selective, mainly affecting the metabolic effects of insulin (effects on muscle and liver) rather than its mitogenic actions (e.g. effects on ovaries). Hyperinsulinaemia is further exacerbated by obesity but can also be present in lean ♀ with PCOS.
- There is also evidence in a number of ♀ with PCOS of insufficient β-cell response to a glucose challenge, which is known to be a precursor to type 2 diabetes mellitus.
- Insulin and IGF-1 receptors are found in abundance in the ovarian stroma and it has been shown that insulin, in the presence of LH, stimulates ovarian production of androgens. This is exaggerated in PCOS.
- Insulin also inhibits SHBG synthesis by the liver with a consequent rise in free androgen levels.

Features

- *Onset of symptoms* Symptoms often begin around puberty, after weight gain, or after stopping the oral contraceptive pill but can present at any time.
- *Oligo/amenorrhoea* (70%) Due to anovulation. These ♀ are usually well-oestrogenized so there is little risk of osteoporosis, unlike other causes of amenorrhoea.
- *Hirsutism* (66%):
  - 25% of ♀ also suffer from acne or ♂-pattern alopecia. Virilization is not a feature of PCOS.
  - There is often a family history of hirsutism or irregular periods. Hirsutism 2° to adrenal or ovarian tumours is usually rapidly progressive, associated with virilization and higher testosterone concentrations.
  - 1% of hirsute ♀ have non-classical congenital adrenal hyperplasia (📖 see Classic presentation, p.308) and this should be excluded particularly in ♀ with significantly raised serum testosterone levels.
- *Obesity* (50%) Symptoms worsen with obesity as it is accompanied by ↑ testosterone concentrations as a result of the associated hyperinsulinaemia. Acanthosis nigricans may be found in 1–3% of insulin resistant ♀ with PCOS.
- *Infertility* (30%) PCOS accounts for 75% of cases of anovulatory infertility. The risk of spontaneous miscarriage is also thought to be higher than the general population

Rule out an androgen-secreting tumour

If there is:
- Evidence of virilization.
- Testosterone >5nmol/L (or >3nmol/L in postmenopausal ♀).
- Rapidly progressive hirsutism.
- *MRI of adrenals and ovaries* will detect adrenal or ovarian tumours >1cm.
- *Selective venous sampling*:
  - Occasionally necessary to locate virilizing tumours undetected by imaging.
  - Blood samples are taken from both adrenal and ovarian veins and from the peripheral circulation.
  - A virilizing tumour is likely if an androgen concentration gradient is detected.

Risks associated with PCOS

Type 2 diabetes mellitus

Type 2 diabetes mellitus is 2–4 × more common in ♀ with PCOS. Impaired glucose tolerance affects 10–30% of ♀ with PCOS and gestational diabetes is also more prevalent. The prevalence of diabetes mellitus is ↑ in ♀ with PCOS independent of weight but is highest in the obese group.

Dyslipidaemia
Several studies have shown an ↑ risk of hypercholesterolaemia, hyper triglyceridaemia and low HDL cholesterol in ♀ with PCOS.

Cardiovascular disease
There is evidence that atherosclerosis develops earlier in ♀ with PCOS. For example ♀ with PCOS have been found to be twice as likely to have coronary artery atherosclerosis compared with controls. However, in epidemiological studies ♀ with PCOS have not been found to have an ↑ mortality from ischaemic heart disease despite their multiple cardiovascular risk factors.

Endometrial hyperplasia and carcinoma
In anovulatory ♀ endometrial stimulation by unopposed oestrogen results in endometrial hyperplasia. Several studies have also shown that this results in a 2–4-fold excess risk of endometrial carcinoma in ♀ with PCOS. However, large epidemiological studies are required to confirm this excess risk.

Investigations

The aims of investigations are 3-fold: to confirm the diagnosis, to exclude serious underlying disorders, and to screen for complications (📖 see Box 53.3).

Confirmation of diagnosis

- *Testosterone concentration:*
  - Performed primarily as a screen for the presence of other causes of hyperandrogenism.
  - ♀ with PCOS may have normal serum testosterone levels and serum androgen concentrations do not necessarily reflect the degree of hirsutism.
- *LH concentration:*
  - Raised in 50–70% of anovulatory patients with reversal of the FSH/LH ratio.
  - The higher the LH level the more likely the risk of anovulation and infertility.
  - Cannot be used alone to diagnose PCOS since it is normal in up to half of affected ♀.
- *SHBG:*
  - Low in 50% of ♀ with PCOS owing to the hyperinsulinaemic state, with a consequent increase in circulating free androgens.
  - Useful indirect marker of insulin resistance.
- Free androgen index:

$$FAI = 100 \times \frac{(total\ testosterone)}{SHBG}$$

- *Pelvic US of ovaries and endometrium:*
  - 91% sensitivity in experienced hands, with transvaginal ultrasound giving the highest yield.
  - Ultrasonic diagnosis of PCOS is made by the presence of >12 follicular cysts between 2–9mm in diameter or ovarian volume >10cm^3.
  - Measurement of endometrial thickness is also useful in the diagnosis of endometrial hyperplasia in the presence of anovulation. Endometrial hyperplasia is diagnosed if the endometrial thickness is >10mm.
  - Transvaginal US will also identify 90% of ovarian virilizing tumours.

Exclusion of serious underlying disease

- *Serum prolactin* In the presence of infertility or oligomenorrhoea.
  - Mild hyperprolactinaemia (up to 2000mU/L) is present in up to 30% of ♀ with PCOS, and dopamine agonist treatment of this may be necessary if pregnancy is desired.
- *17 OH (17OHP) progesterone level:*
  - Used to exclude late onset congenital adrenal hyperplasia.
  - Indicated in those with testosterone concentrations in excess of 5nmol/L or with evidence of virilization.
  - May also perform a Synacthen test looking for an exaggerated rise in 17OHP in response to ACTH in the presence of non-classic 21-hydroxylase deficiency (📖 see Clinical presentation, p.306).

- If the patient is ovulating then all 17OHP measurements should be performed during the follicular phase of the cycle to avoid false +ves.
- *DHEAS and androstenedione concentrations:*
  - Both can be moderately raised in PCOS. DHEAS is a useful adrenal marker of hyperandrogenism. In cases of suspected tumours, levels are usually in excess of 20micromol/L.
  - Do not need to measure routinely in ♀ with PCOS but indicated if serum testosterone >5mmol/L, in the presence of rapidly progressive hirsutism or in the presence of virilization
- *Other:*
  - Depending on clinical suspicion, e.g i) urinary free cortisol or over-night dexamethasone suppression test if Cushing's syndrome is suspected or ii) IGF-1 if acromegaly suspected, but not routinely.

Screening for complications

- *Serum lipids and blood glucose* All obese ♀ with PCOS should have an annual fasting glucose and fasting lipid profile.
- All ♀ with PCOS who fall pregnant should be screened for gestational diabetes.

Management

(📖 see Table 54.1)

Weight loss

Studies have uniformly shown that weight reduction in obese ♀ with PCOS will improve insulin sensitivity and significantly reduce hyperandrogenaemia. Obese ♀ are less likely to respond to antiandrogens and infertility treatment. With a loss of 5% of their starting weight, ♀ with PCOS show improvement in hirsutism, restoration of menstrual regularity, and fertility.

Metformin

In obese and lean insulin resistant ♀ with PCOS, metformin (1g, 2 × daily) improves insulin sensitivity with a corresponding reduction in serum androgen and LH concentrations and an increase in SHBG levels. Metformin may regulate menstruation by improving ovulatory function and thus inducing fertility. Frequency of menstruation may be improved within 3 months of starting therapy. Metformin does not seem to improve response rates to ovulation induction using clomifene or gonadotropins. Experience of metformin in pregnancy is limited so it should be discontinued once pregnancy has been confirmed until further data accrue. However, it does not appear to be teratogenic.

The effects of metformin seem to be independent of weight reduction, although the benefits are greatest when weight reduction occurs in obese ♀. The effect of metformin on weight loss remains unclear. There have been few long-term studies looking at the effect of metformin on hirsutism but it appears that its effects are modest at best and most ♀ with significant hirsutism will require an antiandrogen.

♀ should be warned of its gastrointestinal side-effects. In order to minimize these, they should be started on a low dose (500mg once daily) which may be ↑ gradually to a therapeutic dose over a number of weeks.

Other insulin sensitizers

Troglitazone is a thiazolidinedione, another insulin sensitizer which has shown encouraging effects on menstruation and hyperinsulinaemia in ♀ with PCOS. However, it has been withdrawn from both the UK and USA markets because of liver toxicity. Other thiazolidinediones may in the future be used in the treatment of PCOS but there is insufficient evidence for their current use in PCOS. Furthermore, the thiazolidinediones are associated with unwelcome weight gain and are potentially teratogenic. Their use, therefore, in ♀ seeking fertility is not recommended.

Hirsutism

Pharmacological treatment of hirsutism (Table 54.1) is directed at slowing the growth of new hair but has little impact on established hair. It should be combined with mechanical methods of hair removal such as electrolysis and laser therapy. Therapy is most effective when started early. There is slow improvement over the first 6–12 months of treatment. Patients should be warned that facial hair is slow to respond, treatment is prolonged, and symptoms may recur after discontinuation of drugs. Adequate contraception is mandatory during pharmacological treatment of hirsutism because of possible teratogenicity.

Table 54.1 Pharmacological treatment of hirsutism

Ovarian androgen suppression	Combined oral contraceptive pill, including Dianette® (co-cyprindiol) (low dose cyproterone and ethinylestradiol)
	GnRH analogues
Adrenal androgen suppression	Corticosteroids
Androgen receptor antagonists	Spironolactone
	Cyproterone acetate
	Flutamide
5α-reductase inhibitor	Finasteride
Insulin sensitisers	Metformin
Topical inhibitors of hair follicle growth	Eflornithine

Ovarian androgen suppression
Combined oral contraceptive pill (COCP)
- The oestrogen component increases SHBG levels and thus reduces free androgen concentrations; the progestogen component inhibits LH secretion and thus ovarian androgen production.
- Dianette® (co-cyprindiol), which contains cyproterone acetate (2mg), is preferred. If not tolerated then use COCP containing a progestagen with low androgenic activity e.g. drospirenone (Yasmin®) or norgestimate (Cilest®).
- The effect of the COCP alone on hair growth is modest at best, so it may be combined with an antiandrogen.

GnRH analogues
- Suppress gonadotrophin secretion and thus ovarian androgen production.
- Rarely used. They cause oestrogen deficiency so have to be combined with 'add-back' oestrogen treatment. Also, they are expensive and need to be given parenterally.
- Use is confined to ♀ with severe hyperandrogenism in whom antiandrogens have been ineffective or not tolerated.

Androgen receptor blockers
These are most effective when combined with oral contraceptives. All are contraindicated in pregnancy. They act by competitively inhibiting the binding of testosterone and dihydrotestosterone to the androgen receptor.

Spironolactone
- Antiandrogen of choice particularly in overweight ♀.
- *Dose* 100–200mg a day.
- *Side effects* polymenorrhoea if not combined with the COCP. A fifth of ♀ complain of GI symptoms when on high doses of spironolactone. Potassium levels should be monitored and other potassium-sparing drugs should be avoided.

Cyproterone acetate (CPA)

- A progestagen which also increases *hepatic androgen clearance*.
- *Dose* 25–100mg days 1–10 of the pill cycle in combination with the COCP.
- *Side effects* Amenorrhoea if given alone for prolonged periods or in higher doses. *Progesterone side effects*. Hepatic toxicity rare, but monitoring of liver function 6 monthly is recommended.
- A *washout period* of 3–4 months is recommended prior to attempting conception.

Flutamide

- A potent antiandrogen.
- *Dose* 125–250 mg a day.
- *Side-effects* Dry skin, nausea in 10%. However, there is a 0.4% risk of hepatic toxicity and it should therefore be used with extreme caution.

5α-reductase inhibitors

Block the conversion of testosterone to the more potent androgen, dihydrotestosterone.

- *Finasteride:*
  - *Dose* 2.5–5mg a day. A weak antiandrogen.
  - *Side-effects* No significant adverse effects.
  - Can be used as monotherapy however adequate contraceptive measures are mandatory because of its teratogenicity. In addition, pregnancy should not be attempted until at least 3 months after drug cessation.

Eflornithine 11.5%

- Irreversibly blocks the enzyme ornithine decarboxylase which is involved in growth of hair follicles.
- It is administered as a topical cream on the face and its long-term use reduces new hair growth. Studies have shown its efficacy in the management of mild facial hirsutism following at least 8 weeks of treatment. Treatment should be discontinued if there is no benefit at 4 months. It is not a depilatory cream and so must be combined with mechanical methods of hair removal.
- *Side effects* Skin irritation with burning or pruritus, acne, hypersensitivity.

Amenorrhoea

- A minimum of a withdrawal bleed every 3 months minimizes the risk of endometrial hyperplasia.
- *Treatment:*
  - COCP.
  - Desogestrel is a relatively new progesterone only contraceptive pill with minimal androgenic properties. It may be used to minimize endometrial hyperplasia in amenorrhoeic ♀ with PCOS.
  - Metformin (up to 1g BD)
  - *Alternatives* A progestogen may be added for the latter half of the cycle. However, there is the risk of exacerbating hirsutism. Less androgenic progestogens include medroxyprogesterone e.g. medroxyprogesterone 20mg last 14/7 of 3-month cycle. Norethisterone should be avoided.

Infertility

Ovulation induction regimens are indicated. Obesity adversely affects fertility outcome with poorer pregnancy rates and higher rates of miscarriage so weight reduction should be strongly encouraged.

Metformin

- Use remains controversial but probably does not improve ovulation and pregnancy rates in insulin resistant, particularly overweight, ♀ with PCOS. No reported teratogenic or neonatal complications.
- *Dose* 500mg OD after meals to be ↑ gradually to 1g BD. If ovulation restored following 6 months of treatment then continue for up to 1 year. If pregnancy does not occur then consider other treatments.
- *Side effects* Nausea, bloating, diarrhea, vomiting.

Clomifene citrate

- Inhibits oestrogen negative feedback, ↑ FSH secretion and thus stimulating ovarian follicular growth.
- *Dose* 25–150mg a day from day 2 of menstrual cycle for 5 days.
- *Response rates* 80% of ♀ with PCOS will ovulate, although the pregnancy rate is only 67%. Recent studies have shown that treatment with metformin may improve response to clomifene in resistant cases.
- *Complications* 8% twins, 0.1% higher order multiple pregnancy. Risk of ovarian neoplasia following prolonged clomifene treatment remains unclear, so limit treatment to a maximum of 6 cycles.

Gonadotrophin preparations (hMG or FSH)

- Used in those unresponsive to clomiphene. Low-dose regimes show better response rates and less complications, e.g. 75IU/day for 2 weeks then increase by 37.5IU/day every 7 days as required.
- 94% ovulation rate and 40% conception rate after 4 cycles.
- *Complications* Hyperstimulation, multiple pregnancies.
- Close ultrasonic monitoring is essential.

Surgery

- Laparoscopic ovarian diathermy or laser drilling may restore ovulation in up to 90% of ♀ with cumulative pregnancy rates of 80% within 8 months of treatment. Particularly effective in slim ♀ with PCOS and high LH concentrations.
- *Complications* Surgical adhesions, although usually mild.

In vitro fertilization

- In ♀ who fail to respond to ovulation induction.
- 60–80% conception rate after 6 cycles.

Acne

Treatment for acne should be started as early as possible to prevent scarring. All treatments take up to 12 weeks before significant improvement is seen. All treatments apart from benzoyl peroxide are contraindicated in pregnancy.

Mild-to-moderate acne

Topical benzoyl peroxide 5% Bactericidal properties. May use in conjunction with oral antibiotic therapy to reduce the risk of developing resistance to antibiotics. Side effects: skin irritation and dryness. Add oral antibiotics if no improvement after 2 months of treatment.

Moderate-to-severe acne

- *Topical retinoids* e.g. tretinoin, isotretinoin. Useful alone in mild acne or in conjunction with antibiotics in moderately severe acne. Continue as maintenance therapy to prevent further acne outbreaks. Side effects: irritation, photosensitivity. Apply high factor sunscreen before sun exposure. Avoid in acne involving large areas of skin.
- *Oral antibiotics* e.g. oxytetracycline 500mg BD, doxycycline 100mg OD or minocycline 100mg OD. Response usually seen by 6 weeks and full efficacy by 3 months. Continue antibiotics for 2 months after control is achieved. Prescription usually given for a 3–6-month course. Continue topical retinoids and/or benzoyl peroxide to prevent further outbreaks.
- *Dianette* or *antiandrogens* eg spironolactone may also be effective in treating moderately severe acne.

Severe acne

Isotretinoin is very effective in ♀ with severe acne or acne which has not responded to other oral or topical treatments. Used early it can minimize scarring in inflammatory acne. However, it is highly toxic and can only be prescribed by a consultant dermatologist. Also consider referring ♀ who develop acne in their 30s or 40s and ♀ with psychological problems as a result of acne.

Further reading

Dunaif A (1997). Insulin resistance and polycystic ovary syndrome: mechanism and implications for pathogenesis. *Endoc Rev* **18**(6), 774–800.

Ehrmann DA (2005). Polycystic Ovary Syndrome. *New Engl J Med* **352**, 1223–36.

Ehrmann DA and Rychlik D (2003). Pharmacological treatment of polycystic ovary syndrome. *Semin Reprod Med* **21**(3), 277–83.

Ledger WL and Clark T (2003). Long term consequences of polycystic ovary syndrome. *Royal College of Obsterics and Gynaecology* Guideline number 33.

Lord JM, Flight IHK, and Norman RJ (2003). Insulin sensitizing drugs for polycystic ovary syndrome. *Cochrane Database Syst review* 2003.

Neithardt AB and Barnes RB (2003). The diagnosis and management of hirsutism. *Semin Reprod Med* **21**(3), 285–93.

Nestler JE (2008) Metformin for the treatment of the polycystic ovary syndrome. *N Engl J Med* **358**(1), 47–54.

Pierpoint T, McKeigue PM, Isaacs AJ, *et al.* (1998). Mortality of women with polycystic ovary syndrome at long term follow up. *J Clin Epidemiol* **51**(7), 581–6.

The Rotterdam ESHRE/ASRM-sponsored PCOS consensus workshop group (2004). Revised 2003 Consensus on diagnostic criteria and long-term health risks related to Polycystic ovary syndrome. *Hum Reprod* **19**, 41–7.

Tsilchorozidou T, Overton C, Conway GS (2004). The pathophysiology of polycystic ovary syndrome. *Clini Endocrinol* **60**(1), 1–17.

Congenital adrenal hyperplasia (CAH) in adults

Definition

CAH is an inherited group of disorders characterized by a deficiency of 1 of the enzymes necessary for cortisol biosynthesis.
- >90% of cases are due to 21α-hydroxylase deficiency.
- Wide clinical spectrum, from presentation in neonatal period with salt wasting and virilization to non-classic CAH in adulthood.
- Inherited in an autosomal recessive manner.

Epidemiology

- Wide racial variations, most common in those of Jewish origin.
- Carrier frequency of classic CAH 1:60 in white people.
- Carrier frequency of non-classic CAH 19% in Ashkenazi Jews, 13.5% in Hispanics, 6% in Italians, and 3% in other Caucasian populations.

Pathogenesis

Genetics

- *CYP21* encodes for the 21α-hydroxylase enzyme, located on the short arm of chromosome 6 (chromosome 6p21.3). In close proximity is the *CYP21* pseudogene, with 90% homology but no functional activity.
- 21α-hydroxylase deficiency results from gene mutations, partial gene deletions, or gene conversions in which sequences from the pseudogene are transferred to the active gene, rendering it inactive. There is a correlation between the severity of the molecular defect and the clinical severity of the disorder. Non-classic CAH is usually due to a point mutation (single base change), missense mutations result in simple virilizing disease whereas a gene conversion or partial deletion usually results in presentation in infancy with salt wasting or severe virilization.

Biochemistry

(□ see Fig. 55.1)

21α-hydroxylase deficiency results in aldosterone and cortisol deficiency. There is ACTH oversecretion because of the loss of −ve feedback, and this causes adrenocortical hyperplasia and excessive accumulation of 17-hydroxy progesterone (17OHP) and other steroid precursors. These are then shunted into androgen synthesis pathways resulting in testosterone and androstenedione excess.

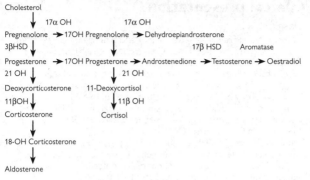

Fig. 55.1 Adrenal steroid biosynthesis pathway.

Clinical presentation

Classic CAH

- Most patients are diagnosed in infancy, and their clinical presentation is discussed elsewhere (☐ see Congenital adrenal hyperplasia, p.564).
- *Problems persisting into adulthood*-sexual dysfunction and subfertility in ♀, particularly in salt wasters. Reconstructive genital surgery is required in the majority of ♀ who were virilized at birth to create an adequate vaginal introitus. With improvement of medical and surgical care, pregnancy rates have improved. Fertility rates of 60–80% have been reported in ♀ with classic CAH.
- In ♂ high levels of adrenal androgens suppress gonadotrophins and thus testicular function. Spermatogenesis may therefore be affected if CAH is poorly controlled. Suboptimally controlled CAH in ♂ also predisposes them to developing testicular adrenal rests. These are always benign but may be misdiagnosed as testicular tumours.

Non-classic CAH

- Due to partial deficiency of 21α-hydroxylase. Glucocorticoid and aldosterone production are normal but there is overproduction of 17OHP and thus androgens.
- Present with hirsutism (60%), acne (33%), and oligomenorrhoea (54%), often around the onset of puberty. Only 13% of ♀ present with subfertility.
- 1/3 of ♀ have polycystic ovaries on US and adrenal incidentalomas or hyperplasia are seen in 40%.
- *Asymptomatic in ♂* The effect of non-classic CAH on ♂ fertility is unknown.

Investigations

Because of the diurnal variation in adrenal hormonal secretion, all investigations should be performed at 9 a.m.

Diagnosis of non-classic CAH—17OHP measurement

Timing of measurement

- Screen in the follicular phase of the menstrual cycle. 17OHP is produced by the corpus luteum, so false +ve results may occur if measured in the luteal phase of the cycle.
- Must be measured at 9 a.m. to avoid false –ve results as 17OHP has a diurnal variation similar to that of ACTH.

Interpretation of result

- <5 nmol/L—normal.
- >15nmol/L—CAH.
- 5–15nmol/L—proceed to ACTH stimulation test. A fifth will have non-classic CAH.

ACTH stimulation test

- Measure 17OHP 60min after ACTH administration.
- An exaggerated rise in 17OHP is seen in non-classic CAH.
- 17OHP level <30nmol/L post-ACTH excludes the diagnosis.
- Most patients have levels >45nmol/L.
- Levels of 30–45nmol/L suggest heterozygosity or non-classic CAH.
- Cortisol response to ACTH stimulation is usually low-normal.

Other investigations

Androgens

- In poorly controlled classic CAH in ♀, testosterone and androstenedione levels may be in the adult ♂ range. Dehydroepiandrosterone sulphate levels are usually only mildly, and not consistently, elevated in CAH.
- Circulating testosterone and, particularly androstenedione, are elevated in non-classic CAH, but there is a large overlap with levels seen in PCOS so serum androgen concentrations cannot be used to distinguish between the disorders.

Renin

- Plasma renin levels are markedly elevated in 75% of patients with inadequately treated classic CAH, reflecting deficient aldosterone production.
- A proportion of ♀ with non-classic CAH may also have mildly elevated renin concentrations.

ACTH

- Greatly elevated in poorly controlled classic CAH.
- Usually normal levels in non-classic CAH.

📖 See Table 55.1 for a list of enzyme deficiencies in CAH.

Table 55.1 Enzyme deficiencies in CAH

Enzyme deficiency	Incidence (per births)	Clinical features
Classic 21α-hydroxylase	1:10 000–1:15 000	Salt wasting, ambiguous genitalia in females, precocious pubarche in males
Non-classic 21α-hydroxylase (partial deficiency)	1:27–1:1000	Hirsutism, oligomenorrhoea in pubertal girls, asymptomatic in boys
11β-hydroxylase	1:100 000	Ambiguous genitalia, virilization, hypertension
3β-hydroxylase	Rare	Mild virilization, salt wasting in severe cases
17α-hydroxylase	Rare	Delayed puberty in females, pseudohermaphroditism in males, hypertension, hypokalaemia

Management

The aims of treatment of CAH in adulthood are:
• To maintain normal energy levels and weight and avoid adrenal crises in all patients.
• To minimize hyperandrogenism and to restore regular menses and fertility in ♀.
• To avoid glucocorticoid over-replacement.
• To treat stress with adequate extra glucocorticoid.

Classic CAH

• *Prednisolone*, total dose 5–7.5 mg/day. Given in 2 divided doses, with a 1/3 of the total dose given on waking (about 7 a.m.) and 2/3 of the dose on retiring. The aim is to suppress the early morning peak of ACTH and thus androgen secretion. The optimum dose is the minimum dose required to normalize serum androgens. Occasional patients who are not controlled on prednisolone may be optimally treated with nocturnal dexamethasone instead (0.25–0.5mg nocte).
• As with other forms of adrenal insufficiency, glucocorticoid doses should be doubled during illness. This is discussed in detail elsewhere (📖 p.260).
• 75% of patients are salt wasters and thus require mineralocorticoid replacement therapy. Fludrocortisone in a dose of 50–200mcg/day is given as a single daily dose. The aim is to keep plasma renin levels in the mid-normal range.
• Bilateral adrenalectomy may very occasionally be considered in patients with severe virilization resistant to conventional therapy.
• *Experimental therapies* Trials have been performed using a combination of low dose hydrocortisone, fludrocortisone, testolactone (an aromatase inhibitor), and flutamide (antiandrogen) in children. This 4-drug regimen appears to improve final height and minimize glucocorticoid side effects with no significant adverse effects. However, long-term effects are currently unknown.
• *Pregnancy*–prior screen patient and partner and give genetic advice. If partner a carrier, 50% risk of affected child 1 in 63 carrier of 21 OH gene).

Non-classic CAH

• *Oligo/amenorrhoea* Glucocorticoid therapy, e.g. noctural dexamethasone 0.25–0.5mg or prednisolone 2.5–5mg/day, may be used. Slightly higher doses may be required to normalize ovulatory function.
• *Hirsutism and acne* May alternatively, and more effectively, be treated using antiandrogens, e.g. cyproterone acetate combined with oral oestrogens (📖 see Management, p.297). Spironolactone should be avoided because of the potential risk of salt wasting and thus hyperreninaemia.
• If plasma renin level is elevated then fludrocortisone given in a dose sufficient to normalize renin concentrations may improve adrenal hyperandrogenism.
• ♂ do not usually require treatment. The occasional ♂ may need glucocorticoids to treat subfertility.

Management of pregnancy in CAH

Indications for prenatal treatment
- *Maternal classic CAH* Screen patient/partner using basal ± ACTH-stimulated 17OHP levels (📖 see Investigations, p.306). If levels elevated, proceed to genotyping. If heterozygote, then prenatal treatment of fetus recommended.
- Previous child from same partner with CAH

Aims of prenatal treatment (📖 see Fig. 55.2)
Prevention of virilization of an affected ♀ fetus.

Treatment (commenced before 10 weeks gestation)
Dexamethasone (20mcg/kg maternal body weight) in 3 divided doses a day crosses the placenta and reduces fetal adrenal hyperandrogenism. Discontinue if ♂ fetus.

Outcome
50–75% of affected ♀ do not require reconstructive surgery.

Complications
- No known fetal congenital malformations or neonanatal complications from dexamethasone treatment.
- Subtle effects of glucocorticoids on neuropsychological function unknown. No significant long-term follow up studies on treated children published to date.
- Maternal complications of glucocorticoid excess e.g. mood swings, weight gain, gestational diabetes and hypertension. Monitor maternal weight, blood pressure, fasting plasma glucose and urinary glucose.

There is debate about whether ♀ with non-classic CAH should be offered prenatal treatment with dexamethasone. There have been no cases of ♀ with non-classic CAH giving birth to a virilized ♀. Additionally, the estimated risk of conceiving an infant with classic CAH is 1:1000. As the risk of fetal virilization is therefore low, dexamethasone treatment of this group of ♀ seems unwarranted. However, these infants should be screened in the neonatal period by measuring 17OHP levels.

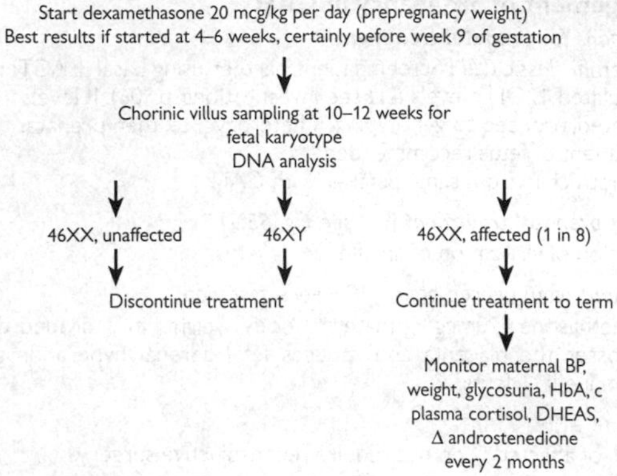

Start dexamethasone 20 mcg/kg per day (prepregnancy weight)
Best results if started at 4–6 weeks, certainly before week 9 of gestation

↓

Chorinic villus sampling at 10–12 weeks for
fetal karyotype
DNA analysis

| 46XX, unaffected | 46XY | 46XX, affected (1 in 8) |

Discontinue treatment   Continue treatment to term

Monitor maternal BP,
weight, glycosuria, HbA, c
plasma cortisol, DHEAS,
Δ androstenedione
every 2 months

Fig. 55.2 Prenatal treatment protocol.

Monitoring of treatment

Annual follow up is usually adequate in adults.

- *Clinical assessment* Look for evidence of hyperandrogenism and glucocorticoid excess. Amenorrhoea in ♀ usually suggests inadequate therapy. Measure BP.
- *17OHP* Aim for a mildly elevated level (about 2 × normal). Normalizing 17OHP will result in complications from supraphysiological doses of glucocorticoids.
- *Plasma renin* Aim for renin in mid-normal range. Hyperandrogenism will be difficult to control if patient is mildly salt-depleted (ACTH production stimulated by hypovolaemia).
- *Androgens* Aim to normalize serum testosterone/androstenedione taken before a.m. steroids.
- *Consider bone density which may be reduced by supraphysiological steroid doses.*

In ♀:

- Good control ensures fertility.
- Testes intermittently checked for masses—adrenal cell rests.

Prognosis

Adults with treated CAH have a normal life expectancy. Improvement in medical and surgical care has also improved QoL for most sufferers. However, there are a few unresolved issues:

* *Height* Despite optimal treatment in childhood, patients with CAH are, on average, significantly shorter than their predicted genetic height. Studies suggest that this may be due to overtreatment with glucocorticoids during infancy.
* *Fertility* Remains reduced in ♀ with CAH, particularly in salt wasters, due to factors including inadequate vaginal introitus and anovulation 2° to both hyperandrogenism and high 17OHP levels. Fertility may also be affected in ♂ with poorly controlled classic CAH.
* *Adrenal incidentalomas and testicular adrenal rest tumours* Benign adrenal adenomas have been reported in up to 50% of patients with classic CAH. ♂ with CAH may develop gonadal adrenocortical rests. These are ACTH-responsive and should be treated by optimizing glucocorticoid therapy. Occasionally adults with nonclassic CAH develop adrenal adenomas or testicular rests and should then be started on steroids.
* *Psychosexual issues* In animal studies, prenatal exposure of genetic ♀ to testosterone during critical periods of development enhances masculine behaviour. ♀ with classic CAH also show an ↑ tendency to ♂ pattern behaviour. A significant number of ♀ with classic CAH, despite adequacy of vaginal reconstruction, are not sexually active.

Further reading

Cabrera MS, Vogiatzi MG, and New MI (2001). Long term outcome in adult males with classic congenital adrenal hyperplasia. *J Clin Endocrinol Metab* **86**(7), 3070–8.

Joint LWPES/ESPE CAH Working Group (2002). Consensus statement on 21-hydroxylase deficiency from the Lawson Wilkins Paediatric Endocrine Society and the European Society for Paediatric Endocrinology. *J Clin Endocrinol Metab* **87**(9), 4048–53.

Merke DP (2008). Approach to the adult with congenital adrenal hyperplasia due to 21-hydroxylase deficiency. *JCEM* **93**, 653–660.

New MI (2006). Extensive clinical experience: nonclassical 21-hydroxylase deficiency. *J Clin Endocrinol Metab.* **91**(11), 205–14. Epub 2006 Aug 15.

New MI, Carlson A, Obeid J, et al. (2001). Prenatal diagnosis for Congenital adrenal hyperplasia in 532 pregnancies. *J Clin Endocrinol Metab* **86**(12), 5651–757.

Ogilvie CM, Crouch NS, Rumsby G, et al. (2006). Congenital adrenal hyperplasia in adults: a review of medical, surgical and psychological issues. *Clin Endocrinol* **64**, 2–11.

Premawaradhana LDKE, Hughes IA, Read GF, et al. (1997). Longer term outcome in females with congenital adrenal hyperplasia: the Cardiff experience. *Clin Endocrinol* **46**, 327–32.

Speiser PW and White PC (2003). Congenital adrenal hyperplasia. *New Engl J Med* **349**(8), 776–88.

Androgen-secreting tumours

Definition

Rare tumours of the ovary or adrenal gland which may be benign or malignant, which cause virilization in ♀ through androgen production.

Epidemiology and pathology

Androgen-secreting ovarian tumours
- 75% develop before the age of 40 years.
- Account for 0.4% of all ovarian tumours. 20% are malignant.
- Tumours are 5–25cm in size. The larger they are, the more likely they are to be malignant. They are rarely bilateral.
- 2 major types:
  - Sex cord stromal cell tumours: often contain testicular cell types.
  - Adrenal-like tumours: often contain adrenocortical or Leydig cells.
- Other tumours, e.g. gonadoblastomas and teratomas, may also on occasion present with virilization.

Androgen-secreting adrenal tumours
- 50% develop before the age of 50 years.
- Larger tumours, particularly >6cm, are more likely to be malignant.

Clinical features

- *Onset of symptoms* Usually recent onset of rapidly progressive symptoms.
- *Hyperandrogenism*
  - Hirsutism of varying degree, often severe (Ferriman–Gallwey score) (☐ see Table 53.2, p.287); ♂-pattern balding and acne are also common.
  - Usually oligo-amenorrhoea.
  - Infertility may be a presenting feature.
- *Virilization* (☐ Box 53.1, p.285) indicates severe hyperandrogenism is associated with clitoromegaly and is present in 98% of ♀ with androgen-producing tumours. Not usually a feature of PCOS.
- *Other:*
  - Abdominal pain.
  - Palpable abdominal mass.
  - Ascites.
  - Symptoms and signs of Cushing's syndrome are present in 50% of ♀ with adrenal tumours.

Investigations

📖 See Fig. 56.1.

Management

Surgery

- Adrenalectomy or ovarian cystectomy/oophorectomy.
- Curative in benign lesions.

Adjunctive therapy

Malignant ovarian and adrenal androgen-secreting tumours are usually resistant to chemotherapy and radiotherapy.

Prognosis

Benign tumours

- Prognosis excellent.
- Hirsutism improves postoperatively, but clitoromegaly, ♂-pattern balding, and deep voice may persist.

Malignant tumours

- *Adrenal tumours* 20% 5-year survival. Most have metastatic disease at the time of surgery.
- *Ovarian tumours* 30% disease-free survival and 40% overall survival at 5 years.

Further reading

Hamilton-Fairley D and Franks S (1997). Androgen secreting tumours. In Sheaves R, Jenkins PJ, Wass JAH (eds.), *Clinical Endocrine Oncology*. Oxford: Blackwell Science, pp.323–9.

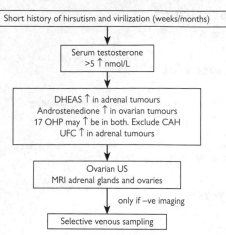

Fig. 56.1 Investigation of androgen-secreting tumours.

Menstrual function disorders—assessment and investigation

Definitions

- *Oligomenorrhoea* is defined as the reduction in the frequency of menses to <9 periods a year.
- 1° *amenorrhoea* is the failure of menarche by the age of 16 years. Prevalence ~0.3%
- 2° *amenorrhoea* refers to the cessation of menses for >6 months in ♀ who had previously menstruated. Prevalence ~3%.

However, the common causes may present with either 1° or 2° amenorrhoea.

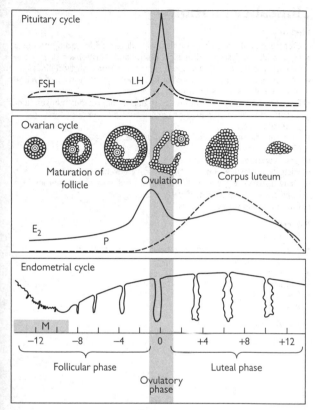

Fig. 57.1 The normal menstrual cycle.

Clinical evaluation

History

- Oestrogen deficiency, e.g. hot flushes, reduced libido, and dyspareunia.
- Hypothalamic dysregulation, e.g. exercise and nutritional history, body weight changes, emotional stress, recent or chronic physical illness.
- In 1° amenorrhoea—history of breast development, history of cyclical pain, age of menarche of mother and sisters.
- In 2° amenorrhoea—duration and regularity of previous menses, family history of early menopause, or familial autoimmune disorders, or galactosaemia.
- Anosmia may indicate Kallman's syndrome.
- Hirsutism or acne.
- Galactorrhoea.
- History suggestive of pituitary, thyroid, or adrenal dysfunction.
- Drug history—e.g. causes of hyperprolactinaemia, chemotherapy, hormonal contraception, recreational drug use.
- Obstetric and surgical history.

Physical examination

- Height, weight, BMI.
- Features of Turner's syndrome or other dysmorphic features.
- 2° sex characteristics.
- Galactorrhoea.
- Evidence of hyperandrogenism or virilization.
- Evidence of thyroid dysfunction.
- Anosmia, visual field defects.

For causes 🕮 see Box 57.1.

Box 57.1 Causes of amenorrhoea

Physiological
- Pregnancy and lactation.
- Postmenopause.

Iatrogenic
- Depomedroxyprogesterone acetate.
- Levonorgestrel-releasing intrauterine device.
- Progesterone-only pill.

Pathological—1°
- Chromosomal abnormalities—50%:
  - Turner's syndrome.
  - Other X chromosomal disorders.
- 2° hypogonadism—25%:
  - Kallmann's syndrome.
  - Pituitary disease.
  - Hypothalamic amenorrhoea.
- Genitourinary malformations—15%:
  - Imperforate hymen.
  - Congenital absence of uterus, cervix, or vagina.
- Other—10%:
  - Androgen insensitivity syndrome.
  - CAH.
  - PCOS.
  - Galactosaemia.

Most causes of 2° amenorrhoea can also cause 1° amenorrhea.

Pathological—2°
- Ovarian—70%:
  - PCOS.
  - Premature ovarian failure.
- Hypothalamic—15%:
  - Weight loss.
  - Excessive exercise.
  - Physical or psychological stress.
  - Craniopharyngioma.
  - Infiltrative lesions of the hypothalamus.
  - Drugs e.g. opiates.
- Pituitary—5%:
  - Hyperprolactinaemia.
  - Hypopituitarism.
  - Isolated gonadotropin deficiency.
- Uterine—5%:
  - Intrauterine adhesions.
- Other endocrine disorders—5%:
  - Thyroid dysfunction.
  - Cushing's syndrome.
    —other causes of hyperandrogenism.

Investigations

📖 See Fig. 57.2.
- Is it 1° or 2° ovarian dysfunction?
  - FSH, LH, oestradiol, prolactin.
- Transvaginal US:
  - Ovarian and uterine morphology—exclude anatomical abnormalities, PCOS, and Turner's syndrome.
  - Endometrial thickness—to assess oestrogen status.
- Other tests depending on clinical suspicion:
  - Induce withdrawal bleed with progesterone (e.g. 10mg medroxyprogesterone acetate bd for 7 days). If a bleed occurs then there is adequate oestrogen priming and endometrial development.
  - Serum testosterone in the presence of hyperandrogenism.
  - Thyroid function tests if any evidence of hyper- or hypothyroidism.
  - Karyotype in ovarian failure or if Turner's syndrome or androgen insensitivity syndrome suspected.
  - MRI of the pituitary fossa if FSH low or in the presence of hyperprolactinaemia.

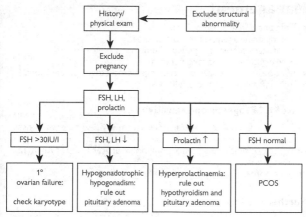

Fig. 57.2 Investigation of amenorrhea.

Management

- Treat underlying disorder, e.g.:
  - Dopamine agonists for prolactinomas.
  - Pituitary surgery for pituitary tumours.
  - Weight gain in anorexia nervosa.
- Treat oestrogen deficiency—oestrogen/progestogen preparations.
- Treat infertility—📖 see p.299

Box 57.2 Progesterone sensitivity

- Skin condition occurs regularly premenstrually—settling with onset of menses.
- Dermatosis includes eczema, pompholyx, urticaria, and erythema multiforme.
- Auto antibodies present (+ve challenge test).

Further reading

Baird DT (1997). Amenorrhoea. *Lancet* **350**, 275–9.

Beswick SJ, Lewis HM, and Stewart PM (2002). A recurrent rash treated by oophrectomy. *QJM* **95**(9), 636–7.

Hickey M and Balen A (2003). Menstrual disorders in adolescence: investigation and management. *Hum Reprod Update* **9**(5), 493–504.

Premature ovarian failure (POF)

Definition

POF is a disorder characterized by amenorrhoea, oestrogen deficiency, and elevated gonadotropins developing in ♀ <40 years, as a result of loss of ovarian follicular function.

Epidemiology

- Incidence – 0.1% of ♀ <30 years and 1% of those <40 years.
- Accounts for 10% of all cases of 2° amenorrhoea.

Causes of POF

- Chromosomal abnormalities (60%):
  - Turner's syndrome.
  - Fragile X syndrome.
  - Other X chromosomal abnormalities.
- Gene mutations:
  - β subunit of FSH.
  - FSH receptor.
  - LH receptor.
- Autoimmune disease (20%).
- Iatrogenic:
  - Chemotherapy.
  - Radiotherapy.
  - Hysterectomy.
- Other:
  - Familial ovarian failure.
  - Galactosaemia.
  - Enzyme deficiencies, e.g. 17-hydroxylase deficiency.
  - Infections, e.g. mumps, CMV, HIV, shigella.
- Idiopathic
  - ?environmental toxin.

Box 58.1 Turner's syndrome

(📖 also see Turner's syndrome, p.546)

- Most common X-chromosome abnormality in ♀, affecting 1: 2500 live ♀ births.
- Result of complete or partial absence of 1 X chromosome.
- *Clinical features* Short stature and gonadal dysgenesis. 90% of affected ♀ have POF.
- *Characteristic phenotype* Webbed neck, micrognathia, low-set ears, high arched palate, widely spaced nipples, and cubitus valgus.
- *Other associated abnormalities* Aortic coarctation and other left-sided congenital heart defects, hypothyroidism, osteoporosis, skeletal abnormalities, lymphoedema, coeliac disease, congenital renal abnormalities, and ENT abnormalities.
- *Diagnosis* Lymphocyte karyotype.
- *Management in adults:*
  - Sex hormone replacement therapy.
  - Treat complications.
- Follow-up:
  - Baseline renal US, thyroid autoantibodies.
  - Annual BMI, BP, TFT, lipids, fasting blood glucose liver function.
  - 3–5-yearly echocardiogram and bone densitometry.
  - Hearing loss 5 years.

Table 58.1 Correlation of karyotype with phenotype

Karyotype	Phenotype
45,X (50%)	Most severe phenotype. High incidence of cardiac and renal abnormalities.
46,Xi(Xq) (20%)	↑ prevalence of thyroiditis, inflammatory bowel disease and deafness.
45,X/46,XX (10%)	Least severe phenotype. ↑ mean height Spontaneous puberty and menses in up to 40%.
46,Xr(X) (10%)	Spontaneous menses in 33%. Congenital abnormalities uncommon Cognitive dysfunction in those with a small ring chromosome.
45,X/46,XY (6%)	↑ risk of gonadoblastoma.
Other (4%)	

Pathogenesis

Failure of normal ovarian follicular response to gonadotrophins with consequent failure of ovarian steroidogenesis. POF is the result of either ovarian follicle depletion or failure of the follicles to function (resistant ovary syndrome). May be distinguished by ovarian US or histologically by ovarian biopsy. Treatment options are the same so invasive techniques looking for the presence of follicles are not indicated.

POF is usually permanent, although ♀ with transient disease have been described. Additionally, <50% of karyotypically normal ♀ with established disease produce oestrogen intermittently and up to a 1/5 of ♀ may ovulate despite high gonadotrophin levels. Spontaneous pregnancy has been reported in 5%.

Clinical presentation

- *Amenorrhoea:*
  - May be 1°, particularly in patients with chromosomal abnormalities.
- *Symptoms of oestrogen deficiency:*
  - Not present in those with 1° amenorrhoea.
  - 75% of ♀ who develop 2° amenorrhoea report hot flushes, night sweats, mood changes, fatigue or dyspareunia; symptoms may precede the onset of menstrual disturbances.
- *Autoimmune disease:*
  - Screen for symptoms and signs of associated autoimmune disorders.
- *Other:*
  - Past history of radiotherapy, chemotherapy, or pelvic surgery.
  - +ve family history in 10% of patients.

Box 58.2 Autoimmune diseases and POF

- Responsible for 20% of all cases of POF.
- A 2nd autoimmune disorder is present in 10–40% of ♀ with autoimmune POF:
  - Addison's disease 10%.
  - Autoimmune thyroid disease 25%.
  - Type 1 diabetes mellitus 2%.
  - Myaesthenia gravis 2%.
  - B12 deficiency.
  - SLE is also more common.
- POF is present in:
  - 60% of ♀ with autoimmune polyglandular syndrome type 1 (📖 see p.254)
  - 25% of ♀ with autoimmune polyglandular syndrome type 2 (📖 see p.255).
- Steroid cell antibodies are +ve in 60–100% of patients with Addison's disease in combination with POF. The presence of +ve steroid cell antibodies in ♀ with Addison's disease confers a 40% risk of ultimately developing POF. Other ovarian antibodies have no predictive value.

Investigation

- *Serum gonadotropins:*
  - Diagnosis is confirmed by serum FSH >40mIU/L on at least 2 occasions at least 1 month apart.
  - Disease may have a fluctuating course with high FSH levels returning to normal and later regain of ovulatory function.
  - LH also elevated, but FSH usually disproportionately higher than LH.
- *Serum oestradiol levels* are usually low.
- *Karyotype:*
  - All ♀ presenting with hypergonadotropic amenorrhoea below age 40 should be karyotyped
  - ♀ with Y chromosomal material should be referred for bilateral gonadectomy to prevent the development of gonadoblastoma.
- *Pelvic US*—to identify normal ovarian and uterine morphology.
- *Transvaginal US:*
  - Ovarian volume and blood flow.
  - Uterine size and anatomy.
- *Bone mineral density*—risk of osteoporosis.
- *Screen for autoimmune disease:*
  - Thyroid and adrenal cortex autoantibodies; if +ve, increases the risk of progression to overt adrenal or thyroid insufficiency.
  - Ovarian antibodies are of no proven clinical value.
  - TSH and fasting blood glucose, FBC.
  - Synacthen test only if adrenal insufficiency is suspected clinically.
  - Other tests as clinically indicated.
- *Ovarian biopsy*—not indicated.

Annual assessment of women with POF

- Assess adequacy of sex hormone replacement therapy:
  - Tolerance and compliance.
  - Side-effects and complications.
  - Persistent symptoms of sex hormone deficiency.
- Address fertility issues.
- Screen for other autoimmune disease (in autoimmune POF):
  - Clinical evaluation.
  - TSH and fasting blood glucose.
  - Synacthen test if clinically indicated.
- Screen for complications:
  - Osteoporosis.
  - Cardiovascular disease.

Management

Sex hormone replacement therapy

- Exogenous oestrogens (HRT) are required to alleviate symptoms and prevent the long-term complications of oestrogen deficiency—osteoporosis and possibly cardiovascular disease. Initial doses depend on the duration of amenorrhoea—if oestrogen deficient for at least 12 months, then start on lowest doses of oestradiol available, to prevent side-effects, but titrate up to full dose within 6 months. If recently amenorrhoeic then full dose may be commenced immediately (🕮 see Table 58.2). Doses used in HRT are not contraceptive and do not suppress spontaneous ovarian follicular activity. HRT should be continued at least until the age of 50 years, the mean age of the natural menopause.
- In non-hysterectomized ♀, a progestagen should be added for 12–14 days a month to prevent endometrial hyperplasia.
- Low-dose androgen replacement therapy may improve persistent fatigue and poor libido despite adequate oestrogen replacement.

Fertility

- A minority of ♀ with POF and a normal karyotype will recover spontaneously. 5% spontaneous fertility rate.
- Oocyte donation and *in vitro* fertilization offer these ♀ their best chance of fertility. Results are promising, with a pregnancy rate of 35% per patient. Results are less good in ♀ with chemotherapy-induced gonadal damage or after pelvic radiotherapy.
- Ovulation induction therapy has been tried but the results have been poor.
- Glucocorticoid therapy has been used in autoimmune POF but efficacy is poor.
- There is currently much research into the removal of functioning ovarian tissue in ♀ prior to undergoing cancer chemotherapy followed by its cryopreservation with the aim of reimplantation at a later stage when fertility is required. Research into this technique is still in its infancy so if considered, subjects and their family must be counselled about the uncertainty of future success rates associated with ovarian cryopreservation.
- Recent improvements in methods of oocyte cryopreservation using rapid freezing in liquid nitrogen (vitrification) have allowed ♀ with high chance of POF (e.g. before chemo/radiotherapy) to store oocytes collected after superovulation. However, this is also experimental and quoted success rates are 20–30% per patient and depend on age and egg quality at time of collection.

Table 58.2 Hormone replacement therapy in POF

Hormone replacement	Dose
Oestrogen	
Conjugated estrogens	1.25mg daily
Estradiol valerate	2–4mg daily
Transdermal estradiol	100mcg twice a week
Progestagen	12–14 days a month:
Norethisterone	1mg
Medroxyprogesterone	10mg
Testosterone	
IM testosterone	50–100mg/month
Testosterone SC implants	50–100mg every 6 months

📖 see Chapter 59, Menopause, pp.340–348 for a full review of hormone replacement therapy.

Prognosis

- Mortality of ♀ with POF may be ↑ 2-fold.
- Oestrogen deficiency leads to:
  - ↑ risk of cardiovascular and cerebrovascular disease.
  - ↑ risk of osteoporosis. Up to 2/3 of ♀ with POF and a normal karyotype have ↓ BMD, with a z score of −1 or less despite at least intermittent hormone replacement therapy. This may be due to a combination of factors including an initial delay in initiating ERT, poor compliance with ERT and oestrogen 'underdosing'.

Further reading

Barlow DH (1996). Premature ovarian failure. *Baillière Clin Ob Gy* **10**(3), 361–84.

Kalantaridou SN, Davis SR, and Nelson LM (1998). Premature ovarian failure. *Endocrinol Metab Clin* **27**(4), 989–1006.

Welte, CK (2008). Primary ovarian insufficiency: a more accurate term for premature ovarian failure. *Clin End* **68**, 499–509.

Menopause

Definition

- The *menopause* is the permanent cessation of menstruation as a result of ovarian failure and is a retrospective diagnosis made after 12 months of amenorrhoea. The average age of ♀ at the time of the menopause is ~50 years, although smokers reach the menopause ~2 years earlier.
- The *perimenopause* encompasses the menopause transition and the first year following the last menstrual period.

Long-term consequences

- *Osteoporosis* During the perimenopausal period there is an accelerated loss of bone mineral density (BMD), rendering postmenopausal ♀ more susceptible to osteoporotic fractures.
- *Ischaemic heart disease (IHD)* Postmenopausal ♀ are 2–3 × more likely to develop IHD than are premenopausal ♀, even after age adjustments. The menopause is associated with an increase in risk factors for atherosclerosis, including less favourable lipid profile, ↓ insulin sensitivity, and an ↑ thrombotic tendency.
- *Dementia* ♀ are 2–3 × more likely to develop Alzheimer disease than men. It is suggested that oestrogen deficiency may play a role in the development of dementia.

Box 59.1 Physiology

The physiology of the menopause remains poorly understood. Ovaries have a finite number of germ cells, with maximal numbers at 20 weeks of intrauterine life. Thereafter, there is a gradual reduction in the number of follicles until the perimenopause when there is an exponential loss of oocytes until the store is depleted at the time of the menopause. Table 59.1 summarizes hormonal changes during the menopausal transition.

Inhibin B and anti-Müllerian hormone (AMH) are ovarian glycoprotiens produced by follicles as they develop from pre-antral to antral stages. Both may participate in ovarian paracrine regulation and, with other molecules, regulate the rate of attrition of follicles. Inhibin B and AMH fall with ovarian ageing, before any detectable rise in FSH and are hence, early markers of incipient ovarian failure and onset of perimenopause. In the early perimenopausal period, FSH levels fluctuate, but the gradual rise in FSH levels maintains oestradiol production by the ovarian follicles. So, contrary to previous belief, average serum oestradiol levels may be high at the onset of the menopause transition, falling only towards the end as the follicles are depleted.

Table 59.1 Hormonal changes during the menopausal transition

	Premenopause (from age 36 years)	Early perimenopause	Advanced perimenopause	Menopause
Menstrual cycle	Regular, ovulatory	Irregular, often short cycles, increasingly anovulatory	Oligomenorrhoea	Amenorrhoea
FSH	Rising but within normal range	Intermittently raised, especially in follicular phase	Persistently ↑	↑↑
Inhibin B	Declining	Low	Low	Very low
E_2	Normal	Normal	Normal/low	Low

Clinical presentation

There are marked cultural differences in the frequency of symptoms related to the menopause; in particular, vasomotor symptoms and mood disturbances are more commonly reported in western countries.

- *Menstrual disturbances* (90%) Cycles gradually become increasingly anovulatory, and variable in length from about 4 years prior to the menopause. Oligomenorrhoea often precedes permanent amenorrhoea. In 10% of ♀, menses cease abruptly with no preceding transitional period.
- *Hot flushes* (40%) Often associated with sweats and skin flushing. Highly variable and are thought to be related to fluctuations in oestrogen concentrations. Tend to resolve spontaneously within 5 years of the menopause.
- *Urinary symptoms* (50%) Atrophy of urethral and bladder mucosa after the menopause and ↓ sensitivity of α-adrenergic receptors of the bladder neck in the perimenopausal period. This may result in urinary incontinence and an ↑ risk of urinary tract infections.
- *Sexual dysfunction* (40%) Vaginal atrophy may result in dyspareunia and vaginal dryness. Additionally, falling androgen levels may reduce sexual arousal and libido.
- *Mood changes* (25–50%) Anxiety, forgetfulness, difficulty in concentration and irritability have all been attributed to the menopause. ♀ with a history of affective disorders are at ↑ risk of mood disturbances in the perimenopausal period.

Evaluation (e.g. if HRT is being considered)

History
- Perimenopausal symptoms and their severity.
- Assess risk factors for cardiovascular disease and osteoporosis.
- Assess risk factors for breast cancer and thromboembolic disease.
- History of active liver disease.

Examination
- BP.
- Breasts.
- Pelvic examination, including cervical smear.

Investigations
- *FSH* levels fluctuate markedly in perimenopausal period and correlate poorly with symptoms. Remember, a raised FSH in the perimenopausal period may not necessarily indicate infertility, so contraception, if desired, should continue until the menopause.
- *Mammography* indicated prior to starting oestrogen replacement therapy only in high risk ♀; otherwise, mammography should be offered as per national screening programme
- *Endometrial biopsy* does not need to be performed routinely, but is essential in ♀ with abnormal uterine bleeding.

Hormone replacement therapy (HRT)

The aim of treatment of perimenopausal ♀ is to alleviate menopausal symptoms. HRT is no longer indicated for the prevention of chronic disease in postmenopausal ♀. However, ♀ who have POF should receive HRT unless there is an absolute contraindication until the age of 50 years.

Benefits of HRT

Hot flushes

Respond well to oestrogen therapy in a dose-dependent manner. Start with a low dose and increase gradually as required to control symptoms. High doses may be required initially (up to the equivalent of 2.5mg conjugated estrogens), particularly in younger ♀ or in those whose symptoms develop abruptly. In 75% of ♀ vasomotor symptoms settle within 5 years so consider stopping HRT after 5 years of treatment. The dose of HRT should be gradually reduced over weeks as sudden withdrawal of oestrogen may precipitate the return of vasomotor symptoms.

In ♀ with a contraindication to HRT, or who are intolerant of it nonhormonal therapies are summarized in Table 59.2.

Urinary symptoms

A trial of HRT, local or systemic, may improve stress and urge incontinence as well as the frequency of cystitis.

Vaginal atrophy

Systemic or local oestrogen therapy improves vaginal dryness and dyspareunia. A maximum of 6 months' use of vaginal cream is recommended unless combined with a progestagen as systemic absorption may increase the risk of endometrial hyperplasia. Estradiol vaginal ring (Estring®) appears to have little stimulatory effect on endometrial tissue and does not increase serum oestradiol concentrations. Concomitant progestagen therapy is therefore not necessary. If oestrogens are contraindicated, then vaginal moisturizers, e.g. Replens®, may help.

Osteoporosis

HRT has been shown to increase bone mineral density in the lumbar spine by 3–5% and at the femoral neck by about 2% by inhibiting bone resorption. There is an associated 30–50% reduction in fracture risk, protection being highest in ♀ on HRT for at least 10 years. The Women's Health Initiative trial (WHI) confirmed that HRT reduces the risk of both hip and vertebral fractures by a 1/3. Timing of initiation of treatment in order to achieve maximal bone protection remains controversial. Evidence suggests that initiation of HRT soon after the menopause is associated with the lowest hip fracture risk but discontinuation of HRT results in bone loss to pretreatment levels.

Colorectal cancer

Observational studies have shown that HRT may protect against colon cancer. This has been confirmed by WHI which showed a 20% reduction in the incidence of colon cancer in HRT users. However, HRT should currently not be prescribed solely to prevent colorectal cancer.

Table 59.2 Alternatives to HRT

Symptom	Management
Vasomotor symptoms	Venlafaxine (75mg od), paroxetine (20mg od) and fluoxetine (20mg od) have been shown to significantly reduce the frequency and severity of hot flushes with minimal side effects. Gabapentin (300mg tds) has also been shown to reduce the frequency and severity of hot flushes. Side effects include dizziness, somnolescence, and weight gain. Megestrol acetate in a dose of 20mg bd also reduces hot flushes by up to 70% but its use is limited by side effects, particularly weight gain. Clonidine is less effective, reducing the occurrence of flushes by 20%, and is often associated with disabling side effects such as dizziness, drowsiness and a dry mouth.
Genitourinary symptoms	Vaginal lubricants e.g. Replens®.
Osteoporosis	Selective oestrogen receptor modulators (SERMS) e.g. raloxifene, however these may exacerbate vasomotor symptoms if present. Bisphosphonates e.g. alendronic acid and risedronate.

Risks of HRT (also 📖 see Box 59.2)

Breast cancer

No personal or family history of breast cancer

There is an ↑ risk of breast cancer in HRT users which is related to the duration of use. The risk increases by 35% following 5 years of use and falls to never-used risk 5 years after discontinuing HRT. For ♀ aged 50 not using HRT, about 45 in every 1000 will have cancer diagnosed over the following 20 years, that is up to age 70. This number increases to 47/1000 ♀ using HRT for 5 years, 51/1000 using HRT for 10 years, and 57/1000 after 15 years of use. The risk is highest in ♀ on combined HRT compared with oestradiol alone. Mortality has not been shown to be ↑ in breast cancer developing in ♀ on HRT.

Family history of breast cancer

The risk of breast cancer may be ↑ 4-fold as a result of the family history, but there is little evidence that the risk is ↑ further by the use of HRT. HRT may be used in these ♀ if severe vasomotor symptoms are present after counselling regarding the above risks.

Past history of breast cancer

Avoid HRT in ♀ with a past history of breast cancer.

Venous thromboembolism (DVT)

HRT increases the risk approximately 3-fold, resulting in an extra 2 cases/10,000 woman-years. The risk is highest in the 1st year of use of HRT and has been shown to be halved by aspirin or statin therapy. This risk is markedly ↑ in ♀ who already have risk factors for DVT, including previous DVT, cardiovascular disease, and within 90 days of hospitalization.

Low risk ♀

- Absolute risk remains small—30 per 100,000 ♀.
- Stop HRT during immobilization or use prophylactic anticoagulation.

Family history of DVT

If HRT is being considered because of severe vasomotor symptoms then do a thrombophilia screen. If +ve, then avoid HRT. ♀ with a +ve family history of thromboembolism are still at a slightly ↑ risk themselves even if the results of the thrombophilia screen are −ve so prescribe HRT cautiously after counselling patient. Transdermal E2 may be preferable.

Past history of DVT/PE

Risk of recurrence is 5% per year so avoid HRT unless on long-term warfarin therapy.

Cerebrovascular disease

HRT has been shown to increase the risk of ischaemic stroke in older ♀, particularly in the presence of atrial fibrillation. HRT should therefore not be used in ♀ with a history of cerebrovascular disease or atrial fibrillation unless they are anticoagulated.

Box 59.2 A summary of contraindications to HRT

Absolute	Relative—seek advice
• Undiagnosed vaginal bleeding.	• Past history of endometrial cancer.
• Pregnancy.	• Family or past history of thromboembolism.
• Active DVT.	• Ischaemic heart disease.
• Active endometrial cancer.	• Cerebrovascular disease.
• Breast cancer.	• Active liver disease.
	• Hypertriglyceridaemia

Endometrial cancer

No ↑ risk in ♀ taking continuous combined HRT preparations. ♀ using sequential combined preparations do not appear to have an ↑ risk of endometrial cancer initially but the risk of endometrial hyperplasia does increase with long-term use (>5 years) despite regular withdrawal bleeds so these ♀ need regular follow up. ♀ with cured stage I tumours may safely take HRT.

Ovarian cancer

HRT may be associated with an ↑ risk of ovarian cancer but the evidence is insufficient at present. A couple of large case-control studies have shown an ↑ risk of ovarian cancer in long term (>10 years) users of unopposed oestrogen replacement therapy. There are few data available on the risk of ovarian cancer in ♀ taking combined HRT. However, studies have also shown that HRT does not have a –ve effect in ovarian cancer survivors.

Gallstones

The risk of gallstones is ↑ 2-fold in HRT users.

Migraine

Migraines may increase in severity and frequency in HRT users. A trial of HRT is still worthwhile if indications are present providing there are no focal neurological signs associated with the migraine. Modification in the dose of oestrogen or its preparation may improve symptoms. Avoid conjugated oestrogens as these are most commonly associated with an increase in the frequency of migraines.

Endometriosis and uterine fibroids

The risk of recurrence of endometriosis or of growth of uterine fibroids is low on HRT.

Liver disease

Use parenteral or transcutaneous oestrogens to avoid hepatic metabolism and monitor liver function in ♀ with impaired liver function tests. Do not use HRT in the presence of active liver disease or liver failure.

Areas of uncertainty with HRT

Cardiovascular disease (CVD)

Data from >30 observational studies suggest that HRT may reduce the risk of developing CVD by up to 50%. However, randomized placebo-controlled trials, e.g. the Heart and Oestrogen-Progestin Replacement Study (HERS) and the WHI trial, have failed to show that HRT protects against IHD. Currently HRT should not be prescribed to prevent cardiovascular disease. However, it may be used cautiously in individual patients with CVD if QoL is significantly reduced from vasomotor symptoms.

Alzheimer disease

Recent evidence suggests that the risk of developing Alzheimer disease may be reduced by up to 50% in ♀ receiving HRT particularly if started early in the menopause. However in ♀ with established Alzheimer disease, there is no evidence to suggest reversal of cognitive dysfunction following initiation of HRT. There is currently insufficient evidence to recommend the use of HRT to prevent Alzheimer disease. In postmenopausal ♀ without dementia HRT may improve certain aspects of cognitive function.

Mood disturbances

There has been a strongly held belief that HRT improves well-being and QoL in perimenopausal and postmenopausal ♀. However, in recent trials where QoL has been assessed, notably HERS and WHI, the improvement in QoL and improved sleep was only seen in ♀ with vasomotor symptoms.

Side effects commonly associated with HRT

- *Breast tenderness* usually subsides within 4–6 months of use.
  If troublesome, use lower oestrogen dose and increase gradually.
- *Mood changes* commonly associated with progestin therapy; manage by changing dose or preparation of progestin.
- *Irregular vaginal bleeding* may be a problem in ♀ on a continuous combined preparation; usually subsides after 6–12 months of treatment. Spotting persists in 10%—may change to a cyclic preparation. 📖 See Box 59.3.

Summary of WHI trial

📖 See Table 59.3.

- Randomized controlled trial of the effects of continuous combined conjugated oestrogen and medroxyprogesterone acetate on healthy postmenopausal ♀, mean follow up 5.2 years.
- Mean age 63 years with 66% of ♀ >60 years of age.
- 70% of participants were overweight or obese and 50% were current or past smokers.
- Absolute risk was highest in the older age group (>65 years).
- Results of WHI cannot be extrapolated to younger HRT users (<55 years of age).
- It is unclear whether different HRT preparations or routes of administration would necessarily have the same benefit/risk profile.

Box 59.3 Who and how to investigate for irregular uterine bleeding

- *Sequential cyclical HRT* 3 or more cycles of bleeding before the 9th day of progestagen therapy or change in the duration or intensity of uterine bleeding.
- *Continuous combined HRT* In first 12 months if bleeding is heavy or extended, if it continues after 12 months of use, or if it starts after a period of amenorrhoea.
- *Endometrial assessment* Essential in ♀ with irregular uterine bleeding. Vaginal US, looking at endometrial thickness, is a sensitive method of detecting endometrial disease. Endometrial thickness of <5mm excludes disease in 96–99% of cases, a sensitivity similar to that of endometrial biopsy. However, specificity is poor so if the endometrium is >5mm (as it will be in 50% of postmenopausal ♀ on HRT) endometrial biopsy will be required to rule out carcinoma.

Table 59.3 Risks and benefits per 10,000 ♀ treated with HRT per year (WHI trial)

Benefits	Number of patients
Hip fractures prevented	5
Colon cancer prevented	6
Adverse events:	
Coronary heart disease	7
Cerebrovascular events	8
Pulmonary embolism	5
Breast cancer (>5 years' use)	8

Dietary phytoestrogens

Phytoestrogens are found in foods such as soy beans, cereals, and seeds. Although they have oestrogen-like activity data from clinical trials are conflicting. It appears that the effect of phytoestrogens on vasomotor symptoms is modest at best. Research does suggest that soy protein has a favourable effect on plasma lipid concentrations and may reduce the risk of cardiovascular disease. However the actual daily dose required is unclear. Finally, data regarding the effect of phytoestrogens on bone loss and breast cancer risk are inconclusive. Phytoestrogen supplements cannot therefore be recommended for the prevention of chronic disease in peri- and post-menopausal ♀ until they are adequately evaluated in clinical trials.

HRT regimens
Estrogen preparations
📖 See Table 59.4. In younger, symptomatic, often perimenopausal ♀, higher doses of oestrogen are often required initially, which can be reduced gradually to the lowest dose effective at controlling symptoms.

Older ♀ who have been amenorrhoeic for over a year should be started on the lowest possible dose of oestrogen.

Route of administration
- *Oral route* is the most popular. Disadvantages:
  - First pass hepatic metabolism means that plasma oestrogen levels are variable, so symptoms do not always respond.
  - May be associated with nausea and may exacerbate liver disease.
  - Must be taken daily so there is no breakthrough of symptoms.
- *Transdermal patches* avoid first pass effect and are thus ideal in ♀ with liver disease or hypertriglyceridaemia. Additionally, patches provide constant systemic hormone levels. However, 10% of ♀ develop skin reactions. Try to avoid moisture and to rotate patch sites to prevent this.
- *Gels* have the advantages of patches but skin irritation is less common.
- *SC implants* have the advantage of good compliance. However, if side-effects develop, implants are difficult to remove. Additionally, may release estradiol for up to 3 years after insertion and cyclical progestagens must be given until oestrogen levels are not detectable.

Progestagen preparations
📖 See Table 59.5 Must be added in non-hysterectomized ♀ to avoid endometrial hyperplasia and subsequent carcinoma.

Sequential cyclical regimen
Give progestagen for a minimum of 10 days a month. Usually given for the first 12 days of each calendar month. Quarterly regimen available—progestagen given for 14 days 4 × a year. However, the risk of endometrial hyperplasia on such a regimen is unknown.

90% of ♀ have a monthly withdrawal bleed. 10% may be amenorrhoeic with no harmful consequences. Bleeding should start after the 9th day of progestagen therapy.

Continuous combined regimen
Lower doses of progestagen are given on a daily basis. Uterine bleeding is usually light in amount but timing is unpredictable. Bleeding should stop in 90% of ♀ within 12 months, the majority in 6 months.

Ideal for older ♀ who do not want monthly withdrawal bleeds. Contraindicated in perimenopausal ♀, as irregular uterine bleeding is more likely and difficult to assess.

Tibolone (2.5 mg a day)

A synthetic steroid with mixed oestrogenic, progestogenic and weak androgenic activities. An alternative form of HRT which does not stimulate the endometrium. It alleviates vasomotor symptoms, may improve mood and libido and is protective against osteoporosis. However its effects on the cardiovascular system and breast tissue and the risk of thromboembolism are unknown. 10% of ♀ may experience vaginal bleeding on tibolone.

Table 59.4 Oestrogen preparations

Preparation	Dose
Conjugated estrogens (PO)	0.625–1.25mg daily
Estradiol valerate (PO)	2mg daily
Estradiol transdermal patch	100mcg twice a week. New patch twice a week
Estradiol gel	1–1.5mg daily
Estradiol subcutaneous implant	25–100mg every 4–8 months. Check serum E_2 prior to implant

Table 59.5 Dosage of progestagen preparations

Progestin	Cyclical dose (d1–12)	Continuous daily dose
Medroxyprogesterone acetate (least androgenic)	10mg	2.5–5mg (higher dose reduces bleeding)
Dydrogesterone	10mg	Unknown
Levonorgestrel	150mcg	Unknown
Norethisterone (most androgenic)	0.7–1mg	0.35–1mg

Androgen replacement therapy

📖 See Box 59.4.

- The major androgens in premenopausal ♀ are androstenedione and testosterone, produced by both the ovaries and adrenal glands. >90% are bound to sex hormone binding globulin and albumin. Androgens are thought to play a role in maintaining bone density and normal sexual and cognitive function in ♀.
- Total and free serum androstenedione and testosterone levels fall by up to 50% after the menopause as a result of both declining ovarian and adrenal androgen production.
- *Indications for androgen replacement therapy* Poor well-being and libido despite adequate oestrogen replacement therapy in ♀ with ovarian failure. Studies suggest that low dose testosterone replacement therapy may enhance libido in addition to improving mood.
- *Mode of administration* SC testosterone implants 50–100 mg every 6–8 months. Testosterone patches (300 mcg/24h) are also available. Always combine with oestrogen therapy.
- *Side effects and possible complications* Hirsutism, acne, or virilization have been reported in approximately 20% of ♀. Adverse changes to lipid profile commonly occur. The effect on cardiovascular risk is unknown. The long term effects of androgen therapy on the endometrium and breast tissue are unknown.

Box 59.4 Monitoring of women receiving androgen replacement therapy

Clinical	Biochemical
• Exclude contraindications:	• Lipid profile
• Polycythaemia.	• Liver function tests.
• Breast or endometrial cancer	
• Assess efficacy.	• FBC (exclude polycythaemia).
• Evaluate side effects.	• S. testosterone.

Further reading

Arlt W (2006). Androgen Therapy in women. *Euro J Endocrinol* **154**, 1–11.

Davis SR *et al* (2008). Testosterone for low libido in postmenopausal women not taking estrogen. *NEJM* **359**, 2005–17.

Humphries KH and Gill S (2003). Risks and benefits of hormone replacement therapy: the evidence speaks. *Can Med Assoc J* **168**, 1001–10.

Million Women Study Collaborators (2003). Breast cancer and hormone-replacement therapy in the Million women Study. *Lancet* **362**, 419–23.

Rymer J, Wilson R, and Ballard K (2003). Making decisions about hormone replacement therapy. *BMJ* **326**, 322–6.

Writing Group for Women's Health Initiative Investigators (2002). Risks and benefits of Estrogen plus progestin in healthy postmenopausal women: principal results from the Women's Health Initiative randomized controlled trial. *JAMA* **288**, 321–33.

Combined oral contraceptive pill (COCP)

Introduction

- Very effective contraception with approximately 5 per 100 users falling pregnant per year.
- *Ethinylestradiol (EE2)*
  - Standard dose is 30mcg, but in older ♀ or those with possible cardiovascular risk factors, 20mcg EE2 may be appropriate.
  - 50mcg of EE2 may be indicated in patients on antiepileptic medication but is otherwise associated with an excess risk of arterial and venous thromboembolism.
- *Progestagen*
  - Commonly used oral contraceptive pills (COCPs) contain 2nd-generation progestagens such as *levonorgestrel* (150–250 mg) and *norethisterone* (1 mg).
  - COCPs containing 3rd-generation progestagens (e.g. *norgestimate* and *desogestrel*) are less androgenic however they may be associated with an ↑ risk of thromboembolism.
  - Yasmin® contains a new progestagen, drospirenone, which is derived from spironolactone. It therefore has antimineralocorticoid activity. It is associated with no weight gain and may have antiandrogenic properties.

For a list of COCP preparations 🕮 see Box 60.1.

COCP side-effects

- Breakthrough bleeding.
- Low mood.
- Nausea.
- Fluid retention and weight gain.
- Breast tenderness and enlargement.
- Headache.
- Reduced libido.
- Chloasma.

Box 60.1 COCP preparations

1st generation
- Norinyl-1®

2nd generation
- BiNovum®
- Brevinor®
- Loestrin 20/30®
- Logynon®
- Microgynon 30/30 ED®
- Norimin®
- Ovranette®
- Ovysmen®
- Synphase®
- TriNovum®

3rd generation
- Cilest®
- Femodene/ED®
- Femodette®
- Katya 30/75®
- Marvelon®
- Mercilon®
- Sunya 20/75®
- Triadene®

4th generation
- Yasmin®

Benefits

Ovarian cancer

The risks of ovarian cancer are halved in ♀ who have been taking the COCP for 5 years or more. This risk reduction persists long after discontinuation of the COCP.

Acne

The COCP reduces free testosterone concentrations by suppressing ovarian production of androgens and by ↑ hepatic SHBG production. COCP with low androgenic progestagens often result in an improvement in acne.

Menstrual disorders

The COCP is associated with reduced menstrual flow and can therefore improve menorrhagia. The COCP also reduces dysmenorrhoea.

Risks

Venous thromboembolism

- The risk of venous thromboembolism in non-pregnant ♀ (5 per 100 000 ♀/year) is ↑ 3-fold in ♀ on the COCP.
- The risk is highest in the first year of use, increases with age, and is ↑ in obese ♀.
- The risk of venous thromboembolism appears to be higher in ♀ taking Dianette® or COCPs containing desogestrel or gestodene.
- ♀ with a family history of thromboembolism should undergo a thrombophilia screen before starting the COCP.

Arterial thrombosis

- There is a 10-fold excess risk of IHD in ♀ smokers over the age of 35 years who are on the COCP. The risk of IHD does not seem to be significantly ↑ in nonsmokers who take low dose COCP.
- The relative risk of ischaemic stroke is only slightly ↑ in ♀ taking low dose COCP. The risk is ↑ in ♀ over the age of 35 years, smokers or in ♀ with hypertension. The risk of haemorrhagic stroke does not seem to be ↑ by taking the COCP.
- Risk of either arterial or venous thrombosis returns to normal within 3 months of discontinuing the COCP.

Hypertension

May be caused by the COCP, and if already present, may be more resistant to treatment.

Hepatic disease

Raised hepatic enzymes may be seen in ♀ on the COCP. The incidence of benign hepatic tumours is also ↑.

Gallstones
The risk of developing gallstones is slightly ↑ by taking the COCP (RR = 1.2).

Breast cancer
- There may be a slightly ↑ risk of breast cancer in ♀ using the COCP (RR = 1.3), particularly in those who began taking the COCP in their teens.
- The risk does not seem to be related to the duration of exposure to the COCP nor to the EE2 dose.
- The relative risk of developing breast cancer returns to normal 10 years after discontinuing the COCP.

Cervical cancer
- The use of COCP appears to be associated with an excess risk of cervical cancer in ♀ who are HPV +ve. The risk increases with the duration of COCP use.
- It is not known whether the risk falls again following the discontinuation of COCP.

Thrombophilia screen
- Antithrombin III.
- Protein C.
- Protein S
- Factor V Leiden.

Table 60.1 OCP contraindications

Absolute	Relative
History of heart disease – ischaemic or valvular	Migraine
Pulmonary hypertension	Sickle-cell disease
History of arterial or venous thrombosis	Gallstones
History of cerebrovascular disease	Inflammatory bowel disease
High risk of thrombosis, e.g. factor V Leiden, antiphospholipid antibodies	Hypertension
Liver disease	Hyperlipidaemia
Migraine if severe or associated with focal aura	Diabetes mellitus
Breast or genital tract cancer	Obesity
Pregnancy	Smokers
Presence of 2 or more relative contraindications	
Age >35 years and a smoker	Otosclerosis
	Family history of thrombosis
	Family history of breast cancer

Consider using a progesterone-only pill in women with contraindications to the combined OCP.

Hormonal emergency contraception

Refers to contraception that a woman can use after unprotected sexual intercourse to prevent pregnancy.

- A single 1.5mg dose of the progestagen levonorgestrel is highly efficacious with a pregnancy rate of between 2–4% if taken within 72h of sexual intercourse. It is most effective the earlier it is taken. The dose is repeated if vomiting occurs within 3h of taking the pill.
- The *mechanism of action* is not clear but is thought to be due to inhibition of ovulation as well as a ↓ likelihood of endometrial implantation.
- *Side effects:* nausea in up to 60% of ♀, vomiting in 10–20%. Consider antiemetic 1h before taking contraception. Other side effects: breast tenderness, fatigue, dizziness.
- *Contraindication*—pregnancy.
- ♀ should be advised to use barrier contraception until their next period.
- 98% of ♀ menstruate within 3–4 weeks of taking levonorgestrel. They should be encouraged to seek medical advice if they do not bleed in that time.
- If pregnancy does occur, levonorgestrel is not known to be teratogenic.

Practical issues

Age and the COCP
- ♀ with no risk factors for arterial or venous thrombosis may continue to use the combined COCP until the age of 50 years.
- Those with risk factors for thromboembolism and IHD should avoid the OCP after the age of 35 years, particularly if they are smokers.
- All ♀ on the COCP after the age of 35 years should be on the lowest effective oestrogen dose (e.g. 20mcg EE2).
- Contraception after the menopause: assume fertile for the 1st year after last menstrual period if >50 years.

Breakthrough bleeding
Causes include:
- Genital tract disease.
- Insufficient oestrogen dose.
- Inappropriate progestagen.
- Missed pill.
- Taking 2 packets continuously.
- Gastroenteritis.
- Drug interactions, e.g. antibiotics, hepatic enzyme inducers.

Antibiotics and the COCP
Broad-spectrum antibiotics interfere with intestinal flora, thereby reducing bioavailability of the COCP. Additional methods of contraception should be used.

COCP and surgery
- Stop COCP at least 4 weeks before major surgery and any surgery to the legs. Do not restart until fully mobile for at least 2 weeks.
- If emergency surgery, then stop COCP and start antithrombotic prophylaxis.

Further reading
Petitti DB (2003). Combination oestrogen-progestin oral contraceptives. *New Engl J Med* **349**, 1443–50.

Testicular physiology

Anatomy

- Normal adult ♂ testicular volume 15–30mL.
- Testicular temperature 2°C lower than rest of body because of scrotal location. This is necessary for normal spermatogenesis.
- 2 main units with differing functions:
  - *Interstitial cells* Comprised of Leydig cells which are found in between the seminiferous tubules and close to the blood vessels. Produce testosterone.
  - *Seminiferous tubules* Make up 90% of testicular volume. Spermatogenesis occurs here, in the presence of high intratesticular concentrations of testosterone. Made up of *germ cells* and *Sertoli cells*. Sertoli cells support spermatogenesis and secrete various hormones, including inhibin and in the embryo, Müllerian inhibitory factor (AMH). The former inhibits FSH secretion from the pituitary gland and the latter is responsible for suppressing ♀ sex organ development during sexual differentiation *in utero*.

📖 See Fig. 61.1 for the testosterone biosynthesis pathway.

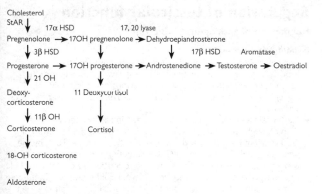

Fig. 61.1 Testosterone biosynthesis pathway.

Regulation of testicular function

Regulation of androgen production

Hypothalamic hormones

- *Gonadotropin releasing hormone (GnRH)* is secreted by the hypothalamus in a pulsatile manner in response to stimuli from the cerebral cortex and limbic system via various neurotransmitters, e.g. endorphins, catecholamines, and dopamine and testicular feedback systems.
- GnRH release initially occurs during sleep in early puberty and then throughout the day in adulthood. It stimulates the secretion of *luteinizing hormone* (LH) and *follicle stimulating hormone* (FSH) by the pituitary gland. The pattern of GnRH secretion is crucial for normal gonadotrophin secretion. Faster pulse frequencies are essential for LH secretion whereas slower frequences favour FSH secretion. Continuous administration of GnRH abolishes both LH and FSH secretion.

Pituitary hormones

- LH binds to Leydig cell receptors and stimulates the synthesis and secretion of testosterone.
- FSH binds to Sertoli cell receptors and stimulates the production of seminiferous tubule fluid as well as a number of substances thought to be important for spermatogenesis.
- Their secretion is regulated by GnRH pulses and through –ve feedback from testicular hormones and peptides.

Testis

- Testosterone is the main androgen produced by the Leydig cells of the testis. Small amounts of androstenedione, DHEA, and dihydrotestosterone (DHT) are also produced. Testosterone has a circadian rhythm with maximum secretion at around 8 a.m. and minimum around 9 p.m.
- Small amounts of oestradiol are also produced in the testis, by the conversion from testosterone. However, most of the circulating oestradiol in ♂ occurs as a result of aromatization of androgens in adipose tissue.
- FSH, in the presence of adequate testosterone levels, stimulates the secretion of inhibin B by Sertoli cells. This in turn acts as a potent inhibitor of FSH secretion.
- The secretion of pituitary gonadotrophins is tightly regulated by testicular function. LH secretion is inhibited by testosterone and its metabolites whereas FSH secretion is controlled by both inhibin B and testosterone. High concentrations of testosterone or of inhibin B results in a –ve feedback inhibition of FSH secretion (📖 see Fig. 61.2).
- Testicular function is also under paracrine control. Inhibin and insulin-like growth factor-1 (IGF-1) act with LH to enhance testosterone production, whereas cytokines inhibit Leydig cell function.

Regulation of spermatogenesis

📖 See Fig. 61.2.

- Both FSH and LH are required for the initiation of spermatogenesis at puberty. LH, by stimulating Leydig cell activity, plays an important part in the early phases of sperm production, when high intratesticular concentrations of testosterone are essential. FSH through its action on the Sertoli cells, is vital for sperm maturation.
- The whole process of spermatogenesis takes approximately 74 days, followed by another 12–21 days for sperm transport through the epididymis. This means that events which may affect spermatogenesis may not be apparent for up to 3 months.

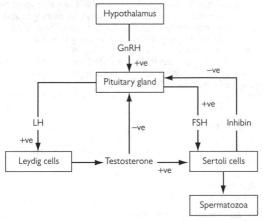

Fig. 61.2 Regulation of spermatogenesis.

Physiology

Testosterone transport

2–4% of circulating testosterone is free and therefore biologically active. The rest is bound to proteins, particularly albumin and sex hormone binding globulin (SHBG).

Testosterone metabolism

- Testosterone is converted in target tissues to the more potent androgen DHT in the presence of the enzyme 5α reductase. There are multiple 5α-reductase isoenzymes; type 2 is the isoenzyme responsible for DHT synthesis in the genitalia, genital skin, and hair follicles. It is therefore essential for normal ♂ virilization and sexual development.
- Both testosterone and DHT exert their activity by binding to androgen receptors, the latter more avidly than testosterone. The androgen receptor is encoded by a gene found on the long arm of the X chromosome (Xq).
- Testosterone may alternatively be converted into oestradiol through the action of the aromatase enzyme, found in greatest quantities in testes and adipose tissue.
- Testosterone and its metabolites are inactivated in the liver and excreted in the urine.

Androgen action

- ♂ sexual differentiation during embryogenesis.
- Development and maintenance of ♂ 2° sex characteristics after puberty.
- Normal ♂ sexual function and behaviour.
- Spermatogenesis.
- Regulation of gonadotropin secretion.

Oestrogen metabolism in males

- Oestradiol daily production rate in ♂: 35–45mcg
- Source of circulating oestradiol:
  - Peripheral aromatization of testosterone 60%.
  - Testes   20%.
  - Peripheral conversion from oestrone   20%.
- 2–3% free oestradiol which is biologically active; the rest is bound to SHBG.

Oestrogen action in males

- Pubertal growth and fusion of the epiphyses.
- Maintenance of bone density.
- Regulation of gonadotropin secretion.

Further reading

De Ronde W, Pols HAP, Van Leeuwen JPTM, et al. (2003). The importance of oestrogens in males. *Clin Endocrinol* **58**(5), 529–42.

Male hypogonadism

Definition

Failure of testes to produce adequate amounts of testosterone, spermatozoa, or both.

Epidemiology

- Klinefelter's syndrome (XXY) (see p. 370) is the most common congenital cause and is thought to occur with an incidence of 2:1000 live births.
- Acquired hypogonadism is even more common, affecting 1:200 ♂.

Evaluation of male hypogonadism

Presentation
- Failure to progress through puberty.
- Sexual dysfunction.
- Infertility.
- Nonspecific symptoms e.g. lethargy, reduced libido, mood changes, weight gain.

The clinical presentation depends on:
- The age of onset (congenital vs. acquired).
- The severity (complete vs. partial).
- The duration (functional vs. permanent).

Secondary hypogonadism

Definition
Hypogonadism as a result of hypothalamic or pituitary dysfunction.

Diagnosis
- Low 9 a.m. serum testosterone.
- Low normal or low LH and FSH, normal inhibin B and anti Müllerian hormone.

Causes
📖 See Box 62.1.

Kallmann syndrome
A genetic disorder characterized by failure of episodic GnRH secretion ± anosmia. Results from disordered migration of GnRH producing neurons into the hypothalamus.

Epidemiology
- Incidence of 1 in 10 000 ♂.
- ♂:♀ ratio = 4:1.

Diagnosis
- Anosmia in 75%.
- ↑ risk of cleft lip and palate, sensorineural deafness, cerebellar ataxia, and renal agenesis.
- Low testosterone, LH, and FSH levels.
- Rest of pituitary function normal.
- Normal MRI pituitary gland and hypothalamus; absent olfactory bulbs may be seen on MRI.
- Normalization of pituitary and gonadal function in response to physiological GnRH replacement.

Genetics
- Most commonly a result of an isolated gene mutation.
- May be inherited in an X-linked (*KAL1*), autosomal dominant *FGFR1* mutation/*KAL2*, or recessive trait.
- *KAL1* gene mutation responsible for some cases of X-linked Kallmann syndrome is located on Xp22.3. It has a more severe reproductive phenotype.
- Mutations of *FGFR1* (fibroblast growth factor receptor 1) gene, located on chromosome 8p11 is associated with the autosomal dominant form of Kallmann syndrome. Affected ♂ have an ↑ likelihood of undescended testes at birth.
- 12–15% incidence of delayed puberty in families of subjects with Kallmann syndrome compared with 1% general population.
- ♂ with autosomal dominant form (*FGFR1* mutation) 50% transmitted to offspring.

Management
- Androgen replacement therapy.
- When fertility is desired, testosterone is stopped and exogenous gonadotropins are administered (📖 see p.410).

Box 62.1 Causes of secondary hypogonadism

- Idiopathic:
  - Kallmann syndrome.
  - Other genetic causes e.g. mutations of *GnRH-R* or *GPR54* genes.
  - Idiopathic hypogonadotrophic hypogonadism (IHH).
  - Fertile eunuch syndrome.
  - Congenital adrenal hypoplasia (*DAX-1* gene mutation).
- Functional:
  - Exercise.
  - Weight changes.
  - Anabolic steroids.
  - Stress – physical/psychological.
  - Systemic illness.
  - Medication and recreational drugs.
- Structural:
  - Tumours eg pituitary adenoma, craniopharyngioma, germinoma.
  - Infiltrative disorders, e.g. sarcoidosis, haemochromatosis.
  - Head trauma
  - Radiotherapy
  - Surgery to the pituitary gland or hypothalamus
- Miscellaneous:
  - Haemochromatosis.
  - Prader–Willi syndrome.
  - Laurence–Moon–Biedl syndrome.

Idiopathic hypogonadotrophic hypogonadism (IHH)
- Congenital form is indistinguishable from Kallmann syndrome apart from the absence of anosmia. >90% of patients are ♂.
- GnRH receptor gene mutation is an uncommon cause of IHH.
- ♂ with acquired IHH may go through normal puberty and have normal testicular size, but present with infertility or poor libido and potency. May be temporary, with normalization of gonadal function after stopping GnRH or testosterone therapy.

Fertile eunuch syndrome
- Incomplete GnRH deficiency. Enough to maintain normal spermatogenesis and testicular growth but insufficient for adequate virilization.
- May require testosterone/hCG for fertility.

Congenital adrenal hypoplasia
- Rare X-linked or autosomal recessive disease caused by a mutation of the *DAX* gene, which is located on the X chromosome.
- Presents with 1° adrenal failure in infancy.
- Hypothalamic hypogonadism is also present.

Structural

- Usually associated with other pituitary hormonal deficiencies.
- In children, craniopharyngiomas are the most common cause. Cranial irradiation for leukaemia or brain tumours may also result in 2° hypogonadism.
- The commonest lesions in adulthood are prolactinomas.

Systemic illness

Severe illness of any kind may cause hypogonadotropic hypogonadism (📖 see Box 62.2).

Drugs

- Anabolic steroids, cocaine and narcotic drugs may all result in 2° hypogonadism.

All drugs causing hyperprolactinaemia (📖 see Box 17.1, p.115) will also cause hypogonadism.

Prader–Willi syndrome

A congenital syndrome affecting 1:25000 births caused by loss of an imprinted gene on paternally derived chromosome 15q11–13.

It should be suspected in infancy in the presence of characteristic facial features (almond eyes, down-turned mouth, strabismus, thin upper lip), severe hypotonia, poor feeding, and developmental delay. The child then develops hyperphagia due to hypothalamic dysfunction resulting in severe obesity. Other characteristic features include short stature, hypogonadotrophic hypogonadism and learning disability.

- Diabetes mellitus type II occurs in 15–40% of adults.

Laurence–Moon–Biedl syndrome

Congenital syndrome characterized by severe obesity, gonadotrophin deficiency, retinal dystrophy, polydactyly, and learning disability.

Box 62.2 Systemic illness resulting in hypogonadism

- Any acute illness (e.g. myocardial infarction, sepsis, head injury).
- Severe stress.
- Haemochromatosis.
- Endocrine disease (Cushing's syndrome, hyperprolactinaemia).
- Liver cirrhosis.
- Chronic renal failure.
- Chronic anaemia (thalassaemia major, sickle cell disease).
- GI disease (coeliac disease, Crohn's disease).
- AIDS.
- Rheumatological disease (rheumatoid arthritis).
- Respiratory disease (e.g. chronic obstructive airways disease, cystic fibrosis).
- Cardiac disease (e.g. congestive cardiac failure).

Primary hypogonadism

Due to testicular failure with normal hypothalamus and pituitary function

Diagnosis

- Low 9 a.m. serum testosterone.
- Elevated LH and FSH, low inhibin B and anti-Müllerian hormone.

Causes

Genetic

Klinefelter's syndrome.

The most common congenital form of 1° hypogonadism. It is thought that a significant number of men with Klinefelter's syndrome are not diagnosed.

- Clinical manifestations will depend on the age of diagnosis. Patients with mosaicism tend to have less severe clinical features.
  - Adolescence:
    —small firm testes (mean 5mL).
    —gynaecomastia.
    —tall stature (↑ leg length).
    —other features of hypogonadism.
    —cognitive dysfunction.
  - Adulthood:
    —reduced libido and erectile dysfunction.
    —gynaecomastia.
    —reduced facial hair.
    —obesity.
    —infertility.
  - Risks:
    —type 2 diabetes mellitus.
    —osteoporosis.
    —thromboembolism.
    —malignancies e.g. extragonadal germ cell tumours. .
- Diagnosis:
  - Karyotyping: 47,XXY in 80%; higher grade chromosomal aneuploidies (e.g. 48,XXXY) or 46,XY/47,XXY mosaicism in the remainder.
  - Low testosterone, elevated FSH and LH.
  - Elevated SHBG and oestradiol.
  - Azoospermia.
- Management:
  - Lifelong androgen replacement.
  - May need surgical reduction of gynaecomastia.
  - Fertility: intracytoplasmic sperm injection (ICSI, 📖 see Chapter 67, Infertility, pp.400–415) using testicular spermatozoa from men with Klinefelter's syndrome has resulted in successful pregnancies. However, couples should be counselled about the ↑ risk of chromosomal abnormalities in offspring.

Other chromosomal disorders

- XX males:
  - Due to an X to Y translocation with only a part of the Y present in one of the X chromosomes.
  - Incidence 1:10 000 births.
  - Similar clinical and biochemical features to Klinefelter's syndrome. In addition, short stature and hypospadias may be present.
- XX/X0 (mixed gonadal dysgenesis):
  - Occasionally phenotypically ♂ with hypospadias and intra-abdominal dysgenetic gonads.
  - Bilateral gonadectomy is essential because of the risk of neoplasia, followed by androgen replacement therapy.
- XYY syndrome:
  - Taller than average, but often have primary gonadal failure with impaired spermatogenesis.
- Y chromosome microdeletions:
  - Causes oligo/azoospermia. Testosterone levels are not usually affected.
- Noonan's syndrome:
  - Autosomal dominant disorder with an incidence of 1:1000 to 1:2500 live births.
  - 46,XY karyotype and 2° external genitalia. However, several stigmata of Turner's syndrome (short stature, webbed neck, ptosis, low set ears, lymphoedema) and ↑ risk cardiac anomalies (valvular pulmonary stenosis and hypertrophic cardiomyopathy). Most have cryptorchidism and 1° testicular failure.

Cryptorchidism

- 10% of 2° neonates have undescended testes, but most of these will descend into the scrotum eventually, so that the incidence of postpubertal cryptorchidism is < 0.5%.
- 15% of cases have bilateral cryptorchidism.

Consequences

- 75% of ♂ with bilateral cryptorchidism are infertile.
- 10% risk of testicular malignancy, highest risk in those with intra-abdominal testes.
- Low testosterone and raised gonadotropins in bilateral cryptorchidism.

Treatment

- *Orchidopexy* Best performed before 18 months, certainly before age 5 years in order to reduce risk of later infertility.
- *Gonadectomy* In patients with intra-abdominal testes, followed by androgen replacement.

Orchitis

- 25% of ♂ who develop mumps after puberty have associated orchitis and 25–50% of these will develop 1° testicular failure.
- HIV infection may also be associated with orchitis.
- 1° testicular failure may occur as part of an autoimmune disease.

Chemotherapy and radiotherapy

- Cytotoxic drugs, particularly alkylating agents, are gonadotoxic. Infertility occurs in 50% of patients following chemotherapy for most malignancies, and a significant number of ♂ require androgen replacement therapy because of low testosterone levels.
- The testes are radiosensitive so hypogonadism can occur as a result of scattered radiation during the treatment of Hodgkin's disease, for example.
- If fertility is desired, sperm should be cryopreserved prior to cancer therapy.

Other drugs

- Sulphasalazine, colchicine and high dose glucocorticoids may reversibly affect testicular function.
- Alcohol excess will also cause 1° testicular failure.

Chronic illness

Any chronic illness may affect testicular function, in particular chronic renal failure, liver cirrhosis, and haemochromatosis.

Testicular trauma

Testicular torsion is another common cause of loss of a testis, and it may also affect the function of the remaining testis.

Box 62.3 Testicular dysfunction—clinical characteristics of male hypogonadism

Testicular failure occurring before onset of puberty
- Testicular volume <5mL.
- Penis <5cm long.
- Lack of scrotal pigmentation and rugae.
- Gynaecomastia.
- High-pitched voice.
- Central fat distribution.
- Eunuchoidism:.
  - Arm span 1cm greater than height.
  - Lower segment >upper segment.
- Delayed bone age.
- No ♂ escutcheon.
- ↓ body and facial hair.

Testicular failure occurring after puberty
- Testes soft, volume <15mL.
- Normal penile length.
- Normal skeletal proportions.
- Gynaecomastia.
- Normal ♂ hair distribution but reduced amount.
- Pale skin, fine wrinkles.
- Central fat distribution.
- Osteoporosis.
- Anaemia (mild).

Clinical assessment

History

- *Developmental history* congenital urinary tract abnormalities, e.g. hypospadias, late testicular descent, or cryptorchidism.
- *Delayed or incomplete puberty.*
- *Infections* e.g. mumps, orchitis.
- *Abdominal/genital trauma.*
- *Testicular torsion.*
- *Anosmia.*
- *Drug history* e.g. sulfasalazine, antihypertensives, chemotherapy, cimetidine, radiotherapy; alcohol and recreational drugs also important.
- *General medical history* Chronic illness, particularly respiratory, neurological and cardiac.
- *Gynaecomastia* Common (☐ see Chapter 64, Gynaecomastia, p.382–386) during adolescence. Recent onset gynaecomastia in adulthood—must rule out oestrogen-producing tumour.
- *Family history* Young syndrome (☐ p.405), cystic fibrosis, Kallmann's syndrome.
- *Sexual history* Erectile function, frequency of intercourse, sexual techniques. Absence of morning erections suggests an organic cause of erectile dysfunction.

Physical examination

- Body hair distribution.
- Muscle mass and fat distribution.
- Eunuchoidism.
- Gynaecomastia.
- Genital examination:
  - *Pubic hair* normal ♂ escutcheon.
  - *Phallus* normal >5cm length and >3cm width.
  - *Testes* size (using Prader orchiometer) and consistency (normal >15m and firm).
  - Look for nodules or areas of tenderness.
- General examination: look for evidence of systemic disease.
  - Assess sense of smell and visual fields.
  - Reflexes.
  - Peripheral pulses.
  - Rectal examination.

Hormonal evaluation of testicular function

Serum testosterone

Diurnal variation in circulating testosterone, peak levels occurring in the early morning. 30% variation between highest and lowest testosterone levels, so 9 a.m. plasma testosterone essential. If level is low, this should be repeated.

Sex hormone binding globulin (SHBG)

- Only 2–4% of circulating testosterone is unbound. 50% is bound to SHBG and the rest to albumin.
- Concentrations of SHBG should be taken into account when interpreting a serum testosterone result. SHBG levels may be affected by a variety of conditions (📖 see Table 62.1).

Gonadotrophins

Raised FSH and LH in 1° testicular failure and inappropriately low in pituitary or hypothalamic hypogonadism. Should always exclude hyperprolactinaemia in 2° hypogonadism.

Oestradiol

Results from the conversion of testosterone and androstenedione by aromatase. 📖 See Table 62.2 for causes of an elevated oestradiol. Request serum oestradiol level if gynaecomastia is present or a testicular tumour is suspected.

Inhibin B and AMH

Gonadal glycoproteins secrete into the circulation. Useful markers of normal testicular functions; low if 1° testicular failure and normal if pituitary/hypothalamic dysfunction.

Other investigations

- Scrotal US (testicular volume/blood flow with Doppler/prescence of hydrocoele etc.).
- Semen analysis (a normal semen analysis is indicative of gonadal health. ♂ with low sperm count should consider sperm cryopreservation to preserve fertility).

Dynamic tests

Of limited clinical value and are thus rarely performed routinely:
- hCG stimulation test:
  - Diagnostic test for examining Leydig cell function.
  - hCG 2000IU IM given on days 0 and 2; testosterone measured on days 0, 2, and 4.
  - In prepubertal boys with absent scrotal testes, a response to hCG indicates intra-abdominal testes. Failure of testosterone to rise after hCG suggests absence of functioning testicular tissue. An exaggerated response to hCG is seen in 2° hypogonadism.

- Clomiphene stimulation test:
  - Used to assess the integrity of the hypothalamo–pituitary testicular axis.
  - A normal response to 3mg/kg (max 200mg) clomiphene daily for 7 days is a 2-fold increase in LH and FSH measured on days 0, 4, 7, and 10.
  - Subnormal response indicates hypothalamic or pituitary hypogonadism but does not differentiate between the 2.

Table 62.1 Factors affecting SHBG concentrations

Raised SHBG	Low SHBG
Androgen deficiency	Hyperinsulinaemia
GH deficiency	Obesity
Ageing	Acromegaly
Thyrotoxicosis	Androgen treatment
Oestrogens	Hypothyroidism
Liver cirrhosis	Cushing's syndrome/glucocorticoid therapy
	Nephrotic syndrome

Table 62.2 Causes of raised oestogens in ♂

Neoplasia
testicular
adrenal
hepatoma
Primary testicular failure
Liver disease
Thyrotoxicosis
Obesity
Androgen resistance syndromes
Antiandrogen therapy.

Further reading

AACE Hypogonadism Task Force. (2002). American Association of Clinical Endocrinologists Medical Guidelines for clinical practice for the evaluation and treatment of hypogonadism in adult male patients–2002 Update. *Endoc Prac* **8**(6), 439–56.

Lanfranco F, Kamischke A, Zitzmann M, *et al.* (2004). Klinefelter's syndrome. *Lancet* **364**, 273–83.

Androgen replacement therapy

Treatment aims

- *Improve libido and sexual function* Testosterone replacement therapy will induce virilization in the hypogonadal ♂ and restores libido and erectile function.
- *Improve mood and well-being* Most studies show an improvement in mood, well-being and QoL following testosterone replacement therapy.
- *Improve muscle mass and strength* Testosterone has direct anabolic effects on skeletal muscle and has been shown to increase muscle mass and strength when given to hypogonadal men. Lean body mass is also ↑ with a reduction in fat mass.
- *Prevent osteoporosis* Hypogonadism is a risk factor for osteoporosis. Testosterone inhibits bone resorption, thereby reducing bone turnover. Its administration to hypogonadal ♂ has been shown to improve bone mineral density and reduce the risk of developing osteoporosis.
- NB *Fertility* is not restored by androgen replacement therapy. ♂ with 2° hypogonadism who desire fertility may be treated with gonadotropins to initiate and maintain spermatogenesis (📖 see p.410). Prior testosterone therapy will not affect fertility prospects but should be stopped before initiating gonadotropin treatment. ♂ with 1° hypogonadism will not respond to gonadotropin or GnRH therapy.

Indications for treatment

- In ♂ with established primary or 2° hypogonadism of any cause.
- 📖 See Box 63.1 for contraindications.

Box 63.1 Contraindications for androgen replacement therapy

Absolute	Relative
• Prostate cancer.	• Benign prostate hyperplasia.
• Breast cancer.	• Polycythaemia.
	• Sleep apnoea

Pretreatment evaluation

Clinical evaluation

History or symptoms of:
- Prostatic hypertrophy.
- Breast or prostate cancer.
- Cardiovascular disease.
- Sleep apnoea.

Examination
- Rectal examination of prostate.
- Breasts.

Laboratory evaluation
- Prostatic specific antigen (PSA) (NB PSA is often low in hypo-gonadal ♂, rising to normal age-matched levels with androgen replacement).
- Haemoglobin and haematocrit.
- Serum lipids.

Box 63.2 Monitoring of therapy

3 months after initiating therapy and then 6–12-monthly:
- Clinical evaluation—relief of symptoms of androgen deficiency and exclude side effects.
- Serum testosterone.
- Rectal examination of the prostate (if >45 years).
- PSA (if >45 years).
- Haemoglobin and haematocrit.
- Serum lipids.

Risks and side effects

Prostatic disease

- Androgens stimulate prostatic growth, and testosterone replacement therapy may therefore induce symptoms of bladder outflow obstruction in ♂ with prostatic hypertrophy.
- It is unlikely that testosterone increases the risk of developing prostate cancer but it may promote the growth of an existing cancer.

Polycythaemia

Testosterone stimulates erythropoiesis. Androgen replacement therapy may increase haemoglobin levels, particularly in older ♂. It may be necessary to reduce the dose of testosterone in ♂ with clinically significant polycythaemia.

Cardiovascular disease

Testosterone replacement therapy may cause a fall in both LDL and HDL cholesterol levels, the significance of which remains unclear. The effect of androgen replacement therapy on the risk of developing coronary heart disease is unknown.

Other

- *Acne*.
- *Gynaecomastia* is occasionally enhanced by testosterone therapy, particularly in peripubertal boys. This is the result of the conversion of testosterone to oestrogens.
- *Fluid retention* may result in worsening symptoms in those with underlying congestive cardiac failure or hepatic cirrhosis.
- *Obstructive sleep apnoea* may be exacerbated by testosterone therapy.
- *Hepatotoxicity* may be induced by oral androgens, particularly the 17α alkylated testosterones.
- *Mood swings*.

Further reading

Handelsman DJ and Zajac JD (2004). Androgen deficiency and replacement therapy in men. *Medical Journal of Australia* **180**, 529–35.

Nieschlag E, Behre HM, Bouchard P, et al. (2004). Testosterone replacement therapy: current trends and future directions. *Hum Reprod Update* **10**(5), 409–19.

Rhoden EL and Morgentaler A (2004). Risks of testosterone replacement therapy and recommendations for monitoring. *New Engl J Med* **350**, 482–92

Table 63.1 Testosterone preparations

Preparation	Dose	Advantage	Problems
IM testosterone esters	250mg every 2–3 weeks. Monitor pre-dose serum testosterone (should be above the lower limit of normal).	2–3 weekly dosage Effective Cheap	Painful IM injection. Contraindicated in bleeding disorders. Wide variations in serum testosterone levels between injections which may be associated with symptoms.
'Nebido'®	1g 3-monthly (after loading dose)	Convenience of infrequent injections	
Testosterone implants	100–600mg every 3–6 months. Monitor predose serum testosterone	Physiological testosterone levels achieved. 3–6-monthly dosing	Minor surgical procedure. Risk of infection and pellet extrusion (3–10%). Must remove pellet surgically if complications of androgen replacement therapy develop.
Transdermal gel (1%)	5–10g gel daily	Physiological testosterone levels achieved. Convenience.	Skin reactions (rare) Possible person to person transfer through direct skin contact.
Transdermal patch	2.5–7.5mg daily	Physiological testosterone levels achieved.	Skin reactions—common.
Oral e.g. testosterone undecanoate and mesterolone (analogue of DHT)	40mg tds 25mg tds	Oral preparations	Highly variable efficacy and bioavailability. Rarely achieves therapeutic efficacy Multiple daily dosing. 17α alkylated testosterones are not used because of the risk of hepatotoxicity.
Buccal testosterone	30mg bd	Physiological testosterone levels achieved	Local discomfort Gingivitis Bitter taste Twice daily dosing

Gynaecomastia

Definition

Enlargement of the ♂ breast as a result of hyperplasia of the glandular tissue to a diameter of >2 cm. 📖 See Fig 64.1. Common, present in up to 1/3 of ♂ <30 years and in up to 50% of ♂ >45 years.
📖 See Box 64.1 for causes.

Box 64.1 Causes of gynaecomastia

- Physiological:
  - Neonatal
  - Puberty— ~50% of boys develop transient gynaecomastia.
  - Idiopathic—~25% of all cases.
- Drugs (possible mechanisms: oestrogen containing, androgen receptor blockers, inhibiting androgen production):
  - Oestrogens, anti-androgens, testosterone.
  - Spironolactone, ACE inhibitors, calcium antagonists, digoxin.
  - Alkylating agents.
  - Alcohol, marijuana, heroin, methadone.
  - Cimetidine.
  - Ketoconazole, metronidazole, antituberculous agents, tricyclic antidepressants, dopamine antagonists, opiates, benzodiazepines.
  - Antiretroviral drugs.
  - Imatinib (chronic myeloid leukaemia).
- Hypogonadism:
  - 1°.
  - 2°.
- Tumours:
  - Oestrogen or androgen producing testicular or adrenal tumours.
  - Human chorionic gonadotropin producing tumours, usually testicular e.g. germinoma; occasionally ectopic e.g. lung.
  - Aromatase producing testicular or hepatic tumours.
- Endocrine:
  - Thyrotoxicosis.
  - Cushing's syndrome.
  - Acromegaly.
  - Androgen insensitivity syndromes.
- Systemic illness:
  - Liver cirrhosis.
  - Chronic renal failure.
  - HIV infection.
  - Malnutrition.

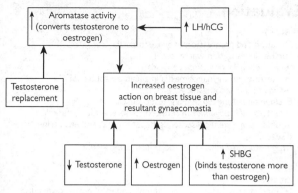

Fig. 64.1 Hormonal influences on gynaecomastia.

Evaluation

History

- Duration and progression of gynaecomastia.
- Further investigation warranted if:
  - Rapidly enlarging gynaecomastia.
  - Recent onset gynaecomastia in a lean postpubertal ♂.
  - Painful gynaecomastia.
- *Exclude underlying tumour*, e.g. testicular cancer.
- *Symptoms of hypogonadism* reduced libido, erectile dysfunction.
- *Symptoms of systemic disease* e.g. hepatic, renal, and endocrine disease.
- *Drug history* including recreational drugs, e.g. alcohol.

Physical examination

- *Breasts*:
  - Pinch breast tissue between thumb and forefinger—distinguish from fat.
  - Measure glandular tissue diameter. Gynaecomastia if >2cm.
  - If >5cm, hard, or irregular, investigate further to exclude breast cancer.
  - Look for galactorrhoea.
- *Testicular palpation*:
  - Exclude tumour.
  - Assess testicular size—?atrophy.
- *2° sex characteristics*.
- Look for evidence of *systemic disease* e.g. chronic liver or renal disease, thyrotoxicosis, Cushing's syndrome, chronic cardiac or pulmonary disease.

Investigations

Baseline investigations

- Serum testosterone.
- Serum oestradiol.
- LH and FSH.
- Prolactin.
- SHBG.
- hCG.
- Liver function tests.

Additional investigations

- If testicular tumour is suspected, e.g. raised oestradiol/hCG: testicular US.
- If adrenal tumour is suspected, e.g. markedly raised oestradiol: dehydroepiandrosterone sulphate; abdominal CT or MRI scan.
- If breast malignancy is suspected: mammography; FNAC/tissue biopsy.
- If lung cancer is suspected, e.g. raised hCG: chest radiograph.
- Other investigations depending on clinical suspicion e.g. renal or thyroid function.

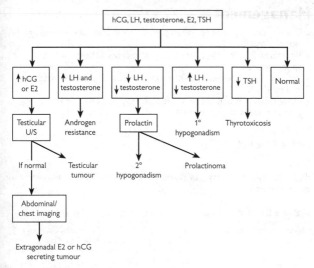

Fig. 64.2 Investigation of gynaecomastia.

Management
- Treat underlying disorder when present. Withdraw offending drugs where possible.
- Reassurance in the majority of idiopathic cases. Often resolves spontaneously.
- Treatment may be required for cosmetic reasons or to alleviate pain and tenderness.
- Drug treatment only partially effective. May be of benefit in treating gynaecomastia of recent onset.

Medical
📖 See Table 64.1.

Surgical
Reduction mammoplasty may be required in ♂ with severe and persistent gynaecomastia.

Table 64.1 Medical treatment of gynaecomastia

Tamoxifen (10–30mg/day)	Antioestrogenic effects. Particularly effective in reducing pain and swelling if used in gynaecomastia of recent onset. A 3-month trial before referral for surgery may be of benefit.
Clomifene (50–100mg/day)	Antioestrogenic. May be effective in reducing breast size in pubertal gynaecomastia.
Danazol (300–600mg/day)	Nonaromatizable androgen. May also reduce breast size in adults. Its use is limited by side effects, particularly weight gain and acne.
Testolactone (450mg/day)	Aromatase inhibitor. May be effective in reducing pubertal gynaecomastia. However, tamoxifen appears to be more effective and better tolerated.
Anastrozole (1mg/day)	Another aromatase inhibitor. Clinical trials have failed to show a beneficial effect on gynaecomastia compared with placebo.

Further reading
Khan HN and Blarney RW (2003). Endocrine treatment of physiological gynaecomastia. *BMJ* **327**, 301–2.

Erectile dysfunction

Definition

The consistent inability to achieve or maintain an erect penis sufficient for satisfactory sexual intercourse. Affects approximately 10% of ♂ and >50% of ♂ >70 years.

Physiology of male sexual function

- The erectile response is the result of the coordinated interaction of nerves, smooth muscle of the corpora cavernosa, pelvic muscles, and blood vessels.
- It is initiated by psychogenic stimuli from the brain or physical stimulation of the genitalia, which are modulated in the limbic system, transmitted down the spinal cord to the sympathetic and parasympathetic outflows of the penile tissue.
- Penile erectile tissue consists of paired corpora cavernosa on the dorsum of the penis and the corpus spongiosum. These are surrounded by fibrous tissue known as the tunica albuginea.
- In the flaccid state, the corporeal smooth muscle is contracted, minimizing corporeal blood flow and enhancing venous drainage.
- Activation of the erectile pathway results in penile smooth muscle relaxation and cavernosal arterial vasodilatation. As the corporeal sinuses fill with blood, the draining venules are compressed against the tunica albuginea so venous outflow is impaired. This results in penile rigidity and an erection.
- Corporeal vasodilatation is mediated by parasympathetic neuronal activation, which induces nitric oxide release by the cavernosal nerves. This activates guanyl cyclase, thereby ↑ cGMP, and causing smooth muscle relaxation.
- Detumescence occurs after the inactivation of cGMP by the enzyme phosphodiesterase, resulting in smooth muscle contraction and vasoconstriction.
- Ejaculation is mediated by the sympathetic nervous system.

Pathophysiology

Erectile dysfunction may thus occur as a result of several mechanisms:
- Neurological damage.
- Arterial insufficiency.
- Venous incompetence.
- Androgen deficiency.
- Penile abnormalities.

Evaluation

History

Sexual history

- Extent of the dysfunction, its duration and progression.
- Presence of nocturnal or morning erections.
- Abrupt onset of erectile dysfunction which is intermittent is often psychogenic in origin.
- Progressive and persistent dysfunction indicates an organic cause.

Symptoms of hypogonadism

Reduced libido, muscle strength and sense of well-being.

Full medical history

- E.g. diabetes mellitus, liver cirrhosis, neurological, cardiovascular or endocrine disease.
- Intermittent claudication suggests a vascular cause.
- A history of genitourinary trauma or surgery is also important.
- Recent change in bladder or bowel function may indicate neurological cause.
- Psychological history.

Drug history

Onset of impotence in relation to commencing a new medication

Social history

- Stress.
- Relationship history.
- Smoking history.
- Recreational drugs including alcohol.

Physical examination

- Evidence of 1° or 2° hypogonadism.
- Evidence of endocrine disorders:
  - Hyperprolactinaemia, thyroid dysfunction, hypopituitarism.
  - Other complications of diabetes mellitus, if present.
- Evidence of neurological disease:
  - Autonomic or peripheral neuropathy.
  - Spinal cord lesions.
- Evidence of systemic disease, e.g.:
  - Chronic liver disease.
  - Chronic cardiac disease.
  - Peripheral vascular disease.
- Genital examination.
  - Assess testicular size—?atrophy.
  - Penile abnormalities, e.g. Peyronie's disease.

📖 See Box 65.1 for causes of erectile dysfunction.

Box 65.1 Causes of erectile dysfunction

- Psychological (20%)
  - Stress, anxiety
  - Psychiatric illness
- Drugs (25%)
  - Alcohol
  - Antihypertensives, e.g.diuretics, ß-blockers, methyldopa
  - Cimetidine
  - Marijuana, heroin, methadone
  - Major tranquillizers
  - Tricyclic antidepressants, benzodiazepines
  - Digoxin
  - Glucocorticoids, anabolic steroids
  - Oestrogens, antiandrogens
- Endocrine (20%)
  - Hypogonadism (primary or secondary)
  - Hyperprolactinaemia
  - Diabetes mellitus (30–50% of ♂ with DM >6 years)
  - Thyroid dysfunction
- Neurological
  - Spinal cord disorders
  - Peripheral and autonomic neuropathies
  - Multiple sclerosis
- Vascular
  - Peripheral vascular disease
  - Trauma
  - Diabetes mellitus
  - Venous incompetence
- Other
  - Haemochromatosis
  - Debilitating diseases
  - Penile abnormalities, e.g. priapism, Peyronie's disease
  - Prostatectomy

Investigation of erectile dysfunction
Baseline investigations
- Serum testosterone.
- Prolactin, LH, and FSH if serum testosterone low.
- Fasting blood glucose.
- Thyroid function tests.
- Liver function tests.
- Renal function.
- Serum lipids.
- Serum ferritin (haemachromatosis).

Additional investigations
Rarely required. To assess vascular causes of impotence if corrective surgery is contemplated:
- *Intracavernosal injection* of a vasodilator, e.g. alprostadil E1 or papaverine. A sustained erection excludes significant vascular insufficiency.
- *Penile doppler ultrasonography* Cavernous arterial flow and venous insufficiency are assessed.

Management

Treat underlying disorder or withdraw offending drugs where possible.

Androgens

This should be 1st-line therapy in ♂ with hypogonadism (🕮 see p.378). Hyperprolactinaemia, when present, should be treated with dopamine agonists and the underlying cause of hypogonadism treated.

Phosphodiesterase (PDE) inhibitors

(🕮 See Table 65.1 and Box 65.2.)

- Act by enhancing cGMP activity in erectile tissue by blocking the enzyme PDE-5, thereby amplifying the vasodilatory action of nitric oxide and thus the normal erectile response to sexual stimulation.
- Trials indicate a 50–80% success rate.

Alprostadil

- Alprostadil results in smooth muscle relaxation and vasodilatation.
- It is administered intraurethrally and is then absorbed into the erectile bodies.
- 60–66% success rate.
- *Side effects* local pain.

Intracavernous injection

- 70–100% success rate, highest in men with non-vasculogenic impotence.
- Alprostadil is a potent vasodilator. The dose should be titrated in 1mcg increments until the desired effect is achieved in order to minimize side-effects.
- Papaverine, a phosphodiesterase inhibitor, induces cavernosal vasodilatation and penile rigidity but causes more side-effects.
- *Side-effects*
  - Priapism in 1–5%. Patients must seek urgent medical advice if an erection lasts >4h.
  - Fibrosis in the injection site in up to 5% of patients. Minimize risk by alternating sides of the penis for injection and injecting a maximum of twice a week.
  - Infection at injection site is rare.
- *Contraindication* Sickle cell disease
- *Injection technique* Avoid the midline so as to avoid urethral and neurovascular damage. Clean the injection site, hold the penis under slight tension and introduce the needle at 90°. Inject after the characteristic 'give' of piercing the fibrous capsule. Apply pressure to injection site after removing the needle to prevent bruising.

Vacuum device

Results are good, with 90% of ♂ achieving a satisfactory erection. The flaccid penis is put into the device and air is withdrawn, creating a vacuum which then allows blood to flow into the penis. A constriction band is then placed on to the base of the penis so that the erection is maintained. This should be removed within 30min.

- *Side-effects* Pain, haematoma.

Penile prosthesis

- Is usually tried in ♂ either reluctant to try other forms of therapy or when other treatments have failed. They may be semi-rigid or inflatable.
- *Complications* Infection, mechanical failure.

Psychosexual counselling

Particularly for ♂ with psychogenic impotence and in ♂ who fail to improve with the above therapies.

Surgical

- Rarely indicated as results are generally disappointing.
- Revascularization techniques may be available in specialist centres.
- Ligation of dorsal veins may restore erectile function temporarily in men with venous insufficiency, although rarely permanently.

Table 65.1 PDE-5 inhibitors

	Sildenafil	Vardenafil	Tadalafil
Dose (mg/day)	50–100	10–20	10–20
Recommended interval between drug administration and sexual activity	60min	30–60min	>30min
Half life (hours)	3–4	4–5	17
Adverse effects (%):			
Headaches	15–30	7–15	7–20
Facial flushing	10–25	10	1–5
Dyspepsia	2–15	0.5–6	1–15
Nasal congestion	1–10	3–7	4–6
Visual disturbance	1–10	0–2	0.1

Box 65.2 PDE-5 inhibitors—contraindications and cautions

Contraindications
- Recent myocardial infarction/stroke.
- Unstable angina.
- Current nitrate use including isosorbide mononitrate/GTN.
- Hypotension (<90/50 mmHg).
- Severe heart failure.
- Severe hepatic impairment.
- Retinitis pigmentosa.
- Ketoconazole or HIV protease inhibitors.

Cautions (reduce dose)
- Hypertension.
- Heart disease.
- Peyronies disease.
- Sickle cell anaemia.
- renal or hepatic impairment.
- Elderly.
- Leukaemia.
- Multiple myeloma.
- Bleeding disorders e.g., active peptic ulcer disease.

Avoid concomitant opiates, including dihydrocodeine—may get prolonged erections

Further reading

Beckman TJ et al (2006). Evaluation and medical management of erectile dysfunction. *Mayo Clinic Proc* **81**, 385–90.

Cohan P and Korenman SG (2001). Erectile dysfunction. *J Clin Endocrinol Metab* **86**, 2391–4.

Fazio L and Brick G (2004). Erectile dysfunction: management update. *Can Med Assoc J* **170**(9), 1429–37.

Testicular tumours

Epidemiology

- 6/100 000 ♂ per year.
- Incidence rising, particularly in North West Europe.
- 📖 See Table 66.1 for classification.

Risk factors

- Cryptorchidism.
- Gonadal dysgenesis.
- Infertility/reduced spermatogenesis.

Table 66.1 Classification of testicular tumours

Tumours		Tumour markers
Germ cell tumours (95%)	Seminoma	None
	Non-seminoma	hCG, α-fetoprotein, CEA
	Mixed	
Stromal tumours (2%)	Leydig cell	
	Sertoli cell	
Gonadoblastoma (2%)		
Other (1%)	Lymphoma	
	Carcinoid	

Prognosis

Seminomas

- 95% cure for early disease. 80% cure for stages II/IV.
- ↑ incidence of 2nd tumours and leukaemias 20 years after therapy.

Non-seminoma germ cell tumours

- 90% cure in early disease, falling to 60% in metastatic disease.
- ↑ incidence of 2nd tumours and leukaemias 20 years after therapy.

Stromal tumours

- Excellent prognosis for benign tumours.
- Malignant tumours are aggressive and are poorly responsive to treatment.

Further reading

Griffin JE and Wilson JD (1998). Disorders of the testes and male reproductive tract. In Wilson JD, Foster DW, Kronenberg HM, Larson PR (eds.), *William's Textbook of Endocrinology*, 9th edn, WB Saunders:Philadelphia, pp.819–76.

Infertility

Definition

- Infertility, defined as failure of pregnancy after 2 years of unprotected regular (2 × week) sexual intercourse, affects approximately 10% of all couples.
- Couples who fail to conceive after 1 year of regular unprotected sexual intercourse should be investigated.
- If there is a known predisposing factor or the ♀ partner is over 35 years of age then investigation should be offered earlier.

Causes

📖 See Boxes 67.1 and 67.2.

- ♀ factors (e.g. PCOS, tubal damage) 35%.
- ♂ factors (idiopathic gonadal failure in 60%) 25%.
- Combined factors 25%.
- Unexplained infertility 15%.

Box 67.1 Causes of female infertility

- Anovulation:
  - PCOS (80% of anovulatory disorders).
  - 2° hypogonadism.
  - Hyperprolactinaemia.
  - Thyroid dysfunction.
  - Hypothalamic disease.
  - Pituitary disease.
  - Systemic illness.
  - Drugs, e.g. anabolic steroids.
  - POF (5% of anovulatory disorders).
- Tubal disorders:
  - Infective, e.g. chlamydia.
  - Endometriosis.
  - Surgery.
- Cervical mucus defects.
- Uterine abnormalities:
  - Congenital.
  - Intrauterine adhesions.
  - Uterine fibroids.

Box 67.2 Causes of male infertility

- Primary gonadal failure:
  - Genetic e.g. Klinefelter's syndrome, Y chromosome microdeletions, immotile cilia/Kartagener syndrome, cystic fibrosis.
  - Congenital cryptorchidism.
  - Orchitis.
  - Torsion or trauma.
  - Chemotherapy and radiotherapy.
  - Other toxins, e.g. alcohol, anabolic steroids.
  - Varicocoele.
  - Idiopathic.
- 2° gonadal failure:
  - Kallman's syndrome (📖 see Secondary hypogonadism, p.366).
  - IHH.
  - Structural hypothalamic/pituitary disease.
- Genital tract abnormalities:
  - Obstructive congenital, infective, postsurgical.
  - Sperm autoimmunity.
- Erectile dysfunction.
- Drugs e.g. spironolactone, corticosteroids, sulfasalazine.
- Systemic disease e.g. cystic fibrosis, Crohn's disease, and other chronic debilitating diseases.

Evaluation

Sexual history

- *Frequency of intercourse* Sexual intercourse every 2–3 days should be encouraged.
- *Use of lubricants* Should be avoided because of the detrimental effect on semen quality.

Female factors

History

- *Age* Fertility declines rapidly after the age of 36 years.
- *Menstrual history*
  - Age at menarche.
  - Length of menstrual cycle and its regularity (e.g. oligo/amenorrhoea).
  - Presence or absence of intermenstrual spotting.
- *Hot flushes* may be indicative of oestrogen deficiency.
- *Spontaneous galactorrhoea* may be caused by hyperprolactinaemia.
- *Hypothalamic hypogonadism* suggested by excessive physical exercise (e.g. running >4 miles/day) or weight loss in excess of 10% in 1 year.
- *Drug history:*
  - Drugs which may cause hyperprolactinaemia (🕮 see Box 17.1, p.115), including cocaine and marijuana.
  - Smoking is thought have an adverse effect on fertility.
  - The use of anabolic steroids may cause 2° hypogonadism.
  - Cytotoxic chemotherapy or radiotherapy may cause ovarian failure.
- *Medical history* diabetes mellitus, thyroid or pituitary dysfunction, and other systemic illnesses.
- Exclude *tubal disease*
  - Recurrent vaginal or urinary tract infections may predispose to pelvic inflammatory disease (PID).
  - Dyspareunia and dysmenorrhoea are often present.
  - Sexually transmitted disease and previous abdominal or gynaecological surgery all predispose to fallopian tube obstruction.
- *2° infertility* Details of previous pregnancies including abortions (spontaneous and therapeutic) and ectopic pregnancies should be ascertained.
- *Family history* Suggestive of risk of POF, PCOS, endometriosis

Physical examination

- *BMI* The ideal BMI for fertility is 20–29.
- *2° sexual characteristics* If absent, look for evidence of Turner's syndrome.
- *Hyperandrogenism* PCOS.
- *Galactorrhoea* Hyperprolactinaemia.
- *External genitalia and pelvic examination.*

Investigations

📖 See Fig. 67.1.

- Assess ovulatory function:
  - In ♀ with regular menstrual cycles—measure a midluteal progesterone (day 21 or approximately 7 days before expected onset of menses).
  - Check serum FSH and LH. In ♀ who are not amenorrhoeic this should be measured on day 2–6 of the menstrual cycle (day 1 = first day of menses). Follicular phase FSH>10 is indicative of reduced ovarian reserve. Ovarian failure is diagnosed if FSH>30.
  - Measure TSH, free T4, and serum prolactin in ♀ with irregular menstrual cycles or who are not ovulating.
- *Karyotype* If 1° ovarian failure is present (raised FSH, LH)
- *Serum testosterone, androstenedione, DHEA, sex hormone binding globulin, and 17OH progesterone* if there is clinical evidence of hyperandrogenism, in the presence of irregular menstrual cycles or if anovulation is confirmed.
- *MRI of the pituitary fossa* in hyperprolactinaemia and hypogonadotropic hypogonadism.
- *Exclude cervical infection* send vaginal discharge for bacteriology and do chlamydia trachomatis serology
- *Pelvic US* assess uterine and ovarian anatomy
- *Assess tubal patency* (refer to specialist multidisciplinary fertility clinic)
  - Hysterosalpingography (HSG) or laparoscopy and dye test (do in the early follicular phase of cycle to avoid doing during pregnancy)
  - Give prophylactic antibiotics if chlamydia status is unknown to avoid postoperative infection.
- *Postcoital test* to assess cervical mucus receptivity to sperm penetration and measurement of *antisperm antibodies* are rarely performed as they are unreliable and the results do not alter management.

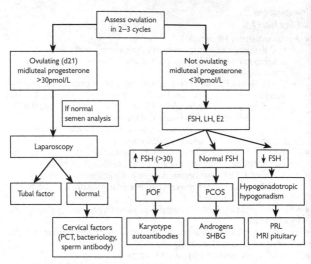

Fig. 67.1 Investigation of ♀ infertility.

Male factors

History and physical examination

- Symptoms of androgen deficiency:
  - Reduced libido and potency.
  - Reduced frequency of shaving.
  - May be asymptomatic.
- *Drug history:*
  - Drug or alcohol abuse and the use of anabolic steroids may all contribute to hypogonadism.
  - Other drugs that may affect spermatogenesis eg sulphasalazine, methotrexate.
  - Cytotoxic chemotherapy may cause 1° testicular failure.
- *History of infection* e.g. mumps, orchitis, sexually transmitted disease or epididymitis.
- *Bronchiectasis* may be associated with epididymal obstruction (Young syndrome) or severe aesthenospermia (immotile cilia syndrome).
- *Testicular injury or surgery* may cause disordered spermatogenesis.
- *2° sex characteristics* may be absent in congenital hypogonadism.
- *Anosmia* Kallmann's syndrome
- *Eunuchoid habitus* (📖 see Box 62.3, p.373) suggestive of prepubertal hypogonadism.
- *Gynaecomastia* may suggest hypogonadism.
- *Testicular size* (using orchidometer):
  - Normal 15–25mL.
  - Reduced to <15mL in hypogonadism.
  - In Klinefelter's syndrome, they are often <5mL.
  - In patients with normal testicular size, suspect genital tract obstruction, e.g. congenital absence of vas deferens.
- Examine rest of *external genitalia* look for penile/urethral abnormalities and epididymal thickening.

Investigations
🕮 See Fig. 67.2.

Semen analysis
Essential in the diagnostic work up of any infertile couple.
• If *normal* (🕮 see Table 67.1) then a ♂ cause is excluded.
• If *abnormal*, then repeat semen analysis approximately 6–12 weeks later.
• Semen collection should be performed after 3 days of sexual
  abstinence. 🕮 See Table 67.1 for interpretation of results.
• If *azoospermia* is present, then rule out obstruction if FSH and
  testosterone concentrations are normal.
• *Asthenospermia*, or immotile sperm, is usually due to immunological
  infertility or infection, e.g. of the prostate (high semen viscosity and pH,
  and leukocytospermia)

FSH, LH, and testosterone levels
• FSH may be elevated in the presence of normal LH and testosterone
  levels and oligospermia. This may be seen in ♂ who are normally
  virilized but infertile as a result of disordered spermatogenesis.
• Low FSH, LH and testosterone concentrations suggest
  2° hypogonadism. An MRI of the pituitary gland and hypothalamus
  is necessary to exclude organic disease.

Further investigations
• *Urinary bacteriology* should be performed in ♂ with leukocytospermia.
• *Scrotal US* may help in the diagnosis of chronic epididymitis. ♂ being
  investigated for infertility are at ↑ risk of testicular tumours.
• *Karyotyping* may be helpful in ♂ with 1° testicular failure. Klinefelter's
  syndrome (47,XXY) is a cause of infertility, and deletions on the long arm
  of the Y chromosome have been found in a significant proportion
  of azoospermic ♂.
• *Sperm antibodies* in semen should not be measured routinely as specific
  treatment is rarely effective.
• *Testicular biopsy* is rarely diagnostic, but may be used to retrieve sperm
  for assisted reproduction techniques in specialist fertility centres.
• *Sperm function tests* are not performed routinely.

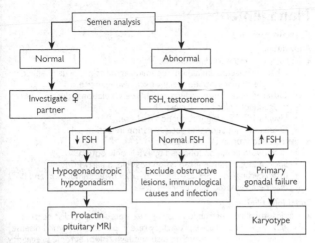

Fig. 67.2 Investigation of ♂ infertility.

Table 67.1 WHO criteria for normal semen analysis[1]

Test	Normal values (fertile)	Nomenclature for abnormal values
Volume	>2mL	Aspermia (no ejaculate)
pH	>7.2	
Total sperm number	>40 × 10⁶/ejaculate	Azoospermia (no sperm in ejaculate)
Sperm concentration	>48 × 10⁶/mL	Oligozoospermia
Motility	>63% progressive motility	Asthenospermia
Morphology	>12% normal forms	Teratospermia
Live sperm	>75%	Necrospermia
Leucocytes	<1 × 10⁶/mL	Leucocytospermia

[1] Reproduced with permission from Guzick DS, Overstreet JW, Factor-Litvak P, et al. (2001). Sperm morphology, motility, and concentration in fertile and infertile men. *New Engl J Med* **345**, 1388–93

Management

Female partner

Anovulation

- *Hypogonadotrophic (WHO class 1):*
  - If hyperprolactinaemic then dopamine agonists are usually effective
  - Lifestyle changes if underweight/excessive exercise.
  - Otherwise, ovulation induction (📖 see Ovulation induction p.412).
- *Normogonadotrophic (WHO class 2):*
  - Usually PCOS: weight reduction if obese.
  - Ovulation induction (📖 see Ovulation induction p.412).
- *Hypergonadotrophic (WHO class 3):*
  - POF ovum donation followed by IVF is only option.
  - Spontaneous transient remission possible in early POF.
  - If still cycling and FSH 15–25IU/L, ovarian hyperstimulation and IVF may be attempted, but poor results.

Tubal infertility

- Surgical tubal reconstruction may be attempted in specialist centres.
- 50–60% 2-year cumulative pregnancy rate in patients with mild disease, but only 10% in more severe disease and high risk of ectopic pregnancy, so IVF may be more appropriate in ♀ with severe disease.
- Cumulative pregnancy rate at least 50% following IVF (20–25% per cycle) unless hydrosalpinx is present. ♀ with hydrosalpinx should be offered salpingectomy prior to IVF to improve success rates.

Endometriosis

- *Minimal/mild:*
  - GnRH agonists, danazol, and progestagens do not improve fertility.
  - Laparoscopic destruction of superficial disease improves pregnancy chances. Resection of ovarian endometriomas may improve ovarian folliculogenesis and thus fertility.
  - Assisted reproductive techniques (ART) (Table 67.2) give pregnancy rate of 25–35% per cycle.
- *Moderate/severe:*
  - Surgery may improve fertility. However, ART often necessary.

Vaginal/cervical factors

Infection Each episode of acute PID causes infertility in 10–15% of cases. *Chlamydia trachomatis* is responsible for half the cases of PID in the developed countries. Treat both partners with antibiotics.

Uterine factors

- *Intracavity fibroids, polyps, uterine septum* can be resected hysteroscopically with high chance of restoring fertility.
- *Intramural fibroids* may also reduce fertility and may require myomectomy.
- *Fibroid embolisation* is not recommended for ♀ wishing fertility as safety in pregnancy not established.

Table 67.2 Assisted reproduction techniques (ART)

Technique	Indications	Pregnancy rates	Notes
Intrauterine insemination (IUI) (usually offered up to 6 cycles)	Unexplained infertility mild oligozoospermia (>2×10⁶ motile sperm) mild endometriosis	<15% per cycle 15%	Washed and prepared motile spermatozoa are injected into the uterine cavity through a catheter just before ovulation. Superovulation may improve success rates but is associated with an increased risk of multiple pregnancy.
In vitro fertilisation (IVF)	Most forms of infertility unless severe male factor. Do not use in women with tubal disease.	20–30% pregnancy rate per cycle. 80–90% delivery rate after 6 cycles in women under the age of 35 years. Success rates markedly reduced after 40 years of age. Babies conceived by IVF have a 2× increased risk of low birth weight and preterm delivery.	After superovulation, ovarian follicles are aspirated under ultrasonic guidance and are fertilised with prepared sperm in vitro. The embryos are then transferred back into the uterine cavity, usually 48 hours after insemination. Luteal support using progesterone supplementation (pessaries or PO) is then provided until pregnancy is confirmed. May adopt a similar technique in women with premature ovarian failure using donated ova which are then fertilised in vitro with partner's sperm. Hormonal support will be required following embryo transfer.
Gamete intrafallopian transfer (GIFT)	Most forms of infertility unless severe male factor.	similar to IVF	Similar to IVF except that retrieved follicles and sperm are injected laparoscopically into a fallopian tube to fertilise naturally. Rarely performed in the UK as it offer's little advantage over IVF.
Intracytoplasmic sperm injection (ICSI)	Male infertility	20–30% per cycle if female partner under 40 years of age. There is a small risk of sex chromosome abnormalities in males (1%) conceived following ICSI.	Viable spermatozoa are injected directly into oocytes retrieved following superovulation. Embryos are then implanted into the uterus. Spermatozoa may be concentrated from an ejaculate or be aspirated from the epididymis or testis in men with obstructive azoospermia.

Male partner
Hypogonadotrophic hypogonadism
- Gonadotrophins: chorionic gonadotrophin 1500–2000IU IM 2 × week. Most also require FSH/hMG 150IU IM 3 × week. Monitor serum testosterone and testicular size. Main side-effect: gynaecomastia.
- *or*
- Pulsatile gonadorelin using a SC infusion pump (📖 see p.414). Dose varies from 25–500ng/kg every 90–120min. Titrate to normalize LH, FSH, and testosterone. Will not work in pituitary disease.
  - Once testes are >8mL, semen analysis every 3–6 months. Takes at least 2 years to maximize spermatogenesis. Normalization of spermatogenesis in 80–90% of ♂.
  - Once spermatogenesis is induced it may be maintained by hCG alone.

Idiopathic semen abnormalities
There is no evidence to suggest that the use of androgens, gonadotropins or antioestrogens help improve fertility in ♂ with idiopathic disorders of spermatogenesis.

Obstructive azoospermia
- Reversal of vasectomy will result in successful pregnancy in up to 50% of cases within 2 years.
- Microsurgery is possible for most other causes with successful pregnancies in 25–35% of couples within 18 months of treatment. During surgery, sperm is often retrieved and stored for possible future intracytoplasmic sperm injection (ICSI).

Varicocoele
Controversial association with ♂ subfertility. Surgical correction is currently not recommended for fertility treatment as there is little evidence that surgery improves pregnancy rates.

Unexplained infertility
Definition
Infertility despite normal sexual intercourse occurring at least twice weekly, normal semen analysis, documentation of ovulation in several cycles, and normal patent tubes (by laparoscopy).

Management
30–50% will become pregnant within 3 years of expectant management. If not pregnant by then, chances that spontaneous pregnancy will occur are greatly reduced and ART should be considered. In ♀ >34 years of age then expectant management is not an option and up to 6 cycles of IUI, or IVF should be considered.

Results
- IUI can achieve a pregnancy rate of 15% per cycle and cumulative delivery rate after several cycles = 50%.
- IVF offers a live birth rate per cycle of >25% in younger ♀, and a cumulative delivery rate approaching 80%. ICSI allows IVF to be offered in severely oligospermia, with pregnancy rates equivalent to standard IVF. Slight increase in congenital malformations after ICSI. Significant risk of multiple pregnancy with any form of ART.

Ovulation induction

Indications
- Anovulation due to:
  - PCOS.
  - Hypopituitarism.
  - Hypogonadotrophic hypogonadism.
- Controlled ovarian hyperstimulation for ART.

Pretreatment assessment
- Exclude thyroid dysfunction and hyperprolactinaemia.
- Check rubella serology.
- Confirm normal semen analysis.
- Confirm tubal patency (laparoscopy, hysterosalpingogram (HSG), or hysterosalping-contrast-sonography (HyCoSy)) prior to gonadotrophin use and/or after failed clomiphene use.
- Optimize lifestyle: maintain satisfactory BMI, exercise in moderation, reduce alcohol intake and stop smoking.
- Baseline pelvic US is essential to exclude ovarian masses and uterine abnormalities prior to treatment.

Clomifene citrate
- *Mode of action:*
  - Binds to oestrogen receptors in hypothalamus, blocking normal −ve feedback thereby ↑ pulse frequency of GnRH. This stimulates FSH and LH release, thereby stimulation the production of 1 or more dominant ovarian follicles.
  - Antioestrogen effect on endometrium, cervix, and vagina.
- *Indications* eugonadotropic anovulation, e.g. PCOS. May also be used in unexplained infertility. Requires normal hypothalamo–pituitary–ovarian axis to work therefore ineffective in hypogonadotrophic hypogonadism.
- *Contraindications* hepatic dysfunction
- *Administration* Start on days 2–5 of menstrual cycle (may have to induce bleed by giving a progestagen for 10 days) and take for a total of 5 days.
- *Dose:*
  - Start on 50mg/day and increase by 50mg every month until midluteal progesterone is >30nmol/L.
  - Spontaneous ovulation should occur 5–10 days after last day of medication.
  - Remain on optimum dose for 6–12 months.
  - Most require 50–100mg/day.
  - Ideally follicle growth should be monitored by regular vaginal US to minimize the risk of multiple pregnancies and ovarian hyperstimulation.
- *Efficacy:*
  - 80–90% ovulate, with conception rates of 50–60% in first 6 ovulatory cycles. May enhance chances of ovulation in non-responders by the administration of 10 000 IU of hCG midcycle (use US guidance; administer hCG when leading follicle is at least 20mm).
  - In overweight ♀ with PCOS who remain anovulatory, the addition of metformin (500mg tds) to clomifene may improve ovulation rates.

- *Side-effects*
  - Hot flushes in 10%, mood swings, depression and headaches in 1%, pelvic pain in 5%, nausea in 2%, breast tenderness in 5%, hair loss in 0.3%, visual disturbances in 1.5%.
  - Ovarian hyperstimulation syndrome (OHSS) in 1%.
  - Multiple pregnancies in 7–10%.
- *Risk of ovarian cancer* Unknown. Infertility is associated with an ↑ risk of ovarian cancer. Additionally, one study suggests a 2-fold ↑ risk of low grade ovarian cancer following long-term clomifene use. Further studies necessary but currently recommended maximum treatment duration is 6–12 months.
- *Tamoxifen* is also an antioestrogen which has similar properties to clomifene. It can be used to induce ovulation with results comparable to clomifene. The dose used is 20–40mg OD for 5–7 days starting on day 2–5 of menstrual cycle.

Ovarian drilling

- Laparoscopic ovarian drilling by laser or diathermy in 4–10 points on the surface of the ovaries may be used in ♀ with PCOS who have failed to conceive on clomifene.
- Its ovulation rate of >80% and pregnancy rate of >60% are comparable to gonadotropin therapy without the risk of multiple pregnancy or ovarian hyperstimulation syndrome. It is most effective in slim ♀ with PCOS with a high LH.
- There is a low risk of pelvic adhesions following ovarian diathermy and a theoretical risk of premature ovarian failure.

Gonadotrophins

- *Indications:*
  - Hypogonadotrophic hypogonadism.
  - ♀ with PCOS who are clomifene resistant.
  - For superovulation as part of ART.
- *Dose and administration* Several regimens available, all require close monitoring with twice weekly oestradiol (E2) measurements and vaginal US. One suggested regime (low dose step-up approach):
  - Start at 50–75IU/day hMG (or FSH) on day 2–4 of the menstrual cycle. On day 7 (or 14) of treatment measure serum E2 and perform a vaginal US. If E2 <200pmol/L and there has been no change in follicle development then increase hMG (or FSH) by 37.5IU. Continue to monitor and increase hMG (or FSH) by 37.5IU (maximum dose 225IU/day) on a weekly basis until there is an ovarian response.
  - If >3 mature follicles (>14mm) develop or E2 >3000 pmol/L then abandon cycle and restart on half-dose hMG/FSH because of risk of OHSS.
  - Otherwise, give hCG at a dose of 5000IU to trigger ovulation when follicle >18mm diameter. May increase to 10 000IU in subsequent cycle if ovulation doesn't occur.
  - May use gonadotrophins for a total of 6 cycles. If unsuccessful then consider ART.
- *Efficacy* 80–85% pregnancy rate after 6 cycles.

- *Side-effects*
  Multiple pregnancy (20%)—OHSS.
- *OHSS:*
  - A potentially fatal syndrome of ovarian enlargement and ↑ vascular permeability with accumulation of fluid in the peritoneal, pleural and pericardial cavities. Occurs during the luteal phase of the cycle, i.e. after hCG stimulation and is more severe if pregnancy occurs due to endogenous hCG production.
  - Mild OHSS occurs in up to 25% of stimulated cycles and results in abdominal bloating and nausea. It resolves with bed rest and fluid replacement. Severe OHSS, associated with hypotension, markedly enlarged ovaries, ascites, and pleural and pericardial effusions, occurs in <0.1%. ♀ need to be hospitalized and resuscitated as there is an ↑ mortality from disseminated intravascular coagulation and pulmonary emboli. Management should be led by an expert reproductive endocrinologist.
  - OHSS is triggered by hCG so is best prevented by witholding hCG during at-risk cycles. Risk factors include the presence of multiple ovarian follicles, PCOS, young age and a previous history of OHSS.
- IVF superovulation should be accompanied by use of a GnRH agonist starting from mid-luteal phase of the preceding cycle (long protocol) or a GnRH antagonist starting in the mid follicular phase of the stimulation cycle (antagonist protocol). These strategies precent premature ovulation before eggs can be collected and significantly improve pregnancy rates

GnRH treatment
- *Indications* Hypothalamic hypogonadism with normal pituitary function.
- *Dose and administration* Pulsatile GnRH using an infusion pump which is worn continuously. This delivers a dose of GnRH every 60–90 min. The dose may be administered either intravenously (2.5–10mcg/90min) or subcutaneously (20mcg/90min).
- *Monitoring:*
  - Monitor E2 levels because risk of hypo-oestrogenaemia if GnRH is given too frequently.
  - Little risk of OHSS or multiple pregnancies so ultrasonic monitoring is not usually necessary.
- *Side-effects* Allergic reaction.
- *Efficacy* Cumulative pregnancy rate of 70–90%.

Cryopreservation, fertility, and cancer treatment
- Chemotherapy and/or radiotherapy for some cancers can adversely affect ♂ and ♀ fertility, resulting in gonadal failure.
- ♂ patients should be offered the chance of sperm cryopreservation and storage prior to commencing cancer treatment so that future fertility may be an option.

- Cryostorage of oocytes and/or ovarian tissue is less successful. However, it should still be offered to ♀ of reproductive age about to embark on cancer treatment if they are well enough to undergo ovarian stimulation and egg retrieval. They should be counselled about the low chance of a successful pregnancy using such techniques. Storage of frozen embryos is more successful but requires the young ♀ cancer patient to already be in a stable relationship with the potential father of her children. Superovulation/IVF with embryo freeing requires a 3–6 week delay in initiation of chemo/radiotherapy which must be sanctioned by the lead oncologist.

Human Fertilisation and Embryology Act (UK)

- A legal framework developed in 1990 to provide guidance on fertility treatment, storage of human eggs, sperm and embryos, and research on human embryos. For example, human eggs and sperm can be stored for a maximum of 10 years and embryos for a maximum of 5 years. Research can only be done on embryos younger than 14 days, no part of genetic make up of the embryo can be altered and the research must be only for the purposes specified in the Act.
- There have been 2 amendments of the Act to date; in 2000 to allow the use of insemination using a dead ♂'s sperm under defined circumstances, and 2001 to allow research into therapeutic cloning. This Act is about to be completely revised (2008).
- The Human Fertilisation and Embryology Authority (HFEA) is a statutory body set up to inspect, monitor and license fertility centres offering IVF, ICSI, and/or donor sperm or egg insemination and to regulate all research involving human embryos. It is also required to keep a register of all IVF treatment cycles and of all children born as a result of IVF or donor sperm or oocytes. The HFEA also provides information to couples seeking fertility treatment or potential donors.
- The HFEA is accountable to the Secretary of State for Health and advises government ministers as required, particularly regarding new developments in fertility technology or research.

Further reading

Braude P and Muhammed S (2003).Assisted conception and the law in the United Kingdom. *BMJ* **327**, 978–81.

Hirsh A (2003). Male subfertility. *BMJ* **327**, 669–72.

Hamilton-Fairley D and Taylor A (2003). Anovulation. *BMJ* **327**, 546–9.

Royal College of Obsterics and Gynaecology (2004). *Fertility assessment and treatment for people with fertility problems.* RCOG, pp.1–208.

Disorders of sexual differentiation

Clinical presentation

- *Infancy* ambiguous genitalia (📖 evaluation is discussed in Ambiguous genitalia, p.561)
- *Puberty:*
  - Failure to progress through puberty (♂ or ♀ phenotype).
  - 1° amenorrhoea in a ♀ phenotype.
  - Virilization of a ♀ phenotype.
- *Adulthood:*
  - Hypogonadism.
  - Infertility.

Evaluation

- *Karyotype* 46,XX vs 46,XY ♂ or ♀
- Imaging:
  - Look for presence of testes or ovaries and uterus.
  - Most easily performed using pelvic US but MRI may be more sensitive in identifying internal genitalia, and abnormally sited gonads in cryptorchidism.

Hormonal evaluation

- LH/FSH.
- Testosterone, androstenedione, SHBG.
- 17-hydroxyprogesterone ± ACTH stimulation (📖 see Investigations, p.306).
- hCG stimulation test (📖 see Clinical assessment, p.375)—to assess the presence of functioning testicular material. Measure testosterone, androstenedione, DHT, and SHBG post-stimulation.
- Others depending on clinical suspicion, e.g. 5-reductase deficiency—check DHT levels before and after hCG stimulation.

For causes 📖 see Box 68.1.

Box 68.1 Causes of disorders of sexual differentiation

(📖 see also Ambiguous genitalia, p.561.)

46,X— undervirilized male
- Gonadal differentiation abnormalities, e.g. gonadal dysgenesis:
  - Cause unknown in the majority.
  - May result from 45,X/46,XY mosaicism or SRY gene mutation.
- Leydig cell abnormalities:
  - Autosomal recessive.
  - Due to inactivating LH receptor gene mutation.
- Biochemical defects of androgen synthesis, e.g.:
  - 3β-HSD, 17α-hydroxylase/17,20-desmolase or 17β-HSD deficiencies.
- Androgen receptor defects:
  - Androgen insensitivity syndrome (p.418).
- 5α-reductase deficiency:
  - Mutation of 5α-reductase type 2 gene.
  - Autosomal recessive inheritance.
  - High testosterone but low DHT concentrations.
  - Phenotype can range from ♀ external genitalia to ♂ with hypospadias. Patients characteristically become virilized after puberty.
- Persistent Müllerian duct syndrome:
  - Müllerian inhibitory substance (MIS), also called anti-Müllerian hormone (AMH), or MIS receptor gene mutation.
- True hermaphrodite.

46,XX—virilized female
- Excess fetal androgens—CAH:
  - 21-OH deficiency (90%).
  - 11B-OH deficiency.
- Excess maternal androgens:
  - Drugs.
  - Virilizing tumours.
- Placental aromatase deficiency.
- 46,XX ♂
  - Due to a Y to X translocation so that the SRY gene is present.
  - Phenotype similar to Klinefelter's syndrome.
- True hermaphrodite.

Androgen insensitivity syndrome

Pathogenesis

- Results from a mutation in androgen receptor gene located on chromosome Xq11–12. Several mutations may occur, inherited in an X-linked recessive fashion. However, approximately 40% of patients have a –ve family history. Major gene deletions result in complete androgen insensitivity but the more common amino acid substitutions can result in any of the phenotypes.
- Incidence 1:20 000–1:64 000.

Clinical features

- *Complete androgen insensitivity (testicular feminization)* results in normal ♀ external genitalia. However the vagina is often shorter than normal and may rarely be absent. No ♂ external sex organs present, but remnants of Müllerian structures are occasionally present. Testes are usually located in the abdomen or in the inguinal canal. There is no spermatogenesis.
- Often present during puberty with 1° amenorrhoea. Height is above ♀ average and breast development may be normal. These patients have a normal ♀ habitus but have little or no pubic and axillary hair. Gender identity and psychological development are ♀.
- *Partial androgen insensitivity* has a wide phenotypic spectrum, ranging from ambiguous genitalia to a normal ♂ phenotype presenting with infertility.
  - Phenotypic ♀ with mild virilization.
  - Reifenstein's syndrome (undervirilized ♂ with gynaecomastia and hypospadias).
  - Infertile ♂.
- 9% risk of seminoma.

Hormonal evaluation

- Testosterone levels are in the normal or often above normal ♂ range. hCG stimulation results in a further rise in testosterone, with little increase in SHBG.
- Oestradiol levels are higher than in normal ♂, but lower than the ♀ average. Oestrogen is produced by the testes and from peripheral aromatization of testosterone.
- LH levels are usually markedly elevated, but FSH is normal.
- Genetic testing is possible in some centres.

Management

- Orchidectomy to prevent malignancy. Exact timing of surgery is controversial but it is usually performed in adolescence after attaining puberty. In phenotypic ♀ with partial androgen insensitivity gonadectomy may be performed before puberty to avoid virilization.
- Oestrogen replacement therapy in phenotypic ♀
- High dose androgen therapy in ♂ with Reifenstein's syndrome may improve virilization.

True hermaphroditism

Pathogenesis

- Unknown. May be familial.
- Affected individuals have both ovarian and testicular tissue, either in the same gonad (ovotestis), or an ovary on one side and a testis on the other. A uterus and a fallopian tube are usually present, the latter on the side of the ovary or ovotestis. Wolffian structures may be present in a 1/3 of individuals on the side of the testis. The testicular tissue is usually dysgenetic although the ovarian tissue may be normal.

Clinical features

- Most individuals have ambiguous genitalia and are raised as ♂, but just under 10% have normal ♀ external genitalia.
- At puberty, 50% of individuals menstruate, which may present as cyclic haematuria in ♂ and most develop breasts.
- Feminization and virilization vary widely. Most are infertile, but fertility has been reported.
- 2% risk of gonadal malignancy, higher in 46,XY individuals.

Evaluation

- 46,XX in 70%, 46,XX/46,XY in 20% and 46,XY in 10%.
- Hypergonadotropic hypogonadism is usual.
- Diagnosis can only be made on gonadal biopsy.

General principles of management

Assignment of gender and reconstructive surgery

Virilized females (female pseudohermaphroditism)

- The majority are brought up as ♀.
- The timing of feminizing surgery remains controversial but is usually deferred until adolescence. The decision should be made on an individual basis, by a multidisciplinary specialist team, the parents and ideally the patient. It appears that a significant number of children who have surgery performed during infancy will require further surgery in their teens. The results of feminizing genitoplasty, which involves clitoral reduction and vaginoplasty, with regard to sexual function are unclear.

Undervirilized males (male pseudohermaphroditism)

- The decision regarding gender reassignment is more complex and depends on the degree of sexual ambiguity in addition to the cause of the disorder and the potential for normal sexual function and fertility.
- Individuals with complete androgen insensitivity are assigned a ♀ sex as they are resistant to testosterone therapy, develop ♀ sexual characteristics, and have a ♀ gender identity. They may require vaginoplasty in adolescence.
- Sex assignment of other forms of ♂ pseudohermaphroditism depends on phallic size. However, the decision should be made by a specialist multidisciplinary team involving parents who should be fully informed.
- A trial of 3 months of testosterone may be used to enhance phallic growth.
- Penile reconstruction and orchidopexy by an experienced urologist may be considered in some patients. Testicular prostheses may be required if orchidopexy is not possible. The optimal procedure and timing of surgery remain controversial and the decision should ideally be made involving the patient when he is old enough to give informed consent. Results of surgery on sexual function are mixed.

Gonadectomy

- ↑ risk of gonadoblastoma in most individuals with abdominal testes. Risk is highest in those with dysgenetic gonads and Y chromosome material. Bilateral gonadectomy should therefore be performed (usually laparascopically).
- Optimal timing of the gonadectomy is unknown. In androgen insensitivity, the risk of gonadoblastoma appears to rise only after the age of 20 years so orchidectomy is recommended in adolescence after attaining puberty. In most other disorders, gonadectomy prior to puberty is recommended.
- Early bilateral orchidectomy should also be performed in 46, XY subjects with 5α-reductase deficiency or 17βHSD deficiency who are being raised as ♀ to prevent virilization at puberty.

Hormone replacement therapy

- Patients with disorders of adrenal biosynthesis, e.g. CAH, require lifelong glucocorticoid and usually mineralocorticoid replacement therapy.
- Most ♂ pseudohermaphrodites and hermaphrodites being raised as ♂ require long-term testosterone replacement therapy.
- Individuals with 5α-reductase deficiency usually receive supra-physiological doses of testosterone in order to achieve satisfactory DHT levels.
- Subjects with androgen insensitivity and ♂ pseudohermaphrodites being raised as ♀ should receive oestrogen replacement therapy to induce puberty and this should be continued thereafter.

Psychological support

- Disorders relating to sexual identity and function require expert counselling.
- Patient support groups are often helpful.

Further reading

Creighton S and Minto C (2001). Managing intersex. *BMJ* **323**, 1264–5.

MacLaughin DT and Donahoe PK (2004). Sex determination and differentiation. *New Engl J Med* **350**, 367–78.

Vogiatzi MG and New MI (1998). Differential diagnosis and therapeutic options for ambiguous genitalia. *Curr Opin Endocrinol Diabet* **5**, 3–10.

Warne GL and Zajac JD (1998). Disorders of sexual differentiation. *Endocrinol Metab Clin North Am* **27**(4), 945–67.

Transsexualism

Definition

A condition in which an apparently anatomically and genetically normal person feels that he or she is a member of the opposite sex. There is an irreversible discomfort with the anatomical gender, which may be severe, often developing in childhood.

Epidemiology

- More common in ♂.
- Estimated prevalence of 1:13 000 ♂ and 1:30 000 ♀.

Aetiology

- Unknown and controversial.
- Some evidence that it may have a neurobiological basis. There appear to be sex differences in the size and shape of certain nuclei in the hypothalamus. ♂ to ♀ transsexuals have been found to have ♀ differentiation of one of these nuclei whereas ♀ to ♂ transsexuals have been found to have a ♂ pattern of differentiation.

Management

Standards of care

- Multidisciplinary approach between psychiatrists, endocrinologists, and surgeons. Patient should be counselled about the treatment options, risks, and implications and realistic expectations should be discussed.
- Endocrine disorders should be excluded prior to entry into the gender reassignment programme—i.e. ensure normal internal and external genitalia, karyotype, gonadotrophins, and testosterone/ oestradiol.
- Psychiatric assessment and follow up is essential before definitive therapy. The transsexual identity should be shown to have been persistently present for at least 2 years to ensure a permanent diagnosis.
- Following this period, the subject should dress and live as a member of the desired sex under the supervision of a psychiatrist. This should continue for at least 3 months before hormonal treatment and 1 year before surgery.
- Psychological follow-up and expert counselling should be available if required throughout the programme, including after surgery.
- In adolescents, puberty can be reversibly halted by GnRH analogue therapy, to prevent irreversible changes in the wrong gender, until a permanent diagnosis is made.

Hormonal manipulation

For contraindications 📖 see Box 69.1.

Male to female transsexuals

- Suppress ♂ 2° sex characteristics: cyproterone acetate (CPA) (100mg/day).
- Induce ♀ 2° sex characteristics:
  - EE2 100mcg/day or estradiol valerate 2mg bd/tds or estradiol patch 100mcg 2 ×/week.
  - Medroxyprogesterone acetate 10mg OD.
- *Aims:*
  - Breast development—maximum after 2 years of treatment.
  - Development of ♀ fat distribution.
  - ↓ body hair and smoother skin. However, facial hair is often resistant to treatment.
  - ↓ muscle bulk and strength.
  - Reduction in testicular size.
  - Hormonal manipulation has little effect on voice.
- Reduce dose of CPA following gender reassignment surgery and discontinue if possible. However, some subjects will require an antiandrogen in order to keep oestradiol doses to a minimum (Table 69.1).
- The dose of oestrogen may be halved after gender reassignment surgery (Table 69.1).
- Change to transdermal oestrogens if >40 years old. Change to HRT doses once >50 years old.
- Adjust oestrogen dose depending on plasma LH and oestradiol levels.
- *Side-effects* (particularly while on high dose EE2+CPA therapy):
  - Hyperprolactinaemia.
  - Venous thromboembolism.
  - Atherosclerosis.
  - Abnormal liver enzymes.
  - Depression.
  - ?↑ risk of breast cancer.

Female to male transsexuals

- Induce ♂ 2° sex characteristics and suppress ♀ 2° sex characteristics: parenteral testosterone (📖 see Table 69.1).
- *Aims:*
  - Cessation of menstrual bleeding.
  - Atrophy of uterus and breasts.
  - Increase muscle bulk and strength.
  - Deepening of voice (after 6-10 weeks).
  - Hirsutism.
  - ♂ body fat distribution.
  - Increase in libido.
- Once sexual characteristics are stable (after approximately 1 year of treatment) and following surgery, reduce testosterone dose based on serum testosterone and LH levels.

- *Side-effects:*
  - Acne (in 40%).
  - Weight gain.
  - Abnormal liver function.
  - Adverse lipid profile.

Box 69.1 Contraindications to hormone manipulation

Feminization	Masculinization
• Prolactinoma.	• Cardiovascular disease.
• Family history of breast cancer.	• Active liver disease.
• Risk of thromboembolism.	• Polycythaemia.
• Active liver disease.	• Cerebrovascular disease.
• Cardiovascular or cerebrovascular disease.	
• Other contraindication to oestrogen therapy (📖 see p.343).	

Gender reassignment surgery
- Performed at least 6–9 months after starting sex hormone therapy.
- A 2nd psychiatric opinion should be sought prior to referral for surgery.
- Usually performed in several stages.

Male to female transsexuals
- Bilateral orchidectomy and resection of the penis.
- Construction of a vagina and labia minora.
- Clitoroplasty.
- Breast augmentation.

Female to male transsexuals
- Bilateral mastectomy.
- Hysterectomy and salpingo-oophorectomy.
- Phalloplasty and testicular prostheses.

Prognosis
- Significantly ↑ morbidity in ♂ to ♀ transsexuals from thromboembolism.
- Hyperprolactinaemia and elevation in liver enzymes are self-limiting in the majority of cases.
- The risk of osteoporosis is not thought to be ↑ in transsexuals.
- There may be a slightly ↑ risk of breast cancer in ♂ to ♀ transsexuals.
- Results from reconstructive surgery, particularly in ♀ to ♂ transsexuals, remain suboptimal.
- There is an ↑ risk of depressive illness and suicide in transsexual individuals.

Box 69.2 Monitoring of therapy
- Every 3 months for first year then every 6 months
- Hormonal therapy is lifelong and so patients should be followed up indefinitely.

Male to female
- Physical examination
- Liver function tests
- Serum lipids and glucose
- LH, oestradiol, prolactin
- PSA (>50 years)
- ?mammogram (>50 years)
- Bone densitometry

Female to male
- Physical examination
- Liver function tests
- Serum lipids and blood glucose
- LH, testosterone
- FBC (exclude polycythaemia)
- Bone densitometry

Table 69.1 Maintenance hormone regimens in the treatment of transsexualism

Feminization (post surgery)	Masculinization (pre and post surgery)
<40 years:	Testosterone 250mg IM every 2 weeks
Ethinylestradiol 30–50mcg od	Transdermal testosterone (gel or patch) 5mg od
estradiol valerate (oral) 2–4mg od	
estradiol valerate (transdermal) 50mcg 2 × /week	
Conjugated estrogens 1.25mg od	
>40 years:	
Transdermal estradiol valerate 50 2 × /week	
May need to continue cyproterone acetate 50mg od or add spironolactone 100–200mg od.	
May need to continue progestagens to maintain libido and augment breast growth.	

Further reading

Gooren LJ, Giltay EJ, and Brunck MC (2008). Long-term treatment of transsexuals with cross-sex hormones: extensive personal experience. *J Clin Endocrinol Metab* **93**(1), 19–25.

Levy A, Crown A, and Reid R (2003). Endocrine intervention for transsexuals. *Clin Endocrinol* **59**, 409–18.

Moore E, Wisniewski A, and Dobs A (2003) Endocrine treatment of transsexual people: a review of treatment regimens, outcomes and adverse effects. *J Clin Endocrinol Metab* **88**(8), 3467–73.

Schlatterer K, von Werder K, Stalla GK (1996). Multistep treatment concept of transsexual patients. *Exp Clin Endocrinol Diabet* **104**, 413–19.

Part 5

Endocrine disorders of pregnancy

Thyroid disorders

Normal physiology

Effect of pregnancy on thyroid function

- *Iodine stores* Fall due to ↑ renal clearance and transplacental transfer to fetus.
- *Thyroid size* Increase in thyroid volume by 10–20% due to hCG stimulation and relative iodine deficiency.
- *Thyroglobulin* Rise corresponds to rise in thyroid size.
- *Thyroid binding globulin (TBG)* Twofold increase in concentration as a result of reduced hepatic clearance and ↑ synthesis stimulated by oestrogen. Concentration plateaus at 20 weeks' gestation, and falls again postpartum.
- *Total T_4 and T_3* ↑ concentrations, corresponding to rise in TBG.
- *Free T_4 and T_3* Small rise in concentration in 1st trimester due to hCG stimulation then fall into normal range. During 2nd and 3rd trimester, FT4 concentration is often just below the normal reference range.
- *Thyroid stimulating hormone (TSH)* Within normal limits in pregnancy. However, suppressed in 13.5% in 1st trimester, 4.5% in 2nd trimester, and 1.2% in 3rd trimester due to hCG thyrotropic effect. +ve correlation between free T_4 and hCG levels and –ve correlation between TSH and hCG levels in first half of pregnancy.
- *Thyrotropin releasing hormone (TRH)* Normal.
- *TSH receptor antibodies* When present in high concentrations in maternal serum may cross the placenta. Antibody titre decreases with progression of pregnancy.

Fetal thyroid function

- TRH and TSH synthesis occurs by 8–10 weeks' gestation and thyroid hormone synthesis occurs by 10–12 weeks' gestation.
- TSH, total and freeT_4 and T_3, and TBG concentrations increase progressively throughout gestation.
- Maternal TSH does not cross the placenta and although TRH crosses the placenta it does not regulate fetal thyroid function. Iodine crosses the placenta and excessive quantities may induce fetal hypothyroidism. Maternal T_4 and T_3 cross the placenta in small quantities and are important for fetal brain development in the 1st half of gestation.

Maternal hyperthyroidism

(📖 see Thyrotoxicosis in pregnancy, p.34)

Incidence

- Affects 0.2% of pregnant women.
- Most are diagnosed before pregnancy or in the 1st trimester of pregnancy.
- In women with Graves' disease in remission, exacerbation may occur in 1st trimester of pregnancy.

Graves' disease

- The commonest scenario is pregnancy in a patient with preexisting Graves' disease on treatment as fertility is low in patients with untreated thyrotoxicosis. Newly diagnosed Graves' disease in pregnancy is unusual.
- Aggravation of disease in 1st trimester with amelioration in 2nd half of pregnancy because of a decrease in maternal immunological activity at that time.
- Symptoms of thyrotoxicosis are difficult to differentiate from normal pregnancy. The most sensitive symptoms are weight loss and tachycardia. Goitre is found in most patients.

Management

- Risks of uncontrolled hyperthyroidism to mother: heart failure/ arryhthmias.
- Antithyroid drugs (ATDs) are the treatment of choice but cross the placenta.
- Propylthiouracil is preferred although the risk of aplasia cutis, a rare fetal scalp defect, with carbimazole is negligible. There is also less transfer to breast milk.
- Avoid β-blockers as they may be associated with fetal growth impairment with prolonged use. Can be used initially for 2–3 weeks while antithyroid drugs take affect.
- Most patients will be on a maintenance dose of ATD. A high dose of ATD may be necessary initially to achieve euthyroidism as quickly as possible (carbimazole 20–40mg/day or propylthiouracil 200–400mg/day) in newly diagnosed patients, then use the minimal dose of ATD to maintain euthyroidism.
- Do not use block-replace regime as higher doses of ATDs required and there is minimal transplacental transfer of T_4, thereby risking fetal hypothyroidism.
- Monitor TFTs every 4–6 weeks.
- Aim to keep FT_4 at upper limit of normal and TSH low-normal.
- In approximately 30% of women ATD may be discontinued at 32–36 weeks' gestation. Consider if euthyroid for at least 4 weeks on lowest dose of propylthiouracil, but continue to monitor TFTs frequently. The presence of a large goitre or ophthalmopathy suggests severe disease and the chances of remission are low so do not stop ATD.
- Risks of neonatal hypothyroidism and goitre are reduced if woman on 200mg propylthiouracil or less (or carbimazole 20mg) in last few weeks of gestation.

- Propylthiouracil (PTU) is secreted in negligible amounts in breast milk. Carbimazole is secreted in higher amounts. Breast feeding is not contraindicated if mother is on < 150mg propylthiouracil or 5mg carbimazole. Give in divided doses after the feeds and monitor neonatal thyroid function.
- Surgical management of thyrotoxicosis is rarely necessary in pregnancy. Only indication: serious ATD complication (e.g. agranulocytosis) or drug resistance. There is a possible ↑ risk of spontaneous abortion or premature delivery associated with surgery during pregnancy.
- Radioiodine therapy is contraindicated in pregnancy and for 4 months beforehand.

Infants born to mothers with Graves' disease
- Risks to fetus of uncontrolled thyrotoxicosis:
  - ↑ risk of spontaneous abortion and stillbirth
  - Intrauterine growth restriction (IUGR)
  - Premature labour
  - Fetal or neonatal hyperthyroidism.
- Follow-up of babies born to mothers on ATDs show normal weight, height, and intellectual function.
- *Fetal hypothyroidism* May occur following treatment of mother with high doses of ATDs (>200mg PTU/day), particularly in the latter half of pregnancy. This is rare and may be diagnosed by demonstrating a large fetal goitre on fetal US in the presence of fetal bradycardia.
- *Fetal hyperthyroidism* May occur after week 25 of gestation. It results in IUGR, fetal goitre, and tachycardia (fetal heart rate >160bpm). It may develop if the mother has high titres of TSH stimulating antibodies (TSAb). Treat by giving mother ATD and monitor fetal heart rate (aim <140bpm), growth and goitre size.
- *Neonatal thyrotoxicosis* Develops in 1% of infants born to thyrotoxic mothers. Due to placental transfer of TSAb. Transient, usually subsides by 6 months, but up to 30% mortality if untreated. Treat with ATD and β-blockers.

Hyperemesis gravidarum (gestational hyperthyroidism)
- Characterized by severe vomiting and weight loss. Cause unknown.
- Begins in early pregnancy (week 6–9 of gestation) and tends to resolve spontaneously by week 20 of gestation.
- Biochemical hyperthyroidism in two-thirds of affected women but T_3 is less commonly elevated. Mechanism: hCG has TSH-like effect, thus stimulating the thyroid gland and suppressing TSH secretion.
- Degree of thyroid stimulation correlates with severity of vomiting.
- No other evidence of thyroid disease, i.e. no goitre, no history of thyroid disease, no ophthalmopathy, and −ve thyroid autoantibodies.
- Antithyroid drugs not required and do not improve symptoms of hyperemesis.

Causes of maternal hyperthyroidism
- Graves' disease (85% of cases).
- Toxic nodule.
- Toxic multinodular goitre.
- Hydatidiform mole.

Maternal hypothyroidism

Prevalence
- 2.5% subclinical hypothyroidism.
- 1–2% overt hypothyroidism.

Risks of suboptimal treatment during pregnancy
- *Spontaneous abortion* Twofold ↑ risk.
- *Pre-eclampsia* 21% of suboptimally treated mothers have pregnancy-induced hypertension (PIH).
- Also, ↑ risk of anaemia during pregnancy and postpartal haemorrhage.
- Risk of impaired fetal intellectual and cognitive development.
- ↑ risk of perinatal death.
- Other risks to fetus those associated with PIH (IUGR, premature delivery, etc).
- The risk of congenital malformations is not thought to be ↑.

Management
- Spontaneous pregnancy in overtly hypothyroid women is unusual as hypothyroid women are likely to have anovulatory menstrual cycles.
- *Levothyroxine therapy* Start on 150mcg. Measure TSH 4 weeks later.
- If already on T_4 before pregnancy, assess TSH at 6–8 weeks gestation, then between weeks 16–20, then again between weeks 28–32 of gestation.
- *Aim* TSH—lower part of normal range; FT4—upper end of normal.
- Increase T_4 dose by 30% (an average of 25–50mcg) when pregnancy confirmed. After delivery, thyroid requirements decrease to prepregnancy levels.
- *NB* Do not give $FeSO_4$ simultaneously with T_4—reduces its efficacy. Separate times for drug ingestion by at least 2h.

Causes of maternal hypothyroidism
- Hashimoto's thyroiditis (most common cause).
- Previous radioiodine therapy or thyroidectomy.
- Previous postpartum thyroiditis.
- Hypopituitarism.

+ve thyroid antibodies but euthyroid
- Twofold excess risk of spontaneous abortion.
- No other complications.
- No risk of neonatal hypothyroidism.
- Risk of PIH not ↑.
- The occasional mother will develop hypothyroidism towards the end of the pregnancy, so check TSH between weeks 28–32 of gestation.
- ↑ risk of postpartum thyroiditis so check TSH at 3 months postpartum.

Postpartum thyroid dysfunction

Prevalence
- 5–10% of women within 1 year of delivery or miscarriage.
- 3 × more common in women with type 1 diabetes mellitus.

Aetiology
- Chronic autoimmune thyroiditis (see Other types of thyroiditis, p.53)

Clinical presentation
- *Hyperthyroidism (32%):*
  - Within 4 months of delivery.
  - The most common symptom is fatigue.
  - Usually resolves spontaneously in 2–3 months.
- *Hypothyroidism (43%):*
  - Develops 4–6 months after delivery.
  - Symptoms may be mild and non-specific.
  - There may be an ↑ risk of post partum depression.
- *Hyperthyroidism followed by hypothyroidism (25%).*
- *Spontaneous recovery* in 80% within 6–12 months of delivery.

Differential diagnosis
- Graves' disease may relapse in the postpartum period. This is differentiated from postpartum thyroiditis by a high uptake on radioiodine scanning.
- Lymphocytic hypophysitis may cause hypothyroidism. However, serum TSH concentrations are inappropriately low.

Investigation
- Thyroid peroxidase antibodies are +ve in 80%.
- Radionuclide uptake scans are rarely necessary. However, there is low uptake during the thyrotoxic phase, differentiating it from Grave's disease where uptake is ↑.

Management
- β-blockers if thyrotoxic and symptomatic until TFTs normalize. Antithyroid medication is unnecessary.
- Levothyroxine if TSH>10 or if TSH between 4–10 and symptomatic.
- No consensus as to how long to treat with thyroxine. Two options:
  - Halve dose at about 12 months postnatal and check TFTs 6 weeks later. If normal, then withdraw T4 and check TFTs 6 weeks later.
  - Withdraw treatment 1 year after completion of family.

Prognosis
- Recurrence in future pregnancies in 70% of women.
- Permanent hypothyroidism develops in up to 50% of women within 10 years. If treatment is withdrawn then annual TSH measurements are essential.

Thyroid cancer in pregnancy

(📖 see Thyroid cancer and pregnancy, p. 79.)

Further reading

Abalovich M, Amino N, Barbour LA, et al. (2007). Management of thyroid dysfunction during pregnancy and postpartum: an Endocrine Society Clinical Practice Guideline. *J Clin Endocrinol Metab* **92**(8 Suppl), S1–47.

Alexander EK, Marqusee E, Lawrence J, et al. (2004). Timing and magnitude of increases in levothyroxine requirements during pregnancy in women with hypothyroidism. *New England Journal of Medicine* **351**(3), 241–9.

Lazarus JH and Kokandi A (2000). Thyroid disease in relation to pregnancy: a decade of change. *Clinical Endocrinology* **53**, 265–78.

LeBeau SO and Mandell SJ (2006). Thyroid disorders during pregnancy. *Endocrine and Metabolism Clinics of North America* **35**, 117–36.

Poppe K and Glinoer D (2003). Thyroid autoimmunity and hypothyroidism before and during pregnancy. *Human Reproduction Update* **9**(2), 149–61.

Stagnaro-Green A (2002). Postpartum thyroiditis. *Journal of Clinical Endocrinology and Metabolism* **87**(9), 4042–7.

Pituitary disorders

Normal anatomical changes during pregnancy

- *Prolactin (PRL)-secreting cells* Marked lactotroph hyperplasia during pregnancy.
- *Gonadotropin-secreting cells* Marked reduction in size and number.
- *TSH and ACTH-secreting cells* No change in size or number.
- *Anterior pituitary* Size increases by up to 70% during pregnancy. May take 1 year to shrink to near pre-pregnancy size in non-lactating women. Gradual slight increase in size with each pregnancy.
- *MRI* Enlarged anterior pituitary gland, but stalk is midline. Posterior pituitary gland may not be seen in late pregnancy.

Normal physiology during pregnancy

- *Serum PRL* Concentrations increase markedly during pregnancy and fall again to pre-pregnancy levels approximately 2 weeks postpartum in non-lactating women.
- *Serum LH and FSH* Undetectable levels in pregnancy and blunted response to GnRH because of −ve feedback inhibition from high levels of sex hormones and PRL.
- *Serum TSH, T_4, and T_3* TSH may be suppressed in the 1st trimester of pregnancy. Free thyroid hormones usually within the normal range.
- *Growth hormone (GH) and IGF-I* Low maternal GH levels and blunted response to hypoglycaemia due to placental production of GH-like substance. IGF-I levels are normal or high in pregnancy.
- *ACTH and cortisol* CRH, ACTH, and cortisol levels are high in pregnancy as both CRH and ACTH are produced by the placenta. In addition, oestrogen-induced increase in cortisol binding globulin (CBG) synthesis during pregnancy will further increase maternal plasma cortisol concentrations. During the latter half of pregnancy there is a progressive increase of ACTH and cortisol levels, peaking during labour. Incomplete suppression of cortisol following dexamethasone suppression test and exagerrated response of cortisol to CRH stimulation. However, normal diurnal variation persists.

Prolactinoma in pregnancy

Effect of pregnancy on tumour size
Risk of significant tumour enlargement (i.e. resulting in visual field disturbances or headaches):
- Microadenoma 1–2%.
- Macroadenoma 15–35%.
- Macroadenoma treated with surgery and/or radiotherapy before pregnancy 4–7%.

Effect of dopamine agonists on the fetus
Bromocriptine
Over 6000 pregnancies have occurred in women receiving bromocriptine in early pregnancy and the incidence of complications in these pregnancies with regards fetal outcome is similar to that of the normal population, indicating that bromocriptine is probably safe in early pregnancy. Data are available on children whose mothers received bromocriptine throughout pregnancy and again the incidence of congenital abnormalities is negligible.

Cabergoline
Also probably safe in early pregnancy, with no ↑ risk of fetal loss or congenital abnormalities but fewer data are available. It is thus recommended that women with prolactinomas seeking fertility should receive bromocriptine to induce ovulation as there is more data on the long-term safety of bromocriptine but cabergoline is being used increasingly as it is better tolerated.

Management
Microprolactinoma
- Initiate dopamine agonist therapy to induce normal ovulatory cycles and fertility.
- Stop bromocriptine as soon as pregnancy is confirmed.
- Assess for visual symptoms and headache at each trimester although the risk of complications is low (<5%). Serum PRL levels are difficult to interpret during pregnancy as they are normally elevated therefore they are not routinely measured.
- MRI is indicated in the occasional patient who becomes symptomatic.
- In the postpartum period, recheck serum PRL level after cessation of breastfeeding. Reassess size of microprolactinoma by MRI only if serum PRL level higher than pre-pregnancy concentrations.
- 40–60% chance of remission of microprolactinoma following pregnancy.

Macroprolactinoma

Management is controversial and must therefore be individualized. Three possible approaches:

- Bromocriptine (because cabergoline does not have a licence in pregnancy) may be used throughout pregnancy to reduce the risk of tumour growth. The patient is monitored by visual fields at each trimester, or more frequently if symptoms of tumour enlargement develop. This is probably the safest and thus preferred approach.
- May use bromocriptine or cabergoline to induce ovulation and then stop it after conception. However, patient must be monitored very carefully during pregnancy with monthly visual field testing.
- If symptoms of tumour enlargement develop or there is a deterioration in visual fields then MRI should be performed to assess tumour growth. If significant tumour enlargement develops then bromocriptine therapy should be initiated.
- Alternatively, the patient may undergo surgical debulking of the tumour and/or radiotherapy before seeking fertility. This will significantly reduce the risk of complications associated with tumour growth. However, this approach may render them gonadotropin deficient. These patients should again be monitored during pregnancy using regular visual fields.
- There is no contraindication to breastfeeding.
- MRI should be performed in the postpartum period in women with macroprolactinomas to look for tumour growth.

Cushing's syndrome

- Pregnancy is rare in women with untreated Cushing's syndrome as 75% of them will experience oligo- or amenorrhoea.
- The diagnosis of Cushing's syndrome is difficult to establish during pregnancy. However, the presence of purple striae and proximal myopathy should alert the physician to the diagnosis of Cushing's syndrome.
- If suspected, the investigation of Cushing's syndrome should be carried out as in the non-pregnant state. However, high urinary free cortisols and non-suppression of cortisol production on a low dose dexamethasone suppression test may be features of a normal pregnancy. The diurnal variation of cortisol secretion is, however, preserved in normal pregnancy.
- Diagnosis is important, as pregnancy in Cushing's syndrome is associated with a high risk of maternal and fetal complications (📖 see Table 71.1).
- Adrenal disease is the most common cause of Cushing's syndrome developing in pregnancy, responsible for over 50% of reported cases.

Management

- *1st trimester:*
  - Offer termination of pregnancy and instigate treatment, particularly if adrenal carcinoma.
  - Alternatively, surgical treatment early in the 2nd trimester.
- *2nd trimester:*
  - Surgery, e.g. adrenalectomy or pituitary adenomectomy. Minimal risk to fetus.
- *3rd trimester:*
  - ↑ risk of diabetes mellitus.
  - Deliver baby as soon as possible (preferably by vaginal delivery to minimize the risk of poor wound healing following a Caesarian section) and instigate treatment.
- Metyrapone used in doses of <2g/day appears to be safe in pregnancy.
- Postoperative glucocorticoid replacement therapy will be required.
- Treatment of Cushing's syndrome in pregnancy may reduce maternal and fetal morbidity and mortality.

Table 71.1 Complications of Cushing's syndrome in pregnancy

Maternal complications	Incidence (%)	Fetal complications	Incidence (%)
Hypertension	70	Spontaneous abortion	12
Diabetes mellitus	27	Perinatal death	18
Congestive cardiac failure	7	Prematurity	60
Poor wound healing	6	Congenital malformations	Low risk; no risk of virilization
Death	4		

Acromegaly

- Fertility in acromegaly is reduced, partly due to hyperprolactinaemia (if present) in addition to secondary hypogonadism. However, there have been several reported cases of pregnancy in acromegaly.
- Acromegaly increases the risk of gestational diabetes and hypertension. However, in the absence of diabetes mellitus there does not appear to be an excess of perinatal morbidity or mortality in babies born to women with acromegaly.
- Significant tumour enlargement occasionally occurs together with enlargement of the normal pituitary lactotrophs, so monthly visual field testing is recommended. It may be treated with bromocriptine until there are more safety data on other forms of treatment. However, treatment may be deferred until after delivery in the majority of patients.
- Few data are available on the use of somatostatin analogues during pregnancy so their routine use is currently not recommended as they cross the placenta. However, there have been a few reports of uneventful pregnancies in patients treated with *octreotide*.

Hypopituitarism in pregnancy

Pre-existing hypopituitarism

- Most commonly due to surgical treatment of and/or radiotherapy for a pituitary adenoma.
- May induce ovulation and thus conception by gonadotrophin stimulation.

Lymphocytic hypophysitis

(📖 see also Lymphocytic hypophysitis, p.178.)

- Rare disorder thought to be autoimmune in origin.
- Characterized by pituitary enlargement on imaging and variable loss of pituitary function.
- Most commonly seen in women in late pregnancy or in the 1st year postpartum.
- Symptoms are due to pressure effects, e.g. visual field defects and headaches, or due to hormonal deficiency.
- Most common hormonal deficiencies:
  - ACTH and vasopressin deficiency.
  - TSH deficiency may also exist.
  - Gonadotrophins and GH levels are usually normal.
  - PRL levels may be mildly elevated in a third, and low in a third.
- *Differential diagnosis:*
  - Pituitary adenoma.
  - Sheehan's syndrome.
- MRI often reveals diffuse homogenous contrast enhancement of the pituitary gland. However, the diagnosis is often only made definitively by pituitary biopsy.
- There is an association with other autoimmune diseases, particularly Hashimoto's thyroiditis.
- Course variable. Pituitary function may deteriorate or improve with time.

Management

- Pituitary hormone replacement therapy as required.
- Surgical decompression if pressure symptoms persist.
- A course of high dose steroid therapy is controversial, with mixed results.

Causes of hypopituitarism during pregnancy

- Pre-existing hypopituitarism.
- Pituitary adenoma.
- Lymphocytic hypophysitis.
- Sheehan's syndrome.

Management of pre-existing hypopituitarism during pregnancy

- *Hydrocortisone* dose may need to be ↑ in the 3rd trimester of pregnancy by 10mg a day as the increase in CBG will reduce the bioavailability of hydrocortisone. Parenteral hydrocortisone in a dose of 100mg IM every 6h should be given during labour and the dose reduced back to maintenance levels in the postpartum period (24–72 hours).
- *Thyroxine* Requirements may increase as pregnancy progresses. Monitor free T_4 each trimester and increase T_4 dose accordingly.
- *GH* There are little data on the effects of GH on pregnancy, but case reports do not suggest a detrimental effect on fetal outcome. However, until more data accrue, GH should be stopped prior to pregnancy. Moreover, as the placenta synthesizes a GH variant, GH therapy is unnecessary.
- *Vasopressin* The placenta synthesizes vasopressinase, which breaks down vasopressin but not desmopressin. Women with partial diabetes insipidus may therefore require desmopressin treatment during pregnancy. Those already receiving desmopressin may require a dose increment during pregnancy. Vasopressinase levels fall rapidly after delivery.

Sheehan's syndrome

Postpartum pituitary infarction/haemorrhage resulting in hypopituitarism. Increasingly uncommon in developed countries with improvements in obstetric care.

Pathogenesis

- The enlarged pituitary gland of pregnancy is susceptible to any compromise to its blood supply.
- Investigations will confirm hypopituitarism.

Risk factors

- Postpartum haemorrhage.
- Type 1 diabetes mellitus.
- Sickle cell disease.

Clinical features

- Failure of lactation.
- Involution of breasts.
- Fatigue, lethargy, and dizziness.
- Amenorrhoea.
- Loss of axillary and pubic hair.
- Symptoms of hypothyroidism.
- Diabetes insipidus is rare.

Management

Pituitary hormone replacement therapy (📖 see Background, p.104).

Further reading

Kovacs K (2003). Sheehan syndrome. *Lancet* **361**, 520–2.

Molitch M (1999). Medical treatment of prolactinomas. *Endocrinology and Metabolism Clinics of North America* **28**(1), 143–69.

Molitch M (2006). Pituitary disorders in pregnancy. *Endocrinology and Metabolism Clinics of North America* **35**, 99–116.

Sam S and Molitch M (2003). Timing and special concerns regarding endocrine surgery during pregnancy. *Endocrinology and Metabolism Clinics of North America* **32**, 337–54.

Adrenal disorders during pregnancy

Normal changes during pregnancy

Changes in maternal adrenocortical function

Markedly ↑ concentrations of all adrenal steroids due to ↑ synthesis and ↓ catabolism.

Feto-placental unit

- *Fetal adrenal gland* DHEAS is produced in vast quantities by the fetal adrenal gland. This is the major precursor for oestrogen synthesis by the placenta. The fetal adrenal gland has a large capacity for steroidogenesis. Stimulus for fetal adrenal gland unknown—possibly hCG or PRL.
- *Placenta* Maternal glucocorticoids are largely inactivated in the placenta by 11βHSD. Maternal androgens are converted to oestrogens by placental aromatase, thus protecting ♀ fetus from virilization.

Addison's disease in pregnancy

- No associated fetal morbidity in women who have pre-existing primary adrenal insufficiency as fetus produces and regulates its own adrenal steroids.
- Management of Addison's disease does not differ in pregnancy.
- Glucocorticoids which are metabolized by placental 11βHSD preferred (i.e. prednisolone or hydrocortisone) to avoid fetal adrenal suppression.
- Increase hydrocortisone dose by about 10mg during the 3rd trimester of pregnancy and at any time in case of intercurrent illness.
- High dose intramuscular hydrocortisone should be given at the time of delivery to cover the stress of labour.
- Doses may be tapered to normal maintenance doses in the postpartum period (🕮 see Box 72.1).
- Addison's disease developing in pregnancy may result in an adrenal crisis, particularly at the time of delivery, because of a delay in diagnosis.
- In early pregnancy vomiting, fatigue, and hyperpigmentation and low BP may be wrongly attributed to pregnancy. However, persisting symptoms should alert the clinician.
- If supected, the diagnosis is confirmed by the presence of low serum cortisol concentrations with failure to rise following ACTH stimulation, and high ACTH levels. However, the normal ranges for serum ACTH and cortisol concentrations have not been established in pregnancy.
- Chronic maternal adrenal insufficiency may be associated with intrauterine fetal growth restriction.
- There is no ↑ risk of developing Addison's disease in the immediate postpartum period.

Box 72.1 Management of adrenal insufficiency during pregnancy

- Hydrocortisone 20–30mg PO in divided doses, as per pre-pregnancy dose.
- Fludrocortisone 50–200mcg PO, as per pre-pregnancy dose.

During uncomplicated labour
- Hydrocortisone 100mg IM 6-hourly for 24h, then reduce to maintenance dose over 72h.
- Keep well hydrated.
- Fludrocortisone may be discontinued while on high doses of hydrocortisone.

Congenital adrenal hyperplasia

- Fertility is reduced, particularly women with the salt-wasting form of CAH.
- Reasons:
  - Inadequate vaginal introitus despite reconstructive surgery.
  - Anovulation as a result of hyperandrogenaemia.
  - Adverse effects of elevated progestagen levels on endometrium.
- 60–80% of women with CAH and an adequate vaginal introitus are fertile.
- Fertility may be maximized by optimal suppression of hyperandrogenism by glucocorticoid therapy (□ see Management, p.308).
- No major complications in pregnancy are known in women with CAH, apart from a possibly ↑ incidence of pre-eclampsia.
- However, women are more likely to require Caesarean section for cephalopelvic disproportion.
- Management is the same as in the non-pregnant woman and steroids are ↑ at the time of delivery as for Addison's disease (□ p.449).
- Monitor serum testosterone and electrolytes every 6–8 weeks.
- Risk to fetus:
  - No risk of virilization from maternal hyperandrogenism as placenta will aromatize androgens to oestrogens.
  - Glucocorticoids do not increase the risk of congenital abnormalities.
  - If partner is a heterozygote or homozygote for CAH then the fetus has a 50% risk of CAH. Prenatal treatment with dexamethasone will then be necessary to avoid virilization of a ♀ fetus (□ see Management of pregnancy in CAH, p.309).

Phaeochromocytoma

- Rare but potentially lethal in pregnancy. Maternal mortality may still be as high as 17%, and 30% fetal mortality if not treated promptly. Highest risk of hypertensive crisis and death is during labour.
- Suspect in women with hypertension, persistent or intermittent, especially in the absence of proteinuria or oedema, hypertension developing before 20 weeks' gestation, or persistent glycosuria.
- Suspect if paroxysmal symptoms are present: palpitations, sweating, headache.
- Prenatal screening in high-risk women e.g. those with a history or family history of MEN-2 or von Hippel–Lindau syndrome.
- Diagnose by 24h urinary catecholamine collection.
- Tumour localization is important—MRI is the imaging of choice in pregnancy.

Management

- α-blockade: phenoxybenzamine Reduces fetal and maternal morbidity and mortality. Appears to be safe in pregnancy. The starting dose is 10mg 12-hourly and is built up gradually to a maximum of 20mg every 8h.
- β-blockade: propranolol Only after adequate α-blockade. May increase the risk of intrauterine fetal growth restriction if started in the 3rd trimester. Give in a dose of 40mg 8-hourly.
- Surgery This is controversial. Some, before 24 weeks' gestation offer surgical removal of phaeochromocytoma (relatively safe following α- and β-blockade). After 24 weeks' gestation, surgery should be deferred until fetal maturity, and then it can be combined with Caesarean section with removal of tumour. Ensure adequate adrenergic blockade before surgery. Often operate after safe delivery of the fetus.

Further reading

Hadden DR (1995). Adrenal disorders of pregnancy. *Endocrinology and Metabolism Clinics of North America* **24**(1), 139–51.

Sam S and Molitch M (2003). Timing and special concerns regarding endocrine surgery during pregnancy. *Endocrinology and Metabolism Clinics of North America* **32**, 337–54.

Calcium and bone metabolism

Calcium and bone physiology

Bone turnover

In order to ensure that bone can undertake its mechanical and metabolic functions it is in a constant state of turnover (see 📖 Fig. 73.1).
- *Osteoclasts*—derived from the monocytic series, resorb bone.
- *Osteoblasts*—derived from the fibroblast-like cells, make bone.
- *Osteocytes*—buried osteoblasts, sense mechanical strain in bone.

Bone mass during life

(📖 see Fig. 73.2)

Bone is laid down rapidly during skeletal growth at puberty. Following this there is a period of stabilization of bone mass in early adult life. After the age of ~40 there is a gradual loss of bone in both sexes. This occurs at the rate of approximately 0.5% annually. However, in ♀ after the menopause there is a period of rapid bone loss. The accelerated loss is maximal immediately after the cessation of ovarian function and then gradually declines over about 10 years until the previous gradual rate of loss is once again established. The excess bone loss associated with the menopause is of the order of 10% of skeletal mass. This menopause-associated loss coupled with higher peak bone mass in ♂ largely explains why osteoporosis and its associated fractures are more common in ♀.

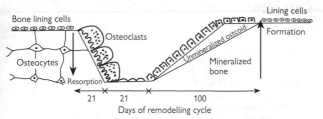

Fig. 73.1 Bone turnover during remodelling cycle.

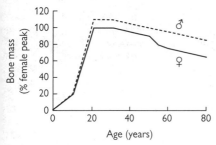

Fig. 73.2 Bone mass and age.

Calcium

Roles of calcium
- Skeletal strength.
- Neuromuscular conduction.
- Stimulus secretion coupling.

Calcium in the circulation
Circulating calcium exists in several forms (📖see Fig. 73.3).
- Ionized—biologically active.
- Complexed to citrate, phosphate etc.—biologically active.
- Bound to protein, mainly albumin—inactive.

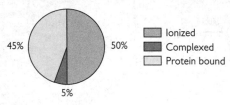

45%   50%

5%

Ionized
Complexed
Protein bound

Fig. 73.3 Forms of circulating calcium.

Investigation of bone

Bone turnover markers

May be useful in:
- Assessing overall risk of osteoporotic fracture.
- Judging response to treatments for osteoporosis.

Resorption markers

- *Collagen crosslinks* These make use of the fact that when collagen is laid down in bone the fibres are held in trimers by covalent links. These links are chemically very stable and are specific to the type of collagen. The excretion of fragments containing these crosslinks is a much better indicator of bone turnover. It can be measured either as the excretion of the linking molecules themselves, known as deoxypyridinoline crosslinks or as small fragments of the ends of the collagen molecule including these crosslinks, known as *telopeptides*. These latter markers can be derived from either the N- or the C-terminal of the collagen molecule and separate assays are available for each. Assays are available for both blood and urine although the former are subject to less error and are to be preferred.
- *Urinary hydroxyproline* relies on the fact that hydroxyproline is unique to collagen and so any hydroxyproline in urine must come from collagen breakdown. Unfortunately, this is not specific to bone (type 1) collagen; furthermore, hydroxyproline is variably metabolized before excretion and so its urinary levels are not a true index of collagen destruction. It has accordingly been superseded.

Formation markers

- *Total alkaline phosphatase* not specific also found in the liver, intestine, and placenta. It is also relatively insensitive to small changes in bone turnover and has only found general use in the monitoring of the activity of Paget's disease.
- *Bone-specific alkaline phosphatase* is more specific but its clinical utility is not yet clear.
- *Osteocalcin* a vitamin K-dependent protein that accounts for about 1% of bone matrix. The serum level of osteocalcin appears to reflect osteoblast activity. However, the results obtained with bone specific alkaline phosphatase and osteocalcin do not always correlate. This is particularly true in Paget's disease where the osteocalcin is frequently scarcely elevated despite the marked increase in bone turnover.
- *P1NP* is a procollagen fragment released from the N terminal as type 1 collagen is laid down. When measured in the serum it is the most sensitive and specific marker of bone formation although its clinical utility is as yet unclear.

Bone imaging

Skeletal radiology

• Useful for:
  • Diagnosis of fracture.
  • Diagnosis of specific diseases (e.g. Paget's disease and osteomalacia).
  • Identification of bone dysplasia.
• Not useful for assessing bone density.

Isotope bone scanning

Bone seeking isotopes, particularly ^{99m}technetium-labelled bisphosphonates, are concentrated in areas of localized ↑ bone cell activity. They are useful for identifying localized areas of bone disease such as fracture, metastasis, or Paget's disease. However, isotope uptake is not selective and so ↑ activity on a scan does not indicate the nature of the underlying bone disease. Hence, subsequent radiology of affected regions is frequently needed to establish the diagnosis.

Isotope bone scans are particularly useful in Paget's disease to establish the extent of skeletal involvement and the underlying disease activity.

Bone mass measurements

📖 See Table 74.1.

Interpretation of results

- The differences in normal ranges between the machines of different manufacturers has led to the practice of quoting bone mass measurements in terms of the number of standard deviations they lie from an expected mean. This can be done in two ways, T score and Z score: 📖 see Table 74.2.
- It is generally accepted a reduction of 1 SD in bone density will approximately double the risk of fracture.
- WHO has developed guidelines for the diagnosis of osteoporosis in postmenopausal ♀ (📖 see Table 74.3).
- No similar criteria have been set in ♂, but the same thresholds are generally accepted.
- For some 2° causes of osteoporosis, particularly corticosteroid use, it has been suggested that the less stringent criterion of T score <−1.5 be used as a treatment intervention threshold.

Bone biopsy

Bone biopsy is occasionally necessary for the diagnosis of difficult patients with metabolic bone disease. This is usually in the context of suspected osteomalacia. Bone biopsy is not indicated for the routine diagnosis of osteoporosis. It is best undertaken in specialist centres.

Table 74.1 Measurement of bone density

Technique	Site	Measures	Radiation	Reproducibility
Dual energy absorptiometry (DXA)	Spine* Femur* Whole body Forearm Calcaneus	Bone mineral per unit area (g/cm2)	~1µSv per site	<1% at spine <2% at femur
Quantitative computed tomography (QCT)	Spine Forearm	True bone mineral density (BMD) (g/cm3)	~50µSv at spine	~1%
Quantitative ultrasound (QUS)	Calcaneus Tibia Fingers	Speed of sound or broadband ultrasound attenuation	Nil	Poor

* Accepted as 'gold standard' measurement.

Table 74.2 T score and Z score

	T score	Z score
Definition	Number of SDs bone density lies from peak mean density for that sex	Number of SDs bone density lies from mean density expected for that sex and age
Significance		Age-independent effect on BMD i.e. secondary osteoporosis
Normal range	Not applicable	−2 – +2

Table 74.3 WHO proposals for diagnosis of postmenopausal osteoporosis

T score	Fragility fracture	Diagnosis
≥−1		Normal
<−1 but ≥−2.5		Low bone mass (osteopenia)
<−2.5	No	Osteoporosis
<−2.5	Yes	Established (severe) osteoporosis

Investigation of calcium, phosphate, and magnesium

Blood concentration

Calcium

The importance of obtaining blood for calcium measurement in the fasting state with little venous stasis has been overstated. It is, however, important to collect blood for the estimation of parathyroid hormone (PTH) and phosphate levels after an overnight fast.

In most clinical situations direct measurement of the ionized calcium concentration is not necessary. However, it is important to correct the measured calcium concentration for the prevailing level of albumin ($\square$see Box 75.1).

Phosphate and magnesium

Measurements of plasma phosphate and magnesium do not normally require to be corrected for plasma proteins. However, phosphate should be measured after an overnight fast.

Box 75.1 Correction of measured calcium concentration

Corrected Ca = measured Ca + 0.02 × (40 − albumin)

where calcium is in mmol/L and albumin in g/L.

Urine excretion

Calcium

A measurment of 24h excretion of calcium is useful for the assessment of the risk of renal stone formation or calcification in states of chronic hypercalcaemia. In other circumstances, particularly the assessment of the cause of hypercalcaemia (1° hyperparathyroidism versus familial hypocal-ciuric hypercalcaemia) an estimate of the renal handling of calcium is more useful. This is most commonly estimated from the ratio of the renal clearance of calcium to that of creatinine in the fasting state (☐see Box 75.2). If all values are in mmol/L the ratio is usually >0.02 in 1° hyperparathy-roidism, values <0.01 are suggestive of hypocalciuric hypercalcaemia.

Other causes of hypocalcium should be excluded eg. renal inefficiency, Vitamin D deficency and same drugs.

Phosphate

A 24h measurement of phosphate excretion largely reflects dietary phos-phate intake and has little clinical utility.

Box 75.2 Calculation of calcium/creatinine excretion ratio

$$CaE = \frac{\text{urine calcium (micromol)}}{\text{urine creatinine (micromol)}} \times \frac{\text{plasma creatinine}}{\text{plasma calcium}}$$

$$= <0.01 \text{ in FHH}$$

$$= >0.02 \text{ in hyperparathyroidism}$$

Calcium-regulating hormones

Parathyroid hormone

Reliable immunoassays for PTH are now available. In general, these are 2-site assays aimed at estimating the concentration of the intact PTH molecule. PTH is relatively labile and specimens require careful handling including early separation from the cells and speedy freezing for storage if the assay is not performed immediately. Since PTH secretion is suppressed by calcium ingestion, it should be measured in the fasting state. The normal range depends on the precise assay employed but typical values are 10–60pg/mL (1–6pmol/L). In African Americans levels are typically higher than in caucasian.

Vitamin D and its metabolites

25OH vitamin D (25OHD)

This is the main storage form of vitamin D and the best measure of vitamin D status. It is relatively stable and samples do not require as speedy handling as PTH. In clinical terms, it is the total vitamin D concentration that is important.

The conventionally accepted normal range is in the region of 5–30ng/mL (roughly 12.5–75nmol/L). However, this normal range was set with the idea of avoiding frank osteomalacia. If the 25OHD is 5–15ng/mL there is likely to be a state of vitamin D insufficiency with elevated PTH concentration and ↑ bone turnover. This can be associated with ↑ risk of fracture, particularly in the elderly.

Low levels of 25OHD can result from a variety of causes (📖 see Vitamin D deficiency, p.498). Likewise, it is unlikely that serious intoxication will occur unless the 25OHD is >100ng/mL. A more pragmatic reference range might be in the region of 20–80ng/mL (50–200nmol/L). (For conversion from ng/mL to nmol/L, multiply by 2.46.)

1,25(OH)₂ vitamin D (1,25(OH)₂D)

Although this is the active form of vitamin D, measurement of its concentration is less often clinically useful than measurement of 25OHD or PTH. It is sometimes useful as a marker of PTH activity and in diseases such as sarcoidosis where there is ↑ extrarenal synthesis of $1,25(OH)_2D$. The normal range is generally accepted as 20–50pg/mL (50–125pmol/L).

Parathyroid hormone related peptide (PTHrP)

It is possible to measure the level of this oncofetoprotein in serum. Although it is raised in many cases of humoural hypercalcaemia of malignancy the diagnosis is usually readily made from other sources (i.e. Ca with suppressed PTH) and this measurement is noncontributory. PTHrP is highly labile and specimens need to be collected into special preservative (Trasylol®) and separated and stored rapidly after venepuncture.

Calcitonin

Calcitonin assays are available but their utility is confined to the diagnosis and monitoring of medullary carcinoma of the thyroid. There is no role for calcitonin measurements in the routine investigation of calcium and bone metabolism.

Hypercalcaemia

Epidemiology

Hypercalcaemia is found in 5% of hospital patients but in only 0.5% of the general population.

Causes

Many different disease states can lead to hypercalcaemia. These are listed by order of importance in hospital practice in Box 76.1. In asymptomatic community-dwelling subjects the vast majority of hypercalcaemia is the result of hyperparathyroidism.

> **Box 76.1 Causes of hypercalcaemia**
>
> *Common*
> - Hyperparathyroidism:
>   - 1°.
>   - Tertiary.
> - Malignancy:
>   - Humoral hypercalcaemia.
>   - Multiple myeloma.
>   - Bony metastases.
>
> *Less common*
> - Vitamin D intoxication.
> - Familial hypocalciuric hypercalcaemia.
> - Sarcoidosis and other granulomatous diseases.
>
> *Uncommon*
> - Thiazide diuretics.
> - Lithium.
> - Immobilization.
> - Hyperthyroidism.
> - Renal failure.
> - Addison's disease.
> - Vitamin A intoxication.

Clinical features

Notwithstanding the underlying cause of hypercalcaemia, the clinical features are similar. With corrected calcium levels <3.0mmol/L it is unlikely that any symptoms will be related to the hypercalcaemia itself. With progressive increases in calcium concentration the likelihood of symptoms increases.

The clinical features of hypercalcaemia are well recognized (listed in Box 76.2): unfortunately, they are non-specific and may equally relate to underlying illness.

Clinical signs of hypercalcaemia are rare. With the exception of band keratopathy, these are not specific. It is important to seek clinical evidence of underlying causes of hypercalcaemia, particularly malignant disease.

In addition to these specific symptoms of hypercalcaemia, symptoms of the long-term consequences of hypercalcaemia should be sought. These include the presence of bone pain or fracture and renal stones. These tend to indicate the presence of chronic hypercalcaemia.

Box 76.2 Clinical features of hypercalcaemia

- Renal:
  - Polyuria.
  - Polydipsia.
- Gastrointestinal:
  - Anorexia.
  - Vomiting.
  - Constipation.
  - Abdominal pain.
- Central nervous system:
  - Confusion.
  - Lethargy.
  - Depression.
- Other:
  - Pruritus.
  - Sore eyes.

Investigation of hypercalcaemia

Confirm the diagnosis

Plasma calcium (corrected for albumin).

Determine the mechanism

- ↑ *PTH* parathyroid overactivity (1° or tertiary hyperparathyroidism, can also occur in familial hypocalciuric hypercalcaemia and in Li therapy due to faulty calcium sensing).
- ↓ *PTH* non-parathyroid cause.
- *Normal PTH:*
  - May imply parathyroid overactivity—incomplete suppression.
  - May imply altered calcium sensor—familial hypocalciuric hypercalcaemia—calcium/creatine excretion ratio will be low.
- Urine calcium to determine calcium/creatinine excretion ratio.

Seek underlying illness (where indicated)

- History and examination.
- Chest x-ray.
- FBC and ESR.
- Biochemical profile (renal and liver function).
- Thyroid function tests (exclude thyrotoxicosis).
- 25OHD and 1,25(OH)$_2$D.
- Plasma and urine protein electrophoresis (exclude myeloma).
- Serum cortisol (short Synacthen® test (exclude Addison's disease)).

To determine end-organ damage

- 24h urine calcium (± urine creatinine for reproducibility).
- Renal tract ultrasound (exclude calculi, nephrocalcinosis).
- Skeletal radiographs (lateral thoracolumbar spine, hands, knees).
- BMD.
- Bone turnover markers.

Hyperparathyroidism

Present in up to 1 in 500 of the general population where it is predominantly a disease of postmenopausal ♀.

The normal physiological response to hypocalcaemia is an increase in PTH secretion. This is termed 2° *hyperparathyroidism* and is not pathological in as much as the PTH secretion remains under feedback control. Continued stimulation of the parathyroid glands can lead to autonomous production of PTH. This in turn causes hypercalcaemia which is termed *tertiary hyperparathyroidism*. This is usually seen in the context of renal disease but can occur in any state of chronic hypocalcaemia such as vitamin D deficiency or malabsorption.

Pathology
- 85% single adenoma.
- 14% hyperplasia.
- Often associated with other endocrine abnormalities, particularly multiple endocrine neoplasia (MEN) types I and II (📖 see Chapter 99, MEN type 1, pp.616–620; Chapter 100, MEN type 2, pp.622–628).
- <1% carcinoma.

Clinical features
- Majority of patients are asymptomatic.
- Features of hypercalcaemia.
- End-organ damage—📖 see Box 76.3.

Natural history
- In majority of patients without end-organ damage disease is benign and stable.
- A significant minority (2–3% per annum) will develop new indications for surgery.
- Excess deaths are due to diabetes and vascular diseases.

Investigation (Box 76.4)
Potential diagnostic pitfalls:
- FHH—differentiate with calcium/creatine excretion ratio (📖 see Familial hypocalciuric hypercalcaemia, p.465,482) (<0.01 in FHH >0.02 in hyperparathyroidism).
- Long-standing vitamin D deficiency where the concomitant osteomalacia and calcium malabsorption can mask hypercalcaemia which becomes apparent only after vitamin D repletion. Consider other causes of a raised PTH (Box 76.5.)
- Drugs associated with hypercalcaemia (e.g. thiazides and lithium).

Investigation is, therefore, primarily aimed at determining the presence of end-organ damage from the hypercalcaemia in order to determine whether operative intervention is indicated.

Box 76.3 End-organ damage in hyperparathyroidism

Bone
- Osteoporosis:
  - Common.
  - Affects all sites but predominant loss is in peripheral cortical bone.
- Radiographic changes:
  - Uncommon.
  - Include subperiosteal resorption, abnormal skull vault, eroded lamina dura (around teeth), and bone cysts.
- Osteitis fibrosa cystica:
  - Rare.
  - Usually with tertiary hyperparathyroidism.

Kidneys
- Renal calculi.
- Nephrocalcinosis.
- Renal impairment.

Joints
- Chondrocalcinosis.
- Pseudogout.

Pancreatitis

Box 76.4 Diagnosis of primary hyperparathyroidism

- Ca > 2.65 mmol (corrected) × 2:
- UE normal:
- Not on lithium or thiazide diuretic
- PTH > 3.0 pmol.
- Urine Ca > 2.5 mmol/day.

Exclusion of underlying condition

- 1° hyperparathyroidism (PHP) can be associated with genetic abnormalities, especially MEN I and II as well as familial hyperparathyroidism.
- These conditions should be sought in patients presenting with PHP and a family history in ≥1 1st-degree relatives or at a young age (<40 years).

Localization of abnormal parathyroid glands

This should only form part of a preoperative assessment and is not indicated in the initial diagnosis of hyperparathyroidism.

- Localization with 2 separate techniques (usually US and ^{99m}Tc-sestamibi) is imperative before minimally invasive parathyroidectomy.
- Otherwise, bilateral neck exploration by an experienced surgeon is optimal in the first instance.
- After failed neck exploration may need other techniques, which include:
  - ^{99m}Tc-sestamibi
  - –thallium/technetium subtraction scanning (less sensitive).
  - CT.
  - US.
- Following failed neck exploration it is often useful to undertake angiography with selective venous sampling—this should be confined to specialist centres.

Box 76.5 Causes of a secondary raised PTH

- GI disorder.
- Renal insufficiency.
- Vitamin D deficiency (25 OHD <20ng/mL).
- Renal hypercalcaemia.
- Drugs (e.g. lithium, thiazides).

Treatment

Surgery

- For indications 📖 see Table 76.1.
- Only by experienced surgeon (>20 procedures per year):
  - *Adenoma* remove affected gland.
  - *Hyperplasia* either:
    —partial parathyroidectomy (perhaps with reimplantation of tissue in more accessible site), *or*
    —total parathyroidectomy with medical treatment for hypoparathyroidism.

Observation

- Suitable for patients with mild disease with no evidence of end-organ damage.
- Such patients can continue for many years without deterioration.
- They require follow up:
  - *Annual* plasma calcium, renal function, BP.
  - *Every 2–3 years* BMD, renal US.
- Any significant deterioration is an indication for surgery.

Medical management

Only indicated if patient not suitable for surgery.
- Hormone replacement therapy:
  - Reduces plasma and urine calcium.
  - Preserves bone mass.
  - Consider the long-term risks (breast cancer, venous thrombosis, heart disease, and stroke).
- Bisphosphonates:
  - Only transient effect on plasma and urine calcium.
  - Preserve bone mass.
- Calcium sensing receptor agonists:
  - Cinacalcet (30 mg t.d) will reduce plasma, but not urinary, calcium concentrations. It increases sensitivity of Calcium sensing receptor decreasing PTH secretion licensed for 2° hyperparathyroidism and parathyroid carcinoma.
  - It is not licensed for use in 1° hyperparathyroidism.

Indications for surgery in primary hyperparathyroidism

It is generally accepted that all patients with symptomatic hyperparathyroidism or evidence of end-organ damage should be considered for parathyroidectomy. This would include:
- Definite symptoms of hypercalcaemia. There is less good evidence that non-specific symptoms such as abdominal pain, tiredness, or mild cognitive impairment benefit from surgery.
- Impaired renal function.
- Renal stones (symptomatic or on radiograph).
- Parathyroid bone disease especially osteitis fibrosis cystica.
- Pancreatitis.

Guidelines for the management of asymptomatic hyperparathyroidism have recently been produced on the basis of a consensus development conference in the USA[1] and following review of evidence in the UK.[2] Although there are some differences between these approaches there is also considerable similarity; many of the differences relate to a perceived ↑ caution in the USA towards leaving patients untreated in the absence of specific evidence of safety.

Table 76.1 Table comparing indications for parathyroidectomy in asymptomatic patients in USA compared with UK

	USA	UK
Plasma calcium	~2.85mmol/L	3.00mmol/L
Urine calcium	10mmol/d	10mmol/d (perhaps)
Creatinine clearance	↓ 30%	Not discused
BMD	T score <–2.5	T score <–2.5
Age	<50	<50

Conservative management

- Patients not managed with surgery require regular follow up.
- Again there is some difference between UK and US recommendations (☐ see Table 76.2).

Table 76.2 Table comparing managements recommendations for patients in USA compared with UK

	UK	USA
Plasma calcium	6 months	6 months
Plasma creatinine	6 months	12 months
BP	6 months	Not mentioned
PTH	12 months	Not mentioned
Urine calcium	12 months	Not recommended
Urine creatinine	12 months	Not recommended
BMD	24–36 months	12 months
Abdominal x-ray / USS	36 months	Not recommended

1 Bilezikian, JP, Watts JT Jr, Fuleihan Gel-H, et al. (2002). Summary statement from a workshop on asymptomatic primary hyperparathyroidism: a perspective for the 21st century. *J Clin Endocrinol Metab* **87**(12), 5353–61.

2 Davies M, Fraser WD, Hoskin DJ (?002). The management of primary hyperparathyroidism. *Clin Endocrinol* (Oxf) **57**(2), 145–55.

Complications of parathyroidectomy

Mechanical
- Vocal cord paresis:
  - Usually transient.
  - May be permanent with extensive exploration, particularly repeated surgery.
  - May require Teflon® injection of vocal cord.
- Tracheal compression from haematoma.

Metabolic (hypocalcaemia)
- Transient:
  - Due to suppression of remaining glands.
  - Usually causes little problem.
  - May sometimes require oral therapy with calcium ± vitamin D metabolites.
- Severe:
  - Due to hungry bones (calcitriol 1mcg/day and oral calcium, e.g. Sandocal-400® 3 × daily may be required for several weeks).
  - Occurs in patients with pre-existing bone disease.
  - Prevent by pretreatment with calcium and vitamin D (1g and 20mcg (800IU) respectively daily) for several weeks—rarely required in practice nowadays. This may worsen hypercalcaemia and must be monitored.
  - May settle with oral therapy but often requires IV calcium.

Outcome after surgery
- <10% fail to become normocalcaemic; of these half will respond to a 2nd operation.
- Relapse occurs in 1/20 patients with adenoma but 1/6 with hyperplasia.
- All patients with parathyroid hyperplasia (including MEN) need indefinite follow-up.
- If the patient is rendered hypoparathyroid by surgery they will need lifelong supplements of calcium ± active metabolites of vitamin D. This can lead to hypercalciuria and the risk of stone formation may still be present in these patients.

Other causes of hypercalcaemia

Hypercalcaemia of malignancy

Mechanism
📖 See Table 76.3.

Clinical features
Hypercalcaemia is usually a late manifestation of malignant disease and frequently indicates the presence of an untreatable tumour load (50% due within 30 days). One exception to this is in small endocrine tumours such as carcinoids and islet cell tumours which can produce humoural mediators of hypercalcaemia (PTHrP) in the absence of significant spread. Hypercalcaemic symptoms are non-specific and frequently difficult to distinguish from those of the underlying disease.

Investigation
📖 see investigation of hypercalcaemia in Clinical features, p.470.

Factors suggesting hypercalcaemia of malignancy include:
- ↑ calcium.
- ↓ PTH.
- Other features of malignant disease.
- ↑ PTHrP—not usually measured in clinical practice.

Steroid suppression test is not usually needed now that modern hormone assays are available. Even when used its sensitivity and specificity are poor.

Treatment
Frequently patients requiring treatment will have severe symptomatic hypercalcaemia. Often emergency treatment is necessary to stabilize the patient before confirmation of the diagnosis of the underlying malignant state can be confirmed. In such circumstances the principles of management are the same as those of severe hypercalcaemia from any cause (📖 see Box 76.6, p.483).

Table 76.3 Types of hypercalcaemia associated with cancer

Type	Frequency	Bone metastases	Causing agent	Tumour type
Local osteolytic	20	Common Extensive	Cytokines Chemokines PTHrP	Breast Myeloma Lymphoma
Humoral	80	Minimal	PTHrP	Sqamous carcinoma Renal Ovarian Endometrial Breast HTLV Lymphoma
1,25OH Vit D	<1	Variable	$1,25(OH)_2D$	Lymphoma
Ectopic PTH	<1	Variable	PTH	Variable

Familial hypocalciuric hypercalcaemia (FHH)

FHH: also known as familial benign hypercalcaemia.
- 2% of all asymptomatic hypercalcaemia.
- Autosomal dominant with virtually complete penetrance.
- Mutation in the calcium-sensing receptor which reduces its sensitivity such that the body behaves as if it were experiencing normocalcaemia even though the plasma calcium level is elevated.
- Generally benign and is not usually associated with symptoms or adverse effects such as renal stones or bone disease.
- Does not usually show any sustained benefit from parathyroidectomy.
- A few adults with FHH have had recurrent pancreatitis. In such cases parathyroidectomy may reduce the frequency of attacks.
- The homozygous state produces severe life-threatening hypercalcaemia soon after birth (neonatal severe hyperparathyroidism). In such cases total parathyroidectomy is life saving.
- Patients have low urine calcium excretion (24h <2.5mmol, fasting calcium/creatine excretion ration <0.01 📖 see Box 75.2, p.465).

Further reading

Pallais JC, Kifor O, Chen YB, *et al.* (2004). Acquired hypocalciuric hypercalcemia due to autoantibodies against the calcium-sensing receptor. *New Engl J Med.* **351**(4), 362–9.

Box 76.6 Management of severe hypercalcaemia

- Vigorous rehydration 200–500ml/hr
- Calciuresis with loop diuretics when nomovolaemia
- Disodium pamidronate 60–90 mg/ alendronic acid 70 mg
- Calcium falls within 12 hours nadix 4–7 days
- Remains normal for 1–3 weeks

1. Stabilize the level of hypercalcemia and prevent any further decline in renal function. This requires the IV infusion of large quantities of 0.9% saline, frequently 3–6L over the first 24h. If there is a danger of salt and water retention a loop diuretic should be added. This is the only role of diuretics in the management of hypercalcaemia. There is no evidence that they lead to sustained reduction in plasma calcium. As they cause intravascular volume depletion they can worsen the situation and so should otherwise be avoided. In very severe renal impairment dialysis might help both stabilize the fluid balance and also assist in the removal of calcium from the plasma.
2. Once the patient is volume replete it is necessary to treat the cause of the hypercalcaemia. The most effective therapy available for this is IV bisphosphonate. Although these agents are specific inhibitors of bone resorption they are frequently beneficial when hypercalcaemia is the result of ↑ tubular reabsorption of calcium brought about by PTHrP production. Several bisphosphonates are available for IV treatment of hypercalcaemia. Plasma calcium will usually fall by about 72h with a nadir at 5 days. Clodronate can be given orally to prolong the duration of effect although it is more usual to retreat with IV bisphosphonate as the calcium rises. IV bisphosphonate therapy is generally well tolerated but a minority of patient may develop ↑ bone pain or a transient pyrexia and flu-like symptoms. Rarer complications include rashes and iritis. Bisphosphonates have been associated with deterioration in renal function. For this reason, they should not be given to patients until adequate rehydration has been administered. In addition, consideration of dose reduction should be made in patients with GFR <30 mL/min.
3. Although the majority of patients will respond to IV bisphosphonates not all will do so. In such cases treatment with calcitonin may be helpful. This is usually given as *salmon calcitonin* and may need to be given as high doses of up to 400IU by IM injection every 6h. In addition to the large volume of injection required this is frequently poorly tolerated with side effects such as flushing and nausea. Some cases of resistant hypercalcaemia will respond to corticosteroid therapy which needs to be given in high doses, such as prednisolone 40mg daily.

Vitamin D intoxication

- The diagnosis is established by the presence of greatly elevated concentrations of 25OHD (>100ng/mL) and 1,25(OH)$_2$D together with suppressed PTH. If calcitriol or alfacalcidol is the offending compound then 25OHD levels will not be elevated.
- In mild cases, particularly when the active vitamin D metabolites are involved, the only treatment necessary is to withdraw the offending treatment and let the calcium levels settle. If the longer-acting vitamin D metabolites are involved then active treatment may be necessary.
  - Patients should first be stabilized with a saline infusion (☐ see Box 76.4, p.483).
  - Following this the traditional management has been to give high dose oral corticosteroids such as prednisolone 40 mg daily. This reduces the vitamin D-stimulated calcium absorption and may have beneficial effects on vitamin D metabolism following intoxication. However, there is now emerging evidence to suggest that bisphosphonates given as for hypercalcaemia of malignancy are equally effective.

Sarcoidosis

- Together with other granulomatous disorders sarcoidosis causes hypercalcaemia by extrarenal production of $1,25(OH)_2D$ in granulomata. This process is not under feedback inhibition, but is substrate regulated. The hypercalcaemia is therefore dependent on vitamin D supply. Patients frequently present with hypercalcaemia in summer or following foreign holidays when the endogenous production of vitamin D is maximal.
- The biochemical picture is of normal 25OHD, raised $1,25(OH)_2D$, and suppressed PTH. In addition, other markers of sarcoid activity such as raised angiotensin converting enzyme (ACE) activity are frequently present.
- Treatment with high-dose corticosteroids as in vitamin D intoxication is generally recommended to control sarcoid activity and to minimize the GI effects of the excess $1,25(OH)_2D$. The antifungal *ketoconazole*, and the antimalarial *chloroquine* (or its derivative, hydroxychloroquine) modulate vitamin D metabolism and have been reported to reduce hypercalcaemia in patients with sarcoidosis. If the calcium levels do not respond to these, there is evidence that bisphosphonates might be useful in this situation.

Further reading

Bilezikian JP, Watts JT Jr, Fuleihan Gel-H, et al. (2002). Summary statement from a workshop on asymptomatic primary hyperparathyroidism: a perspective for the 21st century. J Clinl Endocrinol Metab **87**(12), 5353–61.

Palazzo FF and Sadler GP (2004). Minimally invasive parathyroidectomy. BMJ **328**(7444), 849–50.

Peacock M, Bilezikian JP, Klassen PS, et al. (2005). Cinacalcet hydrochloride maintains long-term normocalcemia in patients with primary hyperthyroidism. J Clin Endocrinol Metab **90**(1), 135-41. Epub 2004 Nov 2.

Stewart AE (2005). Clinical practice. Hypercalcemia associated with cancer. New Engl J Med **352**(4), 373–9.

Hypocalcaemia

Causes

Although hypocalcaemia can result from failure of any of the mechanisms by which plasma calcium concentration is maintained, it is usually the result of either failure of PTH secretion or because of the inability to release calcium from bone. These causes are summarized in Box 77.1.

Box 77.1 Causes of hypocalcaemia

Hypoparathyroidism
- Destruction of parathyroid glands:
  - Autoimmune.
  - Surgical.
  - Radiation.
  - Infiltration.
- Failure of parathyroid development:
  - Isolated, e.g. X-linked.
  - With other abnormalities, e.g. DiGeorge syndrome (with thymic aplasia, immunodeficiency, and cardiac anomalies).
- Failure of PTH secretion:
  - Magnesium deficiency.
  - Overactivity of calcium sensing receptor.
- Failure of PTH action:
  - Pseudohypoparathyroidism—due to G protein abnormality.

Failure of 1,25(OH)$_2$D levels
- Drugs, e.g. ketoconazole.
- Acute pancreatitis.
- Acute systemic illness.

Failure of release of calcium from bone
- Osteomalacia:
  - Vitamin D deficiency.
  - Vitamin D resistance.
  - Renal failure.
- Inhibition of bone resorption:
  - Hypocalcaemic drugs e.g. cisplatin, calcitonin, oral phosphate.
- ↑ uptake of calcium into bone:
  - Osteoblastic metastases (e.g. prostate).
  - Hungry bone syndrome.

Complexing of calcium from the circulation
- ↑ albumin binding in alkalosis.
- Acute pancreatitis:
  - Formation of calcium soaps from autodigestion of fat.
  - Abnormal PTH and vitamin D metabolism.
  - Phosphate infusion.
- Multiple blood transfusion—complexing by citrate.

Clinical features

The clinical features of hypocalcaemia are largely as a result of ↑ neuromuscular excitability. In order of ↑ severity these include:

- Tingling—especially of fingers, toes, or lips.
- Numbness—especially of fingers, toes, or lips.
- Cramps.
- Carpopedal spasm.
- Stridor due to laryngospam.
- Seizures.

The symptoms of hypocalcaemia tend to reflect the severity and rapidity of onset of the metabolic abnormality.

Clinical signs of hypocalcaemia depend upon the demonstration of neuromuscular irritability before this necessarily causes symptoms:

- *Chvostek's sign* is elicited by tapping the facial nerve in front of the ear. A +ve result is indicated by twitching of the corner of the mouth. Slight twitching is seen in up to 15% of normal ♀ but more major involvement of the facial muscles is indicative of hypocalcaemia or hypomagnesaemia.
- *Trousseau's sign* is produced by occlusion of the blood supply to the arm by inflation of a sphygmomanometer cuff above arterial pressure for 3min. If +ve, there will be carpopedal spasm which may be accompanied by painful paraesthesiae.

In addition, there may be clinical signs and symptoms associated with the underlying condition:

- *Vitamin D deficiency* may be associated with bone pain, fractures, or proximal myopathy (📖 see p.498).
- *Hypoparathyroidism* can be accompanied by mental retardation and personality disturbances as well as extrapyramidal signs, cataracts, and papilloedema.
- If *hypocalcaemia* is present during the development of the permanent teeth, these may show areas of enamel hypoplasia. This can be a useful physical sign indicating that the hypocalcaemia is long-standing.

Pseudohypoparathyroidism

- Resistance to parathyroid hormone action.
- Due to defective signalling of PTH action via cell membrane receptor.
- Also affects TSH, LH, FSH, and GH signalling.
- Most commonly caused by autosomal dominant mutation of *GNAS1* gene.
- Significant imprinting:
  - Maternal transmission leads to full blown syndrome of hormone resistance.
  - Paternal transmission causes only phenotypic features of Albright's hereditary osteodystrophy.

Albright's hereditary osteodystrophy

Patients with the most common type of pseudohypoparathyroidism (type Ia) have a characteristic set of skeletal abnormalities known as Albright's hereditary osteodystrophy. This comprises:

- Short stature.
- Obesity.
- Round face.
- Short metacarpals.

Some individuals with Albright's hereditary osteodystrophy do not appear to have a disorder of calcium metabolism. In the past the term *pseudopseudohypoparathyroidism* has been used to describe these. However, it is now clear that these reflect different manifestations of the same underlying genetic defect as a result of imprinting. In the light of the same underlying cellular abnormality, there has been a tendency to avoid the more cumbersome designations and refer to all such patients as having Albright's hereditary osteodystrophy.

Investigation

- Plasma calcium.
- PTH—the presence of a low, or even normal, PTH concentration implies failure of PTH secretion.
- Vitamin D.
- Magnesium may be needed if patient fails to respond.
- Ellsworth–Howard test if pshypoparathyroidism suspected (📖 see Box 77.2)
- In chronic hypocalcaemia skull radiographs will frequently demonstrate calcification of the basal ganglia. As this is of no clinical consequence it is debatable whether the investigation can be justified.

Box 77.2 Modified Ellsworth–Howard test

Method

1. Fast overnight.
2. Give 200mL water every 30min from 6 a.m. to 11 a.m.
3. From 8:30 a.m. collect timed 30min urine samples for phosphate, creatinine, and cAMP.
4. At 8:45 a.m., 10:15 a.m., and 10:45 a.m. collect blood for creatinine and phosphate.
5. At 10:00 a.m. commence 10min infusion of synthetic PTH 1–34, 5 units/kg to a maximum of 200 units.
6. Calculate urinary cAMP excretion as:

$$\text{cAMPE} = [\text{urine cAMP}] \times [\text{plasma creatinine}]/[\text{urine creatinine}]$$

7. Calculate tubular maximum for phosphate reabsorption:

$$\text{TmP/GFR} = ([\text{plasma PO}_4] - P_E)/(1 - 0.01 \times \log_e([\text{plasma PO}_4]/P_E))$$

where $P_E = [\text{urine PO}_4] \times [\text{plasma creatinine}]/[\text{urine creatinine}]$ and all measurements are in mmol/L

or using the nomogram of Walton and Bijvoet ((1975) *Lancet* **2**, 309).

Interpretation

- Patients with a normal response to PTH will demonstrate a brisk increase in cAMP excretion and a decrease in TmP.
- Patients with pseudohypoparathyroidism type I show neither response.
- There is a rarer condition, pseudohypoparathyroidism type II, in which there is a normal cAMP response but a blunted phosphaturic response.
- A similar pattern can be seen in some patients with profound hypocalcaemia due to vitamin D deficiency. It is therefore important to ensure that patients are vitamin D replete before undertaking a PTH infusion test.

Treatment

- *Acute symptomatic hypocalcaemia* is a medical emergency and demands urgent treatment whatever the cause (see Box 77.3).
- Treatment of *chronic hypocalcaemia* is more dependent on the cause.

Chronic hypocalcaemia

Hypoparathyroidism

- In hypoparathyroidism the aim is not to achieve normalization of the plasma calcium, rather to render them asymptomatic with a plasma calcium at, or just below, the normal lower limit. The reason for this is that the renal retention of calcium brought about by PTH has been lost. Thus, any attempt to raise the plasma calcium well into the normal range is likely to result in unacceptable hypercalciuria with the risk of nephrocalcinosis and renal stones.
- In patients with mild parathyroid dysfunction it may be possible to achieve acceptable calcium concentrations by using calcium supplements alone. If used in this way these need to be given in large doses, perhaps as much as 1 g elemental calcium 3 × daily.
- The majority of patients will not achieve adequate control with such treatment. In those cases it is necessary to use vitamin D or its metabolites in pharmacological doses to maintain plasma calcium. The more potent analogues of vitamin D such as *calcitriol* or *alfacalcidol* have the advantage over high-dose calciferol that it is easier to make changes in therapy in response to plasma calcium levels. If hypercalcaemia does occur it settles much more quickly following withdrawal of these compounds than ergocalciferol. The dose of vitamin D is determined by the clinical response but usually lies in the range of 0.5–2mcg of the potent analogues daily. Hypercalcaemia is the main hazard of such therapy. Plasma calcium levels must be checked frequently after any change in therapy and no less than 3-monthly whilst on maintenance.
- It is essential to ensure an adequate intake of calcium as well as vitamin D analogues. In some patients it is necessary to give calcium supplementation, particularly in the young. It is very rarely needed in patients aged >60 years.

Pseudohypoparathyroidism

- The principles underlying the treatment of pseudohypoparathyroidism are the same as those underlying hypoparathyroidism.
- Patients with the most common form of pseudohypoparathyroidism may have resistance to the action of other hormones which rely on G protein signalling. They therefore need to be assessed for thyroid and gonadal dysfunction (because of defective TSH or gonadotrophin action). If these deficiencies are present they need to be treated in the conventional manner.

Vitamin D deficiency

📖 treatment of osteomalacia and vitamin D deficiency is described on p.498.

Overactivity of calcium sensing receptor

This leads to a condition known as autosomal dominant hypocalcaemia. It is a benign condition in which the hypercalcaemia is usually asymptomatic. Treatment should be avoided in the absence of symptoms as elevation of calcium levels even to within the normal range may cause renal impairment.

Box 77.3 Treatment of acute hypocalcaemia

- Patients with tetany or seizures require urgent IV treatment with calcium gluconate (less irritant than the chloride).
  - This is a 10% w/v solution (10mL = 2.25mmol elemental calcium).
  - The solution should always be further diluted to minimize the risk of phlebitis or tissue damage if extravasation occurs.
- Initially, 20mL of 10% calcium gluconate should be diluted in 100–200mL of 0.9% saline or 5% glucose and infused over about 10min.
- Repeat, if symptoms not resolved.
- Care must be taken if the patient has heart disease, especially if taking digoxin, as too rapid elevation of the plasma calcium can cause arrhythmias. In such patients it is advisable to monitor the cardiac rhythm during calcium infusion.
- In order to maintain the plasma calcium give a continuous calcium infusion. 40mL of 10% calcium gluconate should be added to 1L of saline or glucose solution and infused over 24h.
- The plasma calcium should be checked regularly (not less than 6-hourly) and the infusion rate adjusted in response to the change in concentration.
- Failure of the plasma calcium to respond to infused calcium should raise the possibility of hypomagnesaemia. This can be rapidly ascertained by plasma magnesium estimation and, if appropriate, a magnesium infusion commenced (📖 see Treatment, p.504).
- In circumstances where hypoparathyroidism could be predicted (such as block dissection of the neck) infusion of calcium gluconate in an initial dose of 50mL10% solution(~11mmol Ca) diluted in normal saline over 24h should be given to avoid post operative hypocalcaemia. This dose should be adjusted in the light of regular calcium estimations.
- Once oral or NG tube intake is possible calcium and active vitamin D metabolites should be substituted as above.

Further Reading

Shoback, D (2008). Hypoparathyroidism *NEJM* **359**, 391-403.

Rickets and osteomalacia

Definitions

Osteomalacia occurs when there is inadequate mineralization of mature bone. *Rickets* is a disorder of the growing skeleton where there is inadequate mineralization of bone as it is laid down at the epiphysis. In most instances osteomalacia leads to build up of excessive unmineralized osteoid within the skeleton. In rickets there is build up of unmineralized osteoid in the growth plate. This leads to the characteristic radiological appearance of rickets with widening of the growth plate and loss of definition of the ossification centres. These 2 related conditions may coexist.

Clinical features

Osteomalacia
- Bone pain.
- Deformity.
- Fracture.
- Proximal myopathy (depending on the underlying cause).
- Hypocalcaemia (in vitamin D deficiency).

Rickets
- Growth retardation.
- Bone pain and fracture.
- Skeletal deformity:
  - Bowing of the long bones.
  - Widening of the growth plates widening of the wrists, 'rickety rosary' (costochondral junctions enlarged).

Diagnosis

- The diagnosis of osteomalacia is usually based on the appropriate biochemical findings (☐ see Table 78.1).
- The majority of patients with osteomalacia will show no specific radiological abnormalities.
- The most characteristic abnormality is the *Looser's zone* or pseudo-fracture. If these are present they are virtually pathognomonic of osteomalacia.
- If the diagnosis of osteomalacia remains in doubt then bone biopsy may be necessary. This is often the only way of establishing the diagnosis in low turnover conditions such as the toxic osteomalacias.

Box 78.1 Vitamin D resistance

Several different kindreds have been shown to have a defective vitamin D receptor. This is inherited as an autosomal recessive condition. It produces hypocalcaemia and osteomalacia with elevated serum levels of $1,25(OH)_2$ D. Approximately 2/3 of affected individuals have total alopecia. This condition is known as vitamin D-dependent rickets type II. If alopecia is present it is often termed type IIA in contrast to type IIB where hair growth is normal.

Treatment usually requires administration of large doses of active vitamin D metabolites, sometimes reaching doses of 60mcg of calcitriol daily.

Box 78.2 Abnormal vitamin D metabolism

Although liver disease could, in theory, lead to deficient 25-hydroxyla-tion of vitamin D there is so much functional reserve that this is seldom a clinical problem. 2 cases of rickets due to hereditary defects of 25-hydroxylase have been reported.

The most common cause of failure of 1α-hydroxylase is renal failure. Congenital absence of this enzyme leads to a condition known as vitamin D-dependent rickets type I. This is inherited in an autosomal recessive fashion. It leads to profound rickets with myopathy and enamel hypo-plasia. Very large doses of calciferol are needed to heal the bone lesions which, in contrast, will respond to physiological doses of alfacalcidol or calcitriol.

Table 78.1 Biochemical findings and causes of rickets and osteomalacia

	Ca	PO4	Alkaline phosphatase	25OHD	1,25(OH)₂D	PTH	Other
Vitamin D deficiency	↓	↓	↑	↓	↓	↑	
Renal failure	↓	↑	↑	N	↓	↑	↓ GFR
VDDR type I (deficient 1α-hydroxylase)	↓	↓	↑	N	↓	↑	
VDDR type II (deficient vitamin D receptor)	↓	↓	↑	N	↑	↑	
X-linked hypophosphataemia (vitamin D resistant rickets)	N	↓	↑	N	N	N or ↑	
Oncogenic	N or ↓	↓	↑	N	↓	N	May have aminoaciduria, proteinuria
Phosphate depletion	N	↓	↑	N	·	N	↑ urine Ca
Fanconi syndrome	↓ or N	↓	↑	N	↓	N	acidosis, aminoaciduria, glycosuria
Renal tubular acidosis	↓ or N	↓	↑	N	N or ↓	N	Acidosis
Toxic (etidronate, fluoride)	N	N	N	N	N	N	Diagnosed on biopsy

Vitamin D deficiency

Causes

- Poor sunlight exposure:
  - Elderly housebound.
  - Asian women who cover their bodies with clothing.
- Poor diet (especially vegetarians):
  - Malabsorption.
  - ↑ catabolism of vitamin D.
- 2° hyperparathyroidism:
  - Malabsorption.
  - Post gastrectomy.
  - Enzyme-inducing drugs e.g. phenytoin.

Investigation

The diagnosis of vitamin D deficiency is based on the characteristic biochemical abnormalities (☐ see Table 78.1, p.497). Frank osteomalacia is usually associated with very low levels of 25OHD (<5ng/mL) but the associated 2° hyperparathyroidism frequently results in normal or even elevated concentrations of $1,25(OH)_2$ D.

Treatment

- Treatment is best given in the form of ergocalciferol which will restore the biochemistry to normal and heal the bony abnormalities. Although the use of the active metabolites of vitamin D will heal the bony abnormalities it will not correct the underlying biochemical problem and is associated with ↑ risk of hypercalcaemia.
- In adults treatment can be given as a daily dose of ergocalciferol of 20–25mcg (800–1000IU) which is often most easily administered in combination with a calcium supplement. An alternative, which is particularly helpful if poor compliance is suspected, is to give a single large dose of 3.75–7.5 mg (150 000–300 000IU). This is most effectively given as a single oral dose (3–6 × 1.25mg tablets of ergocalciferol) which can be supervised in clinic. It is possible to give a similar dose by IM injection but the absorption from this route is variable.
- Following treatment there usually is a rapid improvement of myopathy and symptoms of hypocalcaemia. Bone pain frequently persists longer and biochemical abnormalities may not settle for several months. Indeed, following the onset of therapy markers of bone turnover such as alkaline phosphatase might even show a transient increase as the osteoid is mineralized and remodelled. Beware hypercalcaemia once the osteomalacia is healed. Calcium concentrations should be monitored and the dose of vitamin D should be reduced if necessary.

X linked hypophosphataemia

- X-linked dominant genetic disorder.
- Severe rickets and osteomalacia.
- Mutation of an endopeptidase gene (*PHEX*).

Clinical features

- The abnormal phosphate levels are often detected early in infancy but skeletal deformities are not apparent until walking commences.
- Typical severe rickets, with short stature and bony deformity.
- Continues into adult life with bone pain, deformity, and fracture in the absence of treatment.
- Proximal myopathy is absent.
- Adults suffer from excessive new bone growth particularly affecting entheses and the longitudinal ligaments of the spinal canal. This can cause spinal cord compression which may need surgical decompression.

Oncogenic osteomalacia

Certain tumours appear to be able to produce FGF23 which is phosphaturic. This is rare and usually occurs with mesenchymal tumours (such as haemangiopericytomas, haemangiomata, or osteoid tumours) but has also been reported with a variety of adenocarcinomas (particularly prostatic cancer) and haematological malignancies (e.g. myeloma and chronic lymphocytic leukaemia). A similar picture can also be seen in some cases of neurofibromatosis. Clinically such patients usually present with profound myopathy as well as bone pain and fracture. Biochemically, the major abnormality is hypophosphataemia but this is usually accompanied by marked reduction in $1,25(OH)_2D$ concentrations. In some patients, other abnormalities of renal tubular function such as glycosuria or aminoaciduria are also present.

- FGF_3 levels are elevated and fall with tumour removal.
- Tumour may be localised by PET or CT.

Complete removal of the tumour results in resolution of the biochemical and skeletal abnormalities. If this is not possible, or if a causal tumour is not identified, treatment with vitamin D metabolites and phosphate supplements (as for X-linked hypophosphataemia) may help the skeletal symptoms.

Fanconi syndrome

The Fanconi syndrome is a combination of renal tubular defects which can result from several different pathologies. In particular there is renal wasting of phosphate, bicarbonate, glucose, and amino acids. The combination of hypophosphataemia with renal tubular acidosis means that osteomalacia is a frequent accompaniment. This can be exacerbated by defective 1α-hydroxylation of vitamin D to its active form. The osteomalacia is treated by correction of the relevant abnormalities. This might involve the administration of phosphate, alkali or $1,25(OH)_2D$ depending on the precise circumstances.

Further reading

Carpenter TO (2003). Oncogenic Osteomalacia—a complex dance of factors. *NEJM* **348**, 1705–1708.

Box 78.3 Causes of hypophosphataemia

- ↓ intestinal absorption:
  - Phosphate binding antacids.
  - Malabsorption.
  - Starvation/malnutrition.
- ↑ renal losses.
  - hyperparathyroidism:
  - 1°.
  - 2°, e.g. in vitamin D deficiency.
  - Renal tubular defects:
  - Fanconi syndrome.
  - X-linked hypophosphataemia.
  - Oncogenic osteomalacia.
  - Alcohol abuse.
  - Poorly controlled diabetes.
  - Acidosis.
  - Drugs:
  - Diuretics.
  - Corticosteroids.
  - Calcitonin.
- Shift into cells:
  - Septicaemia.
  - Insulin treatment.
  - Glucose administration.
  - Salicylate poisoning.

Hypophosphataemia

Phosphate is important for normal mineralization of bone. In the absence of sufficient phosphate osteomalacia results. Clinically the osteomalacia is often indistinguishable from other that are due to other causes, although there may be features that will help distinguish the underlying cause of hypophosphataemia. In addition, phosphate is important in its own right for neuromuscular function and profound hypophosphataemia can be accompanied by encephalopathy, muscle weakness, and cardiomyopathy. It must be remembered that, as phosphate is primarily an intracellular anion, a low plasma phosphate does not necessarily represent actual phosphate depletion. Several different causes of hypophosphataemia are recognized (see Box 78.3).

Treatment

- Mainstay is phosphate replacement, usually Phosphate-Sandoz®, each tablet of which provides 500mg of phosphate.
- Ideally, patients should receive 2–3g of phosphate daily between meals but this is not easy to achieve. All phosphate preparations are unpalatable and act as osmotic purgatives causing diarrhoea.
- Long-term administration of phosphate supplements stimulates parathyroid activity. This can lead to hypercalcaemia, a further fall in phosphate, with worsening of the bone disease due to the development of hyperparathyroid bone disease which may necessitate parathyroidectomy.
- To minimize parathyroid stimulation it is usual to give one of the active metabolites of vitamin D in conjunction with phosphate. Typically, alfacalcidol or calcitriol in a dose of 1–3mcg daily is used.
- Patients receiving such supraphysiological doses of vitamin D metabolites are at continued risk of hypercalcaemia and require regular monitoring of plasma calcium, preferably at least every 3 months. The adequacy of calcitriol replacement can be assessed by maintaining 24h urinary calcium excretion >4–6mmol/day.
- In adults the role of treatment for X-linked hypophosphataemia is probably confined to symptomatic bone disease.
  - There is little evidence that it will improve the long-term outcome.
  - There has even been some evidence that treatment might accelerate new bone formation.
- In children treatment is usually given in the hope of improving final height and minimizing skeletal abnormality—the evidence that it is possible to achieve these goals is conflicting.

Hypomagnesaemia

Introduction

- Low plasma magnesium levels are common in acutely ill patients. Clinical manifestations of this are less common. The most common clinical feature of magnesium deficiency is neuromuscular excitability which is virtually indistinguishable from that associated with hypocalcaemia, which frequently coexists.
- In the presence of magnesium deficiency PTH secretion is defective leading to the presence of, or worsening of hypocalcaemia which will not respond to treatment unless the magnesium deficiency is corrected. In magnesium depletion there is defective transmembrane electrolyte transport. This can cause loss of intracellular potassium and of the renal tubule's ability to retain potassium. Treatment with potassium supplementation is often unsuccessful unless magnesium is replaced at the same time.

Box 79.1 Causes of hypomagnesaemia

- GI losses:
  - Vomiting.
  - Diarrhoea.
  - Losses from fistulae.
  - Malabsorption.
- Renal losses:
  - Chronic parenteral therapy.
  - Osmotic diuresis.
- Diabetes.
- Drugs:
  - Alcohol.
  - Loop diuretics.
  - Aminoglycosides.
  - Cisplatin.
  - Ciclosporin.
  - Amphotericin.
- Metabolic acidosis.
- Hypercalcaemia.
- Other causes:
  - Phosphate depletion.
  - Hungry bone syndrome.

Treatment

Symptomatic magnesium deficiency, especially if associated with hypocalcaemia or hypokalaemia, requires parenteral treatment.

- Although the total deficit may be of the order of 150mmol this should not be replaced immediately.
- Magnesium sulfate 50% solution contains ~2mmol magnesium/mL. Although this can be given by IM injection it is usually more comfortable and controlled to give it by IV infusion. An initial 4–8mmol should be given over 15min followed by a slow infusion of 1mmol/h. The rate of the infusion can be adjusted in the light of the response in plasma magnesium.
- In the presence of renal impairment plasma magnesium can rise quickly and so particular care must be undertaken if magnesium infusion is contemplated in the presence of renal failure.
- After repletion has been achieved intravenously, or in less severe cases, treatment can be continued orally.
- No available oral magnesium supplement is readily available in the UK. Compounds which have been used include the chloride, oxide, and glycerophosphate. In all these instances the dose is frequently limited by the purgative properties of magnesium salts. There is some evidence to suggest that the addition of calcitriol or alfacalcidol might improve magnesium absorption.

Osteoporosis

Introduction

Although the term 'osteoporosis' refers to the reduction in the amount of bony tissue within the skeleton, this is generally associated with a loss of the structural integrity of the internal architecture of the bone. The combination of both these changes means that osteoporotic bone is at high risk of fracture, after even trivial injury. Although most fractures are related to bone mass to some extent the most common osteoporotic fractures are those of the hip, wrist (Colles), and compression fractures of vertebral bodies. Patients who fracture ribs, the upper humerus, leg and pelvis also have a higher incidence of osteoporosis.

Box 80.1 Underlying causes of osteoporosis

- Gonadal failure:
  - Premature menopause (age <45).
  - Hypogonadism in men, e.g. acquired and Klinefelter's syndrome.
  - Turner syndrome.
  - Oestrogen receptor defect.
- Conditions leading to amenorrhoea with low oestrogen (persisting >6months):
  - Hyperprolactinaemia.
  - Anorexia nervosa.
  - Athletic amenorrhoea.
- Endocrine disorders:
  - Cushing's syndrome.
  - GH deficiency.
  - Hyperparathyroidism.
  - Acromegaly with hypogonadism.
  - Hyperthyroidism within 3 years.
  - Diabetes mellitus.
- GI disorders:
  - Malabsorption.
  - Postgastrectomy.
  - Coeliac disease.
  - Crohn's disease.
- Liver disease:
  - Cholestasis.
  - Cirrhosis.
- Neoplastic disorders:
  - Multiple myeloma.
  - Systemic mastocytosis.
- Inflammatory conditions:
  - Rheumatoid arthritis.
  - Cystic fibrosis.
- Nutritional disorders:
  - Parenteral nutrition.
  - Lactose intolerance.

- Drugs:
  - Systemic corticosteroids (when administered for > 3 months).
  - Heparin (when given long term, particularly in pregnancy).
  - Chemotherapy (primarily by gonadal damage).
  - Gonadotrophin-releasing hormone agonists.
  - Ciclosporin.
  - Anticonvulsants (long term).
  - Aromatase inhibition for breast cancer.
  - Androgen deprivation therapy.
- Metabolic abnormalities:
  - Homocystinuria.
- Hereditary disorders.
  - Osteogenesis imperfecta.
  - Marfan syndrome.

Pathology

Osteoporosis may arise from a failure of the body to lay down sufficient bone during growth and maturation; an earlier than usual onset of bone loss following maturity; or an ↑ rate of that loss.

Peak bone mass
- Mainly genetically determined:
  - Racial effects (bone mass higher in Afro-Caribbean and lower in Caucasians.
  - Family influence on the risk of osteoporosis—may account for 70% of variation.
- Also influenced by environmental factors:
  - Exercise—particularly weight-bearing.
  - Nutrition—especially calcium.
- Exposure to oestrogen is also important
  - Early menopause or late puberty (in ♂ or ♀) is associated with ↑ risk of osteoporosis.

Early onset of loss
- Early menopause.
- Conditions leading to bone loss, e.g. glucocorticoid therapy.

Increased net loss
- Ageing:
  - Vitamin D insufficiency.
  - Declining bone formation.
  - Declining renal function.
- Underlying disease states (📖 see Box 80.1, p.509).

Lifestyle factors affecting bone mass
Increase:
Weight-bearing exercise.

Decrease:
- Smoking.
- Excessive alcohol.
- Nulliparity.
- Poor calcium nutrition.

Table 80.1 WHO proposals for diagnosis of postmenopausal osteoporosis

T score	Fragility fracture	Diagnosis
–1		Normal
<–1 but ≥–2.5		Low bone mass (osteopenia)
<–2.5	No	Osteoporosis
<–2.5	Yes	Established (severe) osteoporosis

Epidemiology

- The risk of osteoporotic fracture increases with age. Fracture rates in ♂ are approximately one-half those seen in ♀ of the same age. A ♀ aged 50 has approximately a 1/2 chance of sustaining an osteoporotic fracture in the rest of her life. The corresponding figure for a ♂ is 1/5.
- In the UK each year in ♀ there are in excess of 25 000 vertebral fractures that come to clinical attention together with over 40 000 wrist fractures and 50 000 hip fractures. The latter are a particular health challenge as they invariably result in hospital admission. 1/5 of hip fracture victims will die within 6 months of the injury and only 50% will return to their previous level of independence. It has been estimated that the overall cost of osteoporotic fractures in the UK is £1.7 billion annually.

Box 80.2 Investigations to exclude an underlying cause of osteoporosis

Useful in most patients
- FBC.
- ESR.
- Biochemical profile.
- Renal function.
- Liver function.
- Calcium.
- Thyroid function.
- Testosterone and LH (only in ♂).
- Vitamin D level.

Useful in specific instances
- Oestradiol and FSH (in ♀ where menopausal status not clear).
- Serum and urine electrophoresis (if raised ESR or plasma globulin elevated).
- Endomyscal antibodies (if any suggestion of coeliac disease).
- Other investigations for specific diseases.

Low trauma fractures associated with osteoporosis
Any fracture other than those affecting fingers, toes, or face which is caused by less trauma than a fall from standing height is potentially the result of osteoporosis. Patients suffering such a fracture should be considered for investigation and/or treatment for osteoporosis.

Presentation

- Usually clinically silent until the onset of fracture.
- 2/3 of vertebral fractures do not come to clinical attention.
- Typical vertebral fracture:
  - Sudden episode of well-localized pain.
  - May or may not have been related to injury or exertion.
  - May be radiation of the pain in a girdle distribution.
  - Pain may initially require bed rest but gradually subsides over the following 4–8 weeks: even after this time there may be residual pain at the fracture site.
  - Osteoporotic vertebral fractures only rarely lead to neurological impairment.
- Any evidence of spinal cord compression should prompt a search for malignancy or other underlying cause.
- Following vertebral fracture a patient may be left with persistent back pain, kyphosis, or height loss.
- Although height loss and kyphosis are often thought of as being indicative of osteoporosis they are more frequently the result of degenerative disease. They cannot be the result of osteoporosis in the absence of vertebral fracture.
- Peripheral fractures are also more common in osteoporosis.
- If a bone breaks from a fall from less than standing height that represents a low trauma fracture which might indicate underlying osteoporosis.
- Osteoporosis does not cause generalized skeletal pain.

📖 Fig. 80.1 shows an algorithm for management of osteoporosis in of ♂ and ♀ aged >45 years.

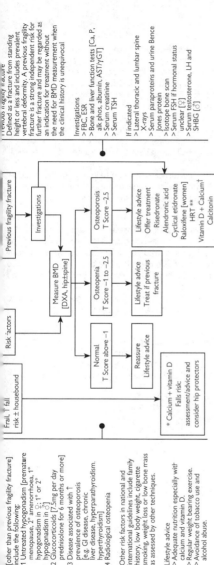

Previous fragility fracture

Defined as a fracture from standing height or less and includes prevalent vertebral deformity. A previous fragility fracture is a strong independent risk for further fracture and may be regarded as an indication for treatment without the need for BMD measurement when the clinical history is unequivocal

Investigations
> FBC, ESR
> Bone and liver function tests [Ca, P, alk phos, albumin, AST/γGT]
> Serum creatinine
> Serum TSH

If indicated
> Lateral thoracic and lumbar spine X-rays
> Serum paraproteins and urine Bence Jones protein
> Isotope bone scan
> Serum FSH if hormonal status unclear [♀]
> Serum testosterone, LH and SHBG [♂]

Frail, ↑ fall risk ± housebound — Risk factors — Previous fragility fracture

Measure BMD [DXA, hip±spine]

Investigations

Normal T Score above −1 → Reassure / Lifestyle advice

Osteopenia T Score −1 to −2.5 → Lifestyle advice / Treat if previous fracture

Osteoporosis T Score −2.5 → Lifestyle advice / Offer treatment / Risedronate / Alendronate / Cyclical etidronate / Raloxifene [women] / HRT ** / Vitamin D + Calcium† / Calcitonin / Calcitriol

* Calcium + vitamin D
Falls risk: assessment/advice and consider hip protectors

[other than previous fragility fracture] include the following:
1 Untreated hypogonadism [premature menopause, 2° amenorrhoea, 1° hypogonadism in ♀; 1° or 2° hypogonadism in ♂]
2 Glucocorticoids [7.5mg per day prednisolone for 6 months or more]
3 Disease associated with ↑ prevalence of osteoporosis [e.g. GI disease, chronic liver disease, hyperparathyroidism.
4 Radiological osteopenia

Other risk factors in national and international guidelines include family history, low body weight, cigarette smoking, weight loss or low bone mass as assessed by other techniques.

Lifestyle advice
> Adequate nutrition especially with calcium and vitamin D.
> Regular weight bearing exercise.
> Avoidance of tobacco use and alcohol abuse.

For men aged < 65 years, specialist referral should be considered.
* Recommended daily dose 0.5–1 g and 800 IU respectively
** HRT: oestrogen in ♀, testosterone in ♂
† Vitamin D and calcium are generally regarded as adjuncts to treatment.
BMD: Bone mineral density
DXA: Dual energy x-ray absorptiometry
HRT: Hormone replacement therapy

Fig. 80.1 Algorithm for medical management of ♂ and ♀ aged >45 years.
Adapted from: Royal College of Physicians and Bone and Tooth society of Great Britain (2000). Osteoporosis: clinical guidelines for prevention and treatment. Update of pharmacological interventions and an algorithm for management. London: Royal College of Physicians, reproduced with permission.

Investigation

Establish the diagnosis

- Plain radiographs are useful for determining the presence of fracture. Apart from this, they are of little utility in the diagnosis of osteoporosis.
- *Bone densitometry* In order to identify the presence of osteoporosis it is important to actually measure the BMD. This is usually carried out at the hip and/or lumbar spine using dual energy x-ray absorptiometry (DXA). The presence of degenerative disease or arterial calcification can elevate the apparent bone density of the spine without adding to skeletal strength. ↑ reliance is therefore being placed on measurements derived from the hip. The scheme for the diagnosis of osteoporosis which was proposed by WHO has generally been accepted for general use (☐ see Table 80.1, p.509).
- Biochemical markers of bone turnover may be helpful in the calculation of fracture risk and in judging the response to antiresorptive therapy but they have no role in the diagnosis of osteoporosis.

Exclude underlying causes

An underlying cause for osteoporosis is present in approximately 1/3 of women and over 1/2 men with osteoporosis. Many of the underlying causes (☐ see Box 80.1, p.506) should be apparent from a careful history and physical examination. A few basic investigations are useful to exclude the more common underlying causes. Other investigations may be needed to exclude other specific conditions.

It is most helpful to target these investigations at those people who have a lower than expected bone mass for their age (Z score <−2).

Monitoring therapy

- Repeat bone densitometry is advocated by some, but controversial.
- Minimum time interval 2 years between scans.
- Effective treatment leads to modest rise (~5% at spine)
- This may be replaced by biochemical markers as assays improve (e.g. P1NP).

Table 80.2 Drug treatments available

Treatment	Treatment	Effective dose	Spine BMD	#	Hip BMD	#
HRT	Oral	2 mg E2	++	?	+	↓[a]
		0.625 mg conjugated estrogens	++	↓	+	?
	Transdermal	50 mcg daily				
SERMs	Raloxifene	60 mg daily	+	↓	+	–
Tibolone		1.25/2.5 mg	+ 2% at 2 yrs	?	+ 2% at 2 yrs	?
Bisphosphonates	Etidronate	400 mg for 14/90 days	+	–/↓	–	–
	Alendronic acid	10 mg daily/ 70 mg weekly	++	↓	+	↓
	Risedronate	5 mg	++	↓	+	↓
	Ibandronic acid	150 mg orally monthly	++	↓	+	–
		3mg IV every 3 months				
	Zoledronic acid	5 mg by slow IV infusion once a year for 3 years	++	↓	++	↓
Calcium and vitamin D		1 g +	+	–/↓	+	↓
		20 mcg (800 IU)				
Calcitonin	SC or IM		+	?	?	?
	Nasal	200 IU daily	+	↓	?	?
Calcitriol		0.25 mcg2x day	+	↓	?	?
Fluoride		Not available in UK	++	↓	+	?
PTH	SC	18 months 20 mg	++		++	

[a] No RCT evidence.

Treatment

Treatments should, whenever possible, be judged by their effect on fracture reduction. Although some treatments are specific to certain clinical situations there are also general measures that apply to all patients with osteoporosis.

In addition to treatments aimed at improving bone mass it must be remembered that fractures can be prevented in other ways. Thus it is prudent to try and minimize the risk of falling by adjusting the home environment and reviewing the need for medications such as hypnotics and antihypertensives. There is conflicting evidence on the use of wearing hip-protecting pads. These can only be recommended in an institutional setting where compliance can be assured.

Lifestyle measures
- Stop smoking.
- Moderate alcohol consumption.
- Encourage weight-bearing exercise:
  - Impact exercise such as skipping or jumping increases bone mass.
  - Lower impact exercise, e.g. walking outdoors for 20min 3 × weekly may reduce fracture risk.
- Encourage well balanced diet.
- Ensure adequate calcium and vitamin D intake.
- If necessary give supplements to achieve calcium intake of 1–1.5g daily.

Choice of therapy
The National Institue of Health and Clinical Excellence (NICE) has produce guidance on the 2° prevention of osteoporotic fractures. In postmenopausal women with a low trauma fracture they recommend:
- Bisphosphonates are cost effective if used in:
  - ♀ >75 without the need for DXA.
  - ♀ between the ages of 65 and 75 with DXA T score of <–2.5.
  - ♀ <65 who have DXA T score of <–3 or <2.5 plus an additional risk factor.
- Raloxifene is recommended for use in the same circumstances as bisphosphonates but only in ♀ who cannot take bisphosphonates because of contraindications or intolerance or in those ♀ who have failed to respond to bisphosphonates.
- Teriparatide is reserved for use in ♀ >65 with very severe osteoporosis (T score –4 or –3.5 + additional risk factor) who have had an inadequate response to antiresorptive therapy.
  - Contraindications: hypercalcaemia, renal impairment, unexplained elevation of alkaline phosphatase, Paget's disease, and prior irradiation.

Glucocorticoid-induced osteoporosis
Glucocorticoid treatment is one of the major 2° causes of osteoporosis. Not all patients receiving steroid treatment do lose bone and it is not clear what determines this. There is some suggestion that patients on corticosteroids may have bones that are more fragile than would be suggested by the BMD. It is often suggested that such patient should be treated at a higher bone density than would be case for other causes of osteoporosis.

The Royal College of Physicians has recently produced guidelines for the management of corticosteroid-induced osteoporosis (Fig. 80.2).

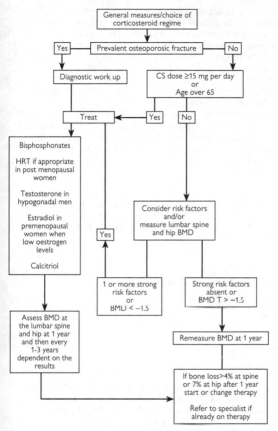

Fig. 80.2 Guidelines for the management of corticosteroid-induced osteoporosis guidelines. Reproduced with permission from the National Osteoporosis Society publication (1998). Guidance on the prevention and management of corticosteroid-induced osteoporosis, Bath.

Complications of therapy

HRT

- Because of adverse effects (breast cancer, venous thromboembolism, coronary disease, and stroke) HRT is no longer recommended as 1° treatment for osteoporosis in normal postmenopausal ♀.
- When a woman is receiving HRT for climacteric symptoms it will provide protection to her skeleton for the duration of treatment.
- Skeletal protection is rapidly lost on cessation of HRT.
- In ♀ with a premature menopause HRT remains the most appropriate means of preventing bone loss in the absence of other contraindications (e.g. breast cancer).
- ♀ who are unable to take conventional HRT might be able to take progestogens alone (e.g. norethisterone 5mg daily); several have been shown to have bone-sparing properties. Tibolone is closely related to the progestogens and has a mixture of oestrogenic, progestogenic, and androgenic effects. It is licensed for the prevention and treatment of osteoporosis.

Bisphosphonates

- Difficult dosing schedules to avoid complexing with calcium in GI tract.
- GI disturbance, including nausea (etidronate and risedronate), oesophagitis (alendronic acid, risedronate ibandronic acid), and diarrhoea (disoduin etidronate).
- ↑ bone pain.
- osteonecrosis of jaw
- possible atrial fibrillation
- flu like symptoms following IV administration

Calcium and vitamin D

Constipation.

Calcitonin

- Parenteral administration.
- Flushing.
- Nausea and diarrhoea.

Side effects less marked following nasal administration. When given in doses of 50–100 units IM or 200 units nasally daily it has analgesic properties and can be used in the management of acute fracture pain.

Calcitriol

Risk of hypercalcaemia and needs regular (ideally 6-monthly) plasma calcium measurements.

Raloxifene

- Similar increase in risk of venous thrombosis as HRT.
- May induce/worsen climacteric symptoms.
- Reduces risk of breast cancer.

Strontium ranelate

- Diarrhoea.
- Venous thromboembolism.

- Strontium is incorporated into bone making bone densitometry difficult to interpret.
- May affect measurement of calcium in plasma.

Teriparatide

- Contraindcations hypercalcaemia, renal impairment unexplained elevation of alkaline phosphatase-Paget's disease, prior irradiation
- Risk of hypercalcaemia is not great and no specific monitoring of treatment is needed.
- Vomiting.
- Leg cramps.
- ↑ risk of osteosarcoma seen in rats given teriparatide for most of their life. It should be avoided in patients with ↑ risk of bone tumours (Paget's disease, raised alkaline phosphatase, previous skeletal radiotherapy).

Box 80.3 Special considerations in men

📖 see algorithm (Fig. 80.1, p.513).
- 2° causes of osteoporosis are more common in ♂ and need to be excluded in all ♂ with osteoporotic fracture.
- Bisphosphonates benefit bone mass in ♂ in a similar way to postmenopausal ♀.
- Hypogonadal ♂ show an improvement in bone mass on testosterone replacement. This can be used as 1° treatment in hypogonadal ♂. However hypogonadal ♂ respond to bisphosphonates as those with normal testosterone levels.

Box 80.4 Special considerations in premenopausal women

- Osteoporosis in premenopausal ♀ is rare but well recognized.
- It is important to exclude underlying causes of bone loss.
- Osteoporosis can very rarely occur in conjunction with pregnancy or lactation. This is frequently self limiting and usually requires little treatment other than calcium supplementation.
- In the absence of a pre-existing fracture, fracture risk is low. Frequently all that is needed is calcium supplementation and lifestyle advice until the menopause when more active therapy is needed to counteract menopausal bone loss.
- In other situations, particularly where fractures are present, most of the therapies that are used in postmenopausal ♀, with the exception of HRT, can be used.
- Some caution needs to be exercised over the use of bisphosphonates in younger people:
  - Teratogenic in animals.
  - Long skeletal retention time making their long-term safety paramount.
  - In such patients it is often worth considering agents such as calcitriol or calcitonin and only using bisphosphonates if these fail.

An alternative strategy is to give no treatment unless there is an osteoporotic fracture if the BMD is stable over 2–4 years.

Causes of increased bone mineral density

Artefacts

- Excess skeletal calcium (lumbar spondylosis, ankylosing spondylitis).
- Extra skeletal calcium (vascular, gallstones).
- Vertebral fracture.
- Radiodense material (surgical implants, strontium).

Focal increase in bone

- Paget's disease.
- Tumours (e.g. haemangioma, Hodgkins, plasmacytoma).

Generalized increase in bone

Acquired osteosclerosis (general osteodystrophy, fluorosis, mastocytosis, hepatitis C, myelofibrosis, acromegaly).

Genetic sclerosing bone dysplasias

- ↓ absorption (e.g. osteopetrosis).
- ↑ formation (e.g. sclerosteosis).
- Disturbed balance of formation and resorption.

Further reading

Black DM, Delmas, PD, Eastell R, *et al.* (2007). Once-yearly zoledronic acid for treatment of post-menopausal osteoporosis. New Engl J Med **356**(18), 1809–22.

Cranney A, Tugwell P, Wells G, *et al.* (2002). Meta-analyses of therapies for postmenopausal osteoporosis. I.Systematic reviews of randomized trials in osteoporosis: induction and methodology. *Endoc Rev* **23**(4), 496–507.

Ebeling PR. (2008). Osteoporosis in men *NEJM* **358**, 1474–82.

Khosla S, et al. (2008). Osteoporosis in men. *Endocrine Reviews* **29**, 441–464.

Meunier PJ, Roux C, Seeman E, *et al.* (2004). The effects of strontium ranelate on the risk of vertebral fracture in women with postmenopausal osteoporosis. *New Engl J Med* **350**(5), 459–68.

Sambrook P and Cooper C (2006). Osteoporosis. *Lancet* **367**(9527); 2010–28.

Paget's disease

Paget's disease is the result of greatly ↑ local bone turnover, which occurs particularly in the middle aged or elderly.

Pathology

- The 1° abnormality in Paget's disease is gross overactivity of the osteoclasts resulting in greatly ↑ bone resorption. This secondarily results in ↑ osteoblastic activity. The new bone is laid down in a highly disorganized manner and leads to the characteristic pagetic abnormality with irregular packets of woven bone being apparent on biopsy and disorganized internal architecture of the bone on plain radiographs.
- Paget's disease can affect any bone in the skeleton but is most frequently found in the pelvis, vertebral column, femur, skull, and tibia. In most patients it affects several sites but in about 20% of cases a single bone is affected (monostotic disease). Typically, the disease will start in one end of a long bone and spread along the bone at a rate of about 1cm per year. Although it can spread within an affected bone it appears that the pattern of disease is fixed by the time of clinical presentation and it is exceedingly rare for new bones to become involved during the course of the disease.
- Paget's disease alters the mechanical properties of the bone. Thus, pagetic bones are more likely to bend under normal physiological loads and liable to fracture. This can take the form of complete fractures which tend to be transverse rather than the more common spiral fractures of long bones. More frequently, fissure or incremental fractures are seen on the convex surface of bowed pagetic bones. These may be painful in their own right but are also liable to proceed to complete fracture. Pagetic bones are also larger than their normal counterparts. This can lead to ↑ arthritis at adjacent joints and to pressure on nerves leading to neurological compression syndromes and, when it occurs in the skull base, sensorineural deafness.

Aetiology of Paget's disease

Unclear. There are 2 major theories:
- Familial:
  - Some genetic associations, especially with sequestomma a 18q.
  - These are not invariable.
- Viral:
  - Inclusion bodies similar to those seen in viral infections are present in pagetic osteoclasts.
  - Some workers have found paramyxoviral (measles or canine distemper) protein or nucleic acid in pagetic bone.
  - Others are not able to replicate this.

Epidemiology

Paget's disease is present in about 2% of the UK population over the age of 55. Its prevalence increases with age and it is more common in ♂ than ♀. Only about 10% of affected patients will have symptomatic disease. It is most common in the UK or in migrants of British descent in North America and Australasia, but rare in Africa. Recent studies in the UK and New Zealand have suggested that the prevalence may be declining with time.

Clinical features

- 90% asymptomatic.
- Most notable feature is pain. This is frequently multifactorial:
    - ↑ metabolic activity of the bone.
    - Changes in bone shape.
    - Fissure fractures.
    - Nerve compression.
    - Arthritis.
- Pagetic bones tend to increase in size or to become bowed (16% cases): bowing can be so severe as to interfere with function.
- Fractures (either complete or fissure) present in 10%.

Investigation

The diagnosis of Paget's disease is primarily radiological.

Radiological features of Paget's disease

- Early disease—primarily lytic:
  - V-shaped 'cutting cone' in long bones.
  - Osteoporosis circumscripta in skull.
- Combined phase (mixed lytic and sclerotic):
  - Cortical thickening.
  - Loss of corticomedullary distinction.
  - Accentuated trabecular markings.
- Late phase—primarily sclerotic:
  - Thickening of long bones.
  - Increase in bone size.
  - Sclerosis.

An isotope bone scan is frequently helpful in assessing the extent of skeletal involvement with Paget's disease. It is particularly important to identify Paget's disease in a weight-bearing bone, because of the risk of fracture. The uptake of tracer depends on the disease activity and isotope bone scans can also be used to assess the response to therapy.

In active disease plasma alkaline phosphatase activity is usually (85%) elevated. An exception to this is in monostotic disease when there may be insufficient bone involved to raise the enzyme levels above normal. Alkaline phosphatase activity responds to successful treatment. There is little advantage in using the more modern markers of bone turnover over the total alkaline phosphatase activity for the monitoring of pagetic activity. A possible exception to this is in patients with liver disease where changes in bone alkaline phosphatase might be masked by the liver isoenzyme.

Complications

- Deafness present in up to 1/2 of cases of skull base Paget's
- Other neurological complications are rare. These can include:
    - Compression of other cranial nerves with skull base disease.
    - *Spinal cord compression* most common with involvement of the thoracic spine and is thought to result as much from a vascular steal syndrome as from physical compression. It frequently responds to medical therapy without need for surgical decompression.
    - Platybasia which can lead to an obstructive hydrocephalus that may require surgical drainage.
- Osteogenic sarcoma:
    - Very rare complication of Paget's disease.
    - Rarely amenable to treatment.
    - Presents with ↑ pain/radiological evidence of tumour, and a mass.
- Any increase of pain in a patient with Paget's disease should arouse suspicion of sarcomatous degeneration. A more common cause however, is resumption of activity of disease.

Pagetic sarcomas are most frequently found in humerus or femur but can affect any bone involved with Paget's disease.

Indications for treating Paget's disease

- Pain.
- Neurological complications (e.g. deafness, spinal cord compression).
- Disease in weight-bearing bones.
- Prevention of long term complications (e.g. bone deformation, osteoarthritis).
- Young patients.
- In preparation for surgery.
- Hypercalcaemia.
- Following fracture.

Treatment

Treatment with agents that decrease bone turnover reduces disease activity as indicated by bone turnover markers and isotope bone scans. There is evidence to suggest that such treatment leads to the deposition of histologically normal bone. Although such treatment has been shown to help pain there is little evidence that it benefits the other consequences of Paget's disease. In particular, the deafness of Paget's disease does not regress after treatment although its progression may be halted. Nonetheless it has become generally accepted to treat patients in the hope that future complications of the disease will be avoided. Typical indications for treatment of Paget's disease are listed in Table 81.1.

The bisphosphonates have become the mainstay of treatment. Calcitonin and plicamycin are no longer used.

Goals of treatment

- Normalize bone turnover.
- Alkaline phosphatase in normal range.
- The more aggressive the initial therapy, the longer the disease remission.
- Minimize symptoms.
- Prevent long-term complications.
- No actual evidence that treatment achieves this.

Monitoring therapy

- Plasma alkaline phosphatase every 6 months.
- Clinical assessment.

Re-treat if symptoms recur with objective evidence of disease recurrence (alkaline phosphatase or +ve isotope scan). If treating for asymptomatic disease re-treat if alkaline phosphatase increases 25% >nadir.

Table 81.1 Biophosphonates licensed in the UK for Paget's disease

Drug	Dose	Duration of treatment	Side-effects
Etidronate	5mg/kg per day orally in middle of 4h fast (max 400mg)	6 months	Nausea Diarrhoea Bone pain ↑ fracture Focal osteomalacia
Pamidronate	3 x 60mg IV infusion or 6 x 30mg IV infusion	Fortnightly interval Weekly interval	Influenza like symptoms ↑ bone pain Iritis
Risedronate	30mg orally, on rising and wait 30min before breakfast	2 months	Increased bone pain Nausea
Tiludronic acid	400mg daily orally in middle of 4h fast	3 months	Nausea Diarrhoea ↑ bone pain
Zoledronic acid	5 mg IV	single dose	Flu-like symptoms, ↑ bone pain

Further reading

Bilezikian, JP, Watts JT Jr, Fuleihan Gel-H, et al. (2002). Summary statement from a workshop on asymptomatic primary hyperparathyroidism: a perspective for the 21st century. *J Clin Endocrinol Metab* **87**(12), 5353–61.

Davies M, Fraser WD, Hosking DJ (2002). The management of primaryhyperparathyroidism. *Clin Endocrinol* (Oxf) **57**(2), 145–55.

Ralston SH, et al (2008). Pathogenous and management of Paget's disease of Core. **372**, 155–163.

Selby PL, Davie MW, Ralston SH, et al. (2002). National Association for the Relief of Paget's Disease: guidelines on the management of Paget's disease of the bone. *Bone* **31**(3), 366–73.

Inherited disorders of bone

Osteogenesis imperfecta

Osteogenesis imperfecta is an inherited form of osteoporosis in which there is a genetic defect in 1 of the 2 genes (*COLIA1* and *COLIA2*) encoding the α-chain of collagen type I collagen production. Several different mutations are recognized and these produce different clinical pictures; these are generally separated into 4 and more recently 7 different types (📖 see Table 82.1).

In addition to the osteoporosis and easy fracture there may also be abnormalities of the teeth (dentigenesis imperfecta), blue sclerae, and hearing loss, hypermobility, and cardiac valvular lesions.

Radiological features include:
• Generalized osteopenia.
• Multiple fractures with deformity.
• Abnormal shape of long bones.
• Wormian bones in skull.

Diagnosis
• Features described in previous section and family history.
• Analysis of collagen type I genes (detect 90%).
• Differential diagnosis includes Brock syndrome, panostotic fibrous dysplasia, hyper- and hypophatasia, and idiopathic juvenile osteoporosis.
• 3 criteria
  • 3 fragility fractures aged <20 years.
  • At least one of: blue sclerae, scoliosis, hearing loss, joint laxity, dentinogenesis imperfecta and family member.
  • Osteoporosis.

Recent studies have demonstrated that infusions of pamidronate lead to ↑ bone mass and reduced fracture incidence in affected children. Patients with milder disease might only be recognized in adulthood; it appears that oral bisphosphonates may be helpful in their management.

Prenatal diagnosis of severe types is possible from US, and genetic counseling should be offered to at-risk families.

Further reading
Rauch F and Glorieux FH (2004). Osteogenesis imperfecta. *Lancet*. **363**(9418), 1377–85.

Table 82.1 Classification of osteogenesis imperfecta

Type	Inheritance	Stature	Teeth	Sclerae	Hearing	Genetic defect
I	AD	Normal	Normal	Blue	Variable loss	Substitution for glycine in COL1A1 and COL1A2
II	AD/AR	Lethal deformity				Rearrangement of COL1A1 and COL1A2
III	AD/AR	(Very short severe scaliosis)	Abnormal	Variable (growth)	Loss common	Glycine substitution is COL1A1 and COL1A2
IV	AD	Mild	Abnormal	Normal	Occasional loss	Point mutations in a2(l) or a1(l)

Part 7

Paediatric endocrinology

Growth and stature

Growth

Regulation of growth

Normal human growth can be divided into 3 overlapping stages (the Karlberg model), each under the control of different factors.

- *Infancy* Growth is largely under nutritional regulation, and wide inter-individual variation in rates of growth is seen. Many infants show significant 'catch-up' or 'catch-down' in weight and length, and by 2 years length is much more predictive of final adult height than at birth.
- *Childhood* Growth is regulated by growth hormone (GH) and thyroxine. It is characterized by alternating periods of mini-growth spurts with intervening stasis, each phase lasting several weeks. However over years, a child will tend to maintain their centile position on height charts with a height velocity between the 25th and 75th centiles.
- *Puberty* The combination of GH and sex hormones promotes bone maturation and a rapid growth acceleration or 'growth spurt'. In both sexes oestrogen eventually causes epiphyseal fusion, resulting in the attainment of final height.

Sex differences

Adult heights differ between ♂ and ♀ by on average 13cm. However, during childhood, onset of the pubertal growth spurt is earlier in ♀, who are therefore on average taller than ♂ between the ages of 10–13 years.

Tempo

Within each sex there may also be marked inter-individual differences in *tempo* of growth (or rate of attainment of final height) and the timing of puberty. Delay or advance of bone maturation is linked with timing of puberty. Constitutional delay in growth and puberty often runs in families, reflecting probable genetic factors. Comparison of *bone age* (estimated from a hand radiograph) with chronological age is therefore an important part of growth assessment.

Final height

Final height is estimated as the height reached when growth velocity slows to <2cm/year and can be confirmed by finding epiphyseal fusion on hand radiograph ± knee radiograph. Final height is largely genetically determined and a target height can be estimated in each individual from their parent's heights.

Assessment of growth

Measurement

- From birth to 2 years old, supine length is measured ideally using a measuring board (e.g. Harpenden neonatometer). 2 adults are needed to ensure that the child is lying straight and legs extended.
- From 2 years old, standing height is measured against a wall-mounted or free-standing stadiometer with the measurer applying moderate upwards neck traction and the child looking forward in the horizontal plane.

- To minimize error in the calculation of height velocity (cm/year), height measurements should be taken at least 6 months apart using the same equipment and ideally by the same person.
- Measurement of *sitting height* and comparison with *leg length* (*standing height – sitting height*) allows an estimate of body proportion.

Growth charts (Figs. 83.1 and 83.2)

Height and weight velocity should be compared to age and sex appropriate reference data by plotting values on standard growth charts (e.g. the UK 1990 Growth Reference, Child Growth Foundation, London, UK).

Mid-parental height (MPH)

MPH is an estimate of the child's genetic height potential and is calculated as

[(mother's height + father's height)/2] + 7 cm (for boys) or – 7 cm (for girls).

It can be used to estimate a child's expected final height, but there is a wide target range (MPH ± 10cm for boys and ± 8.5cm for girls) and it is more commonly used to assess whether the child's current height centile is consistent with genetic expectation.

Bone age

Skeletal maturation proceeds in an orderly manner from the first appearance of each epiphyseal centre to the fusion of the long bones. From chronological age 3–4 years, bone age may be quantified from radiographs of the left hand and wrist by comparison with standard photographs (e.g. Greulich and Pyle method) or by an individual bone scoring system (e.g. Tanner–Whitehouse method). The difference between bone age and chronological age is an estimation of tempo of growth. The initiation of puberty usually coincides with a bone age around 10.5–11 years in girls and 11–11.5 years in boys, although the correlation between bone age and pubertal timing is approximate. Girls reach skeletal maturity at a bone age of 15 years and boys when bone age is 17 years. Thus, bone age allows an estimation of remaining growth potential and can be used to aid in the prediction of final adult height.

Final height prediction

Predictions of final height can be derived from information on current height, age, pubertal status and bone age using calculations described by Tanner and Whitehouse, or Bailey and Pinneau among others (☐ see Further reading, p.549, De Waal *et al.* (1996))

Secular trends

Children's heights ↑ by >1cm in England and by >2cm in Scotland during the period from 1972–94, and similar trends are seen in many other countries. Population growth references used should be appropriate to the population studied and may occasionally need to be updated.

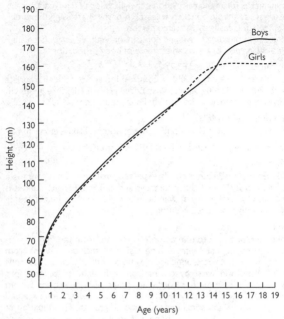

Fig. 83.1 Typical-individual height-attained curves for boys and girls (supine length to the ages of 2; integrated curves of Fig. 83.2)

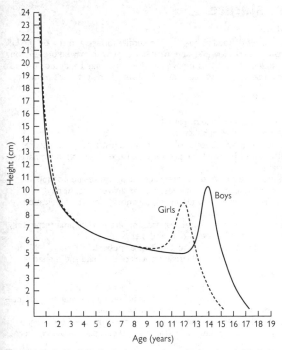

Fig. 83.2 Typical-individual velocity curves for supine length or height in boys and girls. These curves represent the velocity of the typical boy and girl at any given instant.

Short stature

Definition

Short stature is defined as height <2nd centile for age and sex on the UK 1990 growth chart. However, abnormalities of growth may be present long before attained height falls below this level and may be detected much earlier by assessing growth velocity and observing height measurements

Assessment

History

- Who is concerned, child or parents?
- What are the parental heights?
- Has the child always been small, or does the history suggest recent growth failure? Try to obtain previous measurements (e.g. from parents, GP, health visitor, school).
- Ask about maternal illness in pregnancy, drug intake and possible substance abuse in pregnancy, gestation at delivery, size at birth (weight/length/head circumference), childhood illnesses, medication, and developmental milestones.
- Systematic enquiry for headaches, visual disturbance, asthma/respiratory symptoms, abdominal symptoms, and diet.
- Is there a family history of short stature or pubertal delay?
- What are the psychosocial circumstances of the child and the family?

Examination

- Assess height and height velocity over at least 6 months.
- Measure sitting height and derive subischial leg length (standing height – sitting height (cm) if skeletal disproportion suspected)
- Assess for the presence and severity of chronic disease. Low weight-for-height suggests a nutritional diagnosis, GI cause, or other significant systemic disease.
- Pubertal stage using Tanner's criteria.
- Observe for dysmorphic features and signs of endocrinolopathy, presence and severity of chronic disease.
- Measure parents' heights and calculate MPH.

Investigations

- Laboratory tests should include FBC, ESR, electrolytes, thyroid function, calcium, phosphate, antigliadin and antiendomyseal antibodies, IGF-I level, karyotype (of particular importance in girls), and urinalysis.
- These tests may also be clinically indicated: GH provocation testing (e.g. arginine, glucagon, or ITT) (see Table 83.1) with other anterior pituitary function tests, MRI scan with specific reference to the hypothalamus and pituitary, skeletal survey (for bone dysplasia), and very rarely an IGF-1 generation test (☐ for GH resistance, see Growth hormone deficiency, p.540).

Table 83.1 Comparison of GH provocation tests

	Insulin (IV)	Clonidine (oral)	Glucagon (IM)
Age	>10 years	5–10 years Unreliable in puberty and in adulthood	<5 years and in neonates
Advantages	Gold standard Also tests ACTH–cortisol axis	Simple and safe	Safe Also tests ACTH–cortisol axis
Disadvantages	Risk of severe hypoglycaemia but good safety record in experienced centres	Postural hypotension and somnolence	Nausea may last 3–4 h Great care because of late hypoglycaemia

Other agents (e.g. L-dopa or L-arginine) are less commonly used. Measurement of GH levels after exercise has poor sensitivity and specificity for detecting GH deficiency.

Causes

- Genetic short stature
- Constitutional delay in growth and puberty these first 2 together account for ~40% of cases.
- Chronic illness (including untreated coeliac disease, congenital heart disease, chronic renal failure, inflammatory bowel disease).
- Psychosocial deprivation (which may be associated with reversible GH deficiency).
- Small for gestational age (SGA), including intrauterine growth restriction (7.5%).
- Dysmorphic syndromes (e.g. Turner's syndrome, Noonan syndrome, Down syndrome).
- Malnutrition (1°, rare in the UK).
- GH deficiency (8%):
  - Undefined aetiology ('idiopathic', including those with abnormal pituitary morphology on MRI).
  - Congenital malformation in the hypothalamus/pituitary (HP) (e.g. septo-optic dysplasia) or acquired HP disorders (e.g. craniopharyngioma, trauma), the GH-1 gene or the GH releasing hormone receptor gene, or rarely mutations in transcription factors controlling pituitary development.
  - GH resistance (rare genetic mutations in the GH receptor or GH signaling molecules).
  - Endocrine disorders (hypothyroidism, hypoparathyroidism, Cushing's syndrome).
- Skeletal dysplasia (e.g. achondroplasia, hypochondroplasia).
- Metabolic bone disease (e.g. nutritional or hypophosphataemic rickets).

Genetic short stature

Although stature does not follow strict Mendelian laws of inheritance, it does relate to parental height and is probably a polygenic trait. It should be remembered that short parents may themselves have an unidentified dominantly inherited condition (e.g. hypochondroplasia).

Constitutional delay of growth and puberty

Clinical features

- This condition often presents in adolescence but may also be recognized in earlier childhood. Although it is more prevalent in ♂.
- Characteristic features include short stature and delay in pubertal development by >2 standard deviations (SD) and/or bone age delay in an otherwise healthy child. In the adolescent years, short sitting height percentile compared to leg length is typical.
- There is often a family history of delayed puberty.
- Bone age delay may also develop in a number of other conditions, but in constitutional delay, bone age delay usually remains consistent over time and height velocity is normal for the bone age. Final height may not reach target height.
- GH secretion is usually normal, although provocation tests should be primed by prior administration of exogenous sex hormones if bone age is >10 years.

Management

Often only reassurance is necessary. Treatment is sometimes indicated in adolescent boys who have difficulty coping with their short stature or delayed sexual maturation.

- For the younger child with concerns about growth: Low-dose *oxandrolone* (1.25mg/day for up to 12 months, oral). A synthetic derivative of testosterone which has significant growth-promoting but minimal virilizing actions and does not affect final height.
- For the older boy (>14 years) with concerns about puberty: *testosterone* (50–100mg IM, monthly for 3–6 months).
- For the older girl (>13 years) with concerns about puberty: ethinylestradiol (2mcg/d for 3–6 months).

Box 83.1 GH assessment

GH is normally secreted overnight in regular pulses (pulse frequency 180min). Frequently sampled overnight GH profiles are costly and laborious and therefore standardized stimulation tests are more commonly useful. Peak GH <10mcg/L indicates GH deficiency (values >5 and <10mcg/L indicate partial GH deficiency). However, there can be large variation between different assay methods and exact cut-offs must be locally validated. In late pre-puberty there is a physiological blunting of GH secretion and when bone age is >10 years, sex steroid priming (testosterone 100mg IM in boys, or oral ethinylestradiol 20mcg daily for 3 days in either sex) is necessary before GH testing.

A number of different agents may be used to stimulate GH secretion (arginine, insulin, or glucagon, see Table 83.1). All tests should be performed in the morning following an overnight fast, and serial blood samples are collected over 90–180min.

An IGF-1 level should also be measured in the baseline sample, as an additional marker of GH status.

IGF-I generation test

In those with high basal and stimulated GH levels, measurement of IGF-I levels before and following administration of GH (30mcg/kg/day) SC for 4 days allows an assessment of GH sensitivity/resistance. This test is rarely necessary.

Growth hormone deficiency

Primary GH deficiency

1° GH deficiency is usually sporadic, but rarely it may be inherited as autosomal dominant, recessive, or X-linked recessive and may be associated with other pituitary hormone deficiencies. It may represent a defect in homeobox genes (e.g. *Pit1* (leading to GH, TSH, and PRL deficiency), *Prop1* (leading to GH, TSH, PRL, gonadotrophin and later ACTH deficiencies), or *Hesx1*) which control HP development. Mutation in *Hesx1* has been associated with midline defects, such as optic nerve hypoplasia and corpus callosum defects (i.e. 'septo-optic dysplasia'). GH deficiency usually arises because of failure of release of GHRH from the hypothalamus.

Clinical features

- *Infancy* GH deficiency may present with hypoglycaemia. Coexisting ACTH, TSH, and gonadotrophin deficiencies may cause prolonged hyperbilirubinaemia and micropenis. Size may be normal as fetal and infancy growth are more dependent on nutrition and other growth factors than on GH.
- *Childhood* Typical features include slow growth velocity, short stature, ↓ muscle mass and ↑ SC fat. Underdevelopment of the mid-facial bones, relative protrusion of the frontal bones because of mid-facial hypoplasia, delayed dental eruption and delayed closure of the anterior fontanelle may be seen. These children have delayed bone age and delayed puberty.

Secondary GH deficiency

Brain tumours and cranial irradiation

Pituitary or hypothalamic tumours may impair GH secretion and deficiencies of other pituitary hormones may coexist. Cranial irradiation, used to treat intracranial tumours, facial tumours, and acute leukaemia, may also cause GH deficiency. Risk of HP damage is related to total dose administered, fractionation (single dose more toxic than divided), location of the irradiated tissue and age (younger children are more sensitive to radiation damage).

GH secretion is most sensitive to radiation damage, followed by gonadotrophins, TSH, and ACTH. Central precocious puberty may also occur and may mask GH deficiency by promoting growth but will compromise final height if untreated. At-risk children should therefore be screened regularly by careful examination and multiple pituitary hormone testing.

These survivors of childhood cancer may also have other endocrine problems including gonadal damage related to concomitant chemotherapy or radiation scatter, hypothyroidism related to spinal radiation, or glucose intolerance related to total body irradiation. It is recommended that all such patients should undergo endocrine surveillance.

Psychosocial deprivation

Severe psychosocial deprivation may cause reversible disturbance of GH secretion and growth failure. GH secretion improves within 3 weeks of hospitalization or removal from the adverse environment and catch-up growth is often dramatic (see Fig. 83.3), although these children may continue to exhibit other features of emotional disturbance.

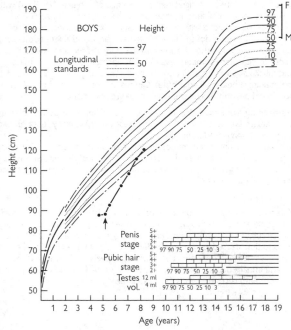

Fig. 83.3 Height of child with psychosocial short stature. Note catch-up on removal, marked by arrow, from parental home. Reproduced from Brook's Clinical Pediatric Endocrinology, Brook C (2001). Blackwell Publishing. With permission from Wiley Blackwell.

Treatment of GH deficiency (Fig. 83.4)

Recombinant human GH has been available since 1985 and is administered by daily SC injection.

- *Dose* The replacement dose for childhood GH deficiency is 25–50mcg/kg/day (~0.7-1.4mcg/m² per day). Catch-up growth is optimized if GH is commenced early. A higher dose can be used in puberty, reflecting the normal elevation in GH levels at Tanner stage 3–4.

- *Side-effects* Local lipoatrophy and benign intracranial hypertension occur rarely. Slipped upper femoral epiphyses are associated with GH deficiency, but the incidence is similar before or after GH treatment. Other pituitary hormone deficiencies may be unmasked by GH therapy and thyroid function should be checked within 4–6 weeks of commencing therapy.
- *Retesting in adulthood* Once final height is achieved, GH secretion should be retested as a significant percentage of subjects (25–80%) with GH deficiency in childhood subsequently have normal GH secretion in adulthood. In those with confirmed GH deficiency, continuation of GH treatment (at a dose of 0.2–0.5mg/day) through the late adolescent years into early adulthood (the *transition* phase) is recommended in order to complete somatic development (increasing lean body mass and muscular strength, reducing fat mass, improving bone density, and maintaining a healthy lipid profile). GH treatment may need to be continued beyond this phase, as adult GH replacement.

The transition from paediatric to adult care is an important time not only to re-evaluate GH status but also to reassess other pituitary function and management of any underying disorder.

It is also recommended that assessment of bone mineral desity, body composition, fasting lipid profile and QoL by questionnaire should be undertaken at this time and repeated at 3–5-yearly intervals for those restarting GH treatment.

GH resistance

GH resistance may arise because of 1° GH receptor defects or post-receptor defects 2° to malnutrition, liver disease, type 1 diabetes, or, very rarely, circulating GH antibodies. *Laron syndrome* is a rare autosomal recessive condition caused by a genetic defect of the GH receptor. Affected individuals have extreme short stature, high levels of GH, low levels of IGF-I and impaired GH-induced IGF-I generation (see Box 83.1, p.539). Treatment with recombinant IGF-I is available.

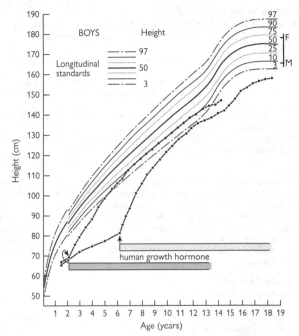

Fig. 83.4 Heights of two brothers with isolated growth-hormone deficiency treated with human GH from ages 6 years and 2 years. Catch-up of older brother is partly by high velocity and partly by prolonged growth and is incomplete. Younger brother shows true complete catch-up. F and M, parents' height centiles; vertical thick line, range of expected heights for family. Reproduced from Brook C (2001). Brook's Clinical Pediatric Endocrinology, Blackwell Publishing. With permission from Wiley Blackwell.

Hypothyroidism (Fig. 83.5)

- Congenital $1°$ hypothyroidism is detected by neonatal screening.
- Hypothyroidism presenting in childhood is usually autoimmune in origin.
- Incidence is higher in girls and those with personal or family history of other autoimmune disease.
- In childhood, hypothyroidism may present with growth failure alone and bone age is often disproportionately delayed. Very rarely, early puberty may occur.
- Investigations show low T_4 and T_3, high TSH, +ve anti-thyroglobulin, and anti-thyroid peroxidase (microsomal) antibodies.
- Replacement therapy with oral levothyroxine ($100mcg/m^2$ per day titrated with thyroid function) results in catch-up growth unless diagnosis is late.

Coeliac disease

More common in children with other autoimmune disorders. Although the classical childhood presentation is an irritable toddler with poor weight gain, diarrhoea, abdominal pain, and distension, in later childhood poor growth with bone age delay may be the presenting feature. Measurement of tissue transglutaminase, antiendomyseal, and antigliadin antibodies are valuable screening tests, but diagnosis needs to be confirmed by small-bowel biopsy. Catch-up growth usually follows commencement of a gluten-free diet.

Skeletal dysplasias

- This heterogeneous group of mostly dominantly inherited disorders includes *achondroplasia* and *hypochondroplasia*.
- These children usually have severe disproportionate short stature and a +ve or suspicious family history.
- Radiological assessment by skeletal survey often allows a specific diagnosis to be made.
- High dose GH therapy has been used in these disorders with variable success. Surgical leg lengthening procedures before and/or after puberty are also an additional option.

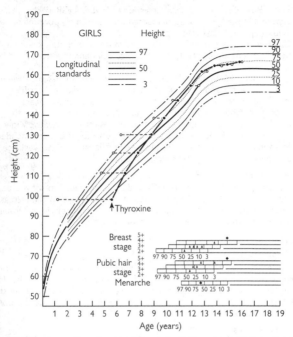

Fig. 83.5 Response of hypothyroid child treated with thyroxine. Solid circles, height for age; open circles, height for bone age. Reproduced from Brook C (2001). Brook's Clinical Pediatric Endocrinology, Blackwell Publishing. With permission from Wiley Blackwell.

Small for gestational age (SGA) and intrauterine growth restriction

- SGA is defined as birth weight and/or length at least 2 SDs below the mean for gestational age. IUGR is defined as growth failure on serial antenatal US scans, and would usually lead to a baby being born SGA. However IUGR in late gestation may result in a baby who is within 2 SD of the mean for birth weight or length.
- 90% of infants with SGA show catch-up growth by age 3 years. 8% of subjects born SGA will remain small at 18 years of age. Catch-up growth is more common in infants with relative sparing of birth length and head circumference (>10th centile).
- In severe IUGR, length and head circumference are also reduced. Severe IUGR may be due to maternal factors such as hypertension in pregnancy, placental dysfunction, or a wide range of chromosomal or genetic conditions in the fetus.

- Silver–Russell syndrome is characterized by severe IUGR, lateral asymmetry, triangular facies, clinodactyly, and extremely poor infancy feeding and postnatal weight gain.
- Children with severe IUGR who do not undergo catch-up growth may have early onset puberty despite bone age delay and therefore achieve a very poor final height.
- Numerous epidemiological studies have shown a relationship between low birth weight and an ↑ risk of a number of disorders in later life, including hypertension, ischaemic heart disease, cerebrovascular disease, metabolic syndrome, and type II diabetes. The risk is ↑ with rapid postnatal weight gain. These associations relate to relatively low birth weight and not exclusively to those born SGA. It is recommended that those born SGA do not require any additional health surveillance above that indicated by clinical circumstances.

Management
GH therapy is used in the SGA/IUGR child who has failed to show catch-up growth by age 4 years GH (at doses of 35–67 µg/kg/day) can increase growth velocity and final height. The effect of GH on later risk of insulin resistance as type 2 diabetes is not known.

Turner's syndrome
(📖 also see Box 58.1, p.327)

Turner's syndrome should always be considered in a girl who is short for her parental target and the classical dysmorphic features may be difficult to identify at younger ages. Karyotype usually confirms the diagnosis, although sufficient cells (>30) should be examined to exclude the possibility of mosaicism.

Clinical features
There may be a history of lymphoedema in the newborn period. Typically, growth velocity starts to decline from 3–5 years old (Fig. 83.6) and gonadal failure combined with a degree of skeletal dysplasia results in loss of the pubertal growth spurt. Mean final height is consistently 20cm below the normal average within each population (143–146cm in the UK). GH secretion is normal although IGF-I levels may be low. 10% progress through puberty spontaneously but only 1% develop ovulatory cycles.

Management
- High dose *GH therapy* (45mcg/kg/day) increases final height, although individual responses are variable. The height gained is related to time on GH treatment, and thus GH therapy should be commenced early: if the diagnosis has been made in early life, treatment is usually started from 3–5 years of age.
- The anabolic steroid *oxandralone* has been used in addition to GH to promote growth from the age of 9 years, but its effect on final height is yet unclear.
- Oral *oestrogen* is commenced between 12–14 years to promote 2° sexual development and pubertal growth. It should be started in low dose (ethinylestradiol 2mcg/day), and gradually ↑ with age. *Progesterone* should be added if breakthrough bleeding occurs or when oestrogen dose reaches 10mcg/day.

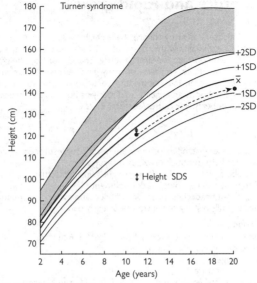

Fig. 83.6 Height SDS for chronological age extrapolated to final height. Reproduced from Brook C, (2001). Brook's Clinical Pediatric Endocrinology, Blackwell publishing. With permission from Wiley Blackwell.

Tall stature and rapid growth

Definition

Although statistically as many children have heights >2 SD above the mean as have heights >2 SD below the mean, referral for evaluation of tall stature is much less common than for short stature. Socially, for boys heights up to 200cm are acceptable, whereas for many girls heights >182cm may be unacceptable. However, tall stature and particularly accelerated growth rates in early childhood can indicate an underlying hormonal disorder, such as precocious puberty. For causes, see Box 83.2.

Assessment

History

- Is tall stature long-standing or does the history suggest recent growth acceleration? Try to obtain previous measurements.
- Enquire about size at birth, infancy weight gain, intellectual development, and neurological development.
- Enquire about headaches, visual disturbance, and evidence of puberty.
- Is there a family history of tall stature or early puberty?

Examination

- Assess height and height velocity over at least 4–6 months.
- Measure sitting height and arm span
- Pubertal stage?
- Dysmorphic features?
- Measure parents' heights and calculate MPH (☐ see Assesment of growth, p.532).

Investigations

The following investigations may be clinically indicated:

- Wrist radiograph for bone age.
- Sex hormone levels (testosterone, oestrogen, androstenedione, DHEAS), baseline and LHRH-stimulated LH and FSH levels.
- Karyotype.
- Serum IGF-I and IGFBP-3 levels.
- Oral glucose tolerance test—GH levels normally suppress to low or undetectable levels (<1mU/L).
- Specific molecular tests for overgrowth syndromes.

Management of tall stature

After excluding abnormal pathology, often only reassurance and information on predicted final height is necessary. In younger children, early induction of puberty using low-dose sex steroids advances the pubertal growth spurt and promotes earlier epiphyseal fusion. In older children already in puberty, high-dose oestrogen therapy in girls, or testosterone in boys, has been used to induce rapid skeletal maturation. However, theoretical side-effects of high-dose oestrogen therapy include thromboembolic disease and oncogenic risk.

Box 83.2 Causes of tall stature in childhood

Normal variants
- Familial tall stature.
- Early maturation (largely familial but also promoted by early childhood nutrition and obesity. Height is not excessive for bone age which is advanced).

Hormonal
- 📖 see Precocious puberty, p.552
- GH or GHRH excess ('pituitary gigantism') resulting from pituitary adenoma or ectopic adenomas is a very rare cause of tall stature (📖 p.124).
- Other hormonal excess, e.g. hyperthyroidism, congenital adrenal hyperplasia (associated with signs of virilization), familial glucocorticoid deficiency.
- Rarely, oestrogen receptor or aromatase deficiencies delay puberty and epiphyseal fusion resulting in tall adult height.

Chromosomal abnormalities
- XXY (Klinefelter's syndrome).
- XYY, XYYY (each 'extra Y' confers on average 13cm additional height).

Other rare syndromes
Overgrowth and dysmorphic features are seen in Marfan's syndrome, homocystinuria, Sotos syndrome, Beckwith–Wiedemann syndrome, and Weaver's syndrome.

Further reading

Carel J.C, Léger J, (2008). Precocious puberty *NEJM* **358**, 2366–2377.

Clayton PE, Cuneo RC, Juul A, et al. (2005). Consensus statement on the management of the GH-treated adolescent in the transition to adult care. *Eur J Endocrinol* **152**, 165–170.

Clayton PE, Cianfarani S, Czernichow P, et al. (2007). Management of the child born small for gestational age child (SGA) through to adulthood: a consensus statement of the International Societies of Paediatric Endocrinology and the Growth Hormone Research Society. *J Clin Endocrinology Metab* Epub 2 January.

Dattani M and Preece M (2004). Growth hormone deficiency and related disorders: insights into causation, diagnosis, and treatment. *Lancet* **363**, 1977–87.

De Waal WJ, Greyn-Fokker MH, Stijnen T, et al. (1996). Accuracy of final height prediction and effect of growth-reductive therapy in 362 constitutionally tall children. *J Clin Endocrinol Metab* **81**, 1206–16.

Growth Hormone Research Society. Consensus guidelines for the diagnosis and treatment of growth (GH) deficiency in childhood and adolescence: summary statement of the GH Research Society. (2000) GH Research Society. *J Clin Endocrinol Metab* **85**, 3990–3.

Saenger P, Wikland KA, Conway GS, et al. (2000). Recommendations for the diagnosis and management of Turner's syndrome. *J Clin Endocrinol Metab* **86**, 3061–9.

Puberty

Normal puberty

Puberty is the sequence of physical and physiological changes occurring at adolescence culminating in full sexual maturity.

Age at onset

Average age at onset of puberty is earlier in girls (~11 years) than in boys (~12 years), but varies widely (~±2 years from the mean age of onset) and is influenced by a number of factors:

- *Historical* Age of menarche has ↓ this century from 17 years in 1900 to 12.8 years today, presumably as a result of improved childhood nutrition and growth.
- *Genetic* Age at onset of puberty is partly familial.
- *Ethnicity* Afro-Caribbean girls tend to have earlier puberty than whites.
- *Weight gain* Earlier puberty is seen in girls who are overweight, whereas girls who engage in strenuous activity and are thin often have delayed puberty.

Hormonal changes prior to and during puberty

- Adrenal androgens (DHEAS and androstenedione) rise 2 years before puberty starts ('adrenarche'). This usually causes no physical changes but occasionally results in early pubic hair and acne ('premature adrenarche').
- Pulsatile secretion of LHRH from the hypothalamus at night is the first step in the initiation of puberty and occurs well before physical signs of puberty. This results in pulsatile secretion of LH and FSH from the pituitary and the gonadotrophin response to LHRH administration reverses from the prepubertal FSH predominance to a higher response in LH levels.

Physical changes

The first indication of puberty is breast development in girls and increase in testicular size in boys. In each sex, puberty then progresses in an orderly or 'consonant' manner through distinct stages (see Table 84.1). Puberty rating by an experienced observer involves identification of pubertal stage; particularly breast development in girls and testicular volume (by comparison with an orchidometer) in boys.

Pubertal growth spurt

↑ oestrogen levels in both boys and girls leads to ↑ GH secretion. Peak height velocity occurs at puberty stage 2–3 in girls and is later in boys, at stage 3–4 (testicular volume 10–12mL).

Table 84.1 The normal stages of puberty ('Tanner stages')

Boys

Stage	Genitalia	Pubic hair	Other events
I	Prepubertal	Vellus not thicker than on abdomen	TV[a] <4mL
II	Enlargement of testes and scrotum	Sparse long pigmented strands at base of penis	TV 4–8mL Voice starts to change
III	Lengthening of penis	Darker, curlier and spreads over pubes	TV 8–10mL Axillary hair
IV	Increase in penis length and breadth	Adult type hair but covering a smaller area	TV 10–15mL Upper lip hair Peak height velocity
V	Adult shape and size	Spread to medial thighs (Stage 6: Spread up linea alba)	TV 15–25mL. Facial hair spreads to cheeks Adult voice

Girls

Stage	Breast	Pubic hair	Other events
I	Elevation of papilla only	Vellus not thicker than on abdomen	
II	Breast bud stage: elevation of breast and papilla	Sparse long pigmented strands along labia	Peak height velocity
III	Further elevation of breast and areola together	Darker, curlier and spreads over pubes	
IV	Areola forms a second mound on top of breast	Adult type hair but covering a smaller area	Menarche
V	Mature stage: areola recedes and only papilla projects	Spread to medial thighs (Stage 6: spread up linea alba)	

[a]TV, testicular volume: measured by size-comparison with a Prader orchidometer.
Adapted with permission from Tanner JM (1962) *Growth at adolescence*, 2nd edn.
Blackwell Scientific Publications, Oxford.

Precocious puberty

Definition
- Early onset of puberty is defined as <8 years in girls and <9 years in boys.
- Gonadotrophin-dependent ('central' or 'true') precocious puberty is characterized by early breast development in girls or testicular enlargement in boys.
- Gonadotrophin-independent puberty occurs due to abnormal peripheral sex hormone secretion, resulting in isolated development of certain 2° sexual characteristics. This may involve autonomous testosterone production in a boy or autonomous oestrogen production in a girl. In addition, testosterone production from the adrenal or an ovarian tumour can induce virilization in a girl.

Assessment of precocious puberty
History
- Age when 2° sexual development first noted.
- What features are present and in what order did they appear? E.g. virilization (pubic, axillary or facial hair, acne, body odour), genital or breast enlargement, galactorrhoea (very rare), menarche, or cyclical mood changes?
- Is there evidence of recent growth acceleration?
- Family history of early puberty?
- Past history of adoption or early weight gain or prior CNS abnormality or insult (e.g. radiation)?

Examination
- Breast or genital and testicular size; degree of virilization (clitoromegaly in girls indicates abnormal androgen levels).
- Neurological examination, particularly visual field assessment and fundoscopy.
- Abdominal or testicular masses.
- Skin (?*café-au-lait* patches—McCune–Albright (📖 see Chapter 93, McCune–Albright syndrome, pp.600–602), or NF-1).
- Assess height and height velocity over 4–6 months.

Investigations
The following investigations may be clinically indicated:
- Wrist radiograph for bone age.
- Thyroid function.
- Sex hormone levels (testosterone, oestrogen, androstenedione, DHEAS).
- LH and FSH levels (baseline and 30, 60min post IV LHRH).
- 17αOH progesterone levels (baseline and 30 and 60min post IV tetracosactide) if congenital adrenal hyperplasia suspected.
- Tumour markers (αFP, βhCG).
- 24h urine steroid profile.
- Abdominal US scan (adrenal glands; ovaries).
- MRI scan (cranial; adrenal glands).

Central precocious puberty

This is due to premature activation of pulsatile LHRH secretion from the hypothalamus and the normal progression in physical changes is maintained ('consonance'). As precocious puberty is defined as occurring younger than 2 SD before the average age, in a normal distribution 2.5% of children will have early onset puberty. In practice, in girls central precocious puberty is more likely to be idiopathic or familial, whereas boys have a greater risk of intracranial or other pathology.

Causes

- Idiopathic or familial.
- Intracranial tumours, hydrocephalus, or other lesions.
- Post cranial irradiation or trauma.
- Intracranial tumours (in particular optic nerve glioma and hypothalamic germinoma), harmotoma, hydrocephalus, and non-specific brain injury (e.g. cerebral palsy).
- May also be triggered by long-standing elevation in sex hormones resulting from any peripheral source or adrenal enzyme defect (e.g. late presenting simple virilizing CAH or inadequately treated CAH).
- Hypothyroidism (elevated TRH stimulates FSH release)—rare.
- Gonadotrophin-secreting tumours (e.g. pituitary adenoma or hepatoblastoma) are rare.

Treatment

Aims of treatment are:

- To avoid psychosocial problems for the child or family.
- To prevent reduced final height due to premature bone maturation and early epiphyseal fusion. A *final height prediction* is often necessary when considering the need for inhibition of puberty. Significant sparing of adult height is only likely to be achieved if presentation occurs and treatment is started ≤6 years of age.

Pituitary LH and FSH secretion can be inhibited by the use of LHRH analogues, e.g. *goserelin* 3.6mg SC monthly or 10.8mg SC 3-monthly, or *triptorelin* 3.75mg SC or deep IM (lower doses if weight <30kg) every 2 weeks for the first 3 injections, then 3–4-weekly thereafter. Treatment efficacy should be monitored regularly by clinical observation and ensuring that LH and FSH levels post IV LHRH remain at low prepubertal levels. The dosing intervals may need to be reduced if there is evidence of inadequate suppression of pubertal development.

Gonadotrophin-independent precocious puberty

At least 2 genetic syndromes have been identified, both resulting in abnormal activation of gonadotrophin receptors independent of normal ligand binding. Thus, in these conditions the gonads autonomously secrete sex hormones and levels of LH and FSH are suppressed by feedback inhibition.

McCune–Albright syndrome

(□ also see Chapter 93, McCune–Albright syndrome, pp.600–602). This is a sporadic condition due to a somatic activating mutation of the GSα protein subunit which affects bones (polyostotic fibrous dysplasia), skin (*café-au-lait* spots) and potentially multiple endocrinopathies.

A number of different hormone receptors share the same G-protein-coupled cyclic AMP second messenger system and hyperthyroidism or hyperparathyroidism may also be present.

All cells descended from the mutated embryonic cell-line are affected, while cells descended from non-mutated cells develop into normal tissues. Thus, the phenotype is highly variable in physical distribution and severity.

Testoxicosis

This is a rare familial condition resulting in precocious puberty only in boys due to an activating LH receptor mutation. Testes show only little increase in size and on biopsy Leydig cell hyperplasia is characteristic. Treatment is by use of androgen receptor blocking agents (cyproterone acetate) and aromatase inhibitors.

Peripheral sex hormone secretion

- Excessive peripheral androgen secretion may occur due to CAH, or androgen-secreting adrenal or gonadal tumours. These children usually have rapid growth, advanced bone age and moderate-to-severe virilization in the absence of testicular or breast development. (Note: a testicular tumour may cause asymmetrical enlargement).
- Peripheral oestrogen production from ovarian tumours are a rare cause of precocious breast development in girls.

Premature thelarche

Premature breast development in the absence of other signs of puberty may present at any age from infancy. Breast size may fluctuate and is often asymmetrical. The cause is unknown, although typically FSH levels (but not LH) are elevated and ovarian US may reveal a single large cyst. Bone maturation, growth rate, and final height are unaffected.

'Thelarche variant'

This is an intermediate condition between premature thelarche and central precocious puberty. The aetiology is unknown. These girls demonstrate ↑ height velocity and rate of bone maturation and ovarian US reveals a more multicystic appearance, as seen in true puberty. There is probably a whole spectrum of presentations between premature thelarche and true precocious puberty. Decision to treat should take into account height velocity and final height prediction as well as the rate of physical maturation and the severity of accompanying pubertal features (e.g. mood swings and difficult behaviour).

'Premature adrenarche' and 'pubarche'

The normal onset of adrenal androgen secretion ('adrenarche') occurs 1–2 years before the onset of puberty. 'Premature' or 'exaggerated' adrenarche is thought to be due to ↑ androgen production or sensitivity and presents with mild features of virilization, such as onset of pubic hair ('pubarche') or acne, in the absence of other features of puberty. Note: clitoromegaly in girls suggests a more severe pathology with excessive androgen production (e.g. CAH or androgen secreting tumour).

The diagnosis is made in the presence of pubic hair and/or axillary hair; the absence of breast/testicular development in children aged <8 years. It is more common in girls.

Management
The management of premature adrenarche usually only requires reassurance after exclusion of other causes as there is no significant impact on final height and onset/progression of puberty. Some of these girls may subsequently develop features of polycystic ovary disease. In these cases treatment should be directed at the presenting feature (e.g. hirsutism, menstrual irregularities).

Delayed/absent puberty

Definition

Delayed puberty is defined as failure to progress into puberty by >2 SD later than the average, i.e. >13 years in girls and >14 years in boys. Clinically, boys are more likely to present with delayed puberty than girls. In addition, some children present with delay in progression from one pubertal stage to the next for >2 years.

Psychological distress may be exacerbated by declining growth velocity relative to their peers. In the long term, severe delay may be a risk factor for ↓ bone mineral density and osteoporosis.

Causes

General

- Constitutional delay of growth and puberty (this is the most common cause; 📖 see Constitutional delay of growth and puberty, p.538).
- Chronic childhood disease, malabsorption (e.g. coeliac disease, inflammatory bowel disease), or undernutrition.

Hypergonadotrophic hypogonadism

Gonadal failure may be:
- Congenital (e.g. Turner's syndrome in girls, Klinefelter's syndrome in boys)
- Acquired (e.g. following chemotherapy, local radiotherapy, infection, torsion).

In these conditions basal and stimulated gonadotrophin levels are raised.

Gonadotrophin deficiency

- Kallman syndrome (including anosmia).
- HP lesions (tumours, post radiotherapy, dysplasia).
- Rare inactivating mutations of genes encoding LH, FSH (or their receptors).

These conditions may also present in the newborn period with micropenis and undescended testes in boys.

Investigation

The following investigations may be clinically indicated:
- LH and FSH levels (basal and post IV LHRH stimulation).
- Plasma oestrogen or testosterone levels.
- Measurement of androgen levels before and after hCG therapy may be used to indicate presence of functional testicular tissue in boys.
- Karyotype.
- Pelvic US in girls to determine ovarian morphology.
- US or MRI imaging in boys to detect an intra-abdominal testes.

It may be difficult to distinguish between constitutional delay and gonadotrophin deficiency, as gonadotrophin levels are low in both conditions. In these cases, induction of puberty may be indicated with regular assessment of testicular growth in boys (which is independent of testosterone therapy) followed by withdrawal of treatment and reassessment when final height is reached.

Management

Depending on the age and concern of the child and parents, short-course exogenous sex steroids can be used to induce pubertal changes. If gonado-trophin deficiency is permanent or the gonads are dysfunctional or absent, then exogenous sex steroids are required to induce and maintain pubertal development (📖 see Constitutional delay of growth and puberty, p.538).

Long-term treatment

See Table 84.2.

Boys

Testosterone (by IM injection) 50mg 4–6-weekly, gradually ↑ to 250mg 4-weekly.

- Monitor penis enlargement, pubic hair, height velocity, and adult body habitus.
- Side-effects include severe acne and rarely priapism.

Girls

Oestrogen (oral). Start at low dose (*ethinyloestradiol* 2mcg daily) and gradu-ally increase.

- Promotes breast development and adult body habitus.
- *Progesterone* (oral) should be added if breakthrough bleeding occurs or when oestrogen dose reaches 10mcg/day.

Table 84.2 Suggested schema for pubertal induction and maintenance in boys and girls

Testosterone dose	Testosterone Interval	Duration	Ethinyloestradiol dose (daily)	Duration
50mg	4 weeks	6 months	2mcg	6 months
100mg	4 weeks	6 months	5mcg	6 months
125mg	4 wecks	6 months	10mcg (+ a progesterone when bleed)	6 months
250mg	3–4 weeks	Onwards	20mcg 'pill'	Onwards

Treatment could be started at age 12–13 years in boys and 11–12 years in girls. Duration for each stage of treatment determined by individual responses

Sexual differentiation

Normal sexual differentiation

Gonadal development

- In the ♂ or ♀ embryo, the bipotential gonad develops as a thickening of mesenchymal cells and coelomic epithelium around the primitive kidney. This *genital ridge* is then colonized by primordial germ cells which migrate from the yolk sac to form the *gonadal ridge*. In the absence of a Y chromosome, the gonad will develop into an ovary.
- In the presence of a normal Y chromosome, immature Sertoli cells, germs cells, and seminiferous tubules can be recognized by 7 weeks, and testis differentiation is complete by 9 weeks. The *SRY* gene is an essential 'sex determining region' on the Y chromosome which signals for testis differentiation.

Internal genitalia

- Embryonic *Müllerian* structures form the uterus, fallopian tubes, and upper 1/3 of the vagina.
- In males, *anti-Müllerian hormone* is secreted by immature Sertoli cells in the testis by 6 weeks, and this causes regression of the Müllerian structures. Leydig cells appear in the testis around day 60, and produce *testosterone* under placental hCG stimulation. Testosterone promotes growth and differentiation of the *Wolffian ducts* to form the epididymis, vas deferens, and seminal vesicles.

External genitalia

- In the absence of any androgen secretion, labia majora, labia minora, and clitoris develop from the embryonic genital swelling, genital fold, and genital tubercle respectively.
- Development of normal ♂ external genitalia requires testosterone production from the testis and its conversion to *dihydrotestosterone* by the enzyme *5α-reductase*. In the presence of dihydrotestosterone, the genital tubercle elongates to form the corpora cavernosa and glans penis, the urethral fold forms the penile shaft, and the labioscrotal swelling forms the scrotum. This process commences around 9 weeks and is completed by 13 weeks. Testicular descent in ♂ occurs in the later $2/3$ of gestation under control of fetal LH and testosterone.

Assessment of ambiguous genitalia

Most cases of ambiguous genitalia present at birth. Involvement of an experienced paediatric endocrinologist and surgeon should be sought as early as possible.

History
- Any maternal medication during pregnancy?
- Are parents consanguineous or is there a family history of ambiguous genitalia?
- Is there a neonatal history of hypoglycaemia or prolonged jaundice?

Examination
- Assess clitoris/phallus size; degree of labial fusion; position of urethra/urogenital sinus (anterior or posterior).
- Are gonads palpable?—Check along line of descent.
- Are there any signs indicating panhypopituitarism?—E.g. midline defects/hypoglycaemia/hypocortisolaemia/prolonged jaundice).
- Dysmorphic features of Turner's syndrome may be seen in XO/XY mosaicism.

Investigations
- Bloods for karyotype, electrolytes, blood glucose, 17αOH progesterone
- US of pelvis and labial folds (for Müllerian structures and gonads).
- Arrange for clinical photographs.
- After 48h old, when the neonatal hormonal surge has decreased, repeat bloods for 17αOH progesterone, cortisol, LH, FSH, and androgen levels. Collect a 2 h urine sample to measure the steroid profile.
- Examination under anesthesia (EUA) and cystogram may be required.

Specific tests
- Short Synacthen® test in a virilized XX (when CAH is suspected) may be required.
- 3-day HCG test in a undervirilized '♂' (testes present or 46, XY) assesses stimulated gonadal production of androgens and may be diagnostic of androgen biosynthesis defects or androgen insensitivity.
- LHRH test examines pituitary gonadotrophin secretion (this test is only informative in the neonatal period).
- Glucagon test examines cortisol and GH secretion.
- Androgen receptor function can be tested on cultured fibroblasts from a genital skin biopsy.
- DNA analysis for androgen receptor mutation, CAH mutations, and androgen biosynthesis mutations.

Disorders of sex development (DSD)

♂ and ♀ internal and external genitalia develop from common embryonic structures. In the absence of ♂ differentiating signals, normal ♀ genitalia develop. Genital ambiguity may therefore occur as a result of chromosomal abnormality, gonadal dysgenesis, biochemical defects of androgen synthesis, inappropriate exposure to external androgens, or androgen receptor insensitivity.

Box 85.1 Definitions

Disorders of chromosomes
Including:
- 45X Turner and variants.
- 47XXY and variants.
- 45X/46XY mixed gonadal dysgenesis.
- 46XX/46XY gonadal chimera.

46XX DSD
Including:
- Disorders of gonadal (ovarian) development.
- Androgen excess.
- Structural disorders e.g. cloacal exstrophy, vaginal atresia.

46XY DSD
Including:
- Disorders of gonadal (testicular) development.
- Disorders in androgen synthesis and action.
- Structural disorders e.g. severe hypospadias, cloacal exstrophy.

46XX DSD

Disorders of ovarian development
Normal ♂ differentiation can occur if the *SRY* gene has been translocated onto an autosome.

Biochemical defects leading to androgen oversecretion
Congenital adrenal hyperplasia (CAH, 21-hydroxylase deficiency most commonly) is the most common cause of ambiguous genitalia in 46, XX.

Maternal hyperandrogenism
- The ♀ fetus may be virilized if maternal androgen levels exceed the capacity of placental aromatase to convert these to oestrogen.
- This may occur due to maternal disease (e.g. CAH, adrenal and ovarian tumours) or use of androgenic medication in pregnancy or rarely placental aromatase deficiency.

46XY DSD

Disorders of testis development
- XY gonadal dysgenesis can be caused by mutations in a number of genes controlling ♂ sexual differentiation, including *SRY, SF-1, WT-1* and *SOX*, and can present with normal external genitalia.
- Early testicular failure resulting from torsion or infarction.

Biochemical defects of androgen synthesis

Rare deficiencies of the enzymes 5α-reductase, 17β-hydroxysteroid dehydrogenase or 3β-hydroxysteroid dehydrogenase which is also associated with glucocorticoid and mineralocorticoid deficiencies are autosomal recessively inherited and may result in variable degrees of undervirilization.

Androgen receptor insensitivity syndrome

(📕 also see Androgen insensitivity syndrome, p.418).

Defects of the androgen receptor gene on the X chromosome, or autosomal post-receptor signalling genes, may result in complete or partial androgen insensitivity.

- *Complete androgen insensitivity* Results in normal ♀ external genitalia and usually only presents with testicular prolapse in childhood or primary amenorrhoea in adolescence.
- *Partial androgen insensitivity* Presentation may vary from mild virilization to micropenis, hypospadias, undescended testes or only ↓ spermatogenesis.

Gonadotrophin defects

- Gonadotrophin deficiency may occur in *hypopituitarism* or may be associated with anosmia (*Kallmann syndrome*). It usually presents with delayed puberty but is an occasional cause of micropenis and undescended testes.
- LH receptor gene defects are rare, and result in complete absence of virilization as the testes are unable to respond to placental hCG.

Anti-Müllerian hormone deficiency or insensitivity

Testes are usually undescended and uterus and fallopian tubes present.

Management of ambiguous genitalia

In the newborn period, the infant should be monitored in hospital for:
- Hypoglycaemia (until hypopituitarism is excluded).
- Salt wasting (until CAH is excluded).

Explain to the parents that the infant appears to be healthy, but has a defect that interferes with determining sex. It is helpful to show the parents the physical findings as you explain this. Advise them to postpone the registration of the birth until after further investigations, and discuss what they will say to relatives and friends. The sex of the baby should be assigned as soon after birth as is practicable given the need for accurate diagnosis.

Sex assignment

Decision on the sex of rearing should be based on the optimal expected outcome in terms of psychosexual and reproductive function. Parents therefore should be allowed discussion with an endocrinologist, a surgeon specializing in urogenital reconstruction, a psychologist, and a social worker. Following the necessary investigations and discussions, early gender assignment optimizes the psychosexual outcome.

Further management
- If ♀ sex is assigned, any testicular tissue should be removed.
- Reconstructive surgery may include clitoral reduction, gonadectomy, and vaginoplasty in girls, and phallus enlargement, hypospadias repair, and orchidopexy in boys. In both sexes multiple-stage procedures may be required.
- Topical or systemic *dihydrotestosterone* may enhance phallus size in ♂ infants and a trial of therapy is sometimes useful before sex assignment.
- Hormone replacement therapy may also be required from puberty into adulthood.
- Continuing psychological support for the parents and children is very important.

Congenital adrenal hyperplasia

(📖 also see Chapter 55, Congenital adrenal hyperplasia in adults, p.302)

A number of autosomally inherited enzyme deficiencies result in cortisol deficiency, excess pituitary ACTH secretion, and adrenal gland hyperplasia.

21-hydroxylase deficiency (>90%)

The most common cause of CAH results in cortisol and mineralocorticoid deficiency, while the build-up of precursor steroids is channelled towards excess adrenal androgen synthesis. Different gene defects in the 21-hydroxylase gene (e.g. deletion, splice site or point mutation) result in different degrees of enzyme dysfunction and thus wide variation in phenotypes.

Clinical features

- Virilization of ♀ fetuses may result in clitoromegaly and labial fusion at birth. 75% have sufficient mineralocorticoid deficiency to cause renal salt-wasting. Because ♂ have normal genitalia at birth, they may present acutely ill in the neonatal period with vomiting, dehydration, collapse, hyponatraemia, and hyperkalaemia. Non-salt-wasting boys present with early genital enlargement, pubarche, and rapid growth.
- If untreated or poorly treated, both sexes may develop pubic hair, acne, rapid height velocity, advanced bone maturation and precocious puberty which may result in very short final height.
- 'Non-classical CAH' is due to milder 21-hydroxylase deficiency, and affected girls present in later childhood or adulthood with hirsuitism, acne, premature/exaggerated adrenarche, menstrual irregularities, and infertility.

11β-hydroxylase deficiency (~5%)

This enzyme, which converts 11-deoxycortisol to cortisol, is the final step in cortisol synthesis. In addition to excess adrenal androgens, the overproduced precursor corticosterone has mineralocorticoid activity. Thus, in contrast to salt wasting in 21-hydroxylase deficiency, these subjects may have hypernatraemia and hypokalaemia. Hypertension is rarely seen in infancy, but may develop during childhood and affects 50–60% of adults.

Specific investigations for CAH

(📖 see also Assessment of ambiguous genitalia, p.561.)

- *Plasma 17αOH progesterone* An elevated level indicates 21-hydroxylase deficiency. It may be difficult to distinguish this from the physiological hormonal surge which occurs in the first 2 days of life. This test should therefore be repeated (together with 11-deoxycortisol) after 48h of age.
- A 24h urine steroid profile (also collected after 48h of age) should confirm the diagnosis and allows detection of the rarer enzyme defects.
- A Synacthen® stimulation test may be required to discriminate between the different enzyme deficiencies.
- Plasma and urine electrolytes may need to be monitored over the first 2 weeks.

- Plasma renin level is also useful to confirm salt wasting in those with normal serum sodium and relatively mild 21-hydroxylase deficiency.

Other rare enzyme deficiencies

- *17α-Hydrolxylase deficiency* Impairs cortisol, androgen, and oestrogen synthesis, but overproduction of mineralocorticoids leads to hypokalaemia and hypertension.
- *3β-Hydroxysteroid dehydrogenase deficiency* Impairs cortisol, mineralocorticoid and androgen biosynthesis. ♂ have hypospadias and undescended testes, however excess DHEA, a weak androgen, may cause mild virilization in ♀.

Steroid acute regulatory protein

- STAR mutation: 46XY sex reversal and severe adrenal failure. Heterozygous defect. Extremely rare.
- CYP11A1 (P450: side-chain cleavage cytochrome enzyme): 46XY sex reversal and severe adrenal failure. Heterozygous defect. Extremely rare.
- P450 oxidoreductase deficiency: Biochemical picture of combined 21-hydroxylase/17α-hydrolxylase/17, 20 Lyase deficiencies. Spectrum of presentation from children with ambiguous genitalia, adrenal failure and the Antley–Bixler skeletal dysplasia through to mildly affected individuals with polycystic ovary syndrome

Management

- *Hydrocortisone* (15 mg/m² per day orally in 3 divided doses). In addition to treating cortisol deficiency, this therapy suppresses ACTH and thereby limits excessive production of adrenal androgens. Occasionally higher doses are required to achieve adequate androgen suppression, however over-treatment may suppress growth.
- In salt losers, initial *IV fluid resuscitation* (10–20mL/kg normal saline), may be required to treat circulatory collapse. Long-term mineralocorticoid replacement (*fludrocortisone* 0.05–0.3mg/day) may have incomplete efficacy, particularly in infancy, and *sodium chloride* supplements are also needed. Up to 10mmol/kg per day may be needed in infancy.
- *Reconstructive surgery* (clitoral reduction, vaginoplasty) Often performed in infancy and further procedures may be required during puberty. Needs experienced surgeon.
- Warn of need for extra steroid during stress.

Monitoring of hormonal therapy

- *Height velocity and bone age* If hydrocortisone therapy is insufficient, growth rate will be above normal and bone age will be advanced. Conversely, if hydrocortisone therapy is excessive, growth is suppressed.
- *17αOHP* Blood levels should be assessed several times each year. Levels should be measured before after each hydrocortisone dose; these may be collected at home by the parents using 'spot' capillary blood samples. In girls and prepubertal boys, androgen levels (testosterone and androstendione) can be measured if there is concern about poor control and/or virilization.

- *Mineralocorticoid and sodium replacement* Should be monitored by measuring plasma electrolytes, and renin levels, and by regular blood pressure assessments.

Genetic advice

- The inheritance of CAH is autosomal recessive and parents should be informed of a 25% risk of recurrence in future offspring.
- If the mutation is identifiable on DNA analysis in the child and parents, chorionic villus sampling may allow prenatal diagnosis.
- Maternal *dexamethasone* therapy from around 5–6 weeks of pregnancy is used to prevent virilization of the ♀ fetus without significant maternal complications.

Further reading

Brook CGD (ed.) (1995). *Clinical Paediatric Endocrinology*, 3rd edn. Blackwell Science, Oxford.

Consensus Statement on 21 hydroxylene deficiency. Joint LWPES/ESPE Working Group (2002). *J Clin Endocrinol Metab* **87**, 4048–53.

Fluck CE, and Miller WL (2006). P450 oxidoreductase deficiency: a new form of congenital adrenal hyperplasia. *Curr Opin Paediatric* **18**, 435–41.

Hochberg Z (ed.) (1998). Practical Algorithms in Pediatric Endocrinology. Karger, Basel.

Hughes IA (1989). *Handbook of Endocrine Investigations in Children*. John Wright & Sons, Bristol, UK

Hughes IA, Houk C, Ahmed SF, *et al.* (2006). Consensus statement on management of intersex disorders. *Arch Dis Child* **91**, 554–63.

Wilkins L (1994). In Kappy MS, Blizzard RM, Migeon CJ (eds.) *The diagnosis and treatment of endocrine disorders in childhood and adolescence*, 4th edn. Charles C Thomas, Springfield, Illinois.

Part 8

Neuroendocrine disorders

The neuroendocrine system

Introduction

- Neuroendocrine cells are found in many sites throughout the body. They are particularly prominent in the GI tract and pancreas, and share a common embryological origin. These cells have the ability to synthesize, store, and release peptide hormones.
- Due to the prevalence of neuroendocrine cells, the majority of neuroendocrine tumours occur within the gastro-entero-pancreatic axis. Of these tumours, >50% are traditionally termed carcinoid tumours and have been usually subclassified into foregut, midgut, and hindgut lesions with the remainder largely comprising pancreatic islet cell tumours.
- Carcinoid and islet cell tumours are generally slow growing.

Further reading

Barakat MT, Meeran K, Bloom SR (2004). Neuroendocrine tumours. *Endocr Relat Cancer* **11**(1), 1–18.

Carcinoid tumours

Definition and classification

- Historically these tumours have been divided into those arising in the foregut, midgut, or hindgut.
- Strictly speaking, carcinoid tumours are serotonin secreting and argentaffin +ve and so the term should be reserved for those typical midgut tumours which fulfill these criteria. Increasingly, the remainder are being classified as neuroendocrine tumours together with their tissue of origin.
- About 85% of carcinoid tumours develop in the GI tract, 10% in the lung, and the rest in various organs such as the thymus or ovary.
- In 30% of patients carcinoid tumours are multiple and associations with other malignancies such as adenocarcinomas of the GI tract and prostate are recognized.

Incidence

The annual incidence of carcinoid tumours is approximately 2.5 per 100,000 population although postmortem studies suggest this may be a significant underestimate.

Carcinoid syndrome

- Only occurs in a subset of patients with carcinoid tumours.
- Occurs when sufficient vasoactive substances are released into the systemic circulation. Consequently, almost all patients with the carcinoid syndrome due to GI tumours have hepatic metastases. In contrast, some bronchial carcinoids may present with classical features of the syndrome without metastatic disease.
- The original description of the syndrome includes flushing, diarrhoea, asthma, right heart valvular lesions, and pellagra-like skin lesions.
- In a published series of patients from Sweden with known GI carcinoids, 84% presented with diarrhoea, 75% with flushing, and 44% with intestinal obstruction. During the course of the illness it was noted that 33% of the patients had carcinoid heart disease and 15% complained of symptoms of wheezing.
- The carcinoid flush may be precipitated by spicy food, hot drinks, alcohol, exercise, and postural changes. The cause of flushing is heterogeneous and results from the release of a variety of vasoactive substances. Acute attacks typically cause a diffuse erythematous flush affecting the face and upper thorax whereas longstanding carcinoid may be associated with a violacious flush and facial telangiectasia.
- A life-threatening carcinoid crisis can be provoked in these patients as a result of anaesthesia or surgical manipulation of the tumour.

Box 87.1 Carcinoid heart disease

- Occurs in two-thirds of patients with the carcinoid syndrome.
- The mechanism is poorly understood.
- Pathologically the lesions are characterized by fibrous thickening of the endocardium in plaques.
- The right side of the heart is typically involved. Thickening and retraction of the tricuspid and pulmonary valve leaflets lead to tricuspid regurgitation in nearly all, and less commonly pulmonary regurgitation, tricuspid stenosis, and pulmonary stenosis. The left side of the heart is involved in <10% of cases.
- Valve replacement can be beneficial but surgery may be associated with significant morbidity and mortality.

---

1 Norheim I, Oberg K, Theodorsson-Norheim, E etal. (1987). Malignant carcinoid tumors: an analysis of 103 patients with regard to tumor localization, hormone production, and survival. *Ann surg.* **206**(2), 115–125.

Diagnostic investigations

Pathology
- Historically carcinoid tumours have been identified by their reaction to silver stains.
- Characterizing the tumour histpathologically is very important and currently includes the use of specific immunohistochemical stains such as chromogranin A, synaptophysin, serotonin, and gastrin.
- Ki67, a marker of cell proliferation, is also used by some centres to guide treatment.

Biochemical investigations
- Urinary 5HIAA (serotonin metabolite) assessment has traditionally been the mainstay of both diagnosis and monitoring. The test offers a specificity of nearly 100% and a sensitivity of 70%.
- Elevated levels are usually only associated with midgut tumours and only once they have metastasized.
- Elevated levels correlate well with symptoms of the carcinoid syndrome and are useful in monitoring response to treatment.
- False +ve tests may result from dietary sources of serotonin (e.g. bananas, avocados, tomatoes, walnuts, pineapples, and chocolate) and interference from drugs (e.g. phenacetin)
- Plasma or platelet serotonin are alternatives to urine testing.
- The most sensitive biochemical marker for neuroendocrine tumours is plasma chromogranin A (false +ve—renal/liver failure, proton pump inhibitors (PPIs), gastritis, inflammatory bowel disease. False −ve— L-dopa, phenothiazines). For carcinoid tumours the sensitivity of the test is nearly 100% but the specificity is lower than for urinary 5HIAA as raised levels are found in most neuroendocrine tumours.
- A plasma gut hormone profile may also be useful for the identification of tumour markers such as gastrin, pancreatic polypeptide, and somatostatin.
- Liver biochemistry is an unreliable marker of hepatic involvement as the alkaline phosphatase may remain in the normal range despite extensive metastatic disease.

Exclude associated inherited syndromes
Carcinoid tumours may rarely be associated with multiple endocrine neoplasia syndrome type 1 (MEN1), von Hippel–Lindau syndrome (VHL), type 1 neurofibromatosis (NF1), and tuberose sclerosis.

Tumour localization and staging

- Imaging with abdominal US, CT, and MRI aims to both localize the 1° tumour and assess the extent of metastatic spread.
- On CT, hepatic carcinoid metastases are usually multifocal, showing enhancement after IV contrast and frequently with low attenuation areas of necrosis. MRI is at least as sensitive as CT with lesions being iso-intense on T1 weighted images but of high signal on T2 weighted images.
- >80% of carcinod tumours have somatostatin receptors and scanning with radiolabelled octreotide can provide very useful information about the localization and extent of metastatic disease. It frequently reveals previously unidentified extrahepatic sites of disease.
- PET scanning, where available, can contribute to tumour localization and staging in difficult cases.

Box 87.2 Monitoring treatment

- Urinary 5HIAA or serum chromogranin A can be useful to monitor response to therapy if these markers were elevated at diagnosis.
- Imaging modalities are also essential to monitor tumour bulk.

Treatment

A multidisciplinary approach to the treatment of these tumours is essential.

Surgical treatment

- In patients with local disease, surgery can be curative but the majority of patients have metastatic disease by the time they seek treatment.
- Even in patients with widespread local disease or distant metastases, surgery may still be of benefit by reducing overall tumour bulk and thereby affording a more favourable response to subsequent non-surgical therapies.
- Surgery may be required to alleviate obstructive intestinal disease.
- Liver transplantation may be considered in a very few selected patients in whom extrahepatic tumour spread and 1° tumour recurrence has been excluded.

Box 87.3 Perioperative management of carcinoid tumours

It may be useful to give IV octreotide in the perioperative period as both anaesthesia and surgery may be associated with the release of various vasoactive peptides which can result in hypotension and bronchospasm leading to a potentially fatal carcinoid crisis.

Medical treatment

Certain symptom specific medical agents can be useful such as loperamide or codeine for diarrhoea.

Somatostatin analogues

- Octreotide and its longer acting analogues reduce the level of biochemical tumour markers in the majority of patients and control symptoms in around 70% of cases. However, radiological evidence of tumour regression with these agents is rare.
- Patient resistance to somatostatin analogues is common after a few years and this potential for tachyphlaxis makes the early use of somatostatin analogues in asymptomatic patients controversial.
- Patients are usually given a test dose of SC octreotide and then generally commenced on the more convenient longer acting analogues. Shortacting SC octreotide tds may be continued until cover with the longer acting analogue is complete.
- A continuous IV infusion of octreotide is the most effective treatment for a carcinoid crisis and is generally given at a rate of 50–100mcg/h.

Hepatic embolization

- Can be performed by surgeons or increasingly by interventional radiologists.
- It is a palliative procedure offering symptom relief by ↓ tumour bulk.
- The duration of improvement may be short lived and occasionally significant side effects such as the hepatorenal syndrome may occur.

External beam radiotherapy

May provide palliation in those with symptomatic bone metastases or spinal cord compression.

Chemotherapy

- Cytotoxic chemotherapy should be considered in patients with advanced, progressive, or uncontrolled symptomatic disease.
- The most promising combination using streptozotocin and 5-fluorouracil (5-FU) produces only short-lasting responses in 10–30% of patients with carcinoid tumours, in contrast to the 50–60% response rate of pancreatic neuroendocrine tumours. Capecitabine (prodrug of 5-FU) can be administered orally and it is hoped that it will offer a more specific antitumour effect.
- Side-effects (e.g. flu-like symptoms, fatigue, weight loss, bone marrow suppression) are generally less severe than with conventional chemotherapy but are still the main limitation to its use.

α-interferon

- There is a good biochemical response rate (about 45%) with clinical improvement of the symptoms of carcinoid syndrome in 70% of patients. Tumour shrinkage has rarely been described.
- A combination of octreotide and α-interferon has been shown to produce biochemical and symptomatic improvement in some patients previously resistant to either drug alone.

Radioactive isotope therapy

- These are relatively new modalities with few long-term data.
- There is increasing evidence to suggest that if a +ve diagnostic uptake scan is obtained then therapeutic treatment with the relevant radionuclide can offer at least significant symptomatic improvement. A few studies have suggested tumour stabilization or regression may be achieved in some cases.

Radiolabelled somatostatin analogues

- Radiolabelled somatostatin analogues such as ^{111}InDTPA octreotide, the newer ^{90}YDOTA octreotide, and ^{177}Lu octreotate which have high affinity for type 2 somatostatin receptors, have been used as therapy. ^{111}InDTPA octreotide has low tissue penetration and stable coupling of α or β emitting isotopes to DTPA octreotide could not be achieved, hence the development of new compounds. ^{90}YDOTA octreotide may result in partial remission in 10–25% of patients while ^{177}Lu octreotate has proved very successful in achieving tumour regression in animal models with encouraging preliminary human studies (remission in 38% and stable disease in 4% at 3 months).
- A new somatostatin analogue (SOM230—pasireotide) with high affinity for receptor subtypes 1, 2, 3, and 5 is currently under evaluation in phase III trials.

Radiolabelled MIBG

- MIBG is structurally related to noadrenaline and after IV injection up to 70% of carcinoid tumours concentrate significant amounts of the compound.
- Limited published data suggest 65–80% of these patients treated with MIBG have palliation of symptoms for varying lengths of time (6–24 months).

Future treatments

Antiangiogenic agents such as inhibitors of vascular endothelial growth factor are currently being evaluated and may be of benefit in preventing tumour progression.

Pellagra

- Rarely pellagra may develop due to nicotinamide deficiency 2° to excessive tryptophan metabolism.
- Nicotinamide supplementation is therapeutic.

Prognosis

- The site of origin and the size of the 1° tumour, together with the extent of metastatic disease, largely determine the prognosis.
- Many carcinoid tumours are indolent and are frequently a postmortem finding having caused no significant symptoms during life.
- Where the disease is confined locally to the region of the 1° tumour the 5-year survival is >90%.
- Individual patients have been reported to live 20–30 years after the diagnosis of metastatic carcinoid tumour but this should not be considered a benign disease. The 5-year survival rate when hepatic metastases are present is approximately 20–40% with a median survival time being about 2 years.
- Increasingly evidence is suggesting that both survival time and quality of life for patients is improved by the use of more active and aggressive therapy.
- The prognosis is greatly influenced by the development of carcinoid heart disease and whether it is then amenable to treatment by heart valve replacement.

Further reading

Kaltsas G, Rockall A, Papadogias D, *et al.* (2004). Recent advances in radiological and radionuclide imaging and therapy of neuroendocrine tumours. *Eur J Endocrinol* **151**(1), 15–27.

Oberg K (2002). Carcinoid tumours: molecular genetics, tumor biology, and update of diagnosis and treatment. *Curr Opin Oncol* **14**(1), 38–45.

Insulinomas

Definitions

- An insulinoma is a tumour of the endocrine pancreas that causes hypoglycaemia through its inappropriate secretion of insulin.
- Unlike other endocrine tumours of the pancreas, where malignancy is common, >90% of insulinomas are benign.
- >80% of insulinomas are solitary, but some are multiple, either simultaneously or consecutively, a situation likely to be associated with MEN1 in approximately 10%.
- Insulinomas are found with equal frequency throughout the head, body and tail of the pancreas.

Incidence

The annual incidence of insulinoma is of the order of 1–2 per million population.

Clinical presentation

- Symptoms of hypoglycaemia may include both adrenergic (e.g. pallor, sweating, tremor, and tachycardia) and neuroglycopaenic (e.g. irritability, confusion, aggression, seizures, and coma) symptoms.
- Patients typically give a history of relief of symptoms with food. Weight gain occurs in at least 30% of patients.

Biochemical investigations

- A laboratory glucose measurement after 3 separate 15h fasts is a reliable initial screening test for insulinoma. A glucose of <2.2mmol/L should be found during symptoms in association with an inappropriately elevated insulin and C-peptide level.
- The presence of sulphonylurea metabolites in the urine or plasma should be excluded and the abuse of exogenous insulin considered.
- In those rare cases where the 15h fasts fail to reveal hypoglycaemia and a diagnosis of insulinoma remains strongly suspected then the gold standard test remains the in-patient supervized 72h fast. The patient must remain active and exercise normally throughout the test. The biochemical criteria are as described for the 15h fasts.

Tumour localization

(📖 see Table 88.1.)

- Islet cell tumours are often small and may not be detected by any imaging technique. The available radiological modalities have a wide reported range of sensitivity which is frequently dependent on the equipment and the operator.
- MRI or spiral CT correctly detects >60% of tumours but preoperative localization can be difficult in tumours <1cm in diameter.
- Arterial stimulation (with calcium or secretin) followed by venous sampling can localize approximately 90% of insulinomas but carries the risks of a more invasive technique.
- Endoscopic US, which requires specialized equipment and expertise, may identify tumours as small as 5mm. The head of the pancreas is visualized with the probe in the duodenum and the body and tail with it in the stomach.
- Intraoperative US using a transducer applied directly to the pancreas improves the sensitivity of US to ~90%.
- Experienced surgeons can frequently identify the lesions intraoperatively by palpation alone and the risk of multiple tumours makes a thorough examination of the whole pancreas essential at operation.
- Somatostatin receptor scintigraphy has been shown to be useful in detecting insulinomas but it is dependent on somatostatin receptor subtype expression by the tumour.

Table 88.1 Radiological localization of pancreatic insulinomas

Localization technique	Reported sensitivity (%)
Transabdominal US	30–61%
Endoscopic US	80%
Intraoperative US	90%
CT	42–78%
MRI	20–100%
Octreotide scanning	68–86%
Pancreatic arteriography	29–90%
Venous sampling	84%

Treatment

- The treatment of choice in all but very elderly or debilitated patients is surgical removal. The perioperative mortality rates are <1% in the hands of an experienced surgeon. The mortality is largely influenced by the incidence of acute pancreatitis and peritonitis.
- Postoperative hyperglycaemia may occur even following partial pancreatectomy.
- Medical treatment to control symptoms may be achieved using a combination of diazoxide and octreotide.
- Radiolabelled somatostatin analogue therapy may induce a biochemical and symptomatic response in patients with malignant insulinomas and some small-scale studies report tumour regression.

Prognosis

- Following removal of a solitary insulinoma, life expectancy is restored to normal.
- Malignant insulinomas, with metastases usually to the liver, have a natural history of years rather than months and symptoms may be controlled with medical therapy or specific antitumour therapy using streptozotocin and 5-FU.
- Average 5 year survival estimated to be approximately 35%.

Gastrinomas

Definitions

- Gastrin, synthesized in the G cells situated predominantly in the gastric antrum, is the principal gut hormone stimulating gastric acid secretion.
- The Zollinger–Ellison (gastrinoma) syndrome is due to the excessive release of gastrin by neuroendocrine tumours of the GI tract and pancreas.
- 85–90% of gastrinomas are located in the pancreatic islets while 10–15% arise from gastrin-producing cells in the duodenum.
- ~60% of patients have metastatic disease at the time of diagnosis.

Prevalence

The estimated prevalence is of the order of 1 per million population.

Clinical presentation

- Patients typically present with peptic and/or oesophageal ulcers that are multiple and refractory to standard medical treatment.
- Complications of peptic ulcer disease such as perforation, haemorrhage, and pyloric stenosis are frequently seen.
- Malabsorption and diarrhoea may be the main presenting complaint in 10–20% of patients and is due to acid-related inactivation of enzymes and mucosal damage in the upper small bowel.
- Up to 25% of gastrinoma patients may have MEN1 and in this context the prevalence of malignant gastrinomas is higher and the long-term survival worse than for sporadic tumours.

Biochemical investigations

- The diagnosis rest on finding an inappropriately elevated fasting plasma gastrin in the presence of ↑ gastric acid secretion.
- Patients should have antisecretory treatment stopped prior to the test (3 days for H_2 blockers and 2 weeks for PPIs) since these drugs are associated with hypergastrinaemia. However, gastrin levels above 250pmol/L are rarely due to PPI therapy alone.
- A gut hormone profile may identify elevated plasma levels of pancreatic polypeptide or other gut hormones.
- The tumour localization techniques described for insulinomas are also relevant for gastrinomas (📖 Tumour localization, p.581).
- Very small tumours or duodenal tumours can be very hard to localize and even small tumours are frequently associated with local lymph node disease.
- Selective arterial angiography may be combined with a provocative test for gastrin release using a bolus of calcium glucanate or secretin for elusive small tumours. 3ml calcium glucanate is injected into the gastroduodenal, superior mesentric, splenic and hepatric artery in turn, with a 5min gap between. After 30 seconds at each site sampling is undertaken.
- For causes of hypergastrinaemia 📖 see Box 89.1.

Box 89.1 Causes of hypergastrinaemia

Low or normal gastric acid production
- H_2 blockers
- PPIs
- Vagotomy
- Hypochlorhydria
- Short gut syndrome
- Renal failure
- Hypercalcaemia

Elevated gastric acid production
- Gastrinoma
- G cell hyperplasia

Treatment

- The treatment of choice is complete surgical tumour removal although this is usually only considered after the tumour has been identified preoperatively.
- Surgery is rarely justified in patients with known hepatic metastases, although some small studies have raised the possibility of benefit from tumour debulking.
- Where preoperative imaging has failed to identify a tumour, the patient is often best maintained on medical therapy with regular imaging to reassess (PPIs need to be given less frequently than H_2 antagonists). Check B_{12} annually.
- Somatostatin analogues do not appear to be more effective at controlling gastric acid hypersecretion and relieving symptoms than PPIs or H_2 blockers.
- The data are currently few but as for insulinomas, radiolabelled somatostatin analogues may be a future treatment option for gastrinomas.
- In patients with MEN1 management is more controversial but the usual policy is to operate when a well-defined tumour can be identified.

Table 89.1 Treatment options for gastrinomas

Medical treatment	Surgery	Palliation
• H_2 blockers	• Tumour resection	• Chemotherapy
• PPIs	• Tumour debulking	• Hepatic artery embolization
• Octreotide	• Liver transplant	

Glucagonomas

Definitions

- Glucagonomas are neuroendocrine tumours that usually arise from the α cells of the pancreas and produce the glucagonoma syndrome through the secretion of glucagon and other peptides derived from the preproglucagon gene.
- The large majority of glucagonomas are malignant, but they are also very indolent tumours and the diagnosis may be overlooked for many years.
- Up to 90% of patients will have lymph node or liver metastases at the time of presentation.
- They are classically associated with the rash of necrolytic migratory erythema.

Incidence

The annual incidence is estimated at 1 per 20 million population.

Clinical presentation

See Table 90.1.
- The characteristic rash—necrolytic migratory erythema—occurs in >70% of cases and usually manifests initially as a well demarcated area of erythema in the groin before migrating to the limbs, buttocks, and perineum.
- Mucous membrane involvement is common with stomatitis, glossitis, vaginitis, and urethritis being frequent features.
- Glucagon antagonizes the effects of insulin, particularly on hepatic glucose metabolism and glucose intolerance is a frequent association (>90%).
- Sustained gluconeogenesis also cause amino acid deficiencies and results in protein catabolism which can be associated with unrelenting weight loss in >60% of patients.
- Glucagon has a direct suppressive effect on the bone marrow resulting in a normochromic normocytic anaemia in almost all patients.
- Up to 20% of glucagonoma patients will have associated MEN1.

Table 90.1 Clinical features of the glucagonoma syndrome

Site	Clinical features
Skin	Necrolytic migratory erythema
Mucous membranes	Angular stomatitis
	Atrophic glossitis
	Vulvovaginitis
	Urethritis
Nails	Onycholysis
Scalp	Alopecia
Metabolism	Glucose intolerance
	Protein catabolism and weight loss
Haematological	Anaemia
	Venous thromboses
Psychiatric	Depression
	Psychosis

Biochemical investigations

- The diagnosis is confirmed on finding raised plasma glucagon levels.
- A gut hormone profile may also show elevated neuroendocrine markers such as pancreatic polypeptide.
- Impaired glucose intolerance and hypoaminoacidaemia may be present.

Tumour localization

- At the time of diagnosis >60% of glucagonomas will have metastasized to the liver and most 1° tumours will be >3cm in diameter.
- These tumours rarely present problems of radiological localization and transabdominal US and CT scanning are usually adequate.
- Small tumours may require more sophisticated imaging techniques (📖 see Tumour localization, p.581). Octreotide scanning probably offers the best means of evaluating the extent of metastatic disease.

Treatment

- Surgery is the only curative therapeutic option, but the potential for a complete cure may be as low as 5%.
- In malignant disease, a surgical cure may still be achieved in those rare cases where the metastases are confined to the liver and the patient is deemed suitable for a liver transplant.
- Somatostatin analogues are the treatment of choice with excellent response rates in treating the necrolytic migratory erythema. They are less effective at reversing the weight loss and have an inconsistent effect on glycaemic control such that diabetes mellitus may need to be managed with insulin therapy.
- If octreotide fails, the rash may be improved using IV amino acids and fatty acids
- Palliative chemotherapy using streptozotocin and 5-FU has been shown to produce a 50% reduction in glucagon levels in 75% of patients but the benefit is frequently only temporary.
- Hepatic artery embolization may result in a dramatic relief of symptoms with remissions of several months recorded.
- As for the other pancreatic islet cell tumours there are preliminary data to suggest that radiolabelled somatostatin analogues may be therapeutic in the glucagonoma syndrome.

VIPomas

Definitions

- In 1958 Verner and Morrison[1] first described a syndrome consisting of refractory watery diarrhoea and hypokalaemia associated with a neuroendocrine tumour of the pancreas.
- The syndrome of watery diarrhoea, hypokalaemia and acidosis (WDHA) is due to secretion of vasoactive intestinal polypeptide (VIP).
- Tumours that secrete VIP are known as VIPomas.
- VIPomas account for <10% of islet cell tumours and mainly occur as solitary tumours.
- >60% are malignant and metastasize to the lymph nodes, liver, kidneys and bone.

Clinical presentation

- The most prominent symptom in most patients is profuse watery diarrhoea which is secretory in nature and therefore rich in electrolytes (Box 91.1).
- Other causes of secretory diarrhoea should be considered in the differential diagnosis (see Box 91.2).
- VIPomas are rare in MEN1 patients, occurring in <1% of cases.

Biochemical investigations

- Elevated levels of plasma VIP are found in all patients with the VIPoma syndrome, although false +ves may occur in dehydrated patients due to diarrhoea from other causes.
- A gut hormone profile may identify other raised tumour markers such as pancreatic polypeptide and aid detection of some other causes of watery diarrhoea e.g. gastrinomas.
- Urinary catecholamine excretion should be assessed, especially in children in whom it is common to find the tumours residing in the adrenal medulla.

Box 91.1 Clinical features of the VIPoma syndrome

- Watery diarrhoea
- Hypokalaemia
- Achlorhydria
- Metabolic acidosis
- Hypercalcaemia
- Hyperglycaemia
- Hypomagnaesaemia
- Facial flushing

Box 91.2 Differential diagnosis of secretory diarrhoea

- Infection e.g. *Escherichia coli* or cholera toxins
- Laxative abuse
- Villous adenoma
- Other gut neuroendocrine tumours e.g. carcinoid tumours or gastrinomas
- Carcinoma of the lung
- Medullary carcinoma of the thyroid
- Systemic mastocytosis
- Immunoglobulin A deficiency

Tumour localization

- The majority of tumours secreting VIP originate in the pancreas while others arise from the sympathetic chain.
- 1° VIPomas have very rarely been reported to arise from a variety of other sites such as the lung, oesophagus, small bowel, colon, and kidney.
- Most patients present with large tumours which can be easily identified by transabdominal US or CT although small tumours may require additional methods of tumour localization as previously discussed (📖 p.581).

Treatment

- Severe cases require IV fluid replacement and careful correction of electrolye disturbances.
- Surgery to remove the tumour is the treatment of 1st choice if technically possible and may be curative in around 40% of patients. Surgical debulking may also be of palliative benefit.
- Somatostatin analogues produce effective symptomatic relief from the diarrhoea in most patients. Long-term use does not result in tumour regression.
- Glucocorticoids in high dosage have also been shown to provide good relief of symptoms.
- A trial of lithium may be warranted in resistant cases and this therapy may be combined with octreotide.
- Chemotherapy using streptozotocin in combination with 5-FU has resulted in response rates of >30%.
- Hepatic artery embolization can offer temporary respite from severe diarrhoea.

Further reading

1 Verner JV and Morrison AB (1958) Islet cell tumor and a syndrome of refractory watery diarrhea and hypokalemia. *Am J Med* **25**(3), 374–380.

Somatostatinomas

Definitions

- Somatostatinomas are very rare neuroendocrine tumours occurring both in the pancreas and in the duodenum.
- >60% are large tumours located in the head or body of the pancreas.
- The clinical syndrome may be diagnosed late in the course of the disease when metastatic spread to local lymph nodes and the liver has already ocured.

Clinical features

See Box 92.1.

- Glucose intolerance or frank diabetes mellitus may have been observed for many years prior to the diagnosis and retrospectively often represents the 1st clinical sign. It is probably due to the inhibitory effect of somatostatin on insulin secretion.
- A high incidence of gallstones has been described similar to that seen as a side-effect with long-term somatostatin analogue therapy.
- Diarrhoea, steatorrhoea, and weight loss appear to be consistent clinical features and may be associated with inhibition of the exocrine pancreas by somatostatin.
- Small duodenal somatostatinomas may occur in association with NF1 (43%) and although these rarely cause the inhibitory clinical syndrome they present with obstructive biliary disease through local spread of the tumour.
- Somatostatinomas are infrequently associated with MEN1 (7%).

Box 92.1 Clinical features of the somatostatin syndrome

- Glucose intolerance/diabetes mellitus (95%)
- Gallstones (68%)
- Diarrhoea and steatorrhoea
- Weight loss (25%)
- Anaemia (14%)
- Hypochlorhydria

Biochemical investigations

- Plasma somatostatin levels will be raised and may also be associated with raised levels of other neuroendocrine tumour markers including ACTH and calcitonin.
- Multisecretory activity is commoner with pancreatic (33%) than with duodenal (16%) somatostatinomas.

Tumour localization

- Transabdominal US and CT scanning may demonstrate the tumour since metastatic disease is often apparent at presentation.
- Additonal methods of tumour localization, as previously described, may also be required (see p.681)

Treatment

- Surgery should be considered as 1st-line treatment as, although a cure is rare, even debulking surgery may result in significant palliation.
- Hepatic embolization can be considered and chemotherapy with streptozotocin and 5-FU may be used to control malignant disease.

Part 9

Inherited endocrine syndromes and multiple endocrine neoplasia (MEN)

McCune–Albright syndrome

Definitions

The syndrome is characterized by:
- Polyostotic fibrous dysplasia.
- Café-au-lait pigmented skin lesions.
- Autonomous function of multiple endocrine glands.

A clinical diagnosis requires 2 of these pathologies.

Genetics

- A genetic but not an inherited condition due to a postzygotic somatic mutation in the gene (GNAS1) that encodes the α chain of the stimulating G protein of adenyl cyclase (GSα mutation). This results in activation of adenyl cyclase.
- The somatic mutation results in mosaicism and consequently the proportion and distribution of affected cells in a tissue will be determined by the precise stage in development at which the mutation occurred.
- Mutational analysis of the GNAS1 gene from affected tissues or blood is available in some centres in the UK.

Clinical features

Polyostotic fibrous dysplasia

- Solitary or multiple expansile bony lesions which can cause fracture deformities and nerve entrapment typically develop before the age of 10 years.
- The femora and the pelvic bones are most frequently affected and radiographs of these bones are useful for screening.
- Osteosarcomas are a rare complication.
- For treatment 📖 see Box 93.1.

Café-au-Lait pigmentation

The lesions are characterized by an irregular border (in neurofibromatosis the border is smooth), do not cross the midline, and tend to be ipsilateral to the bone lesions.

Endocrinopathies— 📖 see Table 93.1

Involvement of other organs

- Hepatobiliary complications such as neonatal jaundice, elevated transaminases and cholestasis are relatively common.
- Cardiomegaly, tachyarrhythmias, and sudden cardiac death may occur.
- Gastrointestinal polyps, splenic hyperplasia, and pancreatitis are reported complications.
- Recognized CNS associations include microcephaly, failure to thrive, and developmental delay.

Table 93.1 Endocrinopathies in McCune–Albright syndrome

Condition	Presentaion	Treatment
Precocious puberty	Frequent initial presentation Typically aged 1–9 years Low gonadotrophins Adults fertile Less frequent in boys	Cyproterone acetate
Thyroid nodules	Present in almost 100% of patients 50% become toxic due to autonomous nodule function	Antithyroid drugs, radio-iodine, surgery
GH secreting pituitary tumours and prolactinomas	Present with features of acromegaly or hyperprolactinaemia	Somatostatin analogues, dopamine agonists, surgery
Cushing's syndrome	Adrenal hyperplasia or adenoma	Adrenalectomy
Hypophosphatemic rickets	↓ phosphate ↓ 1,25 Vit D ↑ ALP Normal calcium, 25 OH Vit D and PTH	Calcitriol, phosphate supplements

Box 93.1 Treatment of polyostotic fibrous dysplasia
- Surgery may be complicated by bleeding and radiotherapy has a limited effect.
- There is some recent evidence to support the use of bisphosphonates, particularly pamidronate, for both symptomatic pain relief and the radiological healing of bone.

Prognosis

- Most patients live well beyond reproductive age.
- Bone deformities may reduce life expectancy.
- Sudden cardiac death is uncommon.

Further reading

Lumbroso S, Paris F, and Sultan C (2002). McCune–Albright syndrome: molecular genetics. *J Paediatr Endocrinol Metab* **15**(3), 875–82.

Spiegel AM and Weinstein LS (2004). Inherited diseases involving g proteins and g protein-coupled receptors. *Annu Rev Med* **55**, 27–39.

Neurofibromatosis

Definitions

- Neurofibromatosis type 1 (NF1) is also known as von Recklinghausen disease and refers to the occurrence of multiple neurofibromas, café-au-lait spots, and Lisch nodules affecting the iris.
- Endocrinopathies are sometimes associated with NF1.
- The prevalence of NF1 is estimated to be 1 in 3500 of the population.
- NF type 2 (NF2) is characterized by the presence of bilateral acoustic neuromas typically resulting in deafness.
- Other features of NF2 include posterior subcapsular cataracts, retinal gliomas, pigmented retinopathy, and gaze palsies.
- NF2 has no common associated endocrinopathies.
- NF2 is rare with an estimated frequency of 1 in 40,000 live births.

NF1

Genetics

- NF1 is a highly penetrant, autosomal dominant condition.
- The NF1 gene is located on chromosome 17 and encodes a GTPase activating protein (Neurofibromin).
- Neurofibromin promotes cleavage of GTP to GDP.

Epidemiology

- The incidence of NF1 is 1 per 3000 of the population.
- NF1 is nearly 100% penetrant but shows variable clinical expression.
- Approximately 50% of cases are sporadic.

Clinical features

- Diagnosis is generally apparent by the age of 1 year.
- The café-au-lait spots become visible shortly after birth (95%) 70% have axillary or grain freckling.
- The multiple cutaneous and subcutaneous neurofibromas appear around puberty (95%).
- Lisch nodules affecting the iris start to appear typically after the age of 5 years (95%).
- The endocrine features are detailed in Box 94.1.
- Learning disabilities occur in 60% of patients with NF1.
- Gliomas may be found in around 15% of patients, most commonly affecting the optic pathways.
- Neurofibrosarcomas complicate around 6% of cases.
- Skeletal dysplasias (e.g. sphenoid wing dysplasia, scoliosis, tibial pseudoarthrosis, pectus excavatum etc.) may be found in up to 5% of cases.
- Vascuar dysplasia may occur with the commonest region affected being the renal vasculature, resulting in renovascular hypertension in up to 3% of cases.

- Macrocephaly (16%), seizures (5%), and short stature (6%) are all reported features of NF1.
- Associated phaeochromocytomas are seen in <5% of NF1 patients.

Box 94.1 Endocrine features of NF1

- Puberty and pregnancy:
  - Both are associated with a change in size of neurofibromas
- Hypothalamus and pituitary:
  - Optic gliomas impinge on adjacent tissues and may affect hypothalamic and/or pituitary function
- Phaeochromocytoma 0.1–5.0%:
  - Serious complication of NF1
  - Uncommon before age 20 years
  - Most commonly adrenal (20% bilateral) but extra adrenal lesions are reported
- Gut neuroendocrine tumours:
  - Found in around 1% of NF1 patients—carcinoid

Further reading

Arun D and Gutmann DH (2004). Recent advances in neurofibromatosis type 1. *Curr Opin Neurol* **17**(2), 101–5.

Rose VM (2004). Neurocutaneous syndromes. *Mo Med* **101**(2), 112–16.

Von Hippel–Lindau disease

Definitions

Characterized by:
- CNS haemangioblastomas.
- Retinal angiomas.
- Renal cysts and carcinomas.
- Phaeochromocytomas.
- Pancreatic neuroendocrine tumours (less common) and pancreatic cysts.
- Occasional endolymphatic sac tumours.
- 📖 See Box 95.1.

Clinical diagnosis established by:
- 2 or more haemangioblastomas.
- A haemangioblastoma and a visual manifestation.
- 1 haemangioblastoma or visual manifestation and a family history of haemangioblastoma.
- The condition occurs in approximately 1 in 36,000 live births.
- The average age of presentation is 27 years and the condition is nearly 100% penetrant by the age of 65 years.
- VHL may be subdivided into type 1 and type 2 disease.
- Type 1 VHL is the commonest form of the disease and is characterized by a tendency to develop tumours in the eyes, brain, spinal cord, kidney, and pancreas.
- Affected family members with VHL type 2 are also susceptible to developing phaeochromocytomas and this may be further subdivided into VHL type 2A (develop phaeocochromocytomas and renal cell carcinomas).

Genetics

- VHL is a highly penetrant autosomal dominant condition.
- The VHL gene is on chromosome 3 and is a tumour suppressor gene.
- Mutations which result in loss of the VHL protein lead to VEGF expression in normoxia as well as hypoxia, thus enhancing the growth of these tumours which are often very vascular.
- Mutational analysis of the VHL gene is available in the UK.
- Genetic testing in affected families is recommended from the age of 5 years.

Box 95.1 Less common manifestations of von Hippel–Lindau disease

• Pancreas	Cysts
	Adenomas
• Epididymis	Cystadenoma
• CNS	Syringomyelia
	Meningioma
• Liver	Adenoma
	Haemangioblastoma
	Cysts
• Lung	Angioma
	Cysts
• Spleen	Angioma

Clinical features

- Retinal angiomas are the initial manifestation of VHL in 40% of patients. They are uncommon before the age of 10 years but continue to develop throughout life. They tend to be peripheral in the retina, appearing as red oval lesions. Bleeding and retinal detachment may occur and treatment is with laser therapy.
- 75% of haemangioblastomas occur in the cerebellum and they are the initial presenting feature in 40% of VHL patients. Treatment is with surgery or radiotherapy.
- Renal carcinoma is the commonest cause of death in VHL patients. By the age of 60 years 70% of VHL patients will be affected, with a mean age of presentation of 44 years. The lesions tend to be multifocal. The management of choice is surgical resection.
- Phaeochromocytomas occur in up to 20% of VHL families and are bilateral in 40% of cases. The frequency of this condition varies widely between families as certain mutations are particularly associated with a high risk of phaeochromocytoma. Regular biochemical screening is essential in these high risk families. Treatment is with α and β blockade followed by surgical resection.
- The majority of pancreatic tumours associated with VHL are non-functioning but they may secrete VIP, insulin, glucagons, or calcitonin. They occur in 10–20% of VHL patients and should be treated expectantly unless, symptomatic, enlarging or >2–3cm.
- Table 95.1 lists the recommended ages to start tests for VHL.

Prognosis

- Until recently, the median survival for a VHL patient was 40–50 years of age with the majority of deaths attributable to renal cell carcinoma.
- Currently the prognosis for individual patients depends upon the location and complications of the tumours but overall is improving as a result of the institution of screening programmes and consequent earlier therapeutic interventions.
- For surveillance in VHL 🕮 see Table 95.2.

Further reading

Kaelin WG Jr (2003). The von Hippel–Lindau gene, kidney cancer and oxygen sensing. *Am Soc Nephrol* **14**(11), 2703–11.

Lonser RR *et al* (2003). Von Hippel-Lindau disease. *Lancet* **361**, 2059–67.

Richard S, Graff J, Lindau J, *et al.* (2005). Von Hippel–Lindau disease. *Lancet* **363**, 1231–4.

Table 95.1 Testing for VHL

Test	Recommended age to start (years)
Palpation (renal and epididymal lesions)	5
Urinalysis	5
24h urinary catecholamines	5
Fundoscopy and fluorescein angiography	5
Cerebral MRI	10
Abdominal MRI for renal, adrenal, and pancreatic lesions	5

Table 95.2 Surveillance in VHL

	Affected	At risk
Annual	Clinical examination	Clinical examination
	Urinalysis	Urinalysis
	24h urinary catecholamines	24h urinary catecholamines
	Fundoscopy	Fundoscopy (aged 5–60 years)
Triennial	Cerebral MRI (to age 50, then 5-yearly)	Cerebral MRI (aged 5–40 years, then 5-yearly to age 60)
	Abdominal MRI	Abdominal MRI (aged 25–65 years)

Carney complex

Definitions

A clinical diagnosis is made by finding 2 of the clinical features listed in 'Clinical presentation' or 1 of these features *plus* either an affected 1st-degree relative or an inactivating mutation in the relevant gene (*PRKARlα*).

Genetics

- Autosomal dominant.
- An inactivating mutation of the *PRKARlα* gene on the long arm of chromosome 17q2 can be identified in approximately 50% of families.

Clinical presentation

- Spotty skin pigmentation.
- Cardiac, skin, or mucosal myxomas.
- Endocrine tumours (🕮 see Box 96.1).
- Psammomatous melanotic schwannoma.

> **Box 96.1 Endocrine tumours associated with Carney complex**
>
> - The commonest endocrine manifestation is 1° pigmented nodular adrenocortical disease (PPNAD) causing Cushing's syndrome.
> - Large cell calcifying Sertoli cell tumour (LCCSCT).
> - GH/PRL secreting pituitary adenoma (also somatotroph/mammotroph hyperplasia).
> - Thyroid adenoma.
> - Ovarian cysts.

Further reading

Sandrini F and Stratakis C (2003). Clinical and molecular genetics of Carney complex. *Mol Genet Metab* **78**(2), 83–92.

Stergiopolous SG, Abu-Asab MS, Tsokos M, *et al.* (2004). Pituitary pathology in Carney complex patients. *Pituitary* **7**, 73–82.

Stratakis CA, Kirschner LS, and Carney JA (2001). Clinical and molecular features of the Carney complex. *J Clin Endocrinol Metab* **86**(9), 4041–6.

Cowden syndrome

Definitions

Estimated to affect 1 in 200,000 individuals.

Genetics

- Autosomal dominant condition.
- Inactivating mutations in the *PTEN* tumour suppressor gene can be identified in approximately 80% of affected probands.

Clinical presentation

Also 📖 see Box 97.1

- The condition is characterized by multiple hamartomas involving organ systems derived from all 3 germ cell layers.
- Patients are also at risk from breast, thyroid, and endometrial carcinomas.
- Thyroid pathology occurs in more >2/3 of patients and the lesions may be multifocal.

Box 97.1 Endocrine features of Cowden syndrome

- Non medullary thyroid carcinomas, especially follicular thyroid carcinoma.
- Multinodular goitre.
- Thyroid adenomas.
- Parathyroid adenomas are extremely rare.

Further reading

Pilarski R and Eng C (2004). Will the real Cowden syndrome please stand up (again)? Expanding mutational and clinical spectra of the PTEN hamartoma tumour syndrome. *J Med Genet* **41**(5), 323–6.

POEMS syndrome

Definitions

Progressive polyneuropathy, organomegaly, endocrinopathy, monoclonal gammopathy, and skin changes (POEMS) is a rare disorder of unclear pathogenesis which is probably mediated by ↑ production of lambda light chains from abnormal plasma cells.

Clinical presentation

- Progressive polyneuropathy.
- Organomegaly, especially hepatosplenomegaly and lymphadenopathy.
- Common endocrinopathies (84%) (multiple in 65%) include hypogonadotrophic hypogonadism (70%—2/3 central, 1/3 1°), hypothyroidism (60%), hypoadrenalism (60%) and diabetes mellitus (50%) hyperprolactinaemia 20%.
- Monoclonal gammopathy.
- Skin changes.

Treatments

Include chemotherapy irradiation and surgery.

Further reading

Dispenzieri A and Gertz MA (2004). Treatment of POEMS syndrome. *Curr Treat Options Oncol* **5**(3), 249–57.

MEN type 1

Definitions

Characterized by:
- Parathyroid tumours/hyperplasia.
- Anterior pituitary adenomas.
- Pancreatic neuroendocrine tumours.

A clinical diagnosis of MEN1 is reached in the presence of 2 out of 3 of these tumours or 1 of these tumours in the context of a family history of MEN1.

The prevalence of MEN1 has been estimated at 1 in 10,000 of the population.

Genetics

- MEN1 is an autosomal dominant condition with an estimated penetrance of 98% by the age of 40 years.
- The *MEN1* gene is located on the long arm of chromosome 11 (11q13) and is a tumour suppressor gene, although the function of the encoded protein, MENIN, is unknown.
- The mutations causing MEN1 are inactivating mutations.
- Many mutations in the *MEN1* gene have been described in affected families and there is no clear genotype–phenotype correlation.
- Mutational analysis is available in the UK, although it is important to note that up to 10% of MEN1 patients will not have mutations identifiable within the coding region of the *MEN1* gene.

Clinical features

- 1° hyperparathyroidism is the commonest presenting feature in MEN1 and occurs in up to 95% of patients with MEN1.
- Pituitary adenomas are found in approximately 30% of MEN1 patients (📖 see Table 99.1).
- The incidence of pancreatic endocrine tumours varies between 30% and 80% in different series (📖 see Table 99.2).
- Other lesions are also associated with MEN1 (📖 see Table 99.3).

Table 99.1 Pituitary tumours in MEN1

Tumour	Frequency
Prolactinoma	60%
Acromegaly	25%
Non-functioning tumour	1%
Cushing's disease	<1%

Table 99.2 Pancreatic tumours in MEN1

Tumour	Frequency
Gastrinoma	60%
Insulinoma	30%
Glucagonoma	2%
VIPoma	<1%
PPoma	<1%
Non-functioning tumour	1%

Table 99.3 Other lesions in MEN1

Tumour	Frequency
Adrenal cortical tumours	5%
Carcinoid tumours	4%
Lipomas	1%
Phaeochromocytoma	0.5%
Malignant melanoma	0.5%
Testicular teratoma	0.5%
Multiple (>3) angiofibromas	75%

Management

Primary hyperparathyroidism

- The hypercalcaemia is frequently mild with an early age of onset and is the first manifestation of the disease in 90% of patients.
- Multiple gland disease (adenomas or hyperplasia) is common, in contrast with sporadic 1° hyperparathyroidism where usually a single adenoma is found.
- No effective medical treatments are currently available and surgical management is the gold standard.
- In view of the potential for multigland disease, total parathyroidectomy with lifelong oral calcitriol replacement should always be considered.
- The timing of surgery in asymptomatic patients with borderline hypercalcaemia is still controversial.

Pituitary adenomas

These are managed with surgery, medical therapies, or radiotherapy as per sporadic pituitary tumours (see p.182).

Pancreatic tumours

- An experienced surgeon is essential if these tumours are to be resected.
- For patients with aggressive disease the pancreas and duodenum together with surrounding lymph nodes may be removed whereas simple enucleation may be sufficient for some lesions.
- Gastrinomas are the major cause of morbidity and mortality in MEN1 patients and these may respond to medical therapy with proton pump inhibitors.

Mutational analysis

The criteria for performing mutational analysis are controversial and vary from centre to centre in the UK. One approach is to recommend assessing the following categories of patient:

- Patients with 2 MEN1 tumours.
- 1st and 2nd-degree relatives of patients with MEN1.
- Consider screening in patients with 1° hyperparathyroidism <40 years of age, particularly in the presence of multigland disease.
- Consider screening in patients with isolated pancreatic neuroendocrine tumours, especially gastrinomas or insulinomas.

Screening

- Screening is relevant for affected patients, asymptomatic mutation carriers, and 1st and 2nd-degree relatives in families with a clinical diagnosis of MEN1 but where a mutation has not been identified.
- Manifestations of MEN1 are very rare before the teenage years but have been described as young as 5 years. Careful parental counselling can encourage some childhood monitoring which ideally should include a careful history for symptoms (e.g. hypoglycaemia) and height and weight assessment in addition to calcium and prolactin measurements.
- Screening involves both a careful clinical history and examination as well as biochemical assessment and imaging modalities (🕮 see Table 99.4).
- Age related penetrance: age 10–7%, 20–52%, 30–87%, 40–98%, 60–100%.

Box 99.1 Prognosis

Malignant pancreatic tumors, especially gastrinomas, are the major cause of mortality in MEN1 but outcomes have been improving with the introduction of appropriate screening programmes for affected and at-risk individuals.

Further reading

Asgharian B, Turner ML, Gibril F, et al. (2004). Cutaneous tumours in patients with multiple endocrine neoplasm type 1 (MEN1) and gastrinomas: prospective study of frequency and development of criteria with high sensitivity and specificity for MEN1. *J Clin Endocrinol Metab* **89**, 5328–36.

Brandi ML Gagel AF, Angeli A, et al. (2001). Guidelines for diagnosis and therapy of MEN type 1 and 2. *J Clin Endocrinol Metab*, **86**(12), 5658–71.

Table 99.4 Screening adults in MEN1

Tumour	Frequency
Calcium, phosphate and PTH	Annual
Basal anterior pituitary function (particularly prolactin and IGF1)	Annual
Fasting gut hormones	Annual
Fasting glucose	Annual
24h urinary 5HIAA and chromogranin A	Annual
MRI abdomen	Annual–3-yearly
MRI pituitary	Baseline

MEN type 2

Definitions

MEN2 may be divided into 3 forms:
- MEN2a comprises familial medullary thyroid carcinoma (FMTC) in combination with phaeochromocytoma and parathyroid tumours.
- MEN2b is defined as the occurrence of familial MTC in association with phaeochromocytoma, mucosal neuromas and a marfanoid habitus.
- FMTC may also occur in isolation.

MEN2a accounts for >75% of all MEN2 cases.

Genetics

- MEN2 is an autosomal dominant condition.
- The C-RET protooncogene, mutations in which cause MEN2, is located on the long arm of chromosome 10 (10q11.2).
- This gene encodes RET which is a transmembrane receptor with an extracellular cysteine-rich domain and an intracellular tyrosine kinase domain.
- The mutations causing MEN2 are activating mutations.
- Different germline mutations cause different clinical syndromes so, in contrast to MEN1, MEN2 shows a strong genotype–phenotype correlation.
- Mutational analysis is available in the UK.
- The C-RET protooncogene is also involved, via inactivating mutations, in the aetiology of Hirschsprung's disease.

Table 100.1 Classification and presentation of MEN2

Pathology	MEN2a	MEN2b	FMTC
MTC	95%	~100%	~100%
Phaeochromocytoma	50%	50%	Not present
Parathyroid neoplasia	20–30%	Not present	Not present
Marfanoid habitus	Not present	75%	Not present
Mucosal neuromas	Not present	10–20%	Not present
Intestinal ganglioneuromatosis	Not present	~40%	Not present

Clinical features—MEN2a

MTC

- MTC is often the initial manifestation and is generally multifocal.
- Phaeochromocytoma and parathyroid disease typically develop later.
- Diagnosis of MTC requires histological analysis which reveals C cell hyperplasia and stromal amyloid.
- Circulating calcitonin levels are generally elevated but hypocalcaemia is not seen.
- With metastatic disease diarrhoea is common (30%).
- Rarely these tumours secrete ACTH resulting in Cushing's syndrome due to ectopic ACTH secretion.

Phaeochromocytoma

- Tend to present later than MTC.
- 50% will be bilateral but malignancy is rare (<10%).
- These lesions must be excluded prior to surgery for any other indication.

Primary hyperparathyroidism

- Generally results from hyperplasia of the glands.
- Hypercalcaemia is typically mild.

Clinical features—MEN2b

- Mucosal neuromas can be found on the distal tongue, conjunctiva, and throughout the gastrointestinal tract.
- A marfanoid habitus is typically evident.
- MTC tends to present earlier than in MEN2a and frequently follows a more aggressive course.

Box 100.1 Pentagastrin test

- Indication borderline basal calcitonin and screening of families with medullary carcinoma (NB calcitonin slightly raised with thyroiditis).
- Patient fasting.
- 0.5mcg/kg pentagastrin IV over 5sec and flush cannula.
- Calcitonin measured at 0, 2, and 10min.
- Elevated basal levels of calcitonin which do not rise with pentagastrin stimulation are seen in children, pregnancy, with some tumours (e.g. carcinoids), pernicious anaemia, thyroiditis, and chronic renal failure.
- Side effects of the test include nausea, flushing, and substernal tightness which typically resolves in <5min.

Stimulated calcitonin	30–100 ng/L:	Follow-up screening recommended
Stimulated calcitonin	100–200 ng/L:	Probable C-cell hyperplasia or early medullary thyroid carcinoma
Stimulated calcitonin	>200 ng/L:	Medullary thyroid carcinoma very likely

Management

MTC

- The definitive treatment is adequate surgery by total thyroidectomy and careful lymph node dissection.
- Postoperative levothyroxine is administered to all patients.
- Tumour spread is usually local but distant metastases do occur.
- Regular postoperative calcitonin assessment (first 3 months, then 6–12-monthly) is used to monitor for disease recurrence.
- MRI, octreotide scanning, and venous catheterization may all be helpful in staging disease recurrence.
- Treatment of recurrent disease responds poorly to radiotherapy or chemotherapy and consequently is generally surgical if appropriate.
- Somatostatin analogues may help symptom control e.g. diarrhoea but do not appear to have an antitumour effect.
- Few data are available to date but therapy with radiolabelled MIBG or somatostatin analogues appears to offer significant symptomatic improvement although tumour stabilization and/or regression was observed only rarely.
- Children with MEN2 should be considered for early prophylactic surgery. This should generally be performed before the age of 5 years and before the age of 1 year in patients with the highest risk mutations.

Phaeochromocytoma

- These tumours are best treated medically with α and β blockade followed by surgical removal.
- The risk of multifocal and/or recurrent disease must be considered.
- Screening has resulted in the earlier detection of these lesions.

Primary hyperparathyroidism

The criteria for diagnosis and the indications for surgery are broadly similar to those for sporadic 1° hyperparathyroidism.

Mutational analysis

- 1st and 2nd-degree relatives of patients with MEN2 and genetic analysis should be performed as early as possible in at-risk children.
- Consider screening in patients with sporadic MTC or sporadic phaeochromocytoma or in patients with mucosal neuromas or other phenotypic features compatible with MEN2b.
- Somatic RET oncogene mutations in confer a worse prognosis in sporadic medullary carcinoma.

Screening

Biochemical and radiological screening is relevant for affected patients, asymptomatic mutation carriers and 1st and 2nd-degree relatives in families with a clinical diagnosis of MEN2 but where a mutation has not been identified (📖 see Table 100.2).

Box 100.2 Prognosis

- Variable.
- Overall 10-year survival rate for MEN2b is 65% and for MEN2a is 80%.
- The prognosis for these patients is improving with earlier screening and intervention.

Further reading

Brandi ML, Gagel AF, Angeli A, et al. (2001). Guidelines for diagnosis and therapy of MEN type 1 and 2. *J Clin Endocrinol Metab* **86**(12), 5658–71.

Carling T. (2005). Multiple endocrine neoplasia syndrome: genetic basis for clinical management. *J Curr Opin Oncol* **17**, 7–12.

Constante G, Meringolo D, Durante C, et al. (2007). Predictive value of serum calcitonin levels for preoperative diagnosis of medullary thyroid carcinoma in a cohort of 5817 consecutive patients with thyroid nodules. *J Clin Endocrinol Metab* **92**(2), 450–5. Epub 2006 Nov 21.

Karges W, Dralle H, Raue F, et al. (2004). Calcitonin measurement to detect medullary thyroid carcinoma in nodular goitre: German evidence-based consensus recommendations. *Exp Clin Endocrinol Diabetes* **112**(1), 52–8.

Marx SJ. (2005). Molecular genetics of multiple endocrine neoplasia types 1 and 2. *J Nat Rev Cancer* **5**, 367–75.

Table 100.2 Screening in MEN2

Test	Frequency
Calcitonin ± pentagastrin stimulation test	Annual
24h urinary catecholamines	Annual
Calcium	Annual
CT/MRI adrenals	Annual–3-yearly

Inherited primary hyperparathyroidism

Definitions

- Parathyroid tumours affect 1 per 1000 population.
- 1° hyperparathyroidism is inherited in up to 10% of patients.

Causes

- MEN1
- MEN2a
- Hyperparathyroidism-jaw tumour syndrome (HPT-JT)
- Familial isolated hyperparathyroidism (FIHP)

HPT-JT

- Autosomal dominant condition.
- Characterized by pathology in 3 main tissues:
  - Parathyroid tumours which show a high penetrance in these patients and in up to 15% of cases will be parathyroid carcinomas.
  - Ossifying fibromas which affect the maxilla and/or mandible in around 30% of HPT-JT patients.
- Renal manifestations may also occur, the commonest are bilateral renal cysts (19% of patients) but also include hamartomas and Wilms' tumours.
- Benign and malignant uterine pathology is seen in up to 75% of women with HPT-JT and reduces reproductive fitness.
- Other tumours have also been reported in these patients including pancreatic adenocarcinomas, testicular mixed germ cell tumours, Hürthle cell thyroid adenomas, and benign and malignant uterine tumours.
- The gene (*HRPT2*), inactivating mutations in which are responsible for HPT-JT, has been identified on the long arm of chromosome 1 and mutational analysis is available in the UK.
- The function of the protein product (parafibromin) encoded by this tumour suppressor gene is unknown.

FIHP

- Affected individuals within a kindred suffer only from 1° hyperparathyroidism as an isolated endocrinopathy.
- In some kindreds mutations in the *MEN1* or *HRPT2* genes have been identified but in the majority the cause is still unknown.

Further reading

Carpten JD, Robbins CM, Villablanca A, *et al* (2002). HRPT2, encoding parafibromin, is mutated in hyperparathyroidism-jaw tumor syndrome. *Nat Genet.* **32**(4), 676–80.

Marx S.J. (2002). Hyperparathyroidism in hereditary syndromes: special expressions and special managements. *J Bone Miner Res.* **17**(2), N37–43.

Inherited renal calculi

Definitions

- Renal calculi affect 12% of ♂ and 5% of ♀ by the 7th decade of life.
- Renal calculi arise due to a reduced urine volume or ↑ excretion of stone-forming components such as calcium, oxalate, urate, cystine, xanthine, and phosphate.
- A variety of causes for renal stones are established (□ see Box 102.1 for general causes of nephrolithiasis) but the commonest aetiology is hypercalciuria.
- Calcium stones account for >80% of all renal calculi.
- Uric acid stones comprise 5–10% of all renal calculi.
- The commonest cause of hypercalciuria is hypercalcaemia and this in turn is most frequently 2° to 1° hyperparathyroidism.
- Nephrolithiasis is frequently a recurrent condition with a relapse rate of 75% in 20 years.
- Features associated with recurrence include early age of onset, +ve family history and lithiasis related to infection or underlying medical conditions.

Genetics

- Renal calculi generally arise from complex multifactorial disease resulting from an interaction between genetic and environmental factors.
- The disorder may be familial in up to 45% of patients.
- The majority of causative genes are probably as yet unidentified and account for much of 'idiopathic' calcium nephrolithiasis.
- Many cases of hypercalciuria are likely to be polygenic but 2 examples of monogenic causes are Dent's disease and autosomal dominant hypocalcaemic hypercalciuria (ADHH).

Dent's disease
- X-linked condition.
- Due to inactivating mutations in a chloride channel (*CLC5*) gene.
- Characterized by hypercalciuria, nephrocalcinosis, β2 microglobinuria, progressive glomerular disease, and mild rickets due to renal phosphate loss in affected ♂.

ADHH
- Autosomal dominant condition.
- Due to activating mutations in the calcium sensing receptor gene.
- May be asymptomatic or present early with neonatal or childhood seizures.

Box 102.1 Causes of renal calculi

- Hypercalciuria.
- Hyperoxaluria.
- Hyperuricosuria.
- Hypocitraturia.
- Urinary tract infection e.g. *Proteus*, *Pseudomonas*, *Klebsiella*.
- 1° renal disease e.g. polycystic kidney disease.
- Drugs e.g. indinavir, diuretics, salicylates, allopurinol, some chemotherapeutic agents.

Box 102.2 Mutational analysis

- Currently largely a research tool.
- Mutations in a variety of genes have been reported to result in renal calculi due to hypercalciuria, hyperoxaluria, cystinuria or hyperuricosuria.
- As these research tests move into the clinical domain then family screening will become increasingly relevant.

Investigation of renal calculi

- 24h urine volume and urine osmolarity (low urine volume raises production of solutes).
- 24h urinary calcium excretion.
- Urine pH.
- Stone composition if possible.
- Exclude causes of hypercalcaemia (hyperparathyroidism, immobilization, or renal tubular acidosis).
- Exclude hypercalciuria (excess chloride, excess sodium, malignancy, sarcoidosis, renal calcium leak and drugs e.g. levothyroxine or loop diuretics).
- Exclude causes of hyperoxaluria (1° hyperoxaluria, vitamin B6 deficiency, short bowel syndrome, and excess dietary oxalates).
- Exclude urinary tract infection.
- Exclude causes of hyperuricosuria (gout, dietary, uricosuric drugs, binge drinking, or myeloproliferative disorders).
- Exclude causes of hypocitraturia—citrate is the 1° agent for removal of excess calcium (renal tubular acidosis, potassium or magnesium deficiency, urinary tract infection, renal failure, and chronic diarrhoea).
- Exclude cysteine (usually genetic in origin) or xanthine (usually 2° to allopurinol treatment) stones.

Management

- Increase fluid intake.
- Appropriate dietary modifications.
- Treat underlying cause.

Further reading

Langman C.B. (2004). The molecular basis of kidney stones. *Curr Opin Paediatr* **16**(2), 188–93.

Thakker R.V. (2004). Diseases associated with the extracellular calcium-sensing receptor. *Cell Calcium* **35**(3), 275–82.

Miscellaneous endocrinology

Hypoglycaemia

Definition (Whipple's triad)

- Plasma glucose of <2.2mmol/L *associated with*
- Symptoms of neuroglycopaenia, *and*
- Reversal of symptoms with correction of glucose levels.

For causes see Box 103.1.

Epidemiology

Uncommon in adults, apart from patients with diabetes being treated with certain agents either alone or in combination (e.g. insulin, sulfonylureas, prandial glucose regulators, thiazolidinediones).

Pathophysiology

Physiology of glucose control

The liver is the major regulator (80–85%) of circulating blood glucose levels in healthy individuals and responds to changes in circulating insulin, GH, cortisol, glucagon, and adrenaline.

- *Postprandial state:* hepatic glucose production is inhibited by both raised glucose and insulin concentrations.
- *Fasting state:* serum glucose falls with consequent fall in insulin secretion, stimulating hepatic efflux of glucose (in the presence of cortisol, GH, and glucagon).
- The brain is dependent on circulating glucose for its energy demands, which are high and comprise up to 50% hepatic glucose output.

Mechanisms of hypoglycaemia

- *Excessive/inappropriate action of insulin or IGF1:* inhibiting hepatic glucose production despite adequate glycogen stores, while peripheral glucose uptake is enhanced.
- *Impaired neuroendocrine response* with inadequate counter-regulatory response (e.g. cortisol or GH) to insulin.
- *Impairment of hepatic glucose production* due to either structural damage or abnormal liver enzymes.

Types of spontaneous hypoglycaemia

- *Fasting hypoglycaemia:* occurs several hours (typically >5h) after food (e.g. early morning, following prolonged fasting or exercise) and almost always indicates underlying disease.
- *Post-prandial (reactive) hypoglycaemia:* occurs 2–5 h after food (🕮 see Post-prandial reactive hypoglycaemia, p. 644).

Symptoms of hypoglycaemia

- *Autonomic (adrenergic) symptoms:* sweats, pallor, tachycardia, tremor, hunger, anxiety.
- *Neuroglycopaenic symptoms:* poor concentration, drowsiness, double vision, irritability, perioral tingling, poor judgement, confusion, violent behaviour, personality change, unexplained collapse, focal neurological signs, seizures, loss of consciousness, and death.

Box 103.1 Causes of hypoglycaemia

- Spontaneous hypoglycaemia.
- Drug induced (commonest cause; both accidental and non-accidental):
  - Anti-diabetic agents used either alone (e.g. insulin, sulfonylureas, prandial glucose regulators) or in combination (e.g. insulin and thiazolidinediones).
  - Alcohol (impairs hepatic gluconeogenesis and is often associated with poor glycogen stores).
  - Quinine can promote hyperinsulinaemia.
  - Salicylates can act by inhibiting hepatic glucose release and ↑ insulin secretion.
- Organ failure and critical illness:
  - Acute liver failure.
  - Chronic renal failure.
- Hormone deficiency:
  - Addison's disease.
  - Isolated ACTH deficiency.
  - GH deficiency.
  - Hypopituitarism.
- Insulinoma:
  - Benign 85%, malignant 15%.
  - Occasionally part of MEN1 (~10%).
- Other tumours:
  - Excessive IGF-II secretion from large mesenchymal tumours (non-islet cell tumour hypoglycaemia (NICH)), e.g. fibrosarcoma, mesothelioma (~ 1/3 are retroperitoneal, 1/3 intra-abdominal, and 1/3 intrathoracic).
  - Hepatocellular carcinoma.
  - Adrenal carcinoma, Phaeochromocytoma.
  - Lymphoma, myeloma, leukaemia.
  - Advanced metastatic malignancy.
- Infection:
  - Septicaemia, e.g. Gram −ve or meningococcal; related to high metabolic requirements, reduced energy intake, and possibly cytokines from the inflammatory process.
  - Malaria.
- Starvation/malnutrition:
  - Anorexia nervosa.
  - Kwashiorkor or marasmus.
- β-cell hyperplasia: very rare in adults.
- Autoimmune:
  - Antibodies to insulin (antibody-bound insulin dissociates leading to elevated free insulin; typically associated with post prandial hypoglycaemia)
  - Insulin receptor activating antibodies (rare, commonest in middle-aged ♀; may require treatment with plasmapheresis or immunosuppression)

- Inborn errors of metabolism:
  - Glycogen storage disease.
  - Hereditary fructose intolerance.
  - Maple syrup disease.
- Hypoglycaemias of infancy and childhood.
- Reactive (post-prandial) hypoglycaemia: see p.644

Clinical features

- Responses to hypoglycaemia are sequential with:
  - Deterioration in neuropsychological performance at plasma glucose 3–3.5mmol/L.
  - Subjective perception of hypoglycaemia at 2.7–2.9mmol/L.
  - EEG changes at 2mmol/L.
- Patients with recurrent hypoglycaemia may not get symptoms until glucose concentrations are very low (so-called 'hypo unawareness'), whilst patients with poorly controlled diabetes mellitus may experience hypoglycaemic symptoms at 'normal' blood glucose levels.
- The majority of symptoms of acute hypoglycaemia are adrenergic, but neuroglycopaenic symptoms occur with subacute and chronic hypoglycaemia.

Investigation of fasting hypoglycaemia

- Glucose strip: unreliable for low glucose concentrations, but if level <4mmol/L a laboratory glucose should be measured.
- Liver and renal function tests.
- Fasting insulin, C-peptide, proinsulin, and glucose during hypoglycaemia (Table 103.1).
- Inappropriately elevated insulin in presence of hypoglycaemia suggests insulinoma or self-administration of insulin or sulfonylurea.
- Presence of C-peptide indicates endogenous insulin release—either insulinoma or sulfonylurea.
- Insulinomas often associated with elevated pro-insulin:insulin ratio.
- Consider assay for presence of sulfonylureas.
- Ethanol concentration.
- Cortisol (± Synacthen® test).
- Fasting β-hydroxybutyrate (elevated in most causes of hypoglycaemia, but suppressed if insulin present e.g. insulinoma, self-administration of insulin or sulfonylureas).
- Consider IGF-I and II: IGF-II may be normal in non-islet cell hypoglycaemia (NICH), but this is in association with suppressed IGF-I and GH; usual IGF-II:IGF-I ratio 3:1, ratio >10 seen in NICH (🕮 see Box 103.2, p.645).
- Chest and abdominal radiographs/CT—? NICH source.
- Consider insulin and insulin receptor antibodies.

Further investigation of fasting hypoglycaemia

- *Glucose and insulin* After 15h fast glucose <2.2mmol/L and insulin >5mU/L is inappropriate. Good screening test if repeated 3 times.
- *72h fast* The most reliable test for hypoglycaemia, (detect 98% patients with insulinoma, compared with 71% at 24h). The patient should remain active. Plasma glucose, insulin, C-peptide and pro-insulin are measured 6-hourly (unless the patient is symptomatic or the glucose level is <3.5mmol/L when measurements are made every 1–2h); the test is terminated if the laboratory glucose <2.2mmol/L or after 72h. β-hydroxybutyrate should be measured at the end of the fast (its presence makes insulinoma unlikely).

- *Exercise test* used to precipitate hypoglycaemia in patients with endogenous hyperinsulinism who might tolerate prolonged periods of fasting.
  - Blood is collected before and at 10min intervals during 30min of intense exercise and for 30min afterwards. Patients with spontaneous hypoglycaemia become exhausted and their glucose concentration falls below 2.2mmol/L
- *Insulin suppression test:*
  - *Rationale* Insulin administration to induce hypoglycaemia should suppress endogenous insulin secretion. C-peptide serves as a measure of endogenous insulin secretion.
  - *Method* IV insulin administered 0.05–0.1U/kg per hour over 2h and measurements of plasma C-peptide and glucose made. Glucose <2.2mmol/L in association with a C-peptide >150pmol/L is inappropriate and suggests the presence of an insulinoma. The test should be terminated at this point. Results are more accurately interpreted using age-matched normative data as the decrease in C-peptide reduces with increasing age.
  - *Caution* Close continual observation is essential as hypoglycaemia may induce seizures or loss of consciousness, and require appropriate emergency treatment. Cortisol deficiency and hepatic dysfunction should be excluded before performing the test.
- *Localization of tumour* (📖 see Tumour localization, p.581) Only performed once an insulinoma is confirmed biochemically. MRI or spiral CT are usually 1st-line investigations (equal sensitivity 50–70%), endoscopic and intraoperative US have an improved resolution and sensitivity but are more invasive.
- *¹¹¹I Octreotide scan* 50% sensitivity, may detect metastases, less good for insulinomas than other pancreatic tumours.
- *Selective angiography* with selective arterial calcium gluconate or secretin stimulation (rarely required). This is performed in centres with experienced radiologists, when biochemically proven insulinomas cannot be visualized on imaging.

Table 103.1 Biochemical features of insulinoma and factitious hypoglycaemia

Plasma marker	Insulinoma	Sulfonylurea	Insulin injection
Glucose	↓	↓	↓
Insulin	↑	↑	↑
C-peptide	↑	↑	↓

Management

Acute hypoglycaemia

- *If conscious* oral carbohydrate (ideally food and a sugary drink) should be administered as soon possible. Glucogel® (formerly known as Hypostop Gel®), a glucose-containing gel, which is absorbed by the buccal mucosa, may be used in drowsy, but conscious, individuals
- *If unconscious* 25–50 ml 25% glucose intravenously into a large vein, followed by a saline flush as the high concentration of glucose is an irritant and may even lead to venous thrombosis. A maintenance infusion of 5% or 10% dextrose is often required thereafter, especially if there is an ongoing risk of recurrent hypoglycaemia (e.g. overdose of a long-acting insulin/analogue).
- 1 mg glucagon IM may be administered if there is no IV access. This increases hepatic glucose efflux, but the effect only lasts for 30min, allowing other means of blood glucose elevation (e.g. oral), before the blood glucose falls again. It is:
  - Ineffective with hepatic dysfunction and if there is glycogen depletion, e.g. ethanol-related hypoglycaemia.
  - Relatively contraindicated in patients with known insulinoma as it may induce further insulin secretion.
  - Ineffective within 3 days following a previous dose of glucagon.
- *2° cerebral oedema:* may complicate hypoglycaemia and should be considered in cases of prolonged coma despite normalization of plasma glucose. Mannitol and or dexamethasone may be helpful.

Recurrent chronic hypoglycaemia

If definitive treatment of the underlying condition is unsuccessful or impossible, symptoms may be alleviated by frequent (e.g. 4-hourly) small meals, including overnight. Diazoxide, administered by mouth, is useful in the management of patients with chronic hypoglycaemia from excess endogenous insulin secretion due to an insulinoma or islet cell hyperplasia.

Further reading

Gama R, Teale, JD, Marks V (2003). Clinical and laboratory investigation of adult spontaneous hypoglycaemia. *J Clin Path* **56**, 641–6.

Service FJ (1997). Hypoglycaemia. *Endoc Metab Clinics N America* **126**(4), 937–52.

Post-prandial reactive hypoglycaemia (PRH)

Definition
Hypoglycaemia following a meal due to an imbalance between glucose influx into (exogenous from food, and endogenous glucose production) and glucose efflux out of the circulation

Pathophysiology and causes
- *Exaggerated insulin response:* related to rapid glucose absorption e.g. post-gastrectomy dumping syndrome. This results in a delayed insulin peak with respect to the peak blood glucose, probably related to an exaggerated GLP-1 (glucagon like peptide-1) response.
- *Incipient diabetes mellitus:* occasionally presents with postprandial hypoglycaemia, possibly related to disordered insulin secretion.
- *Insulin resistance related hyperinsulinaemia:* e.g. obese subjects with or without impaired glucose tolerance.
- *Increased insulin sensitivity:* with deficiency of counter regulatory hormones, glucagon and adrenaline (rapid action), as well as cortisol and growth hormone (delayed action, up to 12h).
- *Impaired glucagon sensitivity and secretion:* in response to hypoglycaemia are involved in the pathogenesis of PRH.
- *Renal glycosuria:* accounts for up to 15% of patients with PRH.
- *Body composition:*
  - 20% of very lean people are prone to PRH.
  - Massive weight reduction increases the risk of PRH.
  - Lower body obesity (esp. in ♀) is associated with high normal insulin sensitivity and PRH.
- *Diet:*
  - High carbohydrate, low fat diet, by ↑ insulin sensitivity.
  - Prolonged very low calorie diets (>2 weeks), by reducing counter - regulatory hormones especially GH.
- *Alcohol:*
  - Inhibits hepatic glucose output.
  - Increases insulin secretion in response to glucose and sucrose.
- Idiopathic.

Investigation
- *Prolonged oral glucose tolerance test:* not physiological, 10% of the normal (asymptomatic) population has a +ve response with blood glucose levels <2.6mmol/L.
- *Hyperglucidic mixed meal test:* more physiological. 47% of patients with suspected PRH have a +ve test vs.1% of asymptomatic subjects.
- *Ambulatory glucose sampling:* gaining favour as it may correlate symptoms with low sugar readings, and improvement of symptoms with recovery from hypoglycaemia.

Management
Diet:
- Frequent, small, low carbohydrate, high protein meals.
- Avoid rapidly absorbed carbohydrates.

- Avoid sugary drinks especially in combination with alcohol.
- Addition of soluble dietary fibres e.g. 5–10g guar gum, or pectin, or hemicellulose per meal, delays absorption and lowers the glycaemic and insulinaemic indices (especially effective in rapid gut transit time).

Drugs:

- Acarbose, an intestinal alpha-glucosidase inhibitor, delays sugar and starch absorption thus reducing the insulin response to a meal.
- Metformin can be useful, 500mg with meals.
- Supplemental chromium is reported to down regulate beta cell activity, and increase glucagon secretion.
- In exceptional cases, with debilitating PRH, diazoxide (side effects water retention, hypertrichosis, digestive disorders), or somatostatin analogues may be required.
- Propranolol and calcium antagonists have been used, however controlled studies are lacking.

Further reading

Brun JF, Fedou C, and Mercier J (2000). Postprandial reactive hypoglycaemia. *Diabet Metab* **26**, 337-351

Gama R, Teale JD, and Marks V (2003). Clinical and laboratory investigation of adult spontaneous hypoglycaemia *J Clin Path* **56**, 641–6.

Box 103.2 Non-islet cell tumour hypoglycaemia (NICH)

- Excess secretion of abnormal IGF-II (big IGF-II) from tumours such as fibrosarcomas and mesotheliomas is associated with hypoglycaemia associated with:
  - Suppressed insulin, c-peptide, and IGF-I.
  - Low growth hormone.
  - Low β-hydroxybutyrate levels.
  - Autonomous IGFBP-II secretion by tumours leads to suppression of GH secretion and therefore reduced IGF-I and IGFBPs and a high IGF-II:IGF-I ratio.
  - IGF-II is usually IGFBP bound, which maintains it within the circulation.
  - IGF-II may therefore remain 'free' in the circulation, with ↑ tissue bioavailability, leading both to suppression of IGF-I and GH and also to hypoglycaemia due to binding and stimulation of insulin receptors.
- Definitive treatment is removal of the tumour.
- High dose glucocorticoids are the most effective medical therapy.
- Therapy with GH replacement stimulates an increase in binding proteins (IGFBP-3) and IGFI and reversal of hypoglycaemia.

Further reading

Teale JD and Wark G (2004). The effectiveness of different treatment options for non-islet cell tumour hypoglycaemia. *Clin Endocrinol* **60**, 457–60.

Obesity

Definition

Obesity is defined as an excess of body fat sufficient to adversely affect health. In the almanac of direct measurements of body fat mass, body mass index (BMI) is a commonly used surrogate marker (see Box 104.1):

- Obesity is often defined in terms of BMI.
- BMI does not take body build into consideration, and thus can be misleading in the presence of large muscle mass.
- Lower cut-off values may be applicable to non-Caucasian ethnic groups.
- Fat distribution: *central (abdominal) obesity ('apple-shape') vs. gluteo-femoral obesity ('pear-shape')*.
- 'Apple-shaped' people have an ↑ cardiovascular risk compared to 'pear-shaped' people.
- Adverse consequences of central obesity may reflect ↑ visceral (intra-abdominal fat) stores, (blood draining into the portal vein may expose the liver directly to the effluent from visceral fat).
- Assess using either waist circumference to hip circumference ratio (WHR) or waist circumference alone (see Boxes 104.2 and 104.3).

Epidemiology

- Rapid increase in both the developed and developing worlds.
- ↑ prevalence of obesity—in 1980, 6% of ♂ and 8% of ♀ in the UK were obese. By 2000, the figures had ↑ to 21% and 21.4% respectively. Now 55% of the population is either overweight or obese.
- Prevalence in children is also ↑ rapidly (15% of 15-year-olds in 2001) with attendant risk of type 2 diabetes. The exact prevalence in childhood is difficult to state precisely because of the lack of a consensus about definition.
- In some ethnic populations, prevalence of overweight is >65%.
- Prevalence varies with age (peak prevalence at 50–70 years) and socio-economic class (14% in social class I, 28% in social class V).

Box 104.1 BMI

BMI (kg/m^2) = weight (kg) / [height (m)]^2

Classification:

BMI (kg/m^2)	WHO class
<18.5	Underweight
18.5–24.9	Healthy
25.0–29.9	Pre-obese (overweight)
30.0–34.9	Obese class I (obese)
35.0–39.9	Obese class II (obese)
>40.0	Obese class III (severely obese)

Box 104.2 WHR and waist circumferences

- Suggested indicators of central obesity (and ↑ cardiovascular risk):

	WHR	**Waist circumference**
♂	>1.0	>102cm
♀	>0.9	>88cm

- Another study suggested a waist circumference <100cm makes insulin resistance unlikely (irrespective of sex).

Box 104.3 Measurement of waist and hip circumferences

Measurements should be recorded over underwear or light clothing. The subject should stand with their arms by their sides.

Waist:

The position of the waist is midway between the lower rib margin and the iliac crest.

1. Identify the bony landmarks in the mid-axillary line.
   a. The lower rib margin (bottom of the rib cage).
   b. The iliac crest (highest bony part of the pelvis).
2. Measure the vertical distance between them. Note the midpoint.
3. Ask the subject to stand with their feet 23–30cm apart.
4. Ensure that the tape measure is at the same level around the body at the midpoint. Gently tighten the tape measure so that it is taut but not too tight.
5. Ask the subject to breathe normally and record the measurement at the end of normal expiration.
6. Record waist circumference.

Hips:

1. Ask the subject to stand with their feet together.
2. The measurer should sit to the side of the subject.
3. The hips should be measured at the maximum extension of the buttocks, ensure the tape is the same level around the body. Tape measure should be taut, but not too tight.
4. Record hip circumference.

Aetiology

Genetic factors

- *Monogenic*: rare.
  - Leptin deficiency/resistance (massive obesity and hyperphagia in early childhood) (see Box 104.4).
  - Prader–Willi (obesity, learning difficulties, chromosome 15).
  - Lawrence–Moon–Biedl (obesity, polydactyly, learning difficulties, retinitis pigmentosa).
  - Melanocortin 4 receptor (MC4R) Box 104.7 p.653 deficiency (obesity, hyperphagia, dominant inheritance.
- *Polygenic*: estimates of heritability range from 40–80%, thus genetic factors play a major role in obesity.

Environmental factors

Excess energy intake or ↓ energy expenditure due to physical inactivity as the major determinants of obesity in genetically susceptible individuals.

Secondary causes

Cushing's disease/syndrome; hypothyroidism; hypothalamic lesions (↑ appetite; consider MRI).

Pathophysiology

- Complex regulation of appetite and energy expenditure. Still not fully understood. Errors likely to cause obesity. Understanding not yet translated into therapeutic modalities (perhaps reflecting that long-term attempts to change one pathway leads to compensatory changes in other pathways).
- *Long-term signals* associated with body-fat stores are provided by leptin and insulin. These circulating molecules also modulate short-term signals that determine meal initiation and termination.
- *Short-term information about hunger and satiety*: include gut hormones, such as cholecystokinin, ghrelin (Box 104.5), and peptide YY_{3-36} (PYY), and signals from vagal afferent neurons within the GI tract that respond to mechanical deformation, macronutrient balance, pH, tonicity, and hormones.
- *Neural and humoral signals*: specific regions of the hypothalamus, brain stem, and neural networks are involved in the regulation of energy homeostasis and are regulated by peripheral signals such as leptin which regulate neuropeptides and neurotransmitters expressed in these brain areas.
- *Fat vs carbohydrates*: overall, close regulation of metabolism and storage of carbohydrates, but not of fat.
- *Weight homeostasis*: overeating increases both fat free mass (FFM) and fat mass (~1kg FFM gain for ~2kg fat gain). FFM is the major determinant of resting energy expenditure ('No, Mrs Smith, you're not fat because you have a slow metabolism').

Box 104.4 Leptin

- 'Hungry hormone'.
- 1st hormone described to be secreted from adipose tissue.
- Encoded by *Lep* gene (chromosome 7q31.3).
- Synthesized in and secreted by adipose tissue.
- Affects the hypothalamus to decrease food intake and increase energy expenditure (by sympathetic activation).
- 1° role in humans may be to indicate nutritional depletion/fasting and for falling leptin levels to indicate insufficient energy reserves for growth and reproduction.
- Exerts potent anti-obesity effects in animals such as the *ob/ob* (leptin deficient) mouse.
- Leptin therapy benefits humans with congenital leptin deficiency and leptin-deficient partial lipodystrophy.
- Most obese humans do not have abnormalities of the leptin gene. Plasma leptin ↑ in obese humans, and obese humans appear to be leptin resistant. Reduced leptin transport to the brain has been suggested as a potential mechanism of leptin resistance in humans.
- Trials in humans with 'polygenic' obesity have been equivocal (high doses of SC leptin leads to more weight loss than placebo, but long-term consequences of supraphysiological doses are unknown; sympathetic activation for weight loss by other agents have unwanted side effects).
- Loss of function mutations in the leptin receptor gene are associated with hyperphagia and early onset obesity; serum leptin levels do not predict leptin receptor mutations.
- Leptin stimulated by glucocorticoids.

Consequences of obesity

- ↑ body fat is associated with ↑ morbidity and mortality, but the causal link is unclear. For example, low cardio-respiratory fitness is an independent predictor of cardiovascular disease, irrespective of body fat.
- Standardized mortality rates rise sharply at BMI of 30 kg/m^2.
- Diseases associated with obesity include:
  - *Type 2 diabetes* (BMI >40 in <55-year-old → ↑ risk 18-fold in ♂, 13-fold in ♀).
  - *Hypertension* (BMI 25–29.9 → ↑ risk 1.6-fold; BMI >40 → ↑ risk 5.5-fold).
  - *Dyslipidaemia* (moderate relationship with total cholesterol, closer relationship with ↑ triglycerides, ↓ HDL-cholesterol).
  - *Cardiovascular disease* (BMI >29 → ↑ risk 4-fold).
  - *Gall bladder disease* (♂, BMI >40 → ↑ risk 21-fold; ♀, BMI >40 → ↑ risk 5-fold).
  - Osteoarthrosis, varicose veins, obstructive sleep apnoea, some cancers (e.g. endometrium, breast, ovary, prostate, colon).
- However, obesity protects against osteoporosis.

Box 104.5 Ghrelin

- Plasma concentrations inversely proportional to degree of obesity.
- Peptide (28 amino acids) from oxyntic cells in the stomach fundus.
- Acts on growth hormone secretagogue receptors to increase the release of growth hormone from the pituitary.
- Also important in energy homeostasis.
- Regulates premeal hunger and meal initiation.
- Circulating ghrelin concentrations increase preprandially and decrease postprandially.
- Ghrelin increases food intake through the stimulation of ghrelin receptors on hypothalamic neuropeptide Y-expressing neurons and agouti-related protein-expressing neurons (💭 see Box 104.6 p.653).
- Patients with Prader–Willi syndrome have disproportionately elevated levels of ghrolin, although the relevance of this finding is unclear at present.

Evaluation of an obese patient

- Weight history from birth onwards (early onset is associated with genetic syndromes).
- Previous treatment/management strategies and their success.
- Current eating habits/activity levels.
- Triggers for eating.
- Family history of obesity.
- Co-morbidities such as cardiovascular disease, diabetes, psychological issues (depression, low self esteem), osteoarthrosis, obstructive sleep apnoea, polycystic ovarian syndrome.
- Assess coexistent cardiovascular risk factors such as smoking and diabetes, family history of cardiovascular disease.
- Look for eruptive xanthomata (hypertriglyceridaemia), acanthosis nigricans (insulin resistance), skin tags (insulin resistance), striae (Cushing's), fat distribution (Cushing's, partial lipodystrophy—probably underdiagnosed).
- Consider 2° cause if additional clinical features:
  - Hypothyroidism (measure TSH).
  - Cushing's syndrome (measure 24h urinary free cortisol and consider dexamethasone suppression testing).
  - Hypothalamic disorder (uncontrolled appetite—MRI).
  - Prader–Willi syndrome.
  - Lawrence–Moon–Biedl syndrome.
- Consider co-existent conditions, e.g. polycystic ovary syndrome.

Investigations

Consider:
- FBC (polycythaemia).
- U&Es.
- LFTs (non-alcoholic steatohepatitis, subsequent cirrhosis).
- Glucose (impaired fasting glucose, diabetes).
- Fasting lipid profile (raised triglycerides, total and LDL-cholesterol, lowered HDL cholesterol).
- TFTs (hypothyroidism).
- Urine dipstick (glycosuria with diabetes, proteinuria with glomerular hyperfiltration)
- ECG (coronary vascular disease, left ventricular hypertrophy).
- Waist and hip circumference.
- Height and weight.

Box 104.6 Neuropeptide Y (NPY)

- Synthesized in the arcuate nucleus of the hypothalamus, and transported axonally to the hypothalamic paraventricular nucleus.
- A potent appetite stimulant and reduces sympathetic output, so reducing energy expenditure.
- ↑ by insulin and glucocorticoids, and ↓ by leptin and oestrogen.
- Genetic studies have not shown any association between the genes for NPY or its receptor in human obesity.

Box 104.7 Melanocortin peptides

- Melanocortin peptides are derived by cleavage from pro-opiomelanocortin (POMC).
- Mutations result in ACTH deficiency, obesity, and pale skin (and no hair in Caucasians).
- Mutations in the receptor (MC4R) are the commonest mongenic causes of obesity found—1% of adults with BMI >30kg/m^2 and 5–6% of overly obese children under the age of 10.
- MC4R mutations are dominantly inherited.

Management

- Weight normalization and maintenance rarely occurs. Even in the best weight management programmes about 10% of weight is lost, but most people regain 2/3 of the lost weight in a year, and 95% of in 5 years.
- A weight loss of 5–10% of the initial body weight reduces the health risks associated with obesity.
- The aims should be modest weight loss maintained for the long term, with treatment methods and goals being decided for each individual after careful assessment of the degree of overweight and any associated co-morbid conditions. See Box 104.9.
- Limited range of treatments available.
- The 1st-line strategy for weight loss and its maintenance is a combination of supervised diet, exercise, and behaviour modification.

Diet

- Diet alone does not usually maintain weight loss, and the majority of dieters regain weight within 3 years.
- Reduce calorie intake to 600 kcal below current intake.
- Reduce fat intake—standard dietary advice is to limit fat intake to 20–35% of total calorie intake. Reduction of fat intake can lead to weight loss, often without a conscious reduction in calorie intake.
- Extreme diets may have problems:
  - *Very low calorie diets* (<600 kcal/day) are used occasionally for up to 26 weeks in specialist centres in combination with high quality proteins (daily intake of 1g/kg of ideal body weight), electrolytes, vitamins, and trace elements. Can produce weight loss of ~2 kg/week (more in 1st week as glycogen-bound fluid is lost). Weight is often regained after stopping the diet. Side effects include fatigue, malaise, electrolyte disturbances.
  - *Very high carbohydrate/low fat diets* have been associated with hypertriglyceridaemia and lower LDL-cholesterol concentrations.
  - *Low carbohydrate/high protein diets* (>25% of calories as protein) have little or no long-term safety data (especially on renal disease, ischaemic heart disease—diets tend to be high in saturated fat and cholesterol). Side effects include constipation, renal stones, ↑ urinary calcium losses. Can be effective in inducing weight loss. Probably work by ↑ sense of satiety, leading to a ↓ calorie intake.

Exercise

- Most effective method of maintenance of weight loss, when combined with calorie restriction and behavioural modification.
- Promotes the preservation of FFM (the major determinant of resting energy expenditure) in the face of weight loss.
- Current recommendations are 20+ min exercise 3–5 times/week.
- Regular exercise induces cardiorespiratory fitness and leads to a beneficial effect on other risk factors, with a reduction in blood pressure and improvement in lipid profile.
- Interestingly, non-voluntary activity ('fidgeting') is a significant determinant of resting energy expenditure. Factors controlling non-voluntary activity are unclear.

Box 104.8 Metabolic syndrome (syndrome X, Reaven's syndrome)

- A clustering of metabolic risk factors: hyperinsulinaemia, impaired glucose tolerance or frank diabetes, ↑ LDL-cholesterol and triglycerides, hypertension, central obesity, and ↓ HDL-cholesterol.
- Associated with ↑ risk of vascular disease. Data suggest that >95% of centrally obese patients have at some risk factors, <50% of subcutaneously obese patients do.
- Different diagnostic criteria exist. A typical definition is 3 of the following criteria:
  - Abdominal obesity (see abdominal circumference cut-off values).
  - Raised plasma triglyceride concentrations.
  - Lowered plasma HDL-cholesterol concentrations.
  - Raised blood pressure.

Box 104.9 Effects of losing weight

- *Diabetes*:
  - Weight loss of 5kg halves the risk of developing type 2 diabetes.
  - Improves glycaemic control.
- *Hypertension*: weight loss of 1kg reduces blood pressure by 1–2mmHg.
- *Dyslipidaemia*: weight loss of 1kg:
  - Lowers LDL-cholesterol by 0.02mmol/L.
  - Lowers triglycerides by 0.015mmol/L.
  - Raises HDL by 0.009mmol/L.
- *Obesity related cancers*: weight loss of 0.5–9kg is associated with a 53% reduction in cancer related deaths.
- *Osteoarthrosis and obstructive sleep apnoea*: weight loss has significant mechanical benefits.
- *Gallstones*: weight loss (or weight gain) can provoke gallstone formation by altering the cholesterol saturation of bile.

Behavioural interventions

- Little data available, but should probably include: self monitoring of behaviour and progress, stimulus control, goal setting, slowing rate of eating, ensuring social support, problem solving, assertiveness, cognitive restructuring (modifying thoughts), reinforcement of changes, relapse prevention, and strategies for dealing with weight regain.
- Formal psychological assessments of patients with eating disorders (a minority of obese patients) is helpful.

Drug treatment

- Should be used in combination with other treatments (exercise, calorie restriction, behaviour modification).
- For patients:
  - At medical risk from obesity (BMI >30kg/m^2); *or*
  - BMI >27 with established co-morbidities (e.g. diabetes, heart disease (not sibutramine), severe respiratory problems, dyslipidaemia).

- Use only after dietary and lifestyle modifications have been unsuccessful (defined as not achieving a 10% weight reduction after at least 3 months of supervised care).
- Not all obese patients respond to drug therapy.
  - Prescribe for no longer than 12 weeks in the first instance.
  - Stop drug treatment if 5% weight reduction not achieved.
  - If a 5% weight loss is attained then may be continued, provided body weight is continually monitored and weight is not regained.
  - Rapid weight regain is common after short-term use of anti-obesity drugs (12 weeks or less).

Fat absorption inhibitors
Orlistat

- Intestinal pancreatic lipase inhibitor; reduces fat absorption.
- Increases dietary fat loss to 30% (compared to <5% on placebo).
- Only use in patients who achieve at least 2.5kg weight loss in 4 weeks using a dietary programme alone (NICE guidelines). This ensures adequate dietary compliance with diet and minimizes GI side effects.
- Average weight loss of 10% per year.
- NICE guidelines:
  - At 3 months, stop if <5% weight loss.
  - At 6 months, stop if <10% weight loss (of initial weight).
  - At 12 months, consider stopping treatment.
- Licensed for use up to 2 years. No long-term safety data yet.
- Contraindications: cholestasis, hepatic dysfunction, malabsorption, pregnancy, breast feeding, concomitant use of fibrate, acarbose, renal impairment (creatinine >150micromol/L), anticoagulation (possible ↓ vitamin K absorption with orlistat).
- No data in patients aged >75 years.
- Start at 120mg od and increase up to 120mg tds with main meals.
- Consider vitamin supplementation (especially vitamin D) if concern about fat-soluble vitamin deficiency.
- Side effects: flatus (24%), oily rectal discharge, fatty stool (20%), faecal urgency (22%), fat soluble vitamin deficiency, incontinence (8%). Side effects limited by dietary fat reduction (to <35% of energy).

Appetite suppressant drugs
Sibutramine

- Centrally acting dopamine, serotonin, and noradrenergic reuptake inhibitor. Also stimulates thermogenesis, ↑ energy use.
- Decreases food intake; increases satiety.
- Cautions: hypertension (>145/90 mmHg), vascular disease.
- Range of drug interactions, including sympathomimetics (e.g. pseudoephedrine, some cough/cold remedies).
- Side effects: nausea, insomnia, dry mouth, constipation, ↑ BP and pulse.
- Monitor BP: stop if BP rises to above 145/90 or if BP rises by more than 10mmHg (systolic or diastolic).
- Monitor heart rate: stop if resting HR increases by ≥10 beats/minute.
- Start at 10mg od. Continue beyond 4 weeks only if 2kg weight loss occurs (can increase dose to 15mg od).

- NICE guidelines: stop if weight loss <5% at 3 months, or if subsequent weight gain of ≥3 kg.
- Not licensed for use beyond 12 months.

Other appetite suppressant drugs such as fenfluramine, dexfenfluramine, and phentermine have been withdrawn because of associations with valvular heart disease and pulmonary hypertension. Phentermine's licence reinstated in Dec 2003; available on a named patient basis for <12 weeks of use (but drug is rarely used)

Rimonabant (now withdrawn)

- Cannabinoid type 1 (CB1) receptor antagonist.
- CB1 receptors:
  - Are 1 of 2 receptors in the endocannabinoid system.
  - Found in many cells, including adipocytes and in the hypothalamus.
- Rimonabant appears to eliminate endocannabinoid-induced hyperphagia and fat accumulation (may also reduce the motivation for nicotine administration, but is not licensed for this indication).
- In phase III trials, rimonabant (20mg od); reduces food intake; induces weight loss (~9kg); reduces waist circumference; increases HDL by 30%; reduces triglycerides by 9%; reduces tobacco dependence (without post-cessation weight gain); reduces the proportion of patients with metabolic syndrome by up to 50%; but has no effect on LDL.
- Phase III studies have a drop out rate of about 10%.
- Side effects: upper respiratory tract infection symptoms, depression (1–10%), anxiety, memory loss, insomnia, diarrhea, nausea, and vomiting.
- Symptoms of upper respiratory tract infection often transient (days).
- Safety data available up to 2 years. No data in patients >75 years old.
- Metabolized by the liver, thus affected by CYP3A4 inhibitors (e.g. ketoconazole, clarithromycin, etc.) and inducers (e.g. carbamazepine).
- ↑ efficacy in Caucasian compared to black patients (?different clearance rate).
- Should not be used in: uncontrolled serious psychiatric illness such as major depression; major liver or renal dysfunction.
- Not for use in combination with antidepressants (no data available).
- ↑ depression and suicidal ideation have been reported in a significant number of patients.

Surgery
Bariatric
- Associated with significant weight loss for at least 8 years.
- Improves QoL, hypertriglyceridaemia, hyperuricaemia, and reduces the incidence of type 2 diabetes.
- Data on benefit to BP and cholesterol concentrations unclear.
- Jejuno-ileal bypass and jaw wiring not as commonly used now.
- Only indicated in severely obese (>100% above ideal weight, BMI >40 or BMI >35 with serious co-morbidities) adults (>18 years).
- Failure to lose weight before surgery is not a contraindication.
- Patients referred from specialist hospital obesity clinic.
- Candidates for surgery should be thoroughly assessed with multidisciplinary assessment (including a biopsychosocial assessment).
- Long-term follow up required.

- *Malabsorptive bariatric surgery:*
  - Shortening the length of gut so that the amount of food absorbed by the body is reduced.
  - Most common procedure now is Roux-en-Y gastric bypass, jejunoileleal or bilio-pancreatic diversions are less common and associated with dumping syndrome or recurrent hypoglycaemia.
- *Restrictive bariatric surgery:*
  - Induces early satiety, limits rate of food intake or both.
  - E.g. laparoscopic gastric banding (permanent reduction in functional capacity of stomach by partitioning off part of the body of the stomach).

Liposuction

- The benefit of liposuction on metabolic parameters is equivocal.
- One study has shown that removal of 10kg SC abdominal adipose tissue by liposuction failed to improve parameters such as BP, plasma glucose, and insulin concentrations.

Further reading

Brennan AM and Mantzoros CS (2006). Drug Insight: the role of leptin in human physiology and pathophysiology—emerging clinical applications. *Nat Clin Pract Endocrinol Metab* **June 2**(6), 318–27.

Kahn R, Buse J, Ferrannini E, *et al.* (2005). The metabolic syndrome: time for a critical appraisal joint statement from the American Diabetes Association and the European Association for the Study of Diabetes. *Diabetes Care* **28**(9), 2289–304.

National Institute for Health and Clinical Excellence (NICE) Clinical guideline 43: Obesity guidance on the prevention, identification, assessment, and management of overweight and obesity in adults and children. ⌨ http://www.nice.org.uk/page.aspx?o=91525

Rucher D, Padwal R, Li SK, *et al.* (2007). Long term pharmacotherapy for obesity and overweight: updated meta-analysis. *BMJ* **335**(7631), 1194–9. Epub 2007 Nov 15.

Sjöström L, Narbo K, Sjöström CD, *et al.* (2007). Effects of bariatric surgery on mortality in Swedish obese subjects. *NEJM* **357**(8), 741–52.

Endocrinology and ageing

Introduction

- Ageing causes changes in many hormonal axes. How much of this change is normal physiology associated with ageing and how much represents true endocrine dysfunction and thus warrants treatment is unclear
- Concomitant disease and polypharmacy are common in the elderly population, with frequent 2° effects upon the endocrine system.

Fluid and electrolyte homeostasis in the elderly

- Elderly patients are particularly prone to fluid and electrolyte disturbances due to changes associated with ageing, concomitant disease, and drug usage.
- Elderly patients have ↓ renal function compared with younger patients:
  - ↓ glomerular filtration rate with creatinine clearance ↓ by 8mL/min/1.73m² per decade after age 30.
  - ↑ renovascular disease.
  - ↓ renal sensitivity to circulating hormones:
    —aldosterone.
    —vasopressin.
    —atrial natriuretic peptide (probable).
  - ↓ ability to dilute or concentrate urine.
- Elderly patients have ↓ renin levels with 2° decreases of aldosterone levels (both basal and stimulated levels). Aldosterone levels may be <50% normal by 70 years of age. ↓ renal sensitivity to aldosterone may result in isolated mineralocorticoid deficiency (distal renal tubular acidosis (type 4) with hyponatraemia, hyperkalaemia, hyperchloraemia, and normal anion gap acidosis); this is more common with diabetes mellitus.

Vasopressin/ADH

- Unlike many other hormones, vasopressin (ADH) responses are potentiated in elderly patients with ↑ release from the neurohypophysis in response to an osmotic stimulus and less effective suppression. Normal vasopressin release is a balance of inhibitory and stimulatory effects at baroreceptors and osmoreceptors. It may be that loss of inhibition with ageing due to degenerative changes results in relatively unopposed stimulation of ADH and a ↓ ability to suppress ADH release.
- In addition, altered renal sensitivity to vasopressin results in ↓ ability to excrete free water.

Hypernatraemia and dehydration

- Perception of thirst is altered in elderly persons (in younger people, thirst is perceived at plasma osmolalities >292mOsm/kg whereas in older people, thirst is perceived at plasma osmolalities >296mOsm/kg). Elderly patients may also be unable to ingest fluids because of other disabilities and/or effects of medications.
- Thus elderly persons are particularly susceptible to dehydration (e.g. during hot summers).

Hyponatraemia

- Particularly common in elderly patients (prevalence of 2–20%). In hospital patients, overall incidence of hyponatraemia (Na <137mmol/L) is 7% but in geriatric facilities is 18–22% with 53% incidence of 1 or more episodes of hyponatraemia at any time during admission to geriatric care facilities. Mortality rates in hospitalized elderly patients with hyponatraemia are high (in patients aged >65 years 16% mortality in those with hyponatraemia compared with 8% without hyponatramia).
- Often associated with medication (e.g. diuretics)
- Commonest electrolyte disturbance in cancer (📖 see SIADH due to ectopic vasopressin production, p.684)
- Symptoms include confusion, lethargy, coma, seizures.
- Overall approach to investigation and management is similar to that of hyponatraemia in younger patients (📖 see Hyponatraemia, p.702).
- Mild idiopathic hyponatraemia is also recognized in elderly patients, without necessarily having sinister cause or consequence, and is thought to be 2° to altered threshold for ADH secretion.

Bone disease

Osteoporosis

Osteoporosis is not an inevitable part of ageing but it is a common disease in elderly people and is associated with high morbidity and mortality in both males and females. 📖 see Osteoporosis, pp.510–520.

Vitamin D deficiency and osteomalacia

- Very common in the elderly.
- Vitamin D insufficiency (evidence of 2° hyperparathyroidism, ↑ bone turnover, BMD loss) occurs at levels of 25OH-vitamin D <50nmol/L.
- Vitamin D deficiency usually defined at levels <25nmol/L (with additional problems of myopathy, ↑ sway, ↓ psychomotor function, and frank osteomalacia).
- Vitamin D deficiency and/or insufficiency is common particularly in elderly institutionalized patients in extreme latitudes and in fracture patients. In a Danish study, 40% of postmenopausal women had vitamin D levels of 25–50nmol/L, with a further 7% with frank deficiency (<25nmol/L). 80% of elderly ♂ and ♀ (aged >65 years) have vitamin D insufficiency. 44% of nursing home patients had severe vitamin D deficiency (25OH vitamin D <12nmol/L). In patients with hip fracture, 75% have vitamin D insufficiency, 25% have vitamin D deficiency, and 5% severe vitamin D deficiency (25OH-vit D< 12.5nmol/L).
- Supplementation with 800IU vitamin D and 1200mg calcium daily in institutionalized elderly patients reduces falls and fractures.
- Supplementation in free-living elderly patients (>65 years of age) also ↓ fracture risk.
- Vitamin D is known to have an antitumour effect with ↓ proliferation, ↑ differentiation of cells, and ↑ apoptosis of malignant cells. Vitamin D may also boost the immune response with further antitumour effect. Vitamin D insufficiency and/or deficiency may contribute to higher rates of malignancy in elderly patients (e.g. breast, colon, and prostate). Therapeutic use of vitamin D in malignant disease is limited by hypercalcaemia.

Primary hyperparathyroidism

- Prevalence of 1° hyperparathyroidism is 10/100 000 in ♀ <40 years old, rising to 190/100 000 in ♀ >65 years old. Half of all cases of 1° hyperparathyroidism occur in ♀ >60 years old.
- Elderly people are more prone to symptoms (weakness, fatigue, confusion) at relatively mild levels of hypercalcaemia (2.8–3.0mmol/L).
- Other causes of hypercalcaemia must be excluded.
- Co-existing vitamin D insufficiency and deficiency is common.
- Management is similar to that described in 📖 Chapter 75, Hypercalcaemia, p.468.
- Surgery is not contraindicated by age alone.

Paget's disease
📖 See Chapter 81, Paget's disease, pp.522–527.

Further reading
Mosekilde L (2005). Vitamin D and the elderly. *Clin End* **62**, 265–81.

GH and IGF-1 in the elderly

- Many of the features of ageing resemble growth hormone deficiency. Changes in body composition include ↓ lean body mass (↓ body water, ↓ muscle mass, and ↓ bone mass) and ↑ total body fat and visceral fat mass, associated with abnormal lipid profile (↑ total and LDL cholesterol, ↑ TGs), insulin resistance, and cardiovascular disease.
- Overall, integrated GH concentrations show a decrease with age with ↓ GH pulse amplitude and duration, but pulse frequency unchanged.
- IGF-I falls with ↑ age (reflected in age-adjusted normative ranges).
- IGF-BP3 falls with age (and is also GH dependent).
- Older patients with GH deficiency related to pituitary disease are usually easily differentiated from other subjects with age-related decline in IGF-I using standard provocative testing (GH response to insulin-induced hypoglycaemia, arginine, or glucagon). Treatment with GH in patients with clear GH deficiency results in ↑ lean body mass and bone mineral density, and ↓ adipose tissue; and possibly psychological and functional improvement.
- Small, frequently open label studies of supraphysiological doses of GH given to healthy older persons have shown that GH may result in improved body composition (improved physiological function has not been observed). Side effects are frequently observed in the treated group (oedema, arthralgias, carpal tunnel syndrome, glucose intolerance) and theoretical concerns of malignancy related to raised IGF-1 levels remain.
- GH is not licensed in the UK for healthy elderly people without clear evidence of GH deficiency.

Gonadal function in the elderly

Women

- The mean age of menopause is 51 years (range 35–58 years) and is defined retrospectively after 12 months of amenorrhea as the permanent cessation of menstruation due to loss of ovarian follicular activity.
  - FSH 10–15 × higher than premenopausal levels.
  - LH 3–5 × higher.
  - Oestrogen 10% of previous level (often lower than ♂ of similar age).
  - Inhibin often undetectable.
- The adrenal gland is the major source of sex steroids postmenopausally, with oestrogen production mainly from aromatization of adrenal androgens (androstenedione) in adipose tissue.
- Low FSH/LH may indicate hypopituitarism, although gonadotrophins may be depressed by serious illness.
- 📖 see Chapter 59, Menopause, p.336 for further discussion.

Men

- ♂ may remain potent and fertile until their death. However, sexual activity, libido, and potency decline gradually and progressively from midlife.
- As with GH, there is an overlap between clinical features of hypogonadism and 'normal ageing' (loss of lean body mass and muscle function, increase in fat mass, loss of virility, loss of libido, and ↓ sexual and overall wellbeing). Functional 2° hypogonadism is common in serious chronic illness, especially when associated with malnutrition and debilitation.
- Normal ranges for testosterone in ♂ of different ages have not been well established.
- Free testosterone levels decrease slowly with age, but there is significant intra- and inter-individual variation. SHBG increases with age. Testicular weight, Leydig cell function, and FSH/LH response to GnRH stimulation all decrease with age.
- The extent to which lower testosterone per se and/or a lower free androgen index explain the age-related decline in sexual function is not clear. Although testosterone levels may be lower than in younger men, testosterone levels are still sufficient for normal libido and sexual function. Profoundly low testosterone levels (<8nmol/L in a 0900 blood sample) in the appropriate clinical setting should prompt investigation for hypoandrogenism. Gonadotrophins should be raised in 1° testicular failure and low levels associated with low testosterone should prompt a search for 2° causes though gonadotrophins may be low because of other serious disease.
- Fat body mass increases more than lean body mass with age; thus there is ↑ aromatization of androgens to oestrogens. The effects of this are unclear.

- Hypoandrogenism may also result from hyperprolactinaemia due to pituitary/hypothalamic disease, renal dysfunction, hypothyroidism, drugs (psychotropic and anti-dopaminergic agents); all more common in the elderly population.

Testosterone therapy

- Few, small studies in elderly ♂, either as replacement in patients with clear hypogonadism or in healthy ♂.
- Data point towards a +ve effect on wellbeing, muscle mass, and strength and ↓ fat mass in elderly patients, with greatest effect in patients with clear hypogonadism.
- Risk of 2° polycythaemia, liver dysfunction (particularly if testosterone taken orally), prostatism, exacerbation of prostate adenocarcinoma, and possibly dyslipidaemia.

Erectile dysfunction

- Common in elderly ♂. 50% of ♂ >60 have erectile dysfunction; 90% of these ♂ have concurrent medical problems or are on medication potentially causing impotence.
- Aetiology often multifactorial:
  - Atherosclerosis—commonest cause with both macro and micro vascular disease.
  - Penile denervation—autonomic neuropathy (most commonly due to diabetes mellitus); pelvic surgery (including prostatectomy—30% of ♂ >75 develop erectile dysfunction after prostatectomy (cf. 7% of younger ♂ after prostatectomy)).
  - Drugs (betablockers, calcium channel antagonists, other antihypertensive agents, psychotropic drugs).
  - Psychogenic.

Delayed/absent ejaculation

- ↑ common with age due to autonomic nerve dysfunction, drugs, previous surgery, and usually the harbinger of erectile dysfunction.
- Evaluation similar to that of younger patients (📖 see Evaluation, p.390).
- Management similar to younger patients; with caveat that phosphodiesterase inhibitors may interact with nitrates and antihypertensive agents.

Fertility

- Spermatogenesis persists into old age.
- There is very little data regarding spermatozoa number, motility, morphology in elderly ♂.
- However, errors in DNA replication increase with age, as reflected in paternal age effects in some genetic disorders.

Adrenal function in the elderly

Cortisol

- Overall, cortisol secretion generally very similar in elderly persons to younger persons.
- Dynamic testing shows more prolonged release of ACTH and cortisol to stress (physiological, insulin-induced hypoglycaemia and/or CRH administration) and slower inhibition of ACTH secretion by cortisol.

Dehydroepiandrosterone sulfate

- DHEA and DHEAS levels peak in humans aged 20–30 years and thereafter decline with age (20% of peak values in ♂ and 30% of peak values in ♀ by age 70 years). Responsiveness to ACTH-stimulated secretion also reduces with age.
- The physiological relevance of the fall of DHEA and DHEAS levels with age is not established.
- Replacement in otherwise healthy elderly patients has not consistently demonstrated improved longevity, well-being, bone density, cognitive function, body mass composition, or cardiovascular status in double-blind placebo-controlled trials, despite many Internet claims to the contrary.

Aldosterone

- 📖 see Fluid and electrolyte homeostasis in the elderly, p.660.

Thyroid disease

Thyroid disease is twice as common in the elderly as in younger patients (see Table 105.1).

Goitre

- Diffuse goitre becomes less frequent with age in both ♂ and ♀ (found in 31% of ♀ aged <45 years compared with 12% of ♀ aged >75 years on clinical examination).
- Multinodular goitre as assessed by both clinical and US examination increases with age (incidence of US-detected multinodular goitre 90% of ♀ >70 years, 60% of ♂ >80 years).
- Management similar to that of multinodular goitre in younger patients (📖 see Multinodular goitre and solitary adenomas, pp.48–51).

Abnormal thyroid function tests

- Concomitant disease and polypharmacy are common in the elderly and may alter the interpretation of results. For example, glucocorticoids (prescribed to 2.5% of the population aged 70–79 years) cause decreased TSH, ↓ thyroid hormone release, ↓ concentration of thyroid hormone binding proteins, ↓ T4 to T3 conversion.
- Sick euthyroid syndrome is more common in the elderly due to frequent concurrent non-thyroidal illness, with reduced free tri-iodothyronine (FT3), ↑ reverse free tri-iodothyronine, and (less commonly) reduced free thyroxine (FT4); with inappropriately normal or suppressed TSH levels.
- 📖 see Table 2.2 (p.9) for effects on thyroid function of drugs frequently prescribed for elderly patients.

Hypothyroidism

- Commonest thyroid problem in elderly people.
- 2–7% of elderly people.
- ♂: ♀ ratio increases with ageing.
- Commonest causes are autoimmune thyroiditis, previous surgery, or radioiodine therapy.
- Only 25% present with classical symptoms of hypothyroidism. An insidious decline in health and mobility is more common than cold intolerance, hair loss, or skin coarsening.
- The elderly are more susceptible to hypothyroid (myxoedema) coma than younger people; it remains rare however.
- Hypothyroidism should be considered in elderly patients with increased CK or transaminases, ↓ Na, macrocytic anaemia, or dyslipidaemia.
- Thyroid replacement therapy should be done cautiously as ischaemic heart disease may be unmasked or exacerbated, e.g. 12.5–25mcg/day of levothyroxine ↑ by 12–25mcg increments every 3–8 weeks until TSH is normalized; similarly liothyronine 5mcg bd with very gradual titration up of doses.
- Total replacement T4 dose is lower in the elderly than in younger patients (in younger patients approximately 1.6mcg/kg is required but older patients require 20–30% less).

- Compliance may be problematic. Supervised therapy or administration using a Dosette® box may help. Alternatively, calculate the total weekly dose of levothyroxine and give 70% of the total dose once a week or 50% of the total dose twice weekly.

Table 105.1 Changes in thyroid-related investigations with ageing

TSH	No significant change; secretion remains pulsatile but loss of physiological nocturnal TSH rise is blunted
T_4	Unchanged overall (both secretion and clearance ↓)
T_3	10–50% decrease; occurs at an earlier age in women than in men
rT_3	↑
Thyroid antibodies	Prevalence ↑ with age; significance uncertain(2% at age 25, 15–32% at age 75)
24h radioactive iodine uptake	Unchanged

Hyperthyroidism

- 2% of elderly people.
- Presentation is often atypical, often with few signs or symptoms.
- Commonly, symptoms are mainly in a single, vulnerable organ system, e.g. depression, lethargy, anxiety, confusion and agitation; muscle wasting and weakness; heart failure, arrhythmias, atrial fibrillation; weight loss; osteoporotic fracture.
- An isolated suppressed TSH concentration is associated with an ↑ cardiovascular mortality and a 3-fold higher risk of atrial fibrillation in the next 10 years. 2–24% of elderly patients with atrial fibrillation are hyperthyroid and 9–35% of elderly patients with hyperthyroidism have atrial fibrillation.
- Underlying cause may be toxic multinodular goitre; Graves' disease.
- Treatment options are similar to those in younger patients (📖 see Treatment p.22).
- Radioactive iodine is favoured because it is definitive and it avoids risks of surgery. Hypothyroidism is common after radioiodine therapy in elderly people.

Thyroid cancer

- Total incidence rate for all thyroid cancers is unchanged but the relative frequencies are altered. Papillary carcinoma is more common in young and middle-aged patients, but the prognosis is poorer in the elderly. Follicular carcinoma is more common with ageing.
- Anaplastic thyroid carcinoma occurs almost exclusively in patients >65 years. It presents with a rapidly-growing hard mass which is often locally invasive and may be associated with metastatic lesions. The prognosis is poor.
- Sarcomas and 1° thyroid lymphomas are more common in elderly patients.
- Overall evaluation and treatment is similar to that of younger patients but accurate preoperative histology is very important as tumours not treated surgically (e.g. anaplastic carcinoma and lymphoma) are relatively more common.

Glucose homeostasis

Elderly patients have impaired glucose homeostasis and are more likely to manifest hyperglycaemia in response to acute illness/stress (e.g. post myocardial infarction).

Further reading

Grimley Evans J, Williams TF, Michel J-P, et al. (eds.) (2000). Oxford Textbook of Geriatric Medicine. Oxford University Press, Oxford.

Vermeulen A (ed.) (1997) Endocrinology of ageing. Ballière's Clin Endocrinol Metab **11**, 223–50.

Endocrinology of critical illness

Endocrine dysfunction and AIDS

Wasting syndrome

Definition

The involuntary loss of >10% of baseline body weight in combination with diarrhoea, weakness, or fever. Wasting is an AIDS-defining condition.

Cause

Unknown, but in part reflects ↓ calorie intake due to anorexia associated with 2° infection. Underlying ↑ resting energy expenditure associated with HIV infection per se. Hypogonadism common in ♂ with wasting syndrome.

Treatment

- *Highly active antiretroviral therapy* (HAART) Associated with overall weight gain, though lean body mass may remain unchanged.
- *Nutritionally based strategies* Adequate caloric intake to meet metabolic demands. Efficacy limited as refeeding generally increases fat body mass with little/less effect on lean body mass.
- *Appetite stimulants* Megestrol acetate increases caloric intake and weight compared to placebo, though most of weight gain due to ↑ fat mass. Dronabinol stimulates appetite but weight gain is minimal.
- *Exercise* Although exercise can increase total and lean body mass in patients with AIDS, its role in patients with wasting syndrome is not known.
- *Androgen therapy* In hypogonadal ♂ patients with wasting syndrome, testosterone increases overall weight and in particular lean body mass. Both IM and transdermal testosterone effective. Testosterone therapy not indicated in eugonadal ♂ with wasting.
- *Growth hormone therapy* Patients with the wasting syndrome generally have GH resistance, as suggested by high serum GH and low IGF-I levels. The most likely cause for this is undernutrition. High dose GH has shown improvements in lean body mass and protein balance in patients with acquired GH deficiency or severe catabolic states. Side effects (peripheral oedema, arthralgias, myalgias) common due to high doses required. GH may improve fat redistribution that occurs with refeeding.
- *Cytokine modulators* Although many inflammatory cytokines are ↑ during acute illness and sepsis, their specific role in wasting syndrome is not known. Thalidomide, a potent inhibitor of TNF, can increase body weight and reduce protein catabolism but has a very high rate of serious side effects and is contraindicated in ♀ of childbearing age due to phocomelia.

Lipodystrophy

- Loss of SC fat particularly in the face, peripheries, and buttocks, in some cases with concomitant subcutaneous fat deposition, particularly in the abdominal area, neck, dorsocervical area ('buffalo hump'). Visceral fat deposition also occurs.
- Associated dyslipidaemia with hypertriglyceridaemia, low HDL cholesterol, insulin resistance, glucose intolerance, and (less commonly) frank diabetes mellitus. ↑ cardiovascular mortality from myocardial infarction.
- Associated with HIV-1 protease inhibitors (PIs), used as part of highly active antiretroviral therapy (HAART). 40% of patients treated with PIs will develop lipodystrophy by 1 year. HIV protease inhibitor-naïve patients have similar body composition and fat distribution to that of non-HIV infected men. Indinavir may be less potent in inducing lipodystrophy than ritonavir and saquinavir.
- Abnormal body composition and hypertriglceridaemia may be part of refeeding phenomenon consequent upon improved wellbeing and loss of anorexia per se.
- Nucleoside reverse transcriptase inhibitors may be associated with fat loss and accumulation also but this may be a separate phenomenon to that seen with PIs.

Management

- Observation in mild cases.
- Very low fat diets and exercise (particular resistance exercise).
- Withdrawal or switching of PIs in some circumstances may be warranted.
- Anabolic agents (testosterone, GH) not effective.
- Liposuction from areas of fat accumulation; fat pad insertions for areas of lipoatrophy also used.
- Standard lipid lowering agents for hypertriglyceridaemia (e.g. gemfibrozil).
- HMG CoA reductase inhibitors metabolized by P4503A4 (which is inhibited by PIs) so risk of myopathy may be ↑.
- Role for thiazolidinediones unclear.

Adrenal
Adrenal insufficiency
Uncommon (<4% of patients with AIDS). In patients with clinical signs suggestive of hypoadrenalism (hyponatraemia, and hypovolaemia) 30% incidence of inadequate response to synacthen.

Causes
- *Infection* Histologically common. Adrenal function usually maintained since 10% of residual adrenal tissue is adequate for normal function
  - CMV (adrenalitis found post mortem in 40–90% of patients dying of AIDS).
  - *Mycobacterium avium intracellulare* (MAI) complex, tuberculosis
  - *Cryptococcus*.
- *Neoplasm* Lymphoma, Kaposi's sarcoma.
- *Haemorrhage*.
- *Drug induced:*
  - Rifampicin induces ↑ hepatic metabolism of corticosteroids. In subjects with already compromised adrenal reserve this may precipitate an Addisonian crisis.
  - Ketoconazole inhibits cortisol synthesis.
  - Megestrol acetate possesses glucocorticoid activity and may cause 2° adrenal insufficiency. Abrupt cessation after long-term treatment may precipitate an adrenal crisis.
- *2° adrenal insufficiency:*
  - Drugs (megestrol acetate).
  - Hypopituitarism 2° to toxoplasmosis, *Cryptococcus*, CMV.
  - Idiopathic anterior pituitary necrosis.

Hypercortisolism
Mild hypercortisolaemia common in all stages of HIV infection, without clinical manifestation of Cushing's syndrome.

Possible causes
- Chronic stress.
- Proinflammatory cytokines.
- Binding protein dysfunction.
- Glucocorticoid resistance.

Gonads

Males

- Testosterone deficiency common in ♂ patients with AIDS (6% of patients with asymptomatic HIV infection compared with 50% of patients with AIDS).
- Hypogonadism is associated with wasting, ↓ muscle mass, fatigue, loss of libido, and impotence. Hypogonadism may be 1° or 2°; up to 75% of patients with hypogonadism have low or inappropriately normal gonadotrophins.

Causes

- *1° hypogonadism*
  - *Testicular destruction/infiltration* due to infection (CMV most commonly, MAI, toxoplasma, TB) or neoplasm (lymphoma, Kaposi's sarcoma, germ cell tumours).
  - *Drug induced* ketoconazole (inhibits steroidogenesis causing lowered testosterone levels); megestrol acetate, other glucocorticoids.
- *2° hypogonadism* due to malnutrition, severe acute illness, destructive disorders of pituitary/hypothalamus (CMV, toxoplasmosis, lymphoma); medications such as megestrol acetate (glucocorticoid-like action causes hypogonadotrophic hypogonadism).

Females

- Hypogonadism in ♀ as evidenced by oligo/amenorrhea less common than in ♂ unless advanced disease. Fertility rates not affected until advanced disease.
- Hypoandrogenism (testosterone, DHEA) common in ♀ with wasting syndrome.

Electrolyte disturbance due to endocrine pertubation in HIV/AIDS

Hyponatraemia

Very common in advanced disease. Due to SIADH in 50%; adrenal insufficiency also a common cause.

Calcium disorders

- *Hypocalcaemia* Common (18% of patients with AIDS). Main cause is vitamin D deficiency. Other causes: severe illness; hypomagnesaemia; altered PTH secretion/metabolism; malabsorption of calcium and vitamin D due to GIT opportunitistic infection; medications (foscarnet [complexes with calcium], pentamidine [induces renal magnesium wasting and 2° PTH deficiency])
- *Hypercalcaemia* Rare. May relate to lymphoma or granulomatous disease.

Thyroid
- Overt thyroid dysfunction is uncommon. Most common thyroid dysfunction is sick euthyroid syndrome (nonthyroidal illness). ↑ thyroid binding globulin often observed (significance unknown).
- Subclinical hypothyroidism may occur during HAART.
- *Infections* Rare; usually postmortem diagnoses. Thyroid function usually euthyroid or sick euthyroid.
  - *Pneumocystis jirovecii (*may also cause a thyroiditis).
  - Mycobacteria.
  - *Cryptococcus neoformans.*
  - *Aspergillosis.*
- *Neoplasm* Rare. Usually eu- or sick euthyroid; may be hypothyroid due to infiltrative destruction.
  - Kaposi's sarcoma.
  - Lymphoma.

Pituitary
- *Anterior hypopituitarism* Very rare.
- *Posterior pituitary dysfunction* causing diabetes indipidus (DI). Common.
- *Infection* Toxoplasmosis, TB.
- *Neoplasm* Cerebral lymphoma.

Cancer

Chemotherapy and radiotherapy may have endocrine effects.

Anticancer chemotherapy

There are 3 types of anticancer chemotherapeutic agents:

- *Cytotoxics* These have no direct hormonal sequelae. Alkylating agents are more likely to induce permanent ♂ sterility (without affecting potency) and in ♀ they may induce premature menopause which may increase the liklihood of osteoporosis.
- *Immunomodulators* Prednisolone in excess causes Cushing's syndrome and acute withdrawal may precipitate adrenal insufficiency. *Cyclophosphamide* in particular may cause early menopause. Thyroid dysfunction has been reported rarely with *tacrolimus* and *interferon-α and -β* therapy.
- *Hormones*
  - *Progestogens* are used in breast cancer; of these, *megestrol acetate* has potent glucocorticoid activity and thus may cause Cushing's syndrome in excess or adrenal insufficiency if abruptly withdrawn.
  - *Aromatase inhibitors* such as *aminoglutethimide* may cause adrenal insufficiency and corticosteroid replacement is necessary.
  - *Trilostane*, which inhibits 3β-hydroxysteroid dehydrogenase, may also cause adrenal insufficiency.
  - *Gonadorelin analogues*, used for prostatic cancer and breast cancer, cause an initial increase in LH levels and then suppression and cause side effects similar to orchidectomy in ♂ and the menopause in ♀.
  - *Antiandrogens* used in prostatic cancer have predictable side effects such as gynaecomastia, hot flushes, impotence, and impaired libido.

Radiotherapy

- Cranial radiotherapy whose field encompasses the hypothalamo–pituitary area may result in hypopituitarism (see Chapter 13, Hypopituitarism, pp.98–102).
- Head and neck irradiation may result in hypothyroidism and hypoparathyroidism.
- After 5 or more years of follow up, 50% of patients treated with radiotherapy only for laryngeal and pharyngeal carcinoma will develop hypothyroidism; combined surgery and radiotherapy results in roughly 90% of patients developing hypothyroidism. The rates for hypoparathyroidism were 88% and 90% respectively.
- Radiotherapy affects the testes dose-dependently. Fertility is affected much more than androgen synthesizing capacity so that most ♂ have normal testosterone levels unless given testicular doses >20–30Gy.
- The effects of radiotherapy to both ovaries is amplified with age. Premature menopause may be elicited by doses >10Gy.

Syndromes of ectopic hormone production

Definition

The secretion into the systemic circulation, of a hormone or other biologically active molecule, by a neoplasm (benign or malignant) that has arisen from a tissue that does not normally produce that hormone or molecule, resulting in a clinically significant syndrome. See Table 106.1 for common syndromes associated with ectopic hormone production.

Table 106.1 Common syndromes associated with ectopic hormone production

Syndrome	Ectopic hormone	Typical tumour types
Hypercalcaemia of malignancy	PTHrP	Squamous cell lung carcinoma
		Other squamous cell carcinoma (skin, oesophagus, head, and neck)
		Renal cell carcinoma
		Breast adenocarcinoma
		Adult T-cell lymphoma associated with HTLV-1
	$1,25(OH)_2$ cholecalciferol	Lymphomas
SIADH	Vasopressin/ADH	Small cell lung carcinoma
		Squamous cell lung carcinoma
		Bronchial carcinoid
		Mesothelioma
		Pancreatic or gut carcinoid
		Adenocarcinoma of the duodenum, pancreas, prostate
		Phaeochromocytoma
		Medullary thyroid carcinoma
		Haematopoietic malignancies (lymphoma, leukaemia)

Syndrome	Ectopic hormone	Typical tumour types
Cushing's syndrome	ACTH (most commonly)	Small cell lung carcinoma
		Thymic carcinoid tumour
		Bronchial carcinoid tumour
		Pancreatic endocrine tumours (including carcinoid tumours)
		Carcinoid tumours of the gut
		Phaeochromocytoma
		Medullary thyroid carcinoma
		Other lung cancers (adenocarcinoma, squamous cell carcinoma)
	CRH (rarely)	Carcinoid tumour
	Ectopic expression of receptors for GIP; LH	Macronodular adrenal hyperplasia
Non-islet cell hypoglycaemia	IGF-2	Mesenchymal tumours
		Mesothelioma
		Fibrosarcomas
Oncogenic osteomalacia	FGF23	Sarcomas
		Haemangiomas
		Fibromas
		Prostate adenocarcinoma
		Osteoblastomas
Male feminization	hCG	Testicular neoplasms (seminomas, teratomas)
		Germinomas
		Choriocarcinomas
Acromegaly	GHRH	Pancreatic islet cell tumours
		Carcinoid tumours
	GH	Lung, pancreatic islet cell tumours

SIADH due to ectopic vasopressin production

Diagnosis

- Hyponatraemia (Na <130mmol/L).
- Dilute plasma (serum osmolality <270mmol).
- Inappropriately concentrated urine (in the face of hyponatraemia and plasma hypoosmolality, any urine osmolality >plasma osmolality is inappropriate).
- Persistant renal Na excretion.
- Euvolaemia (or very mild hypervolaemia).
- Normal renal, adrenal, and thyroid function.

- Plasma urea and uric acid levels can be helpful markers of plasma dilution.
- The commonest tumours causing SIADH are tumours with neuroendocrine features, most commonly small cell lung carcinoma and carcinoid tumours. Small cell lung carcinomas have usually metastasized by the time SIADH is present.
- Lung diseases and neurological disorders (including malignancies) may cause SIADH due to aberrant hypothalamic vasopressin release rather than vasopressin release from the tumour per se. In SIADH due to ectopic hormone secretion, release of vasopressin from the neurohypophysis may be suppressed.
- Other causes of SIADH must be excluded (☐ see Syndrome of inappropriate ADH, p.206).

Management

Hyponatraemia

- The initial management is fluid restriction with daily monitoring of the plasma sodium and osmolality. Hyponatraemia has usually developed gradually, and its correction should be similarly gradual. Fluid restriction to 500mL total fluid intake per day may be needed for several days. Urate levels can be useful as a marker of water intoxication and its resolution. As hyponatraemia is corrected, fluid restriction can be relaxed depending on the plasma sodium. 1500–2000mL/day is usual.
- For patients in whom fluid restriction is insufficient or not possible, demeclocycline (150–300mg tds–qds) can be used to produce a nephrogenic diabetes insipidus to achieve a normal plasma sodium. Demeclocycline can result in photosensitivity and patients should be warned to avoid prolonged exposure to sunlight.
- Life-threatening hyponatraemia (e.g. convulsions) may rarely require hypertonic saline and frusemide; however rapid correction of hyponatraemia may result in central pontine myelinolysis and in the vast majority of cases, water restriction is safe, effective, and sufficient.

Management of the underlying tumour

Curative surgery will also cure the SIADH, as will curative chemotherapy and/or radiotherapy. Chemotherapy and radiotherapy may have an important palliative role as the tumour is usually incurable by the time hyponatraemia is detected.

Humeral hypercalcaemia of malignancy

Hypercalcaemia is a common complication of malignancy; may be due to ectopic hormone secretion (PTHrP; rarely $1,25(OH)_2$ cholecalciferol); cytokine and inflammatory mediators that activate osteoclastic bone resorption (such as IL-6 and RANK-L production by myeloma cells) or due to bone destruction by metastases.

Parathyroid hormone-related peptide (PTHrP)

- PTHrP binds to and activates PTH/PTHrP receptor type 1 resulting in osteoclast-mediated bone resorption and reduced renal excretion of calcium.
- The biochemical picture of hypercalcaemia and hypophosphataemia may be indistinguishable from 1° hyperparathyroidism. However, PTH levels are suppressed in PTHrP-mediated hypercalcaemia (NB. 1° hyperparathyroidism can co-exist with malignancy).
- PTHrP secretion by metastatic cells within bone also causes hypercalcaemia by causing local osteolysis.
- PTHrP can be measured directly and is elevated in 80% of cancer patients with hypercalcaemia.
- Tumours that metastasize to bone are more prone to produce PTHrP than tumours that do not metastasize to bone (50% of 1° breast cancer express PTHrP compared with 92% of metastases of breast cancer to bone). This may be due to induction of PTHrP secretion by the bone microenvironment; alternatively PTHrP production by tumour cells may enhance their ability to metastasize to bone.
- 📖 for tumours associated with humoral hypercalcaemia see Table 106.1, p.682.

Management

- As per normal management of hypercalcaemia (📖 see Other causes of hypercalcaemia, p.468).
- Glucocorticoids may be particularly effective in treatment of hypercalcaemia associated with malignancy. This may be due to direct effects of glucocorticoids on the tumour cells (e.g. haemopoietic malignancies) and/or because of downregulation of production of $1,25(OH)_2$ cholecalciferol.
- Bisphosphonates may also have antitumour effects in myeloma as well as controlling osteoclastic destruction of bone.

Cushing's syndrome due to ectopic ACTH production

- Ectopic ACTH production is responsible for 10–20% of all endogenous Cushing's syndrome.
- Commonest tumour types are those with neuroendocrine features. 50% of ectopic ACTH-secretion is due to small cell lung carcinoma. Carcinoid tumours are also very common (thymic carcinoid 15%; pancreatic endocrine tumours including pancreatic carcinoids 10%; bronchial carcinoid 10%).

Diagnosis

- Despite often extremely high cortisol levels, patients often do not manifest central weight gain, due to the underlying malignant process with its rapid progress and associated cachexia.
- Hypertension, hypokalaemia, metabolic alkalosis, are common features (overwhelming of the 11B-hydroxysteroid dehydrogenase enzyme resulting in exposure of the mineralocorticoid receptor to high circulating glucocorticoids).
- Glucose intolerance, susceptibility to infection, thin skin, poor wound healing, and steroid-associated mood disturbance are all common features.
- Patients may be pigmented due to MSH arising from high POMC levels.
- ACTH levels may be extremely high (usually >100pg/mL).
- In 90% of ectopic ACTH-secreting tumours, high dose dexamethasone testing (2mg qds) shows a failure of cortisol levels to drop to 50% of baseline values, due to a lack of any normal physiological feedback upon ACTH production. However some carcinoid tumours may behave indistinguishably from pituitary-dependent ACTH production. CRH testing and/or inferior petrosal sinus sampling may be necessary to distinguish these conditions.
- Ectopic ACTH-producing tumours can be extremely difficult to localize and may require multiple modalities of imaging.

Management

Excision of the underlying tumour may be possible. Other options include medical management using metyrapone and/or ketoconazole although very high doses may be needed (🕮 see Table 19.3, p.155). Bilateral adrenalectomy with glucocorticoid and mineralocorticoid replacement is also an option.

Macronodular adrenal hyperplasia

- A rare cause of ectopic Cushing's syndrome.
- Most commonly due to synthesis of ectopic GIP receptors in adrenal tissues.
- GIP secretion associated with meals results in activation of adrenal glands and food-related hypercortisolaemia.
- Other ectopic receptors reported include β-adrenergic receptors and LH receptors.

Carcinoid tumours and ectopic hormone production

See p.570 and Table 106.1, p.682.

Liver disease

Sex hormones—males

See Table 106.2.

- Hypogonadism occurs in 70–80% of ♂ with chronic liver disease. There is a combination of 1° testicular failure and failure of hypothalamo–pituitary regulation.
- Alcohol acts independently to produce hypogonadism. There is a combination of 1° testicular failure and failure of hypothalamo–pituitary regulation.
- The effects of elevated oestrogens result in ↑ loss of the ♂ escutcheon, loss of body hair, redistribution of body fat, palmar erythema, spider naevi, and gynaecomastia.
- The ↑ conversion of testosterone and androstenedione to oestrone is attributed at least in part to portosystemic shunting. In addition, the large increase in SHBG concentration will increase the oestrogen/testosterone ratio as testosterone has a higher affinity for SHBG.
- Spironolactone may result in iatrogenic feminization by inhibiting testosterone action.
- There is no evidence that exogenous administration of androgens reverses hypogonadism in chronic liver disease.

Sex hormones—females

See Table 106.2.

- Alcoholism increases the frequency of menstrual disturbances and spontaneous abortion but does not affect fertility.
- Liver dysfunction of whatever aetiology is associated with an early menopause.
- Alcohol rather than liver disease is the prime cause of hypogonadism. Non-alcoholic liver disease is only associated with hypogonadism in advanced liver failure when it is accompanied by encephalopathy and impaired GnRH secretion.
- Plasma testosterone and oestrone concentrations are usually normal, androstenedione concentration is ↑ and dehydroepiandrosterone and dehydroepiandrosterone sulfate levels are reduced.

Thyroid

- The liver synthesizes albumin, T_4-binding prealbumin (TBPA), and T_4-binding gobulin (TBG), all of which bind thyroid hormones covalently and reversibly.
- Thyroid function tests must be interpreted with caution in patients with liver disease. In acute liver disease, e.g. acute viral hepatitis, TBG levels are ↑ which increases the measured total circulating T_4 and T_3 levels. In biliary cirrhosis and chronic active hepatitis TBG may be ↑. In other chronic liver disease and in hepatomas, TBG is also ↑. In severe cases of acute liver disease TBG may be low due to reduced synthesis. The liver deiodinates T_4 to T_3 and this is impaired in liver disease. The T_4 is preferentially converted to rT_3 and there is an increase in the rT_3/T_3 ratio.
- In liver cirrhosis, TBG, T4 and T3 are low.

- Table 106.3 summarizes the changes in TFTs with liver disease. Free T_4 and T_3 assays are essential for the accurate interpretation of thyroid status in liver disease.

Adrenal hormones

- Patients who abuse alcohol may develop a clinical phenotype of Cushing's syndrome with moon facies, centripetal obesity, striae, and muscle wasting, and may have increased plasma cortisol concentrations. This is termed '*pseudo-Cushing's syndrome*'.
- Reversible (on abstention) adrenocorticoid hyperresponsiveness occurs in alcoholics. In liver disease cortisol metabolism may be impaired leading to elevated plasma cortisol levels, loss of diurnal cortisol variation, and failure to suppress with dexamethasone.

Table 106.2 Sex hormone changes in liver disease

Hormone	Level
Testosterone	↓↓
SHBG	↑
Oestrone	↑
Oestradiol	↑/normal
LH	Inappropriately low/normal
FSH	Inappropriately low/normal
Prolactin	↑/normal
IGF-1	↓
IGFBP-3	↓

Table 106.3 Thyroid function changes in liver disease

Hormone	Acute hepatitis	CAH/PBC	Cirrhosis
T_4	↑ ↓	↑	↓
fT_4	↑ →	→	↑
T_3	↓	↑	↓
fT_3	↓	↓	↓
rT_3	↑	→	↑ →
TSH	↑	↑	↑ →
TBG	↑	↑	↓

CAH: chronic active hepatitis
PBC: primary biliary cirrhosis

Further reading

Malik R and Hodgson H (2002), The relationship between the thyroid gland and the liver. *QJ Med* **95**, 559–569.

Renal disease

Calcitriol

There is impaired renal conversion of 25-hydroxyvitamin D_3 to 1,25 $(OH)_2D_3$ in end-stage renal failure (ESRF) leading to metabolic bone disease (see Table 78.1, p.497).

Parathyroid hormone and renal osteodystrophy

- Serum parathyroid hormone PTH secretion is stimulated by low serum calcium in ESRF. This is due to:
  - ↓ renal phosphate clearance (resulting in ↑ cacium/phosphate mineral ion product, precipation of vascular calcification with consequent hypocalcamia triggering PTH release). Vascular calcification is a major contributor to vascular death in ESRF. High phosphate per se may increase PTH secretion directly but evidence of the mechanism for this is lacking.
  - Impaired renal calcitriol secretion.
- As renal function declines, an elevated PTH and a ↓ calcitriol can be detected with creatinine clearance of 50mL/min. This rise in PTH is initially sufficient to maintain the serum calcium in the normal range.
- In ESRF patients are markedly hyperphosphataemic and hypocalcaemic. The degree of hyperparathyroidism progresses inversely with the fall in renal function. Tertiary hyperparathyroidism occurs when PTH secretion becomes autonomous and hypercalcaemia will persist even after renal transplantation.
- Hyperparathyroid bone disease and osteomalacia are the main mechanisms behind the development of high turnover bone disease in renal osteodystrophy. Hypogonadism is also common in both ♂ and ♀ with ESRF. Adynamic bone disease also contributes, probably due to direct toxic effects from urea and other nitrogenous compounds upon bone cells. Renal osteodystrophy causes bone pain and fractures.

Treatment of renal osteodystrophy

- Maintainence of normal phosphate levels with phosphate binders (such as calcium carbonate) and the treatment of osteomalacia. The ↑ use of calcium carbonate has been suggested as the cause of the ↑ incidence of adynamic renal osteodystrophy, but intensive vitamin D therapy and peritoneal dialysis are probably also contributory.
- Alfacalcidol or calcitriol (which do not require renal 1α-hydroxylation) are effective in treating osteomalacia.
- Calcitriol at a dose of 1–2mcg/day is used for established renal osteodystrophy. Lower doses of calcitriol (0.25–0.5mcg/day) are used in early ESRF to prevent the development of renal osteodystrophy.
- Parathyroidectomy is advocated in bone disease uncontrolled by vitamin D therapy or the development of tertiary hyperparathyroidism.
- Cinacalcet acts directly at the calcium sensing receptor to lower PTH secretion. This markedly improves 2° hyperparathyroidism, calcium, and phophate levels, and renal osteodystrophy. Improvement in mortality due to ↓ vascular calcification has not yet been demonstrated.

Prolactin

Hyperprolactinaemia is common in ESRF but is usually mild, i.e. <1000mU/L. The cause is both ↑ secretion and ↓ renal clearance.

Gonadal function

- Hypogonadism—clinical and biochemical—is common in ESRF.
- In ♂, there is impaired pulsatile release of LH, although basal LH levels are usually elevated due to impaired renal clearance. Serum FSH is usually normal or mildly elevated.
- In ♀, levels of oestradiol, progesterone, and FSH are reported to be within the normal range in the early follicular phase but fail to show the usual cyclical changes. Menstrual disturbance is common. Amenorrhoea, polymenorrhoea, and menorrhagia can also occur on dialysis. Infertility is the rule and conception on dialysis is the exception.
- Sexual dysfunction is common in both sexes but has been better studied in ♂. 60% of ♂ have some degree of impotence and examination yields 80% to have testicular atrophy and 14% to have gynaecomastaia.
- Treatment of hypogonadism in ESRF is suboptimal. Testosterone therapy is not associated with any clinical benefit in ♂.

Growth hormone and growth retardation

- Basal GH levels are normal but there is impaired secretion following an adequate hypoglycaemic stimulus in 40–70% of patients with ESRF.
- There is impaired growth in children, particularly during periods of greatest growth velocity and puberty is delayed. This combination leads to short stature. The improved growth velocity after renal transplantation is often too little too late in order to attain a normal stature.
- Recombinant human GH (rhGH) has been shown to be an effective treatment for growth retardation in children with stable chronic renal failure (CRF) and ESRF as well as after renal transplantation.

Thyroid

The 'sick euthyroid' finding is common in CRF (see Sick euthyroid syndrome, p.17).

Adrenal

- The adrenal axis is not impaired clinically by CRF.
- There is evidence of blunted cortisol response to hypoglycaemia but this is not relevant clinically.
- Patients with amyloidosis are at risk of hypoadrenalism due to adrenal amyloid infiltration.

Endocrinology in the critically ill

(📖 See Table 106.4)

ACTH and cortisol

- CRH, ACTH, and cortisol increase rapidly during all forms of acute illness.
- Low albumin and CBG cause free cortisol to be substantially higher.
- This physiological adaptation results in:
  - Provision of substrates for major organ energy expenditure (via catabolism).
  - Haemodynamic advantages (enhanced sensitivity to angiotensin II, ↑ vasopressor and inotropic response to catecholamines.
  - Prevention of an excessive immune response.
- Inflammatory cytokines result in ↑ cortisol metabolism and reduced receptors i.e. peripheral cortisol resistance.
- After moderate-to-severe injuries, plasma cortisol starts to fall after a day or two but only reach normal levels after a week.
- Cortisol is elevated for at least 2 weeks in patients with severe burns.
- Prolonged critical illness results in low CRH and ACTH with a 'normal'or slightly raised cortisol, perhaps driven by an alternative pathway involving endothelin.
- Cortisol deficiency should be suspected in an acutely ill patient with a plasma cortisol of <690nmol/L, or an increment of <250nmol/L on a 250mcg short Synacthen® test.
- Drugs used in intensive care may contribute to adrenal insufficiency by:
  - Reducing cortisol metabolism, e.g. etomidate (frequently used in induction of anathaesia) and ketoconazole.
  - Promoting cortisol metabolism e.g. phenytoin, carbamazepine, and rifampicin

Metabolism

- Hyperglycaemia is common in critical illness (even in non-diabetic subjects) due to ↑ cortisol, catecholamines, GH, and glucagon.
- These hormones and inflammatory cytokines also contribute to insulin resistance.
- IV insulin titrated to maintain normoglycaemia (glucose <6.1mmol/L) reduces mortality by >40%.

TSH and thyroid hormones

- TSH levels usually remain stable in acute injury. Total T_4 and T_3 tend to fall but may remain within the normal range.
- Enhanced thyroid hormone metabolism by ↑ activity of liver deiodinase type 3 (peripheral hormone deactivator).
- With prolonged illness the total T_4 tends to fall below the normal range. The fT_4 remains in the normal range.
- Total and free T_3 levels fall after injury and may remain suppressed for 2–3 weeks after a severe injury. The rT_3 level rises.
- In prolonged critical illness the thyroid function conforms to the 'sick euthyroid syndrome' (📖 see Sick euthyroid syndrome, p.17).

Table 106.4 Endocrine and other changes seen in the ill

Acute illness	
ACTH/CRH	↑↑↑
Albumin/ CBG	↓
Free cortisol	↑↑
Catabolism	↑↑
Immune response	↓
Inflammatory response	↑↑
Cortisol resistance	↑
Glucose	↑
Insulin resistance	↑↑
TSH	→
FT$_4$ and FT$_3$	→ ↓
IGF1, IGFBPs, GHBPs	↓
Prolonged critical illness	
ACTH/CRH	↓↓
Free cortisol	→ or ↑
TSH, total T$_4$	↓
rT$_3$	↑
LH/FSH/T/oestradiol	↓
GH	↓
Response to GHRH	↓

Gonadotrophins and gonadal steroids

In prolonged illness hypogonadotrophic hypogonadism occurs.

Growth hormone

- In critical illness the GH axis is profoundly affected with initially raised GH secretion, but low IGF-1, IGFBPs, and GHBP related to peripheral GH resistance.
- Prolonged critical illness >5–7 days results in low GH and a blunted response to GHRH.
- Recombinant GH was proposed as a beneficial agent for critical illness however the evidence is lacking, and there are reports of a detrimental effect.

Hormone replacement and critical illness

There is no evidence that other than insulin, hormonal supplementation in the critically ill improves outcome.

Further reading

Elleger B, Debaveye Y, and Van den Berghe G (2005). Endocrine interventions in the ICU. *Eur J Intern Med* **16**, 71–82.

Isidori AM, Kaltsas GA, Pozza C, *et al.* (2006). The ectopic adrenocorticotropin syndrome: clinical features, diagnosis, management, and long-term follow-up. *J Clin Endocrinol Metab* **91**(2), 371–7. Epub 2005 Nov 22.

Perioperative management of endocrine patients

Trans-sphenoidal surgery/craniotomy

Preoperative assessment

Confirm the following:

- Anterior and posterior pituitary function normal or on adequate replacement:
  - Short Synacthen® test (note both the 0 and 30min values). And/or normal ACTH/cortiso/< 0900. Note: patients with recent loss of LFTH will have a normal response to SST as adrenal atrophy will not have evolved. If in any doubt, replace with glucocorticoids.
  - FT_4.
  - LH, FSH, oestradiol, or testosterone.
  - Prolactin.
  - Serum and urine osmolality and electrolytes if polyuric.
- Recent (<3 months) MRI pituitary.
- Formal visual field perimetry and visual acuity assessment.
- Document extra-ocular muscle movements.
- Urea and electrolytes (<1 week pre-surgery).
- Group and save serum.
- MRSA screen should be done at least 2 weeks prior to admission for surgery, if the patient has been in hospital within the last year.
- Record therapeutic options discussed with patient, including:
  - Risks of surgery (e.g. CSF leakage, meningitis, bleeding, partial or total hypopituitarism including diabetes insipidus and potential effects on fertility and visual deterioration).
  - Risk of recurrence requiring further surgery or radiotherapy.
  - Warn patients that a sample of fat may be taken from their thigh or abdomen for packing of the pituitary fossa.
  - Reiterate the need for lifelong follow up.
- Ensure antibiotic prophylaxis is given prior to surgery (the precise regimen may vary depending on the centre and patient, e.g. flucloxacillin 500mg qds and amoxicillin 500mg tds PO/IV.; use erythromycin if penicillin-allergic). Some surgeons advocate a prolonged course of antibiotics if CSF leakage occurs, whilst others recommend close surveillance and prompt treatment if concern re: possible meningitis (NB lower threshold for patients with Cushing's disease).
- MRSA +ve patients require prophylaxis with IV vancomycin.
- If steroid deficient, steroid reserve is unknown or if a patient has Cushing's disease (inadequate stress response), give *hydrocortisone* 20 mg orally with morning premedication.

Postoperative (Table 107.1)

- Consider steroid status; if requires steroid cover:
  - Start IM *hydrocortisone (HC)*, 50–100 6–8-hourly, postoperatively.
  - Convert to oral HC (20mg/10mg/10mg) once eating and drinking.
  - After nasal packs removed (following trans-sphenoidal surgery), stop HC (usually <48h).
  - Check 9 a.m. cortisol level the following 2 mornings, having omitted the evening dose for the preceding day. Continue off steroids if asymptomatic, however if symptomatic only omit the evening dose.
- In patients with Cushing's disease, 9 a.m. cortisol (× 2) <50nmol/L indicates cure; occasionally cortisol takes a few days to fall to undetectable levels.
- See Table 107.1 for patients without Cushing's disease:

Table 107.1 Postoperative HC management of patients without Cushing's disease

9 a.m. cortisol level	Action
>550nmol/L	Stay off hydrocortisone
400–550nmol/L	Advise to start hydrocortisone if unwell (give patient supply of oral and parenteral hydrocortisone to take home with appropriate written advice)
<400nmol/L	Start regular oral hydrocortisone (10mg/5mg/5mg)

NB In ♀ patients who have stopped oestrogen replacement therapy <6 weeks before surgery interpret results with caution (potential confounding effect of raised CBG levels).

- If the patient is acutely unwell with postural BP drop when hydrocortisone is stopped, check random cortisol and re-start hydrocortisone without delay.
- Fluid balance—watch for diabetes insipidus:
  - Review the clinical status of the patient at regular intervals (?euvolaemic/hypovolaemic/hypervolaemic).
  - Record fluid input/output assiduously (NB fluid replacement in theatre may be excessive, therefore always include perioperative fluids in fluid balance charts and note sodium content.
  - Check U&Es, plasma and urine osmolalities on a regular basis (at least once daily and more frequently if clinical concerns).
  - Postoperatively, restrict to 2 L total fluid input (IV and PO).
  - Record fluid input/output assiduously.

- If patient becomes polyuric i.e. >200mL/h for ≥3 consecutive hours (in the context of a 2L/24h fluid restriction), then urgently check plasma U&Es, plasma and urine osmolalities, and urinary sodium. While waiting for results allow free fluids; aim to replace the fluid deficit. (NB fluid replacement in theatre may be excessive, always include perioperative fluids in fluid balance sheets).
- If diabetes insipidus confirmed by the results, give a single dose of *desamino-D-arginine vasopressin* (desmopressin) (1mcg SC).
- When fluid deficit has been replaced (usually orally), restart 2–3L fluid restriction (again include IV and PO routes).
- If polyuria recurs, treat as before.
- Regular U&Es, plasma and urine osmolalities required.
- If polyuria continues to recur up to and after 96h postoperatively, consider regular DDAVP orally or intranasally if possible (not if a trans-sphenoidal approach is used).

- Hyponatraemia occurring 1 week after a trans-sphenoidal adenectomy is most commonly due to SIADH; rarely cerebral salt wasting may occur. Check urinary sodium and assess fluid status (cerebral salt wasting causes very high urinary sodium and is associated with dehydration).
- Check thyroid function (FT_4) between day 5 and day 7 postoperatively.
- Check for CSF leakage, bedside test with Glucostix® and send a sample for beta-transferrin/ tau-protein for confirmation.
- Recheck visual acuity and visual field perimetry and eye movements formally prior to discharge.
- Give information to patient including advice on driving:
  - For an ordinary driving licence (group 1 car or motorcycle) a minimum horizontal field of 120 degrees is required as well as no significant defect within the central 20 degrees. For a license to drive a group 2 vehicle (bus or lorry), then normal binocular field is required.
  - If an individual has normal visual fields and acuity, and an uncomplicated trans-sphenoidal operation they may restart to drive once recovered from the surgery (group 1 and group 2 licences).
  - Following a craniotomy group 2 licence holders are suspended for 6 months, however group 1 licence holders can restart driving once recovered providing their vision is satisfactory and there is no history of seizures.
  - All patients should inform their insurance company about the pituitary tumour and pituitary surgery.
- Give information to patient on contact details for the Pituitary Foundation support group, and DVLA:
  - The Pituitary Foundation, 17/18 The Courtyard, Woodlands, Bradley Stoke, Bristol BS12 4NQ. Telephone: 01454 201612.
  - Medical Adviser, The Drivers' Medical Branch, 2 Sandringham Park, Swansea Vale, Llansamlet, Swansea SA6 8QD. Tel: 0870 0600 0301.

Thyroidectomy

Preoperative

- Ensure euthyroidism.
- If surgery is required in the presence of hyperthyroidism, give *potassium iodide* (60mg 3 × a day for 10 days); this reduces thyroid hormone release and probably decreases perioperative blood loss. The radiographic contrast agent iopanoic acid, which is rich in iodine, provides a useful alternative, and has the additional benefit of potently inhibiting the 5-deiodinase thus reducing T_4 to T_3 conversion. Oral *propranolol* (30–120mg 3 × a day) reduces clinical manifestations of thyrotoxicosis.
- Check vocal cord function by indirect laryngoscopy.
- Warn of postoperative risks: recurrent laryngeal nerve damage <1%, keloid scarring, haemorrhage, permanent hypoparathyroidism <0.5%, and hypothyroidism (10% of partial thyroidectomy patients).

Postoperative

- Risk of haemorrhage in first 24h, particularly major haemorrhage deep to the strap muscles leading to airway compression. Watch for stridor, respiratory difficulties, and wound swelling. Drainage from wound drains is unhelpful. Treat by evacuating the haematoma, consider intubation or a tracheostomy. Clip removers and artery forceps should be kept to hand on the ward.
- Recurrent laryngeal nerve damage is permanent in <1% and transient in 2–4%. Patient's voice is often husky for about 3 weeks postoperatively and may be treated with lozenges and humidified air.
- Symptomatic unilateral damage can be treated by stabilization of the affected cord in adduction by submucosal Teflon® injection under direct laryngoscopy.
- Bilateral damage leads to unopposed adductor action of the cricothyroid muscle which causes glottis closure and airway obstruction. Treatment involves reintubation, paralysis, hydrocortisone (100 mg 4 × a day IM for oedema), and extubation at 24h—if that fails, a tracheostomy should be performed.
- If recurrent laryngeal nerve damage is persistent at 9 months, an attempt can be made to resuture the nerve.
- Monitor calcium. Transient hypoparathyroidism is usually evident within 7 days. 📖 see Hypoparathyroism, p.492 for treatment.
- Following total thyroidectomy for malignancy, the patient should be converted to T_3, which should be stopped at least 10 days prior to the postoperative radioiodine uptake scan to allow the TSH to rise (📖 see Follow up of papillary and follicular thyroid carcinoma, p.70). Alternatively recombinant TSH can be used.
- If total thyroidectomy is performed for hyperthyroidism, levothyroxine (~1.5mcg/kg) should be commenced 4–5 days post-operatively, as during the operation, handling of the thyroid results in release of stored thyroid hormones, and levothyroxine has a long t½. Check TSH in 6–8 weeks.
- Following partial thyroidectomy, transient biochemical hypothyroidism may occur during the first 2 months and does not warrant treatment unless the patient is symptomatic or it becomes persistent.

Parathyroidectomy

Parathyroidectomy of 1 or 2 glands undertaken for 1° hyperparathyroidism may result in transient and self-limited hypocalcaemia. Total parathyroidectomy (e.g. for MEN1 or as part of surgical management of advanced head and neck malignancy) may be complicated by severe and permanent hypocalcaemia which may be very difficult to manage.

Postoperative care for patients undergoing parathyroidectomy of 1–2 glands.

- Check calcium, phosphate, magnesium, albumin, on the evening of surgery and daily thereafter. Calcium begins to fall postoperatively after about 4–12h; the nadir is usually reached by 24h. Calcium may recover spontaneously, however 1/3 of patients will require calcium support perioperatively. With the advent of minimally invasive parathryoidectomy and short hospital stays (<24h) many centres advocate prophylactic calcium and vitamin D replacement in all cases in the immediate aftermath of surgery, which is continued until the patient in reviewed 1–2 weeks later in the outpatient clinic.
- *Symptoms of hypocalcaemia* (mainly due to neuromuscular irritability): perioral paraesthesiae, Chovstek's sign, Trousseau's sign, tetany, laryngospasm, bronchospasm, seizures, prolonged QT interval on ECG, extrapyramidal movement disorders, and delirium. Calcium levels often <1.75mmol/L before symptoms manifest, although rapid changes in calcium result in more pronounced symptomatology.
- Magnesium deficiency is common due to previous hyperparathyroidism (causes renal wasting of magnesium). Chronic magnesium deficiency impairs release of PTH and causes functional hypoparathyroidism and hypocalcaemia.

Causes of hypocalcaemia post 1-2 gland removal

- 'Functional hypoparathyroidism' common. Causes: delayed recovery of the other parathyroid glands due to long-term suppression; parathyroid gland ischaemia; parathyroid gland 'stunning' by intraoperative handling; hypomagnesaemia. PTH level will be detectable; phosphate should be normal. Usually spontaneously improves over days to weeks. Management of symptomatic hypocalcaemia (Ca usually <1.8mmol/L) with calcium (up to 2g/day in divided doses). Add in vitamin D/vitamin D metabolites if persistent hypocalcaemia. Replace magnesium as necessary. Gradual withdrawal of therapy to assess recovery.
- 'Hungry bone syndrome' due to extensive skeletal remineralization once skeleton released from PTH excess. Ongoing ↑ ALP, ↓ calcium, ↓ PO₄, ↓ Mg. PTH levels may be normal or high. Pre-existing vitamin D deficiency will exacerbate hypocalcaemia. May require large doses of calcium and vitamin D/vitamin D metabolites for weeks to months.
- *Permanent hypoparathyroidism.* Rare (<2% of cases). Check PTH level after day 3; level will be undetectable (<1pg/mL). Replace with oral calcium and vitamin D/vitamin D metabolites long term.
- *Other complications:*
  - Recurrent laryngeal nerve palsy (<1%).
  - Failure to correct hypercalcaemia.

- Overall both minimally invasive and conventional parathyroidectomy are very safe operations with low morbidity and mortality.

Calcium management following total parathyroidectomy

- Hypocalcaemia is inevitable unless management instituted.
- Pre-emptive treatment is worth considering (e.g. 1α-calcidol 1–2mcg per day—this dose may be insufficient to completely prevent hypocalcaemia but may prevent life-threatening hypocalcaemia and is unlikely to cause serious toxicity in the short term).
- Acute management in patients with life-threatening hypocalcaemia (e.g. Trousseau's sign, laryngospasm, seizures):
  - 10mL of 10% calcium gluconate diluted 1 in 10 in normal saline or dextrose 5% infused into large vein over 10min. Monitor cardiac rhythm.
  - Repeat as necessary to control acute emergency.
  - Patients will need ongoing calcium replacement: 100mL of 10% calcium gluconate in 1L of 5% dextrose or 0.9% sodium chloride infused over 24h (monitor calcium regularly (4–6-hourly) and adjust rate as necessary.
  - Start oral vitamin D analogues and oral calcium.

Vitamin D analogues (1α-calcidol; calcitriol)

- Potent and effective in acute hypocalcaemia due to rapid correction of calcium. Short half-lives allows for rapid and careful titration of dose in response to calcium levels. Narrow therapeutic window (but hypercalcaemia much shorter lived if it develops).
- Dose for dose, calcitriol twice as efficacious as 1α-calcidol (i.e. 1mcg calcitriol equivalent to 2mcg 1α-calcidol). 1α-calcidol can be given down an NG tube.
- Starting doses usually high (e.g. 4–8mcg/day of 1α-calcidol in divided doses) rapidly weaned to maintenance doses (typically 1–2mcg/day 1α calcidol).
- Reassess often (at least every 1–2 days) in early stages of management. Longer term options include ergocalciferol or colecalciferol but hypercalcaemia will be more prolonged if it develops.

Calcium

- 1–2g/daily in divided doses. A maximum daily absorbable dose of calcium is probably 3g day.
- Absorption may vary from different types of calcium salts and may be greater when calcium is given away from food.
- The long-term aim is to manage without calcium just on vitamin D/ vitamin D metabolites.

Long term goal of management is to prevent symptoms of hypocalcaemia without toxicity. Aim for lower half of normal range (2.0–2.3mmol/L) with normal urinary calcium excretion (to minimize risk of nephrolithiasis and nephrocalcinosis.

Phaeochromocytoma

Preoperative

- Check for bilateral disease or metastases: MRI chest and abdomen and an MIBG scan (10% multiple).
- Ensure adequate α- and β-blockade, once the diagnosis is made.
- Start α-blockade before β-blockade (unopposed β-blockade can lead to marked vasoconstriction, ischaemic damage, and hypertension):
  - *α-blockade* Start *phenoxybenzamine* (10–20 mg, orally, 3–4 × day)—an irreversible α-blocker. Adequacy of dosage can be assessed by monitoring the haematocrit and postural drop in (reflects BP vasodilation).
  - Start treatment at least 1 week before surgery, ideally >3 weeks.
  - *β-blockade* start *propranolol* (20–80 mg, orally, 3 × day) at least 48h after initiating phenoxybenzamine.
- Control BP: α- and β-blockers often sufficient, if not add a calcium channel blocker or ACE inhibitor; α-methyltyrosine 1–4g/day (a false catecholamine precursor which inhibits tyrosine hydroxylase, the rate-limiting step for catecholamine synthesis) is rarely used to control BP.
- Some centres advocate the use of additional IV phenoxybenzamine (0.5–1.0mg/kg in 250mL 5% dextrose given over 2h), for the 3 days prior to surgery: (titrate the dose according to the BP; often 0.5mg/kg is sufficient).
- Group and save serum, and cross match 2 units of blood.
- Ensure that the patient is well-hydrated (if necessary use an IV infusion of saline) prior to going to theatre.

Postoperative

- Watch for ↓ BP: sudden withdrawal of catecholamines leads to marked arterial and venous dilatation. This is worsened by inadequate volume loading and should initially be treated with volume replacement rather than by pressor agents.
- If hypertension persists 2 weeks postoperatively, then residual tumour or metastases must be considered.
- Long-term monitoring required as approximately 14% recur.
- If bilateral adrenalectomy performed, see next section.

Bilateral adrenalectomy

- Give hydrocortisone (100mg, 4 × day, IM) postoperatively; this will provide adequate mineralocorticoid as well as glucocorticoid cover. Continue this until eating and drinking (often <48h). Monitor U&Es.
- From day 3, give hydrocortisone PO (double usual replacement dose, e.g. 20mg/10mg/10mg) and add fludrocortisone PO (100mcg daily).
- Long term replacement with hydrocortisone 10/5/5, and fludrocortisone 50–150mcg daily.

Phaeochromocytoma in pregnancy (📖 see p.451)

- Rare condition; may present as paradoxical supine hypertension, with pressure from the gravid uterus causing release of catecholamines, and normal blood pressure in the supine and erect positions.
- Start β-blockade then β-blockade, phenoxybenzamine can cross the placenta but is generally safe for the fetus (may cause perinatal CNS depression and transient hypotension).
- Surgery is more controversial although some authors advocate surgery in the 1st and 2nd trimesters up to 24 weeks' gestation.
- Caesarian section is advocated with a combined tumour resection. Vaginal delivery carries a significant maternal risk.

Syndromes of hormone resistance

Definition

Reduced responsiveness of target organs to a particular hormone, usually secondary to a disorder of the receptor or distal signaling pathways. This leads to alterations in feedback loops and elevated circulating hormone levels.

Thyroid hormone resistance

📖 see Resistance to thyroid hormones, p.39.

Androgen resistance

📖 see Androgen insensitivity syndrome, p.418.

Glucocorticoid resistance

- Autosomal dominant and recessive forms have been described.
- Diminished sensitivity to glucocorticoid leads to reduced glucocorticoid feedback on CRH and ACTH, leading to ↑ CRH, ACTH, and cortisol concentrations.
- The clinical features are not due to excess glucocorticoid as there is reduced peripheral tissue sensitivity. However, elevated ACTH leads to ↑ secretion of mineralocorticoid (e.g. deoxycorticosterone) and androgen (DHEA and DHEAS). This may lead to hypertension and hypokalaemic alkalosis, hirsutism, acne, oligomenorrhea in ♀, and sexual precocity in ♂.
- Glucocorticoid resistance may be differentiated from Cushing's syndrome as despite evidence of ↑ urinary cortisol, abnormal suppression with dexamethasone, and ↑ responsiveness to CRH, the diurnal rhythm of cortisol secretion persists, there are no clinical features of Cushing's syndrome, BMD is normal or ↑, and there is a normal response to insulin induced hypoglycaemia.
- Low-dose dexamethasone treatment (2mg/day) may efficiently suppress ACTH and androgen production.

ACTH resistance

- A rare autosomal recessive disorder where the adrenal cortex fails to respond to ACTH, in the presence of an otherwise normal gland. (mineralocorticoid secretion is preserved under angiotensin II control.)
- The presenting clinical features include hypoglycaemia, which is often neonatal, neonatal jaundice, ↑ skin pigmentation, and frequent infections.
- Occasionally, ACTH resistance is a component of the *triple A syndrome* of alacrima (absence of tears), achalasia of the cardia, and ACTH resistance.
- *Biochemical features:* undetectable or low 9 a.m. cortisol, with grossly elevated ACTH (often >1000ng/mL), and normal renin, aldosterone, and electrolytes, and impaired response to short Synacthen® test.
- *Treatment:* steroid replacement.

Mineralocorticoid resistance

Also known as type 1 pseudohypoaldosteronism, this is a rare inherited disorder which usually presents in children with failure to thrive, salt loss, and dehydration. Both autosomal dominant and recessive forms have been described.

- *Biochemical features*
  - ↓ serum sodium.
  - ↑ serum potassium (hyperkalaemic acidosis).
  - ↑ urinary sodium (despite hyponatraemia).
  - ↑ plasma and urinary aldosterone.
  - ↑ plasma renin activity.
- Diagnosis requires proof of unresponsiveness to mineralocorticoids (no effect of fludrocortisone on urinary sodium).
- Treatment is with sodium supplementation, and carbenoxolone has been used successfully. With time treatment can often be weaned, and salt wasting is unusual following childhood.

Further reading

Charmandari, E, Kino T, Ichijo T, *et al.* (2008). Generalized glucocorticoid resistance: clinical aspects, molecular mechanisms, and Implications of a rare gentic disorder. *JCEM* **93**, 1563–72.

Differential diagnosis of possible manifestations of endocrine disorders

Sweating
- Menopause/gonadal failure.
- Thyrotoxicosis.
- Phaeochromocytoma.
- Acromegaly.
- Hypoglycaemia.
- Diabetes mellitus.
- Autonomic neuropathy (gustatory sweating).
- Renal cell carcinoma.
- Chronic infection (e.g. TB).
- Haematological malignancy (e.g. lymphoma).
- Anxiety.
- Idiopathic.
- Drugs e.g. fluoxetine.

Investigation of sweating
- History.
- Clinical examination.
- Thyroid function tests.
- Serum gonadotrophin levels.
- Blood glucose level.
- Specific investigations according to clinical suspicion.

Management of sweating
- Treat the underlying cause where possible.
- Anti-perspirants.
- Topical aluminium chloride ± ethanol.
- Anticholinergics—glycopyrronium bromide (oral or topical).
- Clonidine—taken at night to avoid sedation.
- Iontophoresis.
- Botulinum toxin A injections into affected areas (inhibits the release of acetyl-choline at the synaptic junction of local nerves).
- Local excision of axillary sweat glands.
- Sympathetic denervation:
  - Video-assisted endoscopic thoracic sympathectomy:
    —excision.
    —radioablation.
  - Sympathotomy (chain disconnection between T2 ganglion and stellate ganglion)

Further reading
Eisenach J, Atkinson J, and Fealey R (2005). Hyperhidrosis:evolving therapies for a well established phenomenon. *Mayo Clin Proc* **80**(5), 657–66.

Palpitations (often associated with sweating)
- Thyrotoxicosis.
- Hypoglycaemia (insulinoma).
- Phaeochromocytoma.

- Anxiety states.
- Cardiac arrhythmia.
- Caffeine excess.
- Alcohol/drug withdrawal.

General malaise, tiredness

- Addison's disease.
- Hypo- or hyperthyroidism.
- Hypogonadism.
- Hypopituitarism/GH deficiency.
- Osteomalacia.
- Diabetes mellitus.
- Cushing's syndrome.
- Anaemia.
- Drugs (prescription and recreational drugs):
  - Anti-histamines.
  - Anti-depressants.
  - Anti-hypertensives (β-blockers, methyl-dopa, clonidine).
  - Neuroleptics.
  - Corticosteroids.
- Malignancy.
- Chronic fatigue syndrome (may be associated with reduced cortisol output both basally and in response to a variety of challenges).
- Chronic illness (cardiac, respiratory, hepatic).
- Fibromyalgia.
- Depression.
- Sleep disorders (obstructive sleep apnoea).
- Infection.
- Musculo-skeletal/neurological disease (mysthaenia gravis).
- Toxins.
- Idiopathic.

Investigation of fatigue

- Careful history taking:
  - Duration, onset, recovery and type of fatigue.
  - Person's usual activity level.
- Clinical examination.
- Serum electrolytes.
- Haemoglobin ± serum ferritin level.
- Inflammatory markers (ESR, CRP).
- Liver function tests.
- Serum calcium and phosphate levels.
- Thyroid function tests.
- Short Synacthen® test.

Further reading

Cleare A (2003). The neuroendocrinology of chronic fatigue syndrome. *Endocrine Reviews* **24**(2), 236–52.

Cornuz J, Guessous I, and Favrat B (2006). Fatigue: a practical approach to diagnosis in primary care *CMAJ* **174**(6), 765–7.

Flushing

- Gonadal failure (with flushing and sweats).
- Drugs.
  - Chlorpropamide.
  - Nicotinic acid.
  - Anti-oestrogens.
  - LHRH agonists.
- Carcinoid (dry flushing—no sweats).
- Mastocytosis.
- Medullary thyroid cancer.
- Anaphylaxis.
- Pancreatic cell carcinoma.
- Phaeochromocytoma (more often pallor).
- Fever.
- Alcohol.
- Autonomic dysfunction.
- Some foods:
  - Fish.
  - Tyramine containing food (cheese).
  - Nitrites (cured meat).
  - Monosodium glutamate.
  - Spicy food.
- Gustatory flushing.
- Benign cutaneous flushing.
- Idiopathic.

Initial evaluation of patients with flushing

- Careful history.
- Physical examination (ideally during a flush although not often possible):
  - Examine skin carefully.
  - Pulse rate.
  - BP.
  - Thyroid examination.
  - Respiratory examination (wheeze).
  - Careful abdominal examination.
  - Urine dipstix.
- Biochemistry:
  - Gonadotrophin levels.
  - 2 × 24h urinary 5HIAA measurements.
  - Serum chromogranin A.
  - 2 × 24h urinary catecholamine measurements.
  - Plasma metanephrines (if high level of suspicion).
  - Serum tryptase level (if suspecting mastocytosis).
  - Calcitonin level (if suspecting medullary thyroid cancer).
  - Plasma VIP (if suspecting pancreatic carcinoma).
  - Immunoglobulin levels (raised IgE may suggest allergies).
- Specific investigations according to suspected diagnosis.

Management of flushing
- Treat the underlying cause.
- Nadolol (non-selective β-blocker) effective in some cases of benign cutaneous flushing.
- Somatostatin analogues can be used to treat flushing associated with carcinoid syndrome.
- Antihistamines may be effective in some histamine-secreting carcinoid tumours.

Further reading

Izikson L, English J, and Zirwas M (2006). The flushing patient:differential diagnosis, workup and treatment. *J Am Acad Derm* **55**(2), 193–208.

Stress and the endocrine system

Definition

Stress may be considered as a state of threatened or perceived as threatened homeostasis. The principal effectors of the stress response are corticotrophin releasing hormone (CRH), glucocorticoids (GCs), catecholamines, arginine vasopressin (AVP) and POMC derived peptides (esp.β-endorphins).

Allostasis is a state of dyshomeostasis occurring due to an inadequate, excessive or prolonged adaptive stress response.

Endocrine effects of stress

Hypothalamo-pituitary axis

- ↑ amplitude of synchronized pulsatile release of CRH and AVP (potent synergistic factor of CRH), into the hypophyseal portal system.
- ↑ stimulated ACTH production.
- ↑ adrenal glucocorticoid and androgen secretion.
- GCs also play a role in termination of the normal stress response by −ve feedback at the pituitary, hypothalamus, and extra hypothalamic regions.

Growth hormone axis

- GCs suppress GH production, and inhibit the effects of IGF-1 (thus, children with anxiety disorders may have short stature).
- CRH increases somatostatin production, inhibiting GH production.
- GH response to IV glucagon is blunted.

Thyroid axis

- GCs reduce the production of TSH, and limit the conversion of T_4 to the more active T_3 by reducing deiodinase activity.
- Somatostatin suppresses both TRH and TSH release.
- 📖 see sick euthyroid syndrome, p.xxx.

Reproductive axis

- CRH reduces GnRH secretion.
- GCs suppress GnRH neurons, pituitary gonadotrophs, and render the gonads resistant to gonadotrophins.
- GCs also render peripheral tissues resistant to oestradiol.
- Chronic stress leads to amenorrhoea in ♀ and low LH and testosterone in ♂.
- Oestrogens increase CRH expression via an oestrogen response element in the promoter region of the CRH gene. This may account for the sex related differences in the stress response and HPA axis activity.
- CRH is produced by the ovary, endometrium, and placenta during the latter half of pregnancy leading to physiological hypercortisolism.

Metabolism

- GCs via their direct effect, and via reduced GH and sex hormone activity, result in muscle and bone catabolism and fat anabolism.
- Chronic activation of the stress system is associated with ↑ visceral adiposity, ↓ lean body mass, and suppressed osteoblastic activity (which may ultimately lead to osteoporosis).
- GCs induce insulin resistance and other features of the metabolic syndrome.

Further reading

Charmandari E, Tsigos C, and Chrousos G (2005). Endocrinology of the stress response. *Annu Rev Physiol* **67**, 259–84.

Alternative or complementary therapy and endocrinology

Introduction

- Many patients use natural products alongside or instead of conventional therapy. Products and information are available from many sources but in particular the Internet.
- Patients need to be asked specifically about usage.
- Hospital pharmacists can be extremely helpful in sourcing information about natural products, including interactions with conventional medicines.
- Quality control of natural products is usually poor, with content ranging anywhere from 0% of stated level to several-fold higher.
- Safety data is often absent or inadequate.
- Discussion of any natural products listed here is not intended **in any way** to imply efficacy or safety of these products or to recommend their usage but rather to illustrate the compounds being promoted for these conditions by alternative information sources.

Alternative therapy used in patients with diabetes mellitus

A major concern with natural products used by patients with diabetes mellitus is of interaction with conventional medicines placing the patient at risk of hypoglycaemia.

Hypoglycaemic agents

These work by ↑ insulin secretion from the pancreas or due to direct insulin-like action at the insulin receptor.

- Banaba (*Lagerstroemia speciosa*)—crepe myrtle. Banaba extracts contain corosolic acid and ellagitannins, which may have direct insulin-like effects at insulin receptors.
- Bitter melon (*Momordica charantia*). Contains a polypeptide with insulin-like effects. Used as juice, powder, extracts, and fried food. Often part of Asian and Indian foods.
- Fenugreek (*Trigonella foenum-gracum*). Used as powder, seeds, or as part of dietary supplement. May enhance insulin release and may also decrease carbohydrate absorption due to laxative effect. May also inhibit platelets and thus increase bleeding diathesis.
- Gymnema (*Gymnema sylvestre*) 'gurmar' in Hindi ('sugar destroying'). Extract 'GS4' also used. May increase endogenous insulin secretion (↑ c-peptide levels noted in users). In some preliminary studies, gymnema improved HbA1c and ↓ insulin or OHA requirements.

Insulin sensitizers

- Cassia cinnamon (*Cinnamomum aromaticum*)—also known as Chinese cinnamon (Cinnamon verum is the usual cinnamon used in the UK although cassia cinnamon may be contained in ground cinnamon mixes). May increase insulin sensitivity and lower fasting blood glucose levels. Appears safe and well tolerated.
- Chromium. Chromium deficiency is associated with impaired glucose tolerance, hyperglycaemia, and ↓ insulin sensitivity. Chromium forms part of a 'glucose tolerance factor' complex and therefore supplements are sometimes labelled 'chromium GTF'. In patients with diabetes and chromium deficiency, addition of chromium improves glycaemic control. However the role of chromium in patients without deficiency is not clear. The American Diabetes Association only recommends chromium usage in patients with documented chromium deficiency. Excessive chromium may cause renal impairment.
- Vanadium. Thought to stimulate hepatic glycogenolysis, inhibit gluconeogenesis, lipolysis, and intestinal glucose transport; increase skeletal muscle glucose uptake, utilization and glycogenolysis. High dose vanadium (taken as vanadyl sulfate) may improve insulin sensitivity and glycaemic control in patients with type 2 diabetes, with large doses of elemental vanadium required for these effects—however, doses >1.8mg/day vanadium may cause renal impairment.
- Ginseng (both Panax ginseng and American ginseng (*Panax quinquefolius*)). Contain ginsenoisides which may improve insulin sensitivity. Efficacy and safety not established.

- Prickly pear cactus (*Opuntia ficus-indica*), also called opuntia or 'nopals' (referring to the cooked leaves of the cactus). Prominent in Mexican folk medicine as a treatment for diabetes. *Opuntia streptacantha* stems may improve glycaemic control either acting as an insulin senstitizer or by slowing carbohydrate absorption; however this is not observed with other prickly pear cactus species.

Carbohydrate absorption inhibitors

- *Soluble fibre.* Increases viscosity of intestinal contents thus slowing gastric emptying time and carbohydrate absorption, resulting in lower postprandial blood glucose levels.
- The following products have some evidence of reducing post prandial blood glucose levels and may also improve total and LDL cholesterol levels in patients. They may also interfere with absorption of drugs, and therefore should not be taken at the same time as conventional medicines:
  - Blond psyllium seed (*Plantago ovata*).
  - Guar gum (*Cyamopsis tetragonoloba*).
  - Oat bran (*Avena sativa*).
  - Soy (*Glycine max*)—contains both soluble and insoluble fibre and may improve insulin resistance, fasting BM, lipid profile, and HbA1c in type 2 diabetes.
- *Insoluble fibre.* Glucomannan (*Amorphophallus konjac*)—can delay glucose absorption.

Other products used by patients with diabetes mellitus

- Alpha-lipoic acid. Anti-oxidant. May improve insulin resistance. May help symptoms of diabetic neuropathy (?mechanism).
- Stevia (*Stevia rebaudiana*)—may enhance insulin secretion. May be toxic.

Alternative therapy used in menopause

Phytoestrogens

- Main types are isoflavones (most potent and most widespread), lignans and coumestans.
- Sources:
  - Isoflavones: legumes (soy, chickpea, garbanzo beans, red clover, lentils, beans). Main active isoflavones are genistein and daidzein.
  - Lignans: flaxseed, lentils, whole grains, beans, many fruits and vegetables
  - Coumestans: red clover, sunflower seeds, sprouts
- Other phytoestrogens: chasteberry (vitex agnus-castus)
- Not structurally similar to oestrogen or to selective oestrogen receptor modulators (SERMs) but contain a phenolic ring that allows binding to oestrogen receptors-α and -β. Effects of binding depend upon ambient oestrogen levels, relative ratio and concentration of ER-α and ER-β; tissue type and location. Relatively much less potent than endogenous oestrogen (by 100–10000-fold).
- Phytoestrogens in vitro stimulate proliferation of normal human breast tissue and of oestrogen-sensitive breast tumour cells. Theoretically, phytoestrogens may stimulate ER+ breast cancer and other oestrogen-sensitive tumours. Phytoestrogens may also antagonize the effects of tamoxifen or other SERMs. Phytoestrogens have not been shown to stimulate endometrial growth; however they are not usually taken with progestogenic compounds. It is not known whether the other serious side effects of conventional oestrogens (e.g. DVT, pulmonary emboli, IHD, stroke) occur with phytoestrogen use. Many sources of phytoestrogens (e.g. coumestans) interfere with warfarin.
- Soy protein (20–60mg/day; containing 34–76mg isoflavones) modestly decreases frequency and severity of vasomotor symptoms in a proportion of menopausal women.
- Synthetic isoflavones (ipriflavone) do not have antivasomotor activity.
- Phytoestrogens from red clover have not shown consistent improvement in vasomotor symptoms. Other sources of phytoestrogens have not shown improvement in menopausal symptoms.
- 📖 for use in osteoporosis see Alternative therapy used by patients with osteoporosis, pp.720–721.

Other compounds with oestrogenic activity

- Kudzu (*Pueraria lobata*).
- Alfalfa (*Medicago sativa*).
- Hops (*Humulus lupulus*).
- Licorice (*Glycyrrhiza glabra*).
- *Panax ginseng* (ginseng)—in vitro evidence of stimulation of breast cancer cells.

Other substances used

- Black cohosh (*Actaea racemosa*, formerly *Cimicifuga racemosa*)—not to be confused with blue cohash and white cohash which are entirely separate plants). Widely used in menopause. Although often advertised as such, black cohash does not bind to oestrogen receptors or have oestrogen effects and little evidence for efficacy for hot flushes.
- Dong quai (*Angelica sinensis*)—not clear if oestrogenic. In vitro evidence of promotion of breast cancer cells.

Alternative therapy used by patients with osteoporosis

Calcium
- Hundreds of preparations available.
- Several types of calcium salts available (including citrate, carbonate, lactate, gluconate, phosphate) with little evidence of superiority of absorption etc. between different compounds, other than calcium citrate useful in patients with low gastric acidity (e.g. on concomitant proton pump inhibitors or H2 antagonists).

Magnesium
- Necessary for release of PTH.
- In itself not effective in treating osteoporosis unless patients are deficient in magnesium.

Fluoride
Increases bone density but not strength—bones less elastic, more brittle—with resultant ↑ fracture rate.

Trace elements
- E.g. manganese, zinc, boron, copper.
- Whilst many trace elements are important for multiple enzyme systems including those in bone, most patients are not deficient and thus supplements have negligible +ve effect upon osteoporosis. Moreover, many minerals in high doses cause serious side effects (e.g. manganese doses >11mg/day can cause extrapyramidal side-effects).

Vitamin D
Multiple preparations available, mainly as ergocalciferol or colecalciferol (vitamin D metabolites require prescription). Tablets containing >200IU Vitamin D require a prescription in the UK.

Isoflavones
- 📖 see Alternative therapy used in menopause, p.718, for more detail about phytoestrogens' mechanism of action.
- Soy protein in doses >80mg/day may improve bone mineral density but no studies of soy have shown improvement in fracture rate. Possible adverse effects upon oestrogen-sensitive tissues such as ER-+ve breast cancer.
- Ipriflavone—semisynthetic isoflavone, produced from daidzein. No oestrogenic effects. No evidence of improved fracture outcome. Some studies of ipriflavone with calcium have reported improved BMD although other studies have not shown an improvement. Ipriflavone can cause serious lymphopaenia (<1 × 10^{9}mL) which may take up to a year to recover.

Tea
- Tea consists of green tea (unfermented), oolong tea (partially fermented), and black tea (completely fermented).

- All teas contain fluoride and have high isoflavonoid content in addition to caffeine.
- Coffee (with a high caffeine content) has been associated with ↑ hip fracture risk. However, tea drinking of all types of has been associated with higher BMD, although no fracture outcome has been reported.

DHEA

📖 see Miscellaneous, p.722.

Wild yam

Wild yam contains diosgenin which is used commercially as a source for DHEA synthesis; however this does not occur in humans.

Other compounds used by patients for osteoporosis

- Flaxseed (alphalinolenic acid and lignans).
- Gelatin.
- Dong quai.
- *Panax ginseng*.
- Alfalfa.
- Licorice.

There is no evidence of a +ve effect upon bone of these compounds.

Miscellaneous

Iodine and the thyroid

- Sources: kelp, shellfish-derived products.
- Effects: iodine-induced goitre or hypothyroidism, particularly in patients with underlying thyroid disease (may have a Wolff–Chaikoff effect in patients with Graves' disease, causing inhibition of iodide organification and thus thyroid hormone production).
- Iodine-induced hyperthyroidism in areas of endemic goitre and iodine deficiency.

DHEA—'elixir of youth'

- Reported to slow or improve changes associated with ageing, including general wellbeing, cognitive function, sexual function, energy levels, body composition, muscle strength, and to aid weight loss and treat the metabolic syndrome.
- Mechanism of action: DHEA is secreted by the adrenal glands and interconverted to DHEAS. Both DHEAS and DHEA are converted to androgens and oestrogens that then act directly at their receptors.
- DHEA and DHEAS may play a role in replacement of adrenal androgens in patients with adrenal insufficiency, resulting in improved wellbeing particularly with respect to sexual function.
- Not proven in controlled trials to improve health in other patients without adrenal insufficiency.
- Risks of androgenic effects in women when taken at high doses (100–200mg/DHEA daily). Theoretical risk of promoting hormone-sensitive cancers such as prostate and breast cancers. DHEA may also interfere with anti-oestrogen effects of anastrazole and other aromatase inhibitors.

Further information

Natural Medicines Comprehensive Database; available at ⬚ www.naturaldatabase.com (requires subscription).

Classification and diagnosis

Background

Diabetes mellitus (DM) is characterized by an elevated blood glucose. The classification of diabetes gives an idea of the underlying cause or defect. Currently 2–6% of the UK population have diabetes but only 1/2 to 2/3 are thought to be diagnosed. Worldwide 189 million people were known to have diabetes in 2003 and this may reach 324 million by 2025.

Diagnosis

DM is a biochemical diagnosis based on fasting and post prandial glucose levels in a 75g OGTT, the venous plasma glucose levels for this are shown in Table 111.1 (p.726). In 1997 the American Diabetes Association (ADA) suggested lowering the normal fasting plasma glucose level to <6.0mmol/L and the diabetic level to >7.0mmol/L. The aim of this was to reduce the need for an OGTT and the 2h post glucose load measurement. A fasting glucose is therefore the diagnostic test of choice and only pregnant ♀ would expect to have a 2h postprandial level checked routinely. A diagnosis of diabetes is made in any symptomatic person with a random blood glucose >11.1mmol/L. Asymptomatic patients or those with intercurrent illness would still require a further abnormal result before a diagnosis of diabetes could be made.

> **Box 111.1 Current classification of diabetes**
>
> *Type 1 (5–25% of cases): pancreatic islet β cell deficiency*
> - Autoimmune – associated with autoantibodies to islet autoantigens (glutamate decarboxylase (GAD), IA-2 and insulin)
> - Idiopathic
>
> *Type 2 (75–95% of cases): defective insulin action or secretion*
> - Insulin resistance.
> - Insulin secretory defect.
>
> *Others*
> - Genetic defects of βcell function:
>   - Maturity onset diabetes of the young (MODY).
>   - Chromosome 20, HNF4β(MODY 1).
>   - Chromosome 7, glucokinase (MODY 2).
>   - Chromosome 12, HNF1α (MODY 3).
>   - Chromosome 13, IPF-1 (MODY 4).
>   —mitochondrial DNA 3242 mutation
>   —mutations associated with neonatal diabetes (KIR6.2, SUR).
>   - Others.
> - Genetic defects of insulin action:
>   - Type A insulin resistance.

- Leprechaunism (type 2 diabetes, intrauterine growth retardation + dysmorphic features).
  - Rabson–Mendenhall syndrome (DM + pineal hyperplasia + acanthosis nigricans).
  - Lipoatrophic diabetes.
  - Others.
- Diseases of the exocrine pancreas:
  - Pancreatitis.
  - Trauma/surgery (pancreatectomy).
  - Neoplasia.
  - Pancreatic destruction, e.g. cystic fibrosis, haemochromatosis.
  - Others.
- Endocrinopathies:
  - Cushing's syndrome.
  - Acromegaly.
  - Phaeochromocytoma.
  - Glucagonoma.
  - Hyperthyroidism.
  - Somatostatinoma.
  - Others.
- Drug or chemical induced.
- Infections:
  - Congenital rubella or cytomegalovirus (CMV).
  - Others.
- Uncommon forms of immune-mediated diabetes:
  - Anti-insulin receptor antibodies.
  - Stiff man syndrome (type 1 diabetes, rigidity of muscles, painful spasms).
  - Others.
- Other genetic syndromes associated with diabetes:
  - Down syndrome.
  - Klinefelter syndrome.
  - Lawrence–Moon–Biedl syndrome.
  - Myotonic dystrophy.
  - Prader–Willi syndrome.
  - Turner syndrome.
  - Wolfram syndrome (or DIDMOAD – diabetes insipidus, DM, optic atrophy + sensorineural deafness).
  - Others.
- Gestational diabetes.

Classification

The first accepted classification of diabetes was drawn up by WHO and modified in 1985 (☐ see Table 111.1). The original classification into insulin dependent DM (IDDM) or type 1 and non-insulin dependent DM (NIDDM) or type 2 is now no longer used but is still seen in non-diabetes literature.

The current classification includes both clinical stage and aetiology and has been used since 1997. The clinical staging is from normal glucose tolerance through impaired glucose tolerance (IGT) and/or impaired fasting hyperglycaemia (IFG) and on to frank DM, which is split into non-insulin requiring, insulin requiring for control, and insulin requiring for survival. The aetiological groups are listed in Box 111.1.

Table 111.1 WHO classification

		Venous plasma glucose (mmol/L)
Normal	Fasting	<6.0
	and	
	2h post-prandial	<7.8
Diabetes	Fasting	>7.0
	or	
	2h post-prandial	>11.1
IGT	Fasting	<7.0
	and	
	2h post-prandial	7.8–11.1
IFG	Fasting	6.0–6.9

Table 111.2 Differences between type 1 and type 2 diabetes

	Type 1 diabetes	Type 2 diabetes
Peak age of onset	12 years	60 years
UK prevalence	0.25%	5–7% (10% of those >65 years of age)
Aetiology	Autoimmune	Combination of insulin resistance, β cell destruction and β cell dysfunction
Initial presentation	Polyuria, polydypsia, and weight loss with ketoacidosis	Hyperglycaemic symptoms but often with complication of diabetes
Treatment	Diet and insulin from outset	Diet with or without oral hypoglycaemic agents or insulin

Genetics

Type 1 patients

The overall lifetime risk in a white population of developing type 1 diabetes is only 0.4%, but this rises to:

- 1–2% if your mother has it.
- 3–6% if your father has it.
- Siblings have about a 6% risk.
- Monozygotic twins have a 36% concordance rate.

Islet cell antibodies are seen in 3% of Oxford schoolchildren but in 40% of monozygotic twins and 6% of siblings of type 1 patients. A genetic predisposition is therefore suggested, but this also highlights the importance of environmental triggers as not all those with antibodies go on to get diabetes. Genetic predisposition accounts for 1/3 of susceptibility to type 1 diabetes.

Although several different regions of the human genome are linked to the development of type 1 diabetes, the most common are the major histocompatibility complex (MHC) antigens/human leukocyte antigens (HLA). >90% of patients with type 1 diabetes in this country have either HLA-DR3, DR4, or both. Certain variants of the *DQB1* or *DQA1* gene result in the expression of susceptible alleles of DR3/DR4. Interestingly this association is not true in all races, notably the Japanese.

There are currently 10 distinct genetic areas (IDDM1–IDDM10) known to be linked to type 1 diabetes; some relate to MHC genes, others to the insulin gene region. MHC antigens commonly found in those with type 1 diabetes, and felt to predispose to it, are B15, B8, and DQ8. The DR2, DQ6, and DQ18 genes appear to be protective. Linkage studies have suggested type 1 susceptibility genes on chromosomes:

- 6q (also known as IDDM5).
- 11p (IDDM2).
- 11q (IDDM4).
- 15q (IDDM3).

These genetic variations may help to explain susceptibility, but their link to the ↑ levels of islet cell antibodies, anti-glutamate decarboxylase (GAD) antibodies, and anti-tyrosine phosphatase antibodies (anti-IA-2 antibodies) often seen soon after diagnosis is less clearly decided. These 3 antibodies, if all are present, give a non-diabetic individual an 88% chance of developing type 1 diabetes in the next 10 years.

Maturity onset diabetes of the young (MODY)

The genes known to be involved in MODY are gradually ↑ as our understanding of insulin signalling and receptors expands.

MODY 1 (HNF4α)

- Accounts for <0.0001% of all type 2 patients and about 5% of cases of MODY.
- Usually presents in adolescence or early adulthood <25 years of age
- Can give severe hyperglycaemia with 20% needing insulin therapy and 40% oral agents
- Results in a high frequency of microvascular complications.
- Inherited as an autosomal dominant with a defect on chromosome 20q resulting in altered activity of the hepatic nuclear factor (HNF)4α gene which is a +ve regulator of HNF1α. This is a transcription factor found in the liver and β cells of the pancreas where it acts as a transactivater of the insulin gene in rat models.

MODY 2 (glucokinase)

- Accounts for <0.2% of type 2 patients and 10–14% of cases of MODY.
- Presents in early childhood
- Gives only mild hyperglycaemia and therefore infrequent microvascular complications with 90% controlled on diet alone and insulin usually only needed when they become pregnant.
- Autosomally dominantly inherited with a defect in the glucokinase gene on chromosome 7 resulting in altered glucose sensing in the β cells of the pancreas and impaired hepatic production of glycogen.

MODY 3 (HNF1α)

- Affects 1–2% of type 2 patients and accounts for 70% of MODY patients.
- Presents in adolescence or early adulthood (peaks around 21 years of age).
- Causes severe hyperglycaemia and frequent microvascular complications; 1/3 require insulin therapy and 1/3 require oral agents.
- Linked to a mutation on chromosome 12q24 which directly alters HNF1 α activity. How this causes type 2 diabetes is not fully understood.

MODY 4 (IPF-1)

- Accounts for <1% of cases of MODY.
- A mutation in transcription factor gene *IPF 1* which in its homozygous form leads to total pancreatic agenesis.
- MODY 5 (HNF1-β).
- Accounts for 3% of cases of MODY.
- Average age of presentation 22 years associated with renal cysts (RCAD—renal cysts and diabetes) often with uterine abnormalities, gout and insulin resistance.

Type 2 patients

In patients with type 2 diabetes the concordance between monozygotic twins for diabetes is much higher (60–100%, vs. 36% for type 1) but the rate amongst dizygotic twins is much less, suggesting a much stronger genetic element in its aetiology than for type 1 diabetes. Unlike patients with type 1 diabetes, however, those with type 2 do not seem to have the same HLA-linked genes. In most families this appears to be polygenic, although the much less common MODY is autosomal dominant but only accounts for a few percent of all type 2 patients. MODY is currently split into 4 types, with type 4 accounting for 15% of cases and currently accounting for those that do not fit into types 1–3, although a chromosome 13 defect in the insulin promoter factor 1 gene may fall into this group.

Other recognized genetic subtypes of type 2 diabetes include *mitochondrial diabetes*, which affects 1–3% of type 2 patients and is maternally transmitted. It is associated with deafness and other neurological abnormalities. *Insulin resistance* is an important part of type 2 diabetes and rare genetic defects causing this are recognized. A 40% reduction in the biological effect of any given insulin molecule is suggested by clamp studies in type 2 patients, but these rarer genetic syndromes may result in a more severe picture.

Further reading

Alberti KGMM, Zimmet PZ, for the WHO consultation (1998). Definition, diagnosis and classification of DM and its complications. Part 1: Diagnosis and classification of DM. Provisional report of a WHO consultation. *Diabet Med* **15**, 539–53.

Alcolado JC and Thomas AW (1995). Maternally inherited DM: the role of mitochondrial DNA defects. *Diabetic Med* **12**(2),102–8.

Hattersley AT (1996). Maturity onset diabetes of the young (MODY). *Baillière Clin Paediatr* **4**(4), 663–80.

Robinson S and Kessling A (1992). Diabetes secondary to genetic disorders. *Baillière Clin Endocrinol Metab* **6**, 867–98.

World Health Organization (1985). *Diabetes Mellitus: Report of a WHO study Group.* (Technical report Series no. 727). World Health Organization: Geneva.

World Health Organization (1999). *Definition, Diagnosis and Classification of Diabetes Mellitus and its complications. Report of a WHO Consultation. Part 1, Diagnosis and Classification of Diabetes Mellitus.* World Health Organization: Geneva.

General management and treatment

Background

After diagnosis all patients with diabetes need to see a dietitian and a diabetes nurse specialist and have a full medical assessment. The first priority is to decide whether this is a person with type 1 or type 2 diabetes as the former needs insulin immediately while the later need initial dietary advice, which should always take into account the patient's circumstances and culture and be individually tailored in order to be achievable.

Assessment of the newly diagnosed patient

History
- Duration of symptoms, e.g. thirst, polyuria, weight loss.
- Possible 2° causes of diabetes, e.g. Acromegaly.
- Family history.
- Presence of complications of diabetes.
- Risk factors for developing complications e.g. smoking, hypertension, hyperlipidaemia.

Examination
- BMI.
- Clues for 2° causes.
- Cardiovascular system—especially BP + peripheral pulses.
- Signs of autonomic and peripheral neuropathy.
- Eyes—for retinopathy.

Investigations
Initial investigations will be modified by the history and examination but as a minimum should include:
- Blood tests for urea and electrolytes, liver and thyroid function, and a full lipid profile
- Urine tests for ketones, macro- and (if –ve) microalbuminuria.
- An ECG in all patients with type 2 diabetes.

Treatment

In patients with type 1 diabetes, insulin therapy is mandatory along with dietary advice and standard diabetes education. The education of all newly diagnosed patients is intended to provide an incentive for good compliance. A full education package should include:

- An explanation as to what diabetes is and what it means to the patient.
- Aims of treatment, e.g. rationale of reducing complications and exact values to aim for.
- Types of—not just drugs but also dietary advice and lifestyle modification such as ↑ physical activity, stopping smoking, and reducing alcohol intake.
- Self monitoring, e.g. both the method(s) of doing this, the reasons for doing it, and what to do with the results.
- An idea of some chronic complications of diabetes and what to look out for, e.g. a podiatrist's input and review is advised, especially for those with type 2 diabetes.
- Advice regarding DVLA, insurance companies, and Diabetes U.K.

All patients with type 2 diabetes should be considered for such an educational package. In most the next step is to try diet, exercise, and weight reduction (if obese, which most will be) before initiating drug therapy if control is not adequate. If this fails to improve control adequately after 3 months, consider oral therapy with *metformin* in the overweight and *sulfonylureas* in the lean if there are no contraindications.

After the initial assessment all patients should be put into a formal review system, whether by their GP or in a hospital diabetic clinic, for further education, maintenance of good control, and complication screening.

Dietary advice

In the overweight patient (e.g. BMI >25) a reduction in total calorie intake to aid weight reduction is also required. A standard diabetic diet should aim to have

- <10% of its energy in the form of saturated fat (<8% if hyperlipidaemic).
- <30% from all fats.
- 50–60% as carbohydrate which is mostly complex high fibre.
- Sugar limited to about 25g/day.
- Sodium content <6g/day in most people or <3g/day if hypertensive.

Alcohol is a significant source of calories, and a reduction in the overweight or hypertriglyceridaemic patient is advisable.

The current 'standard' diet for a person with diabetes is a weight reducing low fat low glycaemic index diet with a reduction in sodium content, as most patients will have type 2 diabetes and are slightly overweight, this needs to be modified to the individual however.

Oral hypoglycaemic agents

Sulfonylureas (Table 112.1)

These agents are used as 1st-line treatment in non-obese patients with type 2 diabetes.
- The 1st generation agents *chlorpropamide*, *tolbutamide*, and *tolazamide* are rarely used today.
- 2nd generation agents such as *glibenclamide*, *gliclazide*, and *glipizide* are now more commonly used.
- 3rd generation agents such as *glimepiride* are also available.

Mode of action

Sulfonylureas act by stimulating a receptor on the surface of β cells, closing a potassium channel, and opening a calcium channel with subsequent insulin release. A doubling of glucose-stimulated insulin secretion can be expected with both 1st and 2nd phase insulin secretion affected. This results in a 1–2% reduction in HbA1c long term.

Side effects

These are hypoglycaemia and weight gain. In the UK Prospective Diabetes Study (UKPDS) the mean weight gain seen after 10 years of therapy was 2.3kg while the incidence of major hypoglycaemic events was 0.4–0.6%/year. The elderly are particularly at risk of hypoglycaemia with the longer acting agents such as glibenclamide and these should be avoided in that age group. Occasional skin reactions, alterations in liver function tests, and minor gastrointestinal symptoms may occur. Also avoid sulfonylureas in porphyria.

Biguanides (Table 112.2)

Metformin is 1st-line therapy in the obese or overweight people with type 2 diabetes and is also used in some insulin-treated, insulin-resistant, overweight subjects to reduce insulin requirements. The UKPDS showed significantly better results from metformin for complications and mortality compared to other therapies in the overweight patient with type 2 diabetes. Although a 1–2 kg weight loss is seen initially, UKPDS data suggests it does not significantly alter weight over a 10-year period.

Mode of action

Metformin works by ↓ hepatic gluconeogenesis and ↑ muscle glucose uptake/metabolism, so ↑ insulin sensitivity. With long term use a 0.8–2.0% reduction in HbA1c can be expected.

Table 112.1 Properties of sulfonylureas

Sulfonylurea	Length of action	Begins working within	Daily dose (mg)
Glibenclamide	16–24h	2–4h	2.5–15
Gliclazide	10–24h	2–4h	40–320
Glipizide	6–24h	2–4h	2.5–20
Chlorpropamide	24–72h	2–4h	100–500
Tolbutamide	6–10h	2–4h	500–2000
Glimepiride	12–24h	2–4h	1–6

Table 112.2 Biguanides and prandial glucose regulators

Drug	Length of action	Begins working within	Daily dose (mg)
Metformin	24–36h	2.5h	500–2000
Repaglinide	4–6h	<1h	0.5–16
Nateglinide	4h	<1h	180–540

Side-effects/contraindications

Contraindicated in patients with renal (creatinine >140nmol/L), hepatic, or cardiac impairment, or who consume significant amounts of alcohol. GI side-effects include nausea, epigastric discomfort, and diarrhoea and occur in up to 1/2 of patients in the first 1–2 weeks of treatment, but are usually transient. If the starting dose is low (e.g. 500mg once daily) most people develop a tolerance to these and are able to take higher doses; <5% are totally intolerant. Rarely skin rashes and lactic acidosis occur. The latter, when seen, is usually in patients with hepatic, renal, or cardiac impairment. Using radiological contrast media with metformin is associated with an ↑ risk of lactic acidosis and therapy should be stopped at the time of or prior to such investigations and restarted 2 days after the test unless renal function has been affected by the procedure in which case delay until this has resolved. Lactic acidosis occurs very infrequently e.g. 0.024–0.15 cases/1000 patient years in a Swedish study. *Phenformin* was used in the past but was withdrawn due to an ↑ risk of lactic acidosis. Although it is known to reduce folic acid and vitamin B_{12} absorption this is not usually a significant problem clinically with metformin.

Prandial glucose regulators (Table 112.2)

These agents can be used in type 2 patients who have inadequate control on diet or metformin, predominantly targeting post prandial hyperglycaemia due to their short duration of action.

Repaglinide, a carbamoylmethyl benzoic acid derivative, is a non-sulfonylurea oral hypoglycaemic agent which stimulates the secretion of insulin from pancreatic β cells. It works on separate parts of the β cell sulfonylurea receptor from the sulfonylureas. Its use results in an approximate 0.6–2% reduction in HbA1c levels. Its very short duration of action reduces the risk of hypoglycaemia compared to some sulfonylureas. It has an insulinotropic effect within 30min of oral administration and a return to normal insulin levels within 4–6h (elimination half-life is around 1h). It should not, however, be used in patients with renal or hepatic impairment and may result in hepatic dysfunction so periodic liver function test monitoring is required.

Nateglinide is a D-phenylalanine derivative with an insulinotropic effect within 15min of oral administration and a return to normal insulin levels by 2h (elimination half-life 1.5h), so reducing the risk of subsequent hypoglycaemia. Efficacy is similar to repaglinide.

α-glucosidase inhibitors

Used in type 2 patients who have inadequate control on diet or other oral agent alone. When taken with food acarbose reduces post prandial glucose peaks by inhibiting the digestive enzyme α-glucosidase which normally breaks carbohydrates into their monosaccharide components, thus retarding glucose uptake from the intestine and reducing postprandial glucose peaks. Some improvement in lipids has also been reported.

These undigested carbohydrates then pass into the large intestine where bacteria metabolize them, which may explain the common side-effects of postprandial fullness/bloating, abdominal pain, flatulence, and diarrhoea.

Starting at 50mg once daily and gradually ↑ the dose at 2–3 weekly intervals to a maximum of 200mg 3 times per day, improves tolerance to this therapy. Less commonly, jaundice and elevated hepatic transaminase levels can also be seen. In the UK PDS adding *acarbose* to other therapies resulted in a further 0.5% drop in HbA1c.

Table 112.3 Oral hypogylcaemic agents: summary

Class	Mechanism of action	Expected reduction in HbA1c (%)
Sulfonylureas	Stimulate pancreatic insulin secretion	1.5–2.5
Biguanides	Increases muscle glucose uptake and metabolism; decreases hepatic gluconeogenesis	0.8–2.0
Prandial glucose regulators	Stimulate pancreatic insulin secretion	0.5–1.9
α-Glucosidase inhibitors	Inhibits a digestive enzyme	0.4–0.7
Thiazolidinediones	Activate PPAR-γ receptor	0.6–1.5

Thiazolidinediones

This class of drugs act as insulin sensitizing agents by activating the peroxisome proliferator activated receptor (PPAR-γ) which stimulates gene transcription for glucose transporter molecules such as Glut 1 and Glut 4. The first of this class was *troglitazone* which was withdrawn soon after its UK launch because of reports of hepatotoxicity but was still used in other countries until newer agents were available. Other agents such as *rosiglitazone* and *pioglitazone*, are available in the UK giving a 0.6–1.5% drop in HbA1c. These do not seem to have the same problem with hepatotoxicity, and there is often an improvement in liver function, especially with non-alcoholic steatohepatitis (NASH). Although the risk of hepatic dysfunction is not high initial checks of liver function and monitoring of liver function test are still currently advised. In view of the more common problem with fluid retention avoidance in heart failure is also strongly suggested. The indication for using these agents varies around the world and in the UK they are used in combining with 2 other oral agents but not with insulin while this combination is licensed in the USA. Recent studies suggest a link with osteoporosis with both the currently available agents and a possible link to cardiovascular disease/myocardial infarction with rosiglitazone which must be considered when selecting patients for these agents. The weight gain seen with both agents is also important when considering the best therapy for any patient.

Indications

Type 2 diabetes, oral combination with metformin or a sulfonylurea or a meglitinide

Dose

- Rosiglitazone 4–8 mg/day (combination metformin and rosiglitazone tablets are also available, either 2mg or 4mg rosiglitazone with 500 mg or 1g metformin per tablet)
- Pioglitazone 15–45mg/day (combination metformin and pioglitazone as 15mg pioglitazone and 850mg metformin per tablet)

Side-effects

- Fluid retention.
- Weight gain.
- Hepatotoxicity.

The incretin system (GLP-1 mimetics and DPP4 inhibitors)

Glucagon like polypeptide-1 (GLP-1) and GI polypeptide (PIP) are hormomes made in the L-cells of the jejunum and ileum in response to a food load entering the GI tract. These incretin hormones stimulates glucose-dependent insulin secretion, suppresses glucagons secretion and slows gastric emptying with an improvement in insulin sensitivity. Exenatide is a GLP-1 mimetic. Dipeptidyl peptidase-4 (DPP-4) breaks down GIP and GLP-1 and this enzyme can be inhibited by oral drugs such as sitagliptin and vildagliptin (i.e. DPP-4 inhibitors) with a resultant 0.4–0.7% reduction in HbA1c over a 12 month period and are weight neutral if not helping to reduce weight. Liver monitoring with vildagliptin is currently recommended. The GLP-1 mimetic exenatide is available and is taken as a twice daily injection of 5mcg or 10mcg per dose with a 0.6–0.8% reduction in HbA1c after 30 weeks' use and a 1.6–2.8kg weight loss over the same period. Several depot preparations of GLP-1 analogues/mimetics are in development.

Indications

- Sitagliptin/vildagliptin—type 2 diabetes, combination with metformin or thiazolidinediones
- Exenatide—type 2 diabetes, combination with metformin or sulphonylurea or both.

Dose

- Sitagliptin 100mg/day orally.
- Vildagliptin 100mg/day orally.
- Exenatide 5–10 mcg twice daily by injection.

Side effects

- Sitagliptin—GI disturbance, upper respiratory tract infection, nasopharyngitis, peripheral oedema.
- Vildagliptin—as sitagliptin + abnormal liver function tests.
- Exenatide:
  - GI upset with nausea, vomiting, abdominal distension, diarrhoea.
  - Headache, dizziness and increase sweating.
  - Injection site reactions.

Insulin

Insulin is required in all patients with type 1 diabetes, and some with type 2, for the preservation of life; in other patients with type 2 diabetes it is needed to achieve better glycaemic/metabolic control or for the relief of hyperglycaemic symptoms. Most insulin is in a biosynthetic human form (from yeast or bacteria) at a standard concentration: U100 (100 units/mL). Some countries still supply U40 and U80 strengths, so care should be taken with patients from abroad. There is also a sizable minority of patients taking bovine or porcine insulins. Bovine insulin is extracted from cattle pancreas and is more antigenic than both human and porcine alternatives and so gives more lipohypertrophy and lipoatrophy.

Insulin can be given by IV or SC routes, and more recently short-acting insulin was also given as an inhaled formulation, but this was recently withdrawn. Standard insulins come as 10mL vials for use with a 0.5mL or 1.0mL syringe or as 3.0mL cartridges for use in pen devices. The insulin itself is un-modified/neutral or mixed with agents such as protamine or zinc to alter its onset of action, peak effect, and duration of action. Analogues of human insulin to give more rapid onset or greater duration of action are also widely available and used. There are >30 types of insulin preparation available, which should allow full 24h cover for a wide variety of lifestyles.

The main problems with all insulin regimens are weight gain and hypoglycaemia. The latter occurring overnight can be troublesome, especially as the patient may not know it has occurred and may just reacts to the morning hyperglycaemia by ↑ their evening insulin dose. Occasional checks of 3 a.m. blood glucose levels may help sort this out. Care with alcohol and adjustments of insulin and pre-bed snacks if nocturnal physical activity such as sex is on the cards will also reduce nocturnal hypos.

Types of insulin

Short-acting (soluble/neutral) insulins

Unmodified or neutral insulins are short acting but are not identical. Humulin® S has an onset 30min after injection with a peak onset at 2–3h and a duration of up to 6–8h. Hypurin® Porcine Neutral has an onset 60min after injection with a peak at 2–5h and a duration of 6–8h. All the soluble human formulations require a 20–30min interval between injecting and eating to be maximally effective.

Insulin analogues

Insulin *lispro* (Humalog®) insulin a*spart* (NovoRapid®) and insulin *glulisine* (Apidra®) have been modified to allow injecting and eating to occur simultaneously as they have a more rapid onset of action and earlier peak effect with peak blood insulin level approximately 1.5–2.5 times that from the same dose of standard neutral human insulin. The duration of action is also shorter at 5h and this may cause problems if there are long gaps between meals

Long-acting analogues insulin g*largine* (Lantus®) and insulin de*temir* (Levemir®), are also available which give a flatter profile with a duration of action of 22–24 hours. These can be used as part of a basal bolus regimen with short-acting analogues or standard soluble insulins. They appear to have less hypoglycaemia than other background insulins and may reduce the risk of nocturnal hypoglycaemia. Their use as a once-daily insulin alone or in combination with oral agents such as glimepiride or the prandial glucose regulators is also proving popular in the elderly type 2 patient.

While insulin glargine has a slightly longer duration of action making it a popular once-daily preparation insulin detemir, because of its albumin binding properties is reported to give less between dose variability in the same individual and with a duration of action of 20–22 hours may be used in similar situations, although a significant proportion of people need to use this twice daily.

Table 112.4 Suggested aims of treatment

Fasting blood glucose	<7mmol/L
HbA1c	<7.2% (or <6.5% in those with significant complications)
Blood pressure	<140/80mmHg
Body mass index	20–25 ideally
Home monitoring	Capillary blood glucose estimations fasting, pre-meal, 2h postprandially and pre bed. These will need to be frequent enough to allow alterations in treatment and assessment of adequate control. Often adequate with 3x week in stable type 2 patients and daily in stable type 1 patients.

Table 112.5 Insulin: summary

Type of insulin	Examples	Peak activity (h)	Duration of action (h)
Insulin analogue	Humalog® (insulin lispro)	0–2	3–4
	(NovoRapid®) Insulin Aspart	1–3	3–4
Short acting	Human Actrapid®	1–3	6–8
	Humulin® S	2–3	6–8
Intermediate acting	Human Insulatard®	2–8	10–16
	Humulin® I	2–8	10–16
	Human Monotard®	3–12	18–24
	Humulin® Zn	4–8	<24
Long acting	Human Ultratard®	6–24	<36

Intermediate acting (isophane) insulins

Insulin action can be extended by addition of protamine to give isophane insulin, with an onset of action 1–2h after injection, a peak at 4–6h, and a duration of action of 8–14h. Different preparations have slightly different profiles when looking at peak effect and maximal insulin concentrations as with soluble preparations.

Biphasic/mixed insulins

Combinations of soluble/neutral or short acting analogues with isophane insulins are extremely popular. The amount of soluble insulin present varies from 10 to 50%, 30% being the most popular. Depending on its mono-components onset is normally at 30min, peak effect 2–6h, and duration 8–12h. Insulin analogue biphasic preparations have an onset, peak, and duration all slightly shorter than these.

Inhaled insulins

An inhaled insulin was available as Exubera®, a short acting insulin taken with meals in the same was as a short-acting or analogue insulin injection, until late 2007.

Insulin regimens

Twice daily free mixing

Historically very popular though now used much more rarely the usual starting regimen was 2/3 isophane, 1/3 soluble, and 2/3 of the total daily dose given pre-breakfast and 1/3 pre-evening meal. The main problems are mixing them, and pre-lunch hypos or hyperglycaemia. If on the same doses twice daily look out for pre-evening meal hyperglycaemia and increase the morning isophane dose to compensate for this, with a reduction in the morning soluble often needed to reduce pre-lunch hypoglycaemia.

Twice daily fixed mixture

Most commonly a 30% soluble/70% isophane mixture but, although this is not ideal for pre-lunch control or alterations in diet and exercise that are not preplanned, it is indicated in type 2 patients with poor control, those with significant osmotic symptoms, and those in whom there is no room to increase oral agents. A suitable starting regimen is a 30/70 mixture with 2/3 pre-breakfast and 1/3 pre-evening meal. The exact doses tend to vary widely depending on insulin sensitivity but a reasonable starting regimen may be 10–15 units pre-breakfast and 5–10 units pre-evening meal.

Basal bolus regimen

Soluble insulin or an insulin analogue given 3 × day pre-meal with a pre-bed isophane or long acting analogue; potentially has more flexibility with meal times, portions, and exercise than the previous regimens. The larger number of injections and the more frequent capillary blood glucose measurements needed makes it less popular with some patients.

If starting as the first type of insulin give 3 equal pre-meal doses and alter as required, e.g. 4–6 units is a reasonable starting dose, with 6–8 units of isophane pre-bed. If converting to a basal bolus regimen from a twice daily biphasic regimen you need to reduce the total daily insulin dose by up to 10%. Initially give 30–50% of the total daily insulin needed as a pre-bedtime isophane or long acting analogue and split the remaining insulin evenly between the meals as soluble or short acting analogue insulin. Once the patient is on this regimen the evening isophane or analogue often needs to be ↑ to maintain adequate fasting sugars.

In patients using short acting insulin analogues, and less often those on standard soluble insulins, a 2 × daily isophane or a long acting analogue is occasionally needed especially if there is a long gap between lunch and the evening meal.

Continuous SC insulin infusion (CSII)

Used in the USA but not as commonly in the UK possibly because of cost issues as well as potential problems with pump failure, ketoacidosis, and cannula site infections, although with improvements in technology these are less common problems now. Soluble insulin or a short acting analogue is given continuously via a SC cannula into the anterior abdomen. National Institute of Clinical Excellence (NICE) guidance on the use of insulin pumps is available and worth reading

Insulin and oral agent mixtures

In type 2 patients several combinations are occasionally used. The 2 most popular are bedtime insulin + daytime tablets, or more frequent insulin + metformin. In the 1st, oral agents continue during the day with a pre-bed isophane or long-acting insulin analogue used to give acceptable fasting sugars pre-breakfast. Although often starting at 10 units/night, doses 5–6 times that are not infrequently needed. This regimen is suitable if someone else such as a district nurse or relative gives the insulin. The 2nd regimen adds up to 2g/day of metformin to any standard insulin regimen to reduce insulin requirements and improve control without the problem of further weight gain often seen if the insulin is continually ↑.

Further reading

Alberti KGMM, Gries FA, et al. (1994). A desktop guide for the management of non-insulin dependent diabetes mellitus (NIDDM): an update. Diabet Med **11**, 899–909.

ADA position statement (1994). Nutrition recommendations and principles for people with diabetes mellitus. Diabet Care **17**, 519–22.

Bailey CJ, Day C, and Campbell IW (2006). A consensus algorithm for treating hyperglycaemia in type 2 diabetes. Brit J Diabet Vasc Dis **6**(4), 147–8

Bailey CJ and Turner's RC (1996). Metformin. New Engl J Med **334**, 574–9.

Campbell IW (1990). Efficacy and limitations of sulphonylurea and metformin. In Bailey CJ, Flatt PR, (eds). New antidiabetic drugs. Smith-Gordon: Nishimura, Japan, pp.33–51.

Diabetes and Nutrition Study Group of the European Association for the Study of Diabetes. Recommendations for the nutritional management of patients with diabetes mellitus (1995). Diabet Nutrit Metab **8**(3), 186–9.

Nissen SE and Wolski K (2007). Effect of rosiglitazone on the risk of myocardial infarction and death from cardiovascular causes. *New Engl J Med* **356**(24), 2457–71. Epub 2007 May 21. Erratum in *New Engl J Med* **357**(1), 100.

Ratner RE (1995). Rational insulin management of insulin-dependent diabetes. In Leslie RDG and Robbins DE (eds) *Diabetes: clinical science in practice*. Cambridge University Press: Cambridge, pp.434–49.

The STOP-NIDDM Trial (2003). Acabose treatment and the risk of Cardiovascular Disease and Hypertension in patients with impaired glucose tolerance. *J Am Med Assoc* **290**, 486–94

UK Prospective Diabetes Study (UKPDS) Group (1998). Intensive blood-glucose control with sulfonylureas or insulin compared with conventional treatment and risk of complications in patients with type 2 diabetes (UKPDS 33) *Lancet* **352**, 837–53.

UK Prospective Diabetes Study (UKPDS) Group (1998). Effect of intensive blood-glucose control with metformin on complications in overweight patients with type 2 diabetes (UKPDS 34) *Lancet* **352**, 854–65.

NICE publications: ⟲ www.nice.org.uk

Type 1 diabetes diagnosis and management of type 1 diabetes in adults Clinical Guideline. July 2004

Type 2 diabetes blood glucose clinical guidelines. September 2002

Type 2 diabetes management of blood pressure and blood lipids clinical guidelines. October 2002

Diabetes (type 1 and 2) inhaled insulin technology appraisal. December 2006

Diabetes (types 1 and 2) long acting insulin analogues. December 2003

Diabetes (type 2) glitazones (review). August 2003

Diabetes (type 1) insulin pump therapy technology appraisal. February 2003

Diabetic eye disease

Epidemiology

Diabetic retinopathy remains the commonest cause of blindness in the working population of developed countries. Currently 2% of the UK diabetic population are thought to be registered blind, giving a person with diabetes a 10–20-fold ↑ risk of blindness. It is suggested that 84 000 of the 7.8 million diabetic North Americans will develop proliferative retinopathy each year and another 95 000 macular oedema.

The prevalence of diabetic retinopathy depends on the duration of diabetes, glycaemic control, BP control, and the racial mix of the group being examined, but about a 30% prevalence for a general diabetic population is often quoted.

In type 1 patients <2% have any lesions of diabetic retinopathy at diagnosis and only 8% have any features of it by 5 years (2% proliferative), but 87–98% have abnormalities 30 years later, 30% of these having had proliferative retinopathy. In type 2 patients 20–37% can be expected to have retinopathy at diagnosis and 15 years later 85% of those on insulin and 60% of those not taking will have abnormalities.

The 4-year incidence for proliferative retinopathy in a large North American epidemiological study was 10.5% in type 1 patients, 7.4% in older onset/type 2 patients taking insulin, and 2.3% in those not on insulin. In the UK currently maculopathy is a more common and therefore more significant sight-threatening complication of diabetes. It is suggested that 75% of those with maculopathy have type 2 diabetes and that there is a 4-year incidence of 10.4% in this group. Although type 2 patients are 10 × more likely to have maculopathy than type 1 patients, 14% of type 1 patients who become blind do so because of maculopathy.

Diabetic retinopathy, like many microvascular complications, is more common in the ethnic minorities than in Caucasians. It should also be remembered that cataracts are more common in people with diabetes and are actually the most common eye abnormality found. These occur in up to 60% of 30–54-year-olds. Other abnormalities to look for include vitreous changes such as asteroid hyalosis which occur in about 2% of patients. These are small spheres or star-shaped opacities seen in the vitreous which appear to sparkle when illuminated under an examining light and do not normally affect vision.

📖 See Box 113.1 for classification.

Box 113.1 Classification and features of diabetic retinopathy

- Background retinopathy (graded as R1 by the National Screening Committee—NSC):
  - Microaneurysms.
  - Haemorrhages.
  - Hard exudates.
- Preproliferative retinopathy (graded as R2):
  - Soft exudates/cotton wool spots.
  - Intra-retinal abnormalities (IRMAs).
  - Venous abnormalities (e.g. venous beading, looping, and reduplication).
- Proliferative retinopathy (graded as R3):
  - New vessels on the disc or within 1 disc diameter of it (NVD).
  - New vessels elsewhere (NVE).
  - Rubeosis iridis (± neovascular glaucoma).
- Maculopathy (graded as M0 if none and M1 if present):
  - Haemorrhages and hard exudates in the macula area.
  - Reduced visual acuity with no abnormality seen.

Other NSC Grades:
- R0—no retinopathy.
- O—other non-diabetic lesions seen (e.g. drusen and macular degeneration).
- P—Evidence of Previous laser therapy/retinal photocoagulation.
- U—Un-grade able or unobtainable, often due to cataracts.

Clinical features and histological features

The classification of diabetic retinopathy is based on ophthalmoscopic examination or retinal photographs but several other changes not seen macroscopically may explain some of these clinical findings.

One of the first histological changes seen is thickening of the capillary basement membrane and loss of the pericytes embedded in it. Both have been linked to hyperglycaemia in experimental models, with sorbitol accumulation and advanced glycation both having a role. In normal retinal capillaries there is a 1:1 relationship between endothelial cells and pericytes. Pericytes may control endothelial cell proliferation, maintain the structural integrity of capillaries, and regulate blood flow. Altering these roles, along with the ↑ blood viscosity, abnormal fibrinolytic activity, and reduced red cell deformity also seen in diabetes may lead to capillary occlusion, tissue hypoxia, and the stimulus for new vessel formation. Exactly how locally produced growth factors, altered protein kinase C, alterations in oxidative stress responses, and alterations in the autoregulation of retinal blood flow combine to cause this remains unclear but is avidly debated.

The natural progression is from background to preproliferative then to proliferative retinopathy/maculopathy, and ultimately sight-threatening disease.

Background retinopathy

Capillary microaneurysms are the earliest feature seen clinically, as red 'dots'. Small intraretinal haemorrhages or 'blots' also occur, as can haemorrhage, into the nerve fibre layer which are often more flame shaped. With ↑ capillary leakage hard exudates, which are lipid deposits, can also be seen.

Preproliferative retinopathy

A *cotton wool spot* is an infarct in the nerve fibre layer which alters axoplasmic transport in ganglion cell neurons giving an oedematous infarct seen as a pale/grey fuzzy edged lesion, which gives it its name. IRMAs are tortuous dilated hypercellular capillaries in the retina which occur in response to retinal ischaemia. A further change seen is alternating dilatation and constriction of veins (venous beading) and other venous alterations such as duplication and loop formation. Overall there are large areas of capillary non-perfusion occurring in the absence of new vessels.

The Early Treatment of Diabetic Retinopathy Study (ETDRS) suggested that certain of these features matter and suggested a '4–2–1' rule:

- 4 quadrants of severe haemorrhages or microaneurysms.
- 2 quadrants of IRMAs.
- 1 quadrant with venous beading.

If you have 1 of these features there is a 15% risk of developing sight-threatening retinopathy within the next year; if 2 are present the risk rises to 45%.

Proliferative retinopathy

New vessels are formed from the retina and can grow along, into, or out from it. A scaffolding for fibrosis then forms. There are 2 forms of new vessels: those on the disc or within 1 disc diameter of the disc (NVD) and new vessels elsewhere (NVE). Both give no symptoms but cause the problems of advanced retinopathy such as haemorrhage, scar tissue formation, traction on the retina, and retinal detachment which actually results in loss of vision. That is why panretinal photocoagulation, which can result in the regression of these new vessels, is used when they are seen.

Diabetic maculopathy

Oedema in the macula area can distort central vision and reduce visual acuity. Any of the above changes can co-exist with maculopathy. The changes seen can be:

- *Oedematous*—clinically it may just be difficult to focus on the macula with a hand-held ophthalmoscope.
- *Exudative*—with haemorrhages, hard exudates, and circinate exudates.
- *Ischaemic*—capillary loss occurs but clinically the macula may look normal on direct ophthalmoscopy but unperfused area will show up on fluorescein angiography.
- Any combination of these.

A ring or circinate pattern of lipid deposits suggest a focal defect which may be treated with focal laser therapy, whereas more diffuse problem may require more extensive treatment with a macula grid of laser.

Eye screening

As so many patients can expect to develop eye complications, some of these are sight threatening, and treatment can reduce this, a suitable screening programme is advisable. In the UK the NSC gives guidance on the protocols for screening, grading of the photographs obtained, and quality assurance of the scheme used. Patients with diabetes should undergo ophthalmic examination eyes at least once a year. A full examination should include the following.

Visual acuity

Use a standard Snellen chart for distance and check each eye separately. Let the patient wear their glasses for the test and if vision is worse than 6/9 also check with a pinhole as this will correct for any refractive (glasses) error. If it does not correct to 6/9 or better consider more careful review; some maculopathy changes cannot be seen easily with a hand-held ophthalmoscope and an ophthalmology review may be needed. Cataracts are a more likely cause, so look carefully at the red reflex. If vision gets worse with a pinhole, assume maculopathy is there until proven otherwise.

High blood glucose readings can give myopia (difficulty in distance vision) and low blood glucose hypermetropia (difficulty in reading), although this is not universal.

Eye examination

- Dilate the pupil before looking into the eye.
  - Use *tropicamide* 1% in most cases as it dilates the pupil adequately in 15–20min and lasts only 2–3h.
  - In those with a dark iris you may also need *phenylephrine* (2.5%) added soon after the tropicamide to give adequate views.
  - The main reasons not to dilate are closed angle glaucoma and recent eye surgery but, as such patients are usually under an eye clinic already, most people are suitable for dilatation.
  - 1% *pilocarpine* drops can be used (although not routinely) if acuity is >6/12 after dilatation. They may speed up reversal and allow driving sooner.
- Once the pupil is dilated, look at the red reflex to check for lens opacities. Examine the anterior chamber, as although rare, rubeosis iridis is important to pick up. The vitreous is examined before examining the retina. When examining the retina use the optic disc as a landmark, follow all 4 arcades of vessels out from it, examine the periphery, and at the end examine the macula as this can be uncomfortably bright through a dilated pupil and if done at the start makes it difficult for anyone to keep their eye still enough to complete the examination adequately.

Retinal photographs

It is said that although consultant diabetologists are more accurate than GPs, they still miss some cases of retinopathy when compared to the gold standard of an ophthalmologist. One way to reduce the 'false −ve rate for a screening programme is to use retinal photography as well as ophthalmoscopy. >90% of people can have good quality photos performed. This was often performed using 35mm slide film although digital images are now of sufficiently good quality, require a less intense flash, and avoid the delay of having to develop film. NSC guidelines now suggest a digital image should be used with a minimum of 27 pixels per degree and a 45 degree field of vision for each of the 2 images taken per eye (1 centered on the macula the other on the optic disc). The photographs/images obtained should then be graded/assessed by a trained observer with a Quality Assurance system to maintain consistency of grading.

When to refer

The physician performing eye screening will need good links with an interested ophthalmologist. Referral will depend on local preferences, but are based on NSC management guidelines as outlined in Box 113.2.

Box 113.2 Reasons for and timing of referral to ophthalmologist

- Immediate referral:
  - R3/proliferative retinopathy, as untreated NVD carries a 40% risk of blindness in <2 years and laser treatment reduces this.
  - Rubeosis iridis/neovascular glaucoma.
  - Vitreous haemorrhage.
  - Advanced retinopathy with fibrous tissue or retinal detachments.
- Early referral (<6 weeks):
  - R2/preproliferative changes.
  - M1/maculopathy, both for non-proliferative retinopathy involving the macula or for any haemorrhages/hard exudates within 1 disc diameter of the fovea.
  - Fall of >2 lines on a Snellen chart (whatever fundoscopy shows).
- Routine referral:
  - Cataracts.
  - Non-proliferative retinopathy with large circinate exudates not threatening the macula/fovea.
- Other categories:
  - R0/no retinopathy—annual screening.
  - R1/background retinopathy—annual screening and inform diabetes care team.

Treatment

Glycaemic control

There is good epidemiological evidence for an association between poor glycaemic control and worsening of retinopathy. The Diabetes Control and Complications Trial (DCCT) looked at intensive glycaemic control in type 1 patients over 6.5 years and showed a 76% reduction in the risk of initially developing retinopathy in the tight glycaemic group compared to the control group. The rate of progression of existing retinopathy was slowed by 54% and the risk of developing severe non-proliferative or proliferative retinopathy was reduced by 47%. The UKPDS looked at type 2 patients over a 9-year period and showed a 21% reduction in progression of retinopathy and a 29% reduction in the need for laser therapy. The long term benefits of improved glycaemic control are therefore clear.

However, the DCCT, the UKPDS, and several previous studies also showed an initial worsening of retinopathy in the first 2 years in the tight/improved glycaemic control groups, and all patients therefore need careful monitoring over this period. The long-term benefits outweigh this initial risk.

Blood pressure control/therapy

There is good evidence for an association between both systolic and diastolic hypertension and retinopathy in type 1 patients, but the link may only be with systolic hypertension in type 2 patients. The UKPDS looked at BP control in type 2 patients and showed that the treatment group, with a mean BP of 144/82 mmHg, when compared to the control group which had a mean of 154/87 mmHg, had a 35% reduction in the need for laser therapy. Adequate BP control, e.g. <140/80 in type 2 patients, is therefore advocated.

Using angiotensin converting enzyme inhibitors (ACEIs) as 1st-line therapy is also suggested with care in those with pre-existing renal disease as these may cause hyperkalaemia and may worsen renal function in those with undiagnosed renal artery stenosis. Experimental evidence suggests these agents may have antiangiogenic effects by altering local growth factor levels as well as any benefit from reducing blood pressure. Studies using *enalapril* and *lisinopril* have both shown a reduction in the progression of retinopathy in type 1 patients.

Lipid control/therapy

Experimental evidence suggests oxidized low-density lipoprotein (LDL)-cholesterol may be cytotoxic for endothelial cells. Epidemiological data also suggests an association between higher LDL cholesterol and worse diabetic retinopathy, especially maculopathy with exudates. A total cholesterol >7.0mmol/L gives a 4-fold greater risk of proliferative retinopathy than a total cholesterol <5.3mmol/L. A worse outcome from laser therapy in those treated for maculopathy has also been seen if hyperlipidaemia is present. Aggressive lipid lowering is therefore advocated, especially in maculopathy.

Antiplatelet therapy

In view of the altered rheological properties of diabetic patients these agents have been tried, but the results are variable. No evidence that they make things worse has been shown, and some studies suggest *aspirin* and *ticlopidine* may slow the progression of retinopathy although the benefit was small.

Lifestyle advice

Although stopping smoking reduces macrovascular risk its effect on retinopathy is less clear. Alcohol consumption and physical activity also show no consistent effect.

Other therapies

The use of agents such as protein kinase-C inhibitors and vascular endothelial growth factor inhibitors (e.g. bevacizumab) are currently being investigated to see if these can delay the progression of diabetic retinopathy and initial studies are encouraging.

Box 113.3 Risk factors for developing/worsening of diabetic retinopathy

- Duration of diabetes.
- Type of diabetes (proliferative disease is more common in type 1 and maculopathy in type 2).
- Poor diabetic control.
- Hypertension.
- Diabetic nephropathy.
- Recent cataract surgery.
- Pregnancy.
- Alcohol (variable results which may be related to the type of alcohol involved, e.g. worse in Scotland than Italy).
- Smoking (variable results but appears worse in young people with exudates and older ♀ with proliferative disease).

Surgical treatment

Laser treatment

- Up to 1500–7000 separate burns, of 100–500microm diameter, each taking about 0.1s to apply, are needed for panretinal or 'scatter' laser photocoagulation. For oedematous/exudative maculopathy a macula grid may use only 100–200 burns of 100–200microm diameter separated by 200–400microm gaps, avoiding the fovea. The ETDRS (Early Treatment Diabetic Retinopathy Study) showed laser therapy was better than no treatment in all visual acuity subgroups, with a 24% blindness rate at 3 years in the non-treated eyes compared to a 12% rate in the treated group.
- Laser therapy is usually performed as 3–4 sessions of outpatient treatment on conscious patients. Topical local anaesthetic drops allow a contact lens to be placed on the cornea and are often all that is needed. In some patients, however, as this procedure may be slightly uncomfortable, a retro-orbital injection (performed through the inside of the lower eyelid) can be given to anaesthetize the eye.
- The laser energy is absorbed by the choroid and the pigment epithelium which lie below the neurosensory layer which also absorbs the energy/heat and is destroyed.
- In patients with severe proliferative retinopathy, pan-retinal photocoagulation reduces visual loss (i.e. an acuity >1/60 or worse) by >80% while a macula grid reduces visual loss in maculopathy by >50%.
- Laser treatment aims to prevent further visual loss, especially in maculopathy, not to restore vision, and the distinction must be emphasized to all patients requiring treatment. The benefits from laser therapy currently outweigh the risks, which include accidental burns to the fovea if the eye moves during therapy, a reduction in night vision and, in a small number, interference with visual field severe enough to affect the ability to drive.

Vitrectomy

If the vitreous contains scar tissue, haemorrhage, or any opacity, a vitrectomy to remove it may help restore vision and allows the chance for intraoperative laser treatment or a better view for postoperative laser therapy. It can also help reduce retinal traction and allows retinal reattachment to be performed. A success rate at restoring vision of 70% is seen but the risk of worsening vision, detaching the retina, or worsening lens opacities should also be considered.

Cataract extraction

This is a common procedure with a slightly higher complication rate than in the non-diabetic population. Approximately 15% of patients undergoing a cataract extraction can be expected to have diabetes. A large lens implant should be considered, especially if laser therapy is going to be needed subsequently. Worsening of maculopathy after cataract extraction is also a risk which needs careful monitoring.

Further reading

British Multi-Centre Study Group (1983). Photocoagulation for diabetic maculopathy. *Diabetes* **32**, 1010–16.

Early Treatment Diabetic Retinopathy Study Research Group (1985). *Arch Ophthalmol* **103**, 1796–1806.

Scottish Intercollegiate Guidelines Network (2001). Management of Diabetes. ⊕ http://www.sign. ac.uk/guidelines/fulltext/55/index.html

Useful addresses

Action for Blind People, 14–16 Verney Road, London SE16 3DZ. Tel: 020 7732 8771

Partially Sighted Society, Queen's Road, Doncaster DN1 2NX. Tel: 01302 323132

Royal National Institute for the Blind, 224 Great Portland Street, London, W1N 6AA. Tel: 020 7388 1266

Useful web sites

⊕ www.diabetic-retinopathy.screening.n\hs.uk www.nscretinopathy.org.uk

⊕ www.nice.org.uk (Type 2 diabetes retinopathy clinical guideline February 2002)

Diabetic renal disease

Background

Diabetic nephropathy is now a major cause of premature death in patients with all types of diabetes. Approximately 1/6 patients entering most renal replacement programs in developed countries will now have diabetes, at least 50% having type 2 diabetes.

Definition

Diabetic nephropathy is defined as albuminuria (albumin excretion rate >300 mg/24h, which equates to a 24h urinary protein >0.5g) and declining renal function in a patient with known diabetes who does not have a urinary tract infection, heart failure, or any other renal disease. This is usually associated with systemic hypertension, diabetic retinopathy, or neuropathy, and in the absence of these the diagnosis needs to be carefully evaluated. 📖 See Box 114.1.

Epidemiology

Microalbuminuria has a prevalence of 6–60% of patients with type 1 diabetes, after 5–15 years duration of diabetes. Diabetic nephropathy will occur in up to 35% of patients with type 1 diabetes, more commonly in ♂ and in those diagnosed <15 years of age with a peak incidence approaching 3%/year 16–20 years after onset of diabetes. Of those type 1 patients who develop proteinuria 2/3 will subsequently develop renal failure. In the UK 15% of all deaths in diabetic patients <50 years old are due to nephropathy.

In type 2 patients there are more obvious racial differences, with up to 25% of Caucasians and 50% of Asians expected to develop nephropathy giving a prevalence in a general clinic of 4–33%. The duration of diabetes before development of clinical nephropathy is also often shorter in type 2 than in type 1 patients. This may be due to an initial delay in diagnosis of type 2 diabetes.

Box 114.1 Definitions

- *Proteinuria*—urinary protein >0.5g/24h.
- *Albuminuria*—urinary albumin excretion rate >300mg/24h or >200mcg/min.
- *Microalbuminuria*—urinary albumin excretion rate 30–300mg/day or 20–200mcg/min.

Making the diagnosis

A urine +ve on dip testing for protein (i.e. >0.5mg/L protein or >300mg/L albumin) suggests diabetic nephropathy. A timed urine collection either overnight or over 24h will confirm proteinuria or albuminuria, but other causes of proteinuria must be excluded before labeling this diabetic nephropathy. Proteinuria from non-diabetic renal disease occurs in up to 10% of type 1 and 30% of type 2 patients. Urinary tract infections, acute illness, heavy exercise, and cardiac failure are the most common causes to exclude. The absence of hypertension or diabetic retinopathy would also question the diagnosis, and confirmation from a renal biopsy may be required.

If the urine is standard dip test –ve for albumin, microalbuminuria should be looked for. The implementation group for the St Vincent Declaration recommend that all patients with –ve protein on conventional urinalysis are annually screened for micro-albuminuria. A urinary albumin:creatinine ratio >2.5mg/mmol in ♂ and >3.5mg/mmol in ♀ or a +ve urine dip test (urine albumin >20mcg) should be followed by a timed urine collection repeated 3 × with at least 2 abnormal.

Pathology

Although macroscopically there is an increase in kidney size, microscopically there is thickening of the glomerular basement membrane, expansion of glomerular supporting tissues (the mesangium) and fibrotic changes in both efferent and afferent arterioles. If localized this is termed *nodular glomerular sclerosis* (Kimmelsteil–Wilson nodules) and if more widespread, *diffuse glomerular sclerosis*.

The thickened basement membrane initially results in an alteration in its electrical charge but not in pore size, which allows ↑ passage of albumin into the glomerular ultrafiltrate seen clinically as microalbuminuria.

Box 114.2 False +ves for microalbuminuria

- Exercise.
- Urinary tract infection.
- Menstruation.
- Semen.

Pathogenesis

Hyperglycaemia

As with all microvascular diabetic complications, hyperglycaemia has been implicated in the pathogenesis of diabetic nephropathy via metabolic alterations. The DCCT showed a reduction in the development of microalbuminuria in patients with better glycaemic control, which would support this. The UK PDS showed similar improvements. These metabolic alterations may be due to sorbitol accumulation from the polyol pathway, due to the accumulation of advanced glycation end-products (AGE) or to an as yet unknown mechanism.

AGE have been linked to the extracellular matrix accumulation known to occur in nephropathy. The use of aminoguanidine to block renal AGE accumulation and an associated slowing in the progression of albuminuria and mesangial expansion would support their role in the pathogenesis of nephropathy. The evidence for the polyol path-way's importance comes from aldose reductase inhibitor trials, the results of which are more variable. Ongoing studies (e.g. Action 1 and Action 2 for aminoguanidine) will examine whether any agents are useful clinically.

Haemodynamic alterations

↑ intraglomerular pressures can be associated with elevations in systemic blood pressure (85% of type 1 patients with nephropathy are hypertensive), ↑ vasoactive hormones (e.g. angiotensin-II, endothelin) or altered levels of specific growth factors (e.g. TGF-β, IGF-I, and VEGF). Hormonal and growth factor alterations have been suggested as important in the initial hyperfiltration phase seen in type 1 patients who progress to nephropathy, and a role for angiotensin-II in the accumulation of extracellular matrix has also been postulated. Whether these changes are 2° to or independent of hyperglycaemia is not certain.

Genetic predisposition

There is an increase in red blood cell sodium–lithium counter-transport activity in nephropathic patients and their parents in some populations, and an ↑ incidence of hypertension in the relatives of diabetic patients with nephropathy. An association between nephropathy and polymorphisms of the ACE gene has also been noted.

Smoking

A consistent link between cigarette smoking and nephropathy has been known for some time, but an aetiological mechanism is not yet known.

Natural history

In 20–40% of type 1 diabetic patients there is initially a period of glomerular hyperfiltration. The 1st sign of nephropathy, however, is microalbuminuria, usually occurring 5–15 years after the onset of type 1 diabetes but possibly present at the time of diagnosis in those with type 2 diabetes. Associated with this is often the development of hypertension, a reduction in high-density lipoprotein (HDL)-cholesterol and an increase in LDL-cholesterol and triglycerides.

This progresses to the next stage of frank proteinuria or albuminuria, which has a peak incidence ~17 years after the diagnosis of type 1 diabetes. This is the start of overt nephropathy, as in both type 1 and type 2 patients an approximate $10mL/min^{-1}$ $1.73 \, m^{-2}$ reduction in glomerular filtration rate occurs each year once the albumin excretion rate has reached 300mg/day, although in some patients the deterioration may be more rapid, and treatment may reduce it. Once serum creatinine concentration reaches 200micromol/L, a fall of 1mL/min per month in glomerular filtration rate is then expected. This leads to end-stage renal failure (ESRF) with uraemia and potentially death 7–10 years after onset of albuminuria. A plot of the reciprocal of creatinine against time demonstrates a relatively straight line showing the projected rate of deterioration.

Patients with diabetes and persistent proteinuria/albuminuria have a high mortality, due to cardiovascular disease in 40% of cases. Nephropathy carries a 20–100 × greater mortality than in age-matched diabetic patients without proteinuria. 📖 See Box 114.3.

Box 114.3 Risk factors for development of microalbuminuria

- duration of diabetes.
- poor long term glycaemic control.
- hypertension.
- dyslipidaemia.
- hyperfiltration.
- parents with renal disease.

Treatment

Treatment options for ESRF are either renal dialysis (haemodialysis or ambulatory peritoneal dialysis) or renal transplantation, but life expectancy with either is no better than with some common malignancies. Several other therapies can, however, delay the progression to this stage.

Blood pressure

Controlling hypertension reduces the progression to microalbuminuria and from this to albuminuria and subsequent progression to ESRF. BP should be reduced to <130/85mmHg with avoidance of hypotension, although if proteinuria is >1g/day a better target is <120/75mmHg. Weight loss, alcohol restriction, and reduced salt intake help, but drugs are usually needed to achieve this.

Studies show benefits from β-blockers, furosemide, hydralazine, and calcium channel blockers, but the ACEIs are currently the preferred 1st-line agent in both microalbuminuric and albuminuric patients as they also have an effect on kidney function independent of their hypotensive action. Several studies suggest, however, that more than one agent will be required to control BP adequately.

Large studies with several ACEIs have confirmed their benefit in hypertensive patients by delaying the progression of microalbuminuria to albuminuria and then to ESRF. There is no documented benefit in treating normotensive patients without microalbuminuria. Captopril (50mg 2 × day) for 2 years in type 1 patients with micro-albuminuria reduced progression to albuminuria by 68%. Enalapril (10mg daily) given to type 2 patients with microalbuminuria for 5 years reduced progression to albuminuria by 67%. When used for 4 years in type 1 patients with nephropathy, captopril (50mg 2 × day) reduced the risk of death, dialysis, and transplantation by 50% and slowed the reduction in creatinine clearance.

The EUCLID study looked at treating normotensive microalbuminuric type 1 patients. In this study lisinopril reduced the albumin excretion rate by nearly 20% compared to placebo but there was a 3mmHg lower BP in the treatment group. From this it is suggested that normotensive type 1 patients be treated with ACEIs. An enalapril study in normotensive type 2 patients showed similar results.

Angiotensin II receptor antagonists can also reduce progression of microalbuminuria and end stage renal failure from trials with losartan (RENAAL) and irbesartan (IDNT, IRMA-II).

NICE has published guidance on the management of BP in people with type 2 diabetes while the Association of British Clinical Diabetologists (ABCD) also provides algorithms for the agents to use to help control BP in these people.

Glycaemic control

Correction of hyperglycaemia can reverse glomerular basement membrane thickening and mesangial changes. Studies looking at progression to microalbuminuria and subsequent progression to frank albuminuria (e.g. the Steno 1 and II Studies, the KROC Study) also suggest a clinical benefit from improving glycaemic control. In the DCCT tight glycaemic control of type 1 patients was shown to reduce progression to microalbuminuria by 30% and subsequent progression to albuminuria by 54%. Not all trials confirm this (e.g. the Micro-albuminuria Collaborative Study Group Trial) and not all patients with good control in the above trials gained benefit.

Even so, the current treatment aim is to normalize or significantly reduce HbA1c (<7.2%) while avoiding any weight gain or hypoglycaemia associated with the ↑ used of both oral agents and insulin needed to do so.

Dietary protein restriction

High dietary protein can damage the kidney by ↑ renal blood flow and intraglomerular pressures in experimental situations. For microalbuminuric type 1 patients reducing dietary animal protein intake in small studies appears to reduce both hyperfiltration and micralbuminuria, and the benefit in more severe renal impairment is more evident. In type 2 patients the UK PDS showed an initial reduction in microalbuminuria with dietary modification which may in part be related to protein reduction. A dietary protein content <0.8 g/kg is suggested.

Lipid lowering

Although diabetic nephropathy is not shown to reduce the progression of microalbuminuria to albuminuria or renal failure, these patients have a significant dyslipidaemia and a high cardiovascular mortality and require careful lipid monitoring and aggressive treatment. The use of aspirin for similar reasons is also advisable. NICE clinical guideline for the management of blood lipids can be found on their web site (🖰 www.nice.org.uk).

Further reading

Ahmad J, Siddiqui MA, and Ahmad H (1997). Effective postponement of diabetic nephropathy in normotensive type 2 diabetic patients with microalbuminuria. *Diabet Care* **20**, 1576–81.

Diabetes Control and Complications Trial Research Group (1993). The effect of intensive treatment of diabetes on the development of microvascular complications of DM. *New Engl J Med* **329**, 304–9.

Diabetes Control and Complications Trial Research Group (1995). Effect of intensive therapy on the development and progression of diabetic nephropathy in the DCCT. *Kidney Int* **42**, 1703–20.

EUCLID Study Group (1997). Randomized placebo-controlled trial of lisinopril in normotensive patients with insulin-dependent diabetes and normoalbuminuria or microalbuminuria. *Lancet* **349**, 1787–92.

Laffel LMB, McGill JB, Dans DJ on behalf of the North American Microalbuminuria Studsy Group (1995). The beneficial effect of angiotensin converting enzyme inhibition with captopril on diabetic nephropathy in normotensive IDDM patients with microalbuminuria. *Am J Med* **99**, 497–504.

Lewis EJ, Hunsicker LG, Bain RP, *et al.* (1993). The effect of angiotensin converting enzyme inhibition on diabetic nephropathy. *New Engl J Med* **329**, 1456–62.

Microalbuminuria Captopril Study Group (1996). Captopril reduces the risk of nephropathy in IDDM patients with microalbuminuria. *Diabetologia* **39**, 587–93.

NICE (2002). Type 2 diabetes–renal disease Clinical Guidelines. NICE: London. ⌖ www.nice.org.uk

NICE (2002). Type 2 Diabetes–management of blood pressure and blood lipids, Clinical Guidelines. NICE: London. ⌖ www.nice.org.uk

Ravid M, Brosch D, Levi Z *et al.* (1998). Use of enalapril to attenuate decline in renal function in normotensive, normalbuminuric patients with type 2 DM. *Ann Int Med* **128**, 982–8.

UK Prospective Diabetes Study Group (1998). Intensive blood glucose control with sulphonylureas or insulin compared with conventional treatment and risk of complications in patients with type 2 diabetes (UKPDS 33). *Lancet* **352**, 837–53.

UK Prospective Diabetes Study Group (1998). Tight blood pressure control and risk of macrovascular and microvascular complications in type 2 diabetes: UKPDS 38. *BMJ* **317**, 703–13.

UK Prospective Diabetes Study Group (1998). Efficacy of atenolol and captopril in reducing risk of macrovascular and microvascular complications in type 2 diabetes: UKPDS 39. *BMJ* **317**, 713–20.

Diabetic neuropathy

Definition

Involvement of cranial, peripheral, and autonomic nerves may be found in patients with diabetes, and termed diabetic neuropathy; this usually suggests a diffuse, predominantly sensory peripheral neuropathy. The effects on nerve function can be both acute or chronic as well as being transient or permanent. The consequences of neuropathy include:

- Neuropathic ulcers, usually on the feet.
- Charcot arthropathy.
- Altered sensation (both pain and ↑ sensitivity to normal sensation).
- Impotence (with autonomic neuropathy).

📖 See box 115.1 for classification.

> **Box 115.1 Classification of diabetic neuropathies**
>
> - Sensory neuropathy:
>   - Acute.
>   - Chronic.
> - Autonomic neuropathy.
> - Mononeuropathy:
>   - Entrapment neuropathy.
>   - External pressure palsies.
>   - Spontaneous mononeuropathy.
> - Proximal motor neuropathy (diabetic amyotrophy).

Pathology

Diabetic neuropathy is one of the microvascular complications of diabetes. Pathologically distal axonal loss occurs with focal demyelination and attempts at nerve regeneration. The vasa nervorum often shows basement membrane thickening, endothelial cell changes, and some occlusion of its lumen. This results in slowing of nerve conduction velocities or a complete loss of nerve function. Both metabolic and vascular changes have been implicated in its aetiology.

Pathogenesis

Hyperglycaemia is probably the underlying cause of the histological and functional changes. Several possible mechanisms have been suggested:

- Overloading of the normal pathways for glucose metabolism resulting in ↑ use of the polyol pathway which leads to ↑ levels of sorbitol and fructose and ↓ levels of myoinositol and glutathione. This may result in more free radical damage and also lowers nitric oxide levels, so altering nerve blood flow. Experimental models using aldose reductase inhibitors which can improve some aspects of diabetic neuropathy add some weight to this theory.
- Possible accumulation of AGE (via non-enzymatic glycation) may also have a role to play, as could the hypercoagulable state and altered blood rheology known to occur in all patients with diabetes. Aminoguanidine, which blocks AGE formation, when used in animal studies can increase both nerve conduction velocities and nerve blood flow in diabetic subjects, strengthening the role of AGE accumulation in this process.
- In the more acute neuropathies, acute ischaemia of the nerves due to vascular abnormalities has been suggested as the cause but again the underlying reason why this should occur is still unclear. Insulin-induced 'neuritis' may occur when insulin therapy is started and blood glucose levels fall.
- Other potential aetiological factors include changes in local growth factor production and oxidative stress.

Further work is needed to clarify the exact role of each of the above mechanisms. In the meantime, studies showing improvements in neuropathy associated with good diabetic control strengthen the argument for the role of hyperglycaemia and offers us a treatment option while we await other therapies.

Peripheral sensorimotor neuropathy

Although hyperglycaemia can alter nerve function and often gives some sensory symptoms at diagnosis, correcting the hyperglycaemia can often resolve these. Chronic sensorimotor neuropathy, on the other hand, is the most common feature of peripheral nerve involvement seen in patients with diabetes. The exact prevalence of diabetic neuropathy varies in most studies because of the different definitions and examination techniques used. For example, sensitive nerve conduction studies can show up to 80% of patients have abnormal results. In more normal practice, however, 20–30% of unselected patients can be expected either to have symptomatic neuropathy or have abnormalities on examination which are clinically significant. But at least 50% of these patients are asymptomatic. This will increase with increasing duration of diabetes, so although 7–8% of type 2 patients may have abnormalities at diagnosis, 50% can be expected to have them 25 years later.

Box 115.2 Features of peripheral sensorimotor neuropathy

- Usually insidious onset with numbness or paraesthesia, often found on screening rather than as a presenting problem.
- Starts in the toes and on the soles of the feet then spreads up to mid shin level, mostly in a symmetrical fashion. Less often it also involves the fingers and hands.
- Affects all sensory modalities and results in reduced vibration perception thresholds, pinprick, fine touch, and temperature sensations.
- ↓ vibration sensation and absent ankle reflexes are often the 1st features found. Another risk factor for ulceration is inability to feel a 10g monofilament.
- Less often the skin is tender/sensitive to touch (hyperaesthesia) or frank pain can occur.
- Painful neuropathy affects up to 5% of a general clinic population. This pain may be sharp, stabbing or burning in nature, and at times very severe.
- There may also be some wasting of the intrinsic muscles of the foot with clawing of the toes.

Mononeuropathies

Peripheral mononeuropathies and cranial mononeuropathies are not uncommon. These may be spontaneous or may be due to entrapment or external pressure. Of the peripheral mono-neuropathies median nerve involvement and carpal tunnel syndrome may be found in up to 10% of patients and require nerve conduction studies and then surgical decompression. Entrapment of the lateral cutaneous nerve of the thigh is also seen more commonly in those with diabetes, giving pain over the lateral aspect of the thigh. Common peroneal nerve involvement causing foot drop and tarsal tunnel syndrome are also recognized but less common.

Cranial mononeuropathies usually occur suddenly and have a good prognosis. Palsies of cranial nerves III and VI are the most common seen, but these are not a common problem in patients with diabetes. In the IIIrd nerve palsy sparing of the pupillary responses is usual. Spontaneous recover is slow over several months and no treatment apart from symptomatic help such as an eye patch is needed. Unlike entrapment neuropathies where decompression may help, no effective treatment is currently available in most of these cases with spontaneous mononeuropathies.

Proximal motor neuropathy (diabetic amyotrophy)

This is an uncommon but disturbing condition to have, mostly affecting ♂ in their 50s with type 2 diabetes. It presents with severe pain and paraesthesia in the upper legs, and is felt as a deep aching pain which may be burning in nature and can keep patients awake at night, put them off eating, and result in marked cachexia. This, with proximal muscle weakness and wasting of the quadriceps in particular, can be very debilitating. The lumbar sacral plexus lower motor neurons are affected and improvement is usually spontaneous over 3–4 months. Before making this diagnosis, however, consider other causes such as malignancies and lumbar disc disease.

Oral antidiabetic agents may play a part in the aetiology of this problem and conversion to insulin therapy is advised, although the anorexia experienced when the pain is severe can make this difficult. Although recovery happens over a few months only 50% recover fully, but no other treatment is currently known to improve on this.

Examination

- Mandatory at diagnosis and at least yearly in all asymptomatic patients.
- Test vibration, fine touch (with a 10g monofilament), and reflexes as a minimum. Using a neurothesiometer or biosthesiometer gives a more quantitative measure of vibration than a 128Hz tuning fork. Inability to feel the vibrating head at >25V in the toes is associated with a significant risk of neuropathic ulceration and should be considered a sign of 'at risk' feet.

Differential diagnoses
- Uraemia.
- Vitamin B_{12} deficiency.
- Infections (e.g. HIV and leprosy).
- Toxins (e.g. alcohol, lead, mercury).
- Malignancy.

Treatment
- *For all patients* Review by a podiatrist and if indicated an orthotist to give education on foot care and suitable footwear is advised. If followed by regular chiropody review this can help prevent some problems developing.
- *Asymptomatic patients* No drugs are yet available, in the past aldose reductase inhibitors such as *tolrestat* have been advocated for this indication by some but a recent Cochrane review suggests no benefit above placebo.
- *Painful neuropathy* Initially try capsaicin 0.075% topically to the affected area, being careful to avoid normal skin because this chili pepper extract, which depletes sensory nerve terminals of substance P, can be uncomfortable when applied to normal skin. It can take several weeks to be effective and may induce tingling and so worsening of symptoms initially. In some patients simple analgesics such as *paracetamol* or opiates such as *tramadol* have been shown to help. In more severe cases tricyclic antidepressants are the 1st-line treatment of choice with *imipramine* 20–100mg at night being less sedative than *amitriptyline* 25–75mg. Although agents such as *carbamazepine*, *phenytoin*, and *paroxetine* have less anticholinergic effects, they are also not as effective and are therefore used as second line. G*abapentin* and *pregabalin* however are well tolerated and more effective and are usually used before the other anticonvulsants and antidepressants. If the pain is severe and like an electric shock, anticonvulsants such as *carbamazepine* and *phenytoin* may however be effective.
- A more recent addition to the therapy for painful neuropathy is *Duloxetine* which is licenced as a 2nd or 3rd line agent. It is a combined serotonin and noradrenaline reuptake inhibitor, comparative trials against other agents are not current available, but it is effective compared to placebo in over half of people.
- *Hyperaesthesia* Occlusive dressings such as Opsite® may prove helpful. For more severe pain, oral agents are needed.
- *More recent studies* with agents such as the protein kinase C inhibitors show more encouraging results and treatment with these agents may soon be available.

General treatments

Specific treatments for each form of neuropathy have already been discussed, but there is some evidence for more general therapies.

- Poor diabetic control appears to be associated with worsening neuropathy and improving glycaemic control is advocated in any patient, especially if neuropathy is present.
- The use of evening primrose oil in rats and preliminary human studies suggests this may improve some aspects of diabetic neuropathy. The mechanism by which this works is not certain but it does increase production of cyclo-oxygenase-mediated prostanoids such as prostacyclin which could act as a vasodilator and so improve nerve blood supply.
- Other more specific vasodilators have also been examined, with blockers and ACEIs showing particularly useful results in experimental settings.
- An alternative approach is not to try to improve the underlying problem but to alter the body's response to it. Nerve growth factor (NGF) and IGF-I have been examined for their ability to cause nerve regeneration and growth, and NGF in particular looks potentially very interesting. Other such agents are also under investigation such as the protein kinase C β inhibitors and studies with these are encouraging.

Autonomic neuropathy

The commonest effect of autonomic neuropathy is erectile dysfunction which affects 40% of ♂ with diabetes. Only a small number develop the severe GI and bladder dysfunction. The recent interest in *sildenafil* has highlighted this. Abnormal autonomic function tests can be expected in 20–40% of a general diabetic clinic population. The ↑ problems during surgery from cardiac involvement should be remembered.

Clinical features

- Impotence.
- Postural hypotension—giving dizziness and syncope in up to 12%.
- Resting tachycardia or fixed heart rate/loss of sinus arrhythmia—in up to 20%.
- Gustatory sweating—sweating after tasting food.
- Dysphagia with delayed gastric emptying, nausea/vomiting.
- Constipation/diarrhoea.
- Urinary retention/overflow incontinence.
- Anhidrosis—absent sweating on the feet is especially problematic as it increases the risk of ulceration.
- Abnormal pupillary reflexes.

Assessment

At least annually check:

- Lying and standing BP (measure systolic BP 2min after standing; normal is <10mmHg drop, >30mmHg is abnormal).
- Pupillary responses to light.

Other less commonly performed tests to consider if the diagnosis is uncertain or in high risk patients include:

- *Loss of sinus arrhythmia* Measure inspiratory and expiratory heart rates after 5s of each (<10 beats/min difference is abnormal, >15 is normal).
- *Loss of heart rate response to Valsalva manoeuvre* Look at the ratio of the shortest R–R interval during forced expiration against a closed glottis compared to the longest R–R interval after it (<1.2 is abnormal).
- *BP response to sustained hand grip* Diastolic BP prior to the test is compared to diastolic BP after 5min of sustaining a grip equivalent to 30% of maximal grip. A diastolic BP rise >16mmHg is normal, <10mmHg is abnormal. A rolled up BP cuff to achieve the required hand grip may be used.
- For *gastric symptoms* consider a radioisotope test meal to look for delayed gastric emptying.

Treatment

This is based on the specific symptom and is usually symptomatic only. In all patients improvement in diabetic control is advocated in case any of it is reversible, but this is not usually very helpful or effective.

Postural hypotension

- May be exacerbated by drugs such as diuretics, vasodilators, and tricyclic antidepressants.
- Mechanical measures such as sleeping with the head elevated and wearing support stockings may help.
- Ensure an adequate salt intake.
- *Fludrocortisone* 50mcg once daily initially and ↑ as required up to 400mcg may be helpful, but beware of hypertension or oedema.
- *Desmopressin* and *octreotide* have also been used.

Impotence (☐ see *Erectile dysfunction, p.388*)

Libido is not normally affected and pain is also unusual, so look for hypogonadism and Peyronie's if they are present. Autonomic neuropathy is the likely cause but many drugs, especially thiazides and beta-blockers, can also cause it, as can alcohol, tobacco, cannabis, and stress. These should be assessed by direct questioning. Examination should include:

- Genitalia and 2° sexual characteristics.
- Peripheral pulses—as vascular insufficiency may play a part.
- Lower limb reflexes and vibration thresholds—to confirm that neuropathy is present.

Biochemical screening should at least include:

- Prolactin.
- Testosterone.
- Gonadotrophins (LH/FSH).

Exacerbating factors such as alcohol and antihypertensive drugs should be modified. The main therapies are:

- Oral therapies include; *sildenafil* (start at 25–50mg, increase to 100mg if needed and taken 1h prior to sexual intercourse, *vardenafil* (start at 10mg, ↑ to 20mg if needed and taken 25–60min prior to sexual intercourse), *tadalafil* (start at 10mg ↑ to 20mg if needed and taken 30min to 12h prior to sexual intercourse).
- Intraurethral *alprostadil* (start at 125mcg, increase to 250 or 500mcg if needed).
- Intracavernosal *alprostadil* (trial dose is 2.5mcg, treatment is 5–40mcg).
- Vacuum devices.

None of these is ideal. Sildenafil, although an oral therapy, is effective in only 60% of those with diabetes and is contraindicated with severe heart disease and those on nitrates, which rules many out.

Gastroparesis

Delayed gastric emptying can cause recurrent hypoglycaemic episodes. Promotilic agents can also help. Treatment options:

- *Cisapride* (10mg pre-meals/3–4 × day)—now withdrawn in the UK.
- *Metoclopramide* (5–10mg pre-meals/3 × day).
- *Domperidone* (10–20mg pre-meals).

- *Erythromycin*—acts as a motilin agonist to increase gastric emptying but may make patients feel nauseated so of limited use.
- *Surgery*—gastric drainage procedures should not be undertaken lightly.

Large bowel involvement

Constipation is treated with standard bulking and softening laxatives. The episodic diarrhoea is more troublesome, and treatment for this may include:

- *loperamide* (2mg 4 × day) or codeine phosphate (30mg 4 × day)
- antibiotics in case of bacterial overgrowth, such as *erythromycin* 250mg 4 × day for 7 days, or tetracycline 250mg 2 × day for 7 days
- Other agents such as *clonidine* and *ondansetron* have also shown some benefit.

Neuropathic bladder

Sacral nerve involvement can cause bladder abnormalities with reduced sensations of bladder fullness and ↑ residual volume after micturition. Regular toileting initially may help but intermittent self-catheterization or a long-term catheter may be required.

Anhidrosis

Dry feet can cause cracks in the skin and act as a site for infection. Emollient creams may help prevent this.

Further reading

Boulton AJM, Gries FA, and Jervell LA (1998). Guidelines for the diagnosis and outpatient management of diabetic peripheral neuropathy. *Diabet Med* **15**(6), 508–14.

NICE (2004). Type 1 diabetes. Diagnosis and management of type 1 diabetes in adults Clinical Guideline July 2004. NICE: London ⊕ www.nice.org.uk

NICE (2004). Type 2 diabetes. Prevention and management of foot problems Clinical Guideline January 2004. NICE: London ⊕ www.nice.org.uk

Macrovascular disease

People with diabetes have a significantly greater risk of coronary heart disease, cerebrovascular disease, and peripheral vascular disease than the non-diabetic population. Most people with diabetes will die from 1 of these (75% of patients with type 2). It has been suggested that a diagnosis of type 2 diabetes equates to a cardiovascular risk equivalent to ageing 15 years.

Epidemiology

The exact prevalence and incidence of macrovascular disease and its outcomes will vary depending on the age, sex, and ethnic mix of the patients being assessed. In general cardiovascular disease accounts for 75% of deaths in type 2 patients and 35% in type 1 patients. Although the atheroma seen is histologically the same as in a non-diabetic population, it tends to be more diffuse and progresses more rapidly. It also occurs at an earlier age and affects both sexes equally: ♀ therefore seem to lose their natural premenopausal advantage.

- Overall peripheral vascular disease occurs in up to 10% of patients and they have up to 15-fold greater risk of needing a non-traumatic amputation than the non-diabetic population.
- Thromboembolic cerebrovascular events occurs in up to 8%, which is a 2–4-fold ↑ risk compared to the non-diabetic population and accounts for 15% of deaths in type 2 patients.
- The risk of having a myocardial infarction is also ↑ 2–4 times. ♀ seem particularly at risk of cardiovascular disease compared to the non-diabetic population.

Patients with type 1 diabetes have half the rate of coronary heart disease, 1/3 the rate of cerebrovascular disease, and 2/3 the rate of peripheral vascular disease compared to type 2 patients, but their rate of all these is greater than that for the non-diabetic population. ♂ and ♀ are equally affected, with the incidence rates for ischaemic heart disease about 6 times that of both cerebrovascular and peripheral vascular disease.

Secondary prevention
- Stop smoking.
- Aspirin.
- β-blockers.
- Lipid lowering drugs.

Pathogenesis

Atherosclerosis has a well known set of risk factors, such as smoking and family history, all of which still apply in a diabetic population. Some factors, however, are more common in those with diabetes and may also confer a greater risk to the diabetic population. These include:

- *Glycaemic control* In patients with type 1 diabetes worsening levels of hyperglycaemia, as suggested by higher average HbA1c levels are said to relate to the degree of disease present. In those with type 2 diabetes this association is less clear cut, although the UKPDS does suggest this is also the case as better glycaemic control was associated with a trend for fewer myocardial infarctions.
- *Hypertension* More common in both type 1 and type 2 patients and results in vascular endothelial injury so predisposing to atheroma formation. The UKPDS suggests BP control is a more important individual risk factor than glycaemic control.
- *Hyperlipidaemia* Common: e.g. hyperinsulinaemia in insulin-resistant type 2 patients causes reduced HDL-cholesterol, elevated triglycerides (and VLDL), and smaller denser and therefore more atherogenic LDL-cholesterol.
- *Obesity* An independent risk factor, more common in type 2 patients. Central obesity in particular is more atherogenic.
- *Insulin resistance* or elevated circulating insulin/proinsulin-like molecule levels are known to increase the risk of atherosclerosis in both diabetic and non-diabetic populations. This may be linked to impaired endothelial function.
- *Altered coagulability* Circulating fibrinogen, platelet activator inhibitor (PAI)-1 and von Willebrand factor levels are ↑ and platelets are less deformable. This may be more prothrombotic, but the exact significance remains uncertain.

The UKPDS has shown the major risk factors for coronary heart disease in type 2 patients to be elevated LDL-cholesterol, ↓ HDL-cholesterol, hypertension, hyperglycaemia, and smoking. Exactly why these risk factors are commonly seen/linked in the same patient, particularly type 2 diabetic patients, is uncertain. Several hypotheses have been put forward, but none as yet explains them all adequately. However, each suggests an element of genetic susceptibility mixed with environmental effects. A genetic predisposition to insulin resistance, for example, may combine with poor intrauterine nutrition to produce a low birthweight infant with a susceptibility to vascular disease and diabetes later in life. But other factors must be involved, as not all those who later develop diabetes and vascular disease were small at birth.

Lipid abnormalities found in patients with diabetes

Hyperlipidaemia in a patient with diabetes, at any level of cholesterol, is associated with a greater risk of macrovascular disease than in a non-diabetic population. Patients with diabetes may have altered activity of insulin-dependent enzymes such as lipoprotein lipase which results in delayed systemic clearance of certain lipids. This, combined with altered hepatic production of apoprotein-B containing lipoproteins, gives a more atherogenic profile.

Usual findings are of ↑ triglyceride containing lipoproteins, chylomicrons, and VLDL. Although more common in the insulin-resistant type 2 patients this can also be seen in type 1 patients as can a low HDL-cholesterol (HDL$_2$ especially). Other atherogenic changes include a tendency to develop small dense LDL cholesterol particles and a greater tendency to oxidative damage which renders them even more atherogenic. Lipoprotein (Lpa) levels are also often raised.

Even so, other common 1° causes of hyperlipidaemia, such as familial hypercholesterolaemia or familial combined hyperlipidaemia, should not be missed. Screening for 2° causes of hyperlipidaemia such as hypothyroidism or drug induced (alcohol, thiazides, and β blockers in particular) is also strongly advised.

Management

In all patients the 1st treatment is dietary modification. In a patient who is actually following a good diabetic diet, however, there is often not much room for improvement.

Other standard advice should also be given:

- Stop smoking—reduces risk of death by about 50% over a 15-year period.
- Reduce weight if overweight/obese.
- Increase physical activity.

While the reductions in mortality, re-infarction, and stroke in the major lipid lowering trials such as the 4S study (Scandinavian Simvastatin Survival Study), CARE (Cholesterol and Recurrent Events Trial), LIPID (Long-term Intervention with Pravastatin in Ischaemic Disease), and WOSCOPS (West of Scotland Coronary Prevention Study) are all very impressive, the diabetic subgroups show as good if not better reductions although the numbers in each were relatively small (🕮 see table 116.1). In 4S, for example, the simvastatin-treated diabetic subgroup (4.5% of those in the study) had a 23% rate of major coronary events compared to 45% in the diabetic placebo group, while the nondiabetic simvastatin group had 19% and the placebo non-diabetic group had 27%. On the basis of this it is suggested that if 100 patients with diabetes who have angina or are post myocardial infarction are treated with simvastatin for 6 years, 24 of the 46 expected coronary deaths and non-fatal myocardial infarctions can be prevented.v

Table 116.1 Lipid reduction studies

	4S	WOSCOP	CARE	LIPID
Type of study	2° prevention of CHD	1° prevention of CHD	2° prevention of CHD	2° prevention of CHD
Duration of study (years)	6	5	5	6
Number studied	4444	6595	4159	9014
Mean total cholesterol (mmol/L) (range)	6.8 (5.5–8.0)	7.0 (>6.5)	5.4 (<6.2)	(4.0–7.0)
Age range (years)	35–70	45–64	21–75	31–75
% men	81	100	86	83
% with diabetes	4.5	1	17	8.6
Treatment	Simvastatin 20–40mg daily	Pravastatin 40mg daily	Pravastatin 40mg daily	Pravastatin 40mg daily
Event reduction for major coronary events	34% for non-diabetics 55% for diabetics	31% overall	23% for non-diabetics 25% for diabetics	23% overall

More recent lipid lowering trials including larger numbers of people with diabetes such as CARDS (Collaborative Atorvastatin Diabetes Study) and ASPEN (Atorvastatin Study for the Prevention of Endpoints in Non-insulin dependent diabetes) again show significant benefit but the Anglo-Scandinavian Cardiac Outcomes Trial- lipid lowering arm (ASCOT-LLA) was not quite so encouraging.

Once the above lifestyle measures have been implemented, consider the need for drug therapy. In the past the Sheffield tables, New Zealand tables, or the Joint British Societies Coronary Risk Prediction Chart (📖 see Fig. 122.1, p821) were used to determine risk in 1° prevention but any person with diabetes is now though of as such a high risk group secondary prevention target with a total cholesterol target <4.0mmol/L, an LDL <2.0mmol/L and an HDL >1.0mmol/L are now advocated Remember that a fit patient with diabetes has a similar risk when compared to a non-diabetic of the same age and sex who has also had a coronary event. Other targets are advocated by many, especially for those patients post coronary artery bypass grafting or post angioplasty. Triglycerides should be brought <1.5mmol/L, as above this atherogenic lipoprotein changes are said to occur.

In those with mixed hyperlipidaemia, consider a fibrate or a statin licenced for this indication. A fibrate will reduce triglycerides by 30–40% and LDL-cholesterol by 20% while a statin would reduce triglycerides slightly less (10–15%) and LDL-cholesterol slightly more (25–35%). Fibrates also alter the LDL-cholesterol to its less atherogenic form. The choice of agent must be tailored to the individual patient. For hypercholesterolaemia alone a statin is 1st choice, as in the non-diabetic patient, and in severely resistant patients combination therapy with statins, ezetimibe, fibrates, and less often resins may be required. Combination statin and ezetimibe may reduce LDL more effectively than increasing the statin dose alone.

Treatment aims for lipids

- Total cholesterol <4.0mmol/L.
- LDL cholesterol <2.0mmol/L.
- Aim to have triglycerides <1.5mmol/L.

Box 116.1 Investigations

Take a full history and carefully examine the patient. In all patients then check:
- Dip test urine for protein.
- Serum urea, electrolytes, and creatinine (and creatinine clearance if creatinine is raised).
- Fasting lipids.
- ECG (for left ventricular hypertrophy and signs of ischaemia).

Also consider:
- The need for a chest radiograph for signs of heart failure/cardiomegaly.
- An echocardiogram.
- Cortisol + dexamethasone suppression test.
- Catecholamines.
- Renin/aldosterone.

Hypertension

Epidemiology

Hypertension is twice as common in the diabetic population as in the non-diabetic population, and standard ethnic differences in the prevalence of hypertension still hold true. It is known that hypertension worsens the severity of and increases the risk of developing both microvascular and macrovascular disease. Using a cut-off of >160/90mmHg, hypertension occurs in:

- 10–30% of patients with type 1 diabetes.
- 20–30% of microalbuminuric type 1 patients.
- 80–90% of macroalbuminuric type 1 patients.
- 30–50% of Caucasians with type 2 diabetes.

Using the UKPDS suggested target of 140/80, hypertension is even more common.

Pathogenesis

- *Type 1 patients* Hypertension is strongly associated with diabetic nephropathy and microalbuminuria and occurs at an earlier stage than that seen in many other causes of renal disease. This may in part be linked to a genetic predisposition also giving ↑ activity in red blood cell sodium–lithium counter-transport activity which leads to ↑ peripheral vascular resistance. Insulin may also have a suppressive effect on renin release, so giving hyporeninaemic hypoaldosteronism.
- *Type 2 patients* Hypertension is associated with insulin resistance and hyperinsulinaemia; again, this may be genetically mediated. Hyperinsulinaemia can directly cause hypertension by ↑ sympathetic nervous system activity, ↑ proximal tubule sodium resorption, and stimulating vascular smooth muscle cell proliferation. Hyperglycaemia also has an antinatriuretic effect and with hyperinsulinaemia leading to hypokalaemia which results in both glucose and sodium reabsorption being ↑ all increases the potential for hypertension.

Management

Treatment aim

The current recommendation is for all patients with diabetes to have a blood pressure <140/80mmHg. The hypertension study in the UKPDS highlights the benefits for type 2 patients of such a treatment level on mortality, diabetes related end-points, and microvascular end-points. In this a 10/5mmHg difference in BP was associated with a 34% risk reduction in macrovascular end-points, a 37% risk reduction in microvascular end-points, and a 44% risk reduction in stroke. The Hypertension Optimum Treatment (HOT) study again suggests a target of <140/80mmHg although in those who already have significant end-organ damage a lower target is advocated by some (<130/80).The Anglo-Scandinavian Cardiac Outcomes Trial–Blood Pressure Lowering Arm (ALLHAT–BPLA) reinforced the role of calcium channel blockers and angiotensin coverting enzyme inhibitors (ACEI) in combination.

Predisposing conditions
Other conditions which can cause both hypertension and hyperglycaemia should be considered, e.g. Cushing's syndrome, acromegaly, and phaeochromocytoma.

End-organ damage
Look for evidence of end-organ damage (eyes, heart, kidneys, and peripheral vascular tree in particular).

Assessment of cardiac risk factors
Look for associated risk factors for coronary heart disease.

Treatment

General
Once this initial assessment is complete, modify other risk factors such as glycaemic control, smoking, and dyslipidaemia. Then look at:
- Weight reduction if obese.
- Reduced salt intake (<6 g/day).
- Reduced alcohol intake (<21 units/week in ♂, <14 in ♀).
- Exercise (20–40min of moderate exertion 3–5 ×/week).

Pharmacological
After this, start drug therapy for the hypertension. Most agents currently available will drop systolic BP by no more than 20mmHg at most. Remember that in the UKPDS BP study, 1/3 of those achieving the tight BP targets we are now aiming for required 3 or more drugs to do so. Recently the NICE guidelines for BP treatment were updated and now advocate an 'A/CD' approach. That is starting with 'A', an ACEI (or an angiotensin II receptor blocker/antagonist if the ACEI is not tolerated) and then adding in either a 'C'/calcium channel blocker or a 'D'/thiazide type diuretic with an alpha blocker, a beta blocker or further diuretic therapy then added if this fails to reduce BP adequately.
- In the presence of microalbuminuria or frank proteinuria, always consider an ACEI 1st line, or an angiotensin II receptor antagonist if not tolerated.
- In Afro-Caribbean diabetics a diuretic may also be needed to improve the efficacy of the ACEI as these and β-blockers are less effective than calcium channel blockers and diuretics in these patients.
- Several agents, such as high dose thiazides and β-blockers, can, however, worsen diabetic control, mask hypoglycaemia, and exacerbate dyslipidaemia so tailor the drugs chosen to each patient. Interestingly a recent review of data from the Nurses Health Study (NHS I and II) and the Health Professionals Follow-up study (HPFS) suggested that while these agents may increase the risk of developing diabetes it may not be associated with an ↑ risk of cardiovascular or total mortality, which may be related to BP control but is not certain.
- In those with angina a β-blocker has added benefits
- In those with peripheral vascular disease vasodilators such as the calcium channel blockers may be beneficial.

Box 116.2 Management of acute myocardial infarction

Patients with diabetes are more likely to have a myocardial infarction and more likely to die from it than the non-diabetic population. This may be due to a greater likelihood of myocardial pump failure. Several studies highlight this:

Trial and outcome examined	Non-diabetic subgroup	Diabetic subgroup
ISSI-2: Non-streptokinase 4-year mortality	27%	41%
GUSTO: In-hospital mortality	6.2%	10.6%
GISSI-2: Re-infarction rates	14%	30%

Up to 20–40% of patients admitted to hospital with a myocardial infarction will have hyperglycaemia, many of whom will not have previously diagnosed diabetes.

As in the non-diabetic population, streptokinase, aspirin, and acute angioplasty have proven benefits. The previous contraindication for thrombolysis in those with proliferative diabetic retinopathy has been questioned by many. Tight glycaemic control (blood glucose 7–10mmol/L) using IV glucose and insulin for at least 24h followed by SC insulin, as used in the DIGAMI study, also has benefits. In this study, patients with an admission blood glucose >11.0mmol/L who were treated with this regimen had a 7.5% absolute risk reduction in mortality at 1 year and an 11% risk reduction at 3.5 years compared to the control group (i.e. 33% mortality with treatment vs. 44% in controls at 3.5 years). This equates to 1 life saved for every 9 treated with this regimen. The exact reason for this is unclear.

- It is suggested that all patients with a blood glucose >11mmol/L benefit from such treatment whether previously known to have diabetes or not. Using an admission HbA1c to detect those with undiagnosed or stress-related hyperglycaemia can be useful, but should not result in withholding the acute treatment of this hyperglycaemia in such patients. It may, however, help to identify those who may be troubled by hypoglycaemia and may not therefore be suitable for SC insulin or sulfonylureas in the intermediate or long term.

- Using ACEIs early after myocardial infarction gives a 0.5% absolute risk reduction in 30-day mortality and a 4–8% risk reduction over 15–50 months in a general population. Analysis of the diabetic subgroup in the GISSI-3 study showed a 30% relative risk reduction in 6-week mortality for the diabetics (8.7% vs. 12.4%) compared to a 5% reduction for non-diabetics. In view of the greater proportion of diabetics with poor left ventricular function after myocardial infarction compared to the non-diabetic population, this difference is very important.

Further reading

Hanssen L, Zanchetti A, Carruthers SG *et al.* (1998). Effects of intensive blood pressure lowering and low dose aspirin in patients with hypertension: principal results of the Hypertension Optimun Treatment (HOT) randomised trial. *Lancet* **351**, 1755–62.

Malmberg K for the DIGAMI (DM, Insulin Glucose Infusion in Acute Myocardial) study group (1997). Prospective randomized study of intensive insulin treatment on long term survival after acute myocardial infarction in patients with DM. *BMJ* **314**, 1512–15.

NICE (2006). Hypertension: management of hypertension in adults in primary care. NICE clinical guidelines 34 (partial update of NICE clinical guideline 18), June 2006. NICE: London. www.nice.org.uk

NICE Clinical Guideline CG 66 (May, 2008). Type 2 diabetes: the management of type 2 diabetes. Management of blood pressure and lipids. www.nice.org.uk

Pyorala K, Pedersen TR, Kjekshus J *et al.*(1997). Cholesterol lowering with simvastatin improves prognosis of diabetic patients with coronary heart disease. *Diabetes Care* **20**, 614–20.

Taylor EN Hu FB, and Curhan GC (2006). Antihypertensive medications and the risk of incident type 2 diabetes. *Diabetes Care* **29**, 1065–70

UKPDS Group (1998). Tight blood pressure control and risk of macrovascular and microvascular complications in type 2 diabetes: UKPDS 38. *BMJ* **317**, 703–13.

UKPDS Group (1998). Efficacy of atenolol and captopril in reducing the risk of acrovascular and microvascular complications in type 2 diabetes: UKPDS 39. *BMJ* **317**, 713–20.

Zuanetti G, Latini R, Maggioni AP, *et al.* (1997). Effect of the ACE inhibitor lisinopril in diabetic patients with acute myocardial infarction. Data from GISSI-3 Study. *Circulation* **96**, 4239–45.

Diabetic foot

📖 See Table 117.1, Box 117.1 and 117.2.

Risk factors for foot ulcer development

Several features/factors are thought to predispose to ulcer formation, and awareness of these may highlight 'at risk' patients for education and other preventive strategies. These ulcers can occur anywhere on the foot, but the tips of claw/hammer toes and over the metatarsal heads are the most frequent sites. The risk factors/features include:

- *Peripheral neuropathy* (seen in up to 80% of diabetic patients with foot ulcers) reduces awareness of pain and trauma caused by footwear and foreign bodies in shoes. Look for reduced monofilament sensation (e.g. reduced to a 10g monofilament) and reduced vibration perception thresholds (e.g. reduced sensation to a 128Hz tuning fork for <10s or >25V with a biosthesiometer), suggesting at risk feet.
- *Autonomic neuropathy* leading to anhidrosis can dry out the skin and cause it to crack, so allowing a portal of entry for infection. These feet are often warm and dry with distended veins.
- *Motor neuropathy* can result in altered foot muscle tone, wasting of small muscles, raising of the medial longitudinal arch, and clawing of the toes which can put more pressure through the metatarsal heads and heels so predisposing to callus and ulcer formation. Electrophysiology can help examine this, but is too invasive for widespread routine use.
- *Peripheral vascular disease* (seen in up to 10% of patients) and *microvascular circulatory disease* leads to local ischaemia, ↑ the potential for ulcer formation and can delay wound healing when ulceration occurs. Always examine peripheral pulses and consider doppler studies if abnormal. An ankle:brachial artery ratio of >1.1 suggests arterial disease (a ratio of the BP in the ankle and the arm measured while at rest).
- *Duration of diabetes* relates to the presence of the above factors but is often quoted as an independent risk factor, as is ↑ age. But type 2 diabetes may be present and undiagnosed for some time.
- The presence of *other microvascular complications* such as nephropathy and retinopathy is also a risk factor for foot ulcer development.
- *Previous ulceration* is another important risk factor, and anyone with previous problems deserves very careful monitoring/follow up.
- *Lack of diabetes monitoring* and lack of previous examinations of the feet are also recognized risk factors.
- *Mechanical, chemical or thermal trauma/injury* is often the predisposing factor, and any profession or pastime that increases the risk of these is a risk factor.

Table 117.1 Epidemiology of foot ulceration in the UK

Prevalence of foot ulceration	5–10%
Number of people with diabetes developing foot ulcers	14 000–42 000
Proportion of people with diabetes undergoing lower limb amputation	1%
Number of people with diabetes undergoing lower limb amputation per year	2000
Annual NHS expenditure on diabetes foot-related care	£13 million

Box 117.1 Clinical features of diabetic feet

Neuropathic feet
- Warm.
- Dry skin.
- Palpable foot pulses.
- No discomfort with ulcer.
- Callus present.

Ischaemic feet
- Cold/cool.
- Atrophic/often hairless.
- No palpable foot pulses
- More often tender/painful.
- Claudication/rest pain
- Skin blanches on elevation and reddens on dependency.

Box 117.2 Wagner's classification of diabetic foot lesions[1]

- Grade 0—high-risk foot, no ulcer present.
- Grade 1—superficial ulcer, not infected.
- Grade 2—deep ulcer with or without cellulitis but no abscess or bone involvement.
- Grade 3—deep ulcer with bone involvement or abscess formation.
- Grade 4—localized gangrene (toe, forefoot, heel).
- Grade 5—gangrene of the whole foot.

1. Wagner FW, O'Neal LW (1983). Algorithms of diabetic foot care. In Levin ME, O'Neil LW, (eds). *The Diabetic Foot*, 2nd edn. Mosby Yearbook: St Louis, pp.291–302. Copyright Elsevier, reproduced with permission.

Treatment

This is a multidisciplinary problem requiring collaboration between interested diabetologists, diabetes nurse specialists, podiatrists, orthotists, vascular surgeons, plastic surgeons, and occasionally orthopaedic surgeons.
Treatment is aimed at several distinct areas, namely:

- At-risk feet with no current ulceration.
- Treating existing ulcers.
- Treating infected ulcers.
- Treating osteomyelitis.
- Treating vascular insufficiency.

At-risk feet with no current ulceration

When at-risk feet are identified in any patient with diabetes, standard
advice should be given and this will need to be repeated/reinforced regularly. This advice would usually include:

- General advice on nail care, hygiene and care with footwear—often
  best from the chiropodist.
- Reinforce the need for regular daily examination of the feet by the
  patient or carer.
- Consider regular podiatry/chiropody review as well as self-monitoring.
  Also reinforce the need for more urgent review if the patient discovers
  problems.
- Consider the need for modification of footwear or special footwear if
  there are abnormalities with foot posture or problems with pressure
  loading on certain parts of the foot. Padded socks can also reduce
  trauma. Advise the patient to examine shoes before putting them on,
  wear lace-ups or shoes with lots of room for the toes and avoid ill-fitting
  fashion shoes. In some people protective toecaps can prove very useful.
- Avoid walking barefoot.

At the moment no other therapy is advocated in this group of patients,
but, as discussed in the neuropathy section, good diabetic control is
important and other agents may be useful in the future such as aldose
reductase inhibitors, inhibitors of non-enzymatic glycation, and various
growth factors.

Existing ulcers

All ulcers should be considered deep and involving bone until proved otherwise. Also:

- *Optimize diabetic control.*
- *Reduction of oedema* is important to aid healing.
- *Regular debridement* of callus and dead tissue/skin is important for both
  neuropathic and ischaemic ulcers. Debridement is usually best with a
  scalpel and forceps although chemical agents (such as *varidase*, which
  contains streptokinase) can occasionally help. But, as these agents
  can also damage healthy tissue, use under careful supervision. More
  recently the use of sterile maggots has been shown to be effective.
  After debridement apply dressings but change these regularly. Be
  careful that tight dressings do not impair a poor circulation further and
  that thick dressings or quantities of sticky tape to hold them on do not
  cause their own skin trauma or pressure effects.

- *Infection control* Infection may be localized but any evidence of deeper infection or sinus formation raises the possibility of osteomyelitis. Systemic symptoms of an infection may be minimal as may pain/tenderness in the foot itself, so be suspicious of more severe infection than you can see in everyone. The organisms may be ordinary skin commensals given a port of entry but send swabs for culture and think of *Staphylococcus aureus* or streptococci as likely organisms.
  - If a sinus is present, probe it and if down to bone assume there is osteomyelitis. Culture anything you get out. Plain radiographs may show bone erosion or destruction with osteomyelitis; radioisotope scans using technetium can show ↑ uptake with both infection and Charcot arthropathy. The use of MRI scanning can be useful to differentiate in this situation.
  - If infection is present use triple therapy with *flucloxacillin* (500mg 4 × daily), *ampicillin/amoxicillin* (500mg 3 × daily) and *metronidazole* (200mg 3 × daily) or consider using *amoxicillin/ clavulanic acid* (250/125mg 3 × daily) or *ciprofloxacin* (500–750mg 2 × daily) and *clindamycin* (300–450mg 2 × daily) depending on the organisms grown and patient tolerability. This will need to be IV/rectal initially if the infection is severe and for the deeper infections several months of therapy may be needed. If osteomyelitis is present consider using *ciprofloxacin* or *sodium fusidate* which have better bone penetration and again use for several months. Linezolid is also a useful therapy as a 2nd or 3rd-line agent but care with hepatic and renal impairment and the need to monitor for potential thrombocytopenia, anaemia or pancytopenia may limit its use.
  - In some patients this approach fails to control osteomyelitis adequately and resection/amputation is required, so regular liaison with an interested surgeon is imperative.
- *Reducing trauma* and *pressure relief* in neuropathic ulcers Padded socks can reduce sheer stress and trauma. Suitable shoes and insoles can help to relieve pressure to allow healing to occur as long as unnecessary walking is minimized. If this is not enough a pneumatic boot/Aircast boot or a total contact cast may be needed. These allow the patient to be mobile but take the weight away from the ulcerated area or foot and put all the weight/pressure through to the calf instead. The involvement of both chiropodists and orthotists is therefore essential.
- *Revascularization* Always consider coexistent vascular disease in a neuropathic foot or predominantly ischaemic ulcers/feet. Vascular bypass grafting/reconstruction or angioplasty can give excellent results with a 70–95% limb salvage rate often quoted. The improved blood supply will also help healing of existing ulcers and may negate the need for amputation or allow the area requiring resection to be minimized. If vascular intervention is unsuccessful or not possible then amputation is required, preferably as a below-knee procedure to give a better mobilization potential postoperatively.

Box 117.3 The Charcot foot

Epidemiology

This is a relatively rare complication of diabetes: an average district general hospital clinic will have 3–10 patients with this problem.

Pathogenesis

It is suggested that blood flow increases due to sympathetic nerve loss. This causes osteoclast activity and bone turnover to increase, so making the bones of the foot more susceptible to damage. Even minor trauma can therefore result in destructive changes in this susceptible bone.

Clinical features

The most likely site is the tarsal–metatarsal region or the metatarsophalangeal joints. Initially it gives a warm/hot, swollen, and often uncomfortable foot, which may be indistinguishable from cellulitis and gout. Peripheral pulses are invariably present and peripheral neuropathy is evident clinically.

Plain radiographs will be normal initially and later show fractures with osteolysis and joint reorganization with subluxation of the metatarsophalangeal joints and dislocation of the large joints of the foot. Isotope scans with technetium are abnormal from early on, but differentiation from infective or other inflammatory causes can be difficult. MRI scanning may prove more useful for this in the future as may 111indium-labelled white cell studies if infection is suspected.

Eventually, in the untreated patient, 2 classic deformities are seen:
- A 'rocker bottom' deformity due to displacement and subluxation of the tarsus downwards.
- Medial convexity due to displacement of the talonavicular joint or tarsometatarsal dislocation.

Management

If diagnosed early, immobilization may help prevent joint destruction. Exactly how best to do this is not agreed but using a non-walking plaster cast or an Aircast type of boot is needed for at least 2–3 months while bone repair/remodelling is going on. Some advocate immobilization for anything up to a year. The recent use of bisphosphates to speed this up by reducing osteoclast activity is interesting and already under further evaluation.

Further reading

Boulton AJM (2003). Foot problems in patients with DM. In Williams G and Pickup JC (eds.), *Textbook of Diabetes*, 3rd edn. Blackwell Science: Oxford.

A National Clinical Guideline recommended for use in Scotland by the Scottish Intercollegiate Network (SIGN) (1997). *Management of Diabetic Foot Disease*. (available from SIGN Secretariat, 9 Queen Street, Edinburgh, EH2 1JQ). ⏂ www.sign.ac.uk/guidelines/

NICE (2004) NICE clinical guidance, Type 2 diabetes–footcare. NCIE: London. ⏂ www.nice.org.uk

Wagner FW (1983). Algorithms of diabetic foot care. In Levin ME, O'Neil LW (eds). *The Diabetic Foot*, 2nd edn. Mosby Yearbook: St Louis, pp.291–302.

Diabetes and pregnancy

Background

0.27% of ♀ who become pregnant have previously known diabetes accounting for 0.10% of live births, and 2–3% of pregnant ♀ have a diagnosis of gestational diabetes made during their pregnancy. In both cases there are risks both to the mother and the fetus, with an historical fetal abnormality rate of up to 30% or 12× that of the background population often being quoted. The increasing proportion of ♀ with type 2 diabetes among diabetes pregnancies should also be looked for.

Risks

Fetal

With greater emphasis on improving glycaemic control, a 2.5–3-fold ↑ congenital malformation rate in mothers with previously known diabetes and a 1.8-fold increase in those without, compared to the non-diabetic population, is more realistic now. Cardiac, renal, and neural tube defects occur, particularly sacral agenesis. Hyperglycaemia in the first 8 weeks of fetal life, during organogenesis, is thought to be the underlying cause. This explains the lower rate in those with gestational diabetes which classically occurs later than this, but not completely. Alterations in oxygen free radicals, myosinositol, and arachidonic acid metabolism and alterations in zinc metabolism have also been implicated.

The most common problem seen in the infant is macrosomia (in 8–50%), which can result in birth trauma and an ↑ intervention rate. As well as causing obesity, fetal hyperinsulinaemia also accelerates skeletal maturation, delays pulmonary maturation, and causes ↑ growth of insulin-sensitive tissues giving hypertrophy of the liver and heart. These infants also have an ↑ risk of hypoglycaemia, seen transiently in up to 50%, and jaundice, with rates of 6–50% quoted, and up to 50% of these requiring phototherapy. Polycythaemia is also seen.

Maternal

Maternal problems include an ↑ risk of infection and of preeclampsia, which is 2–3 times as likely to occur as in a non-diabetic mother. In ♀ with Type 1 diabetes a 3 fold ↑ prevalence of thyroid dysfunction both during the pregnancy and post partum needs to be remembered and screened for.

Inheritance of diabetes

If the background rate of diabetes is 0.15%, the infant of a diabetic mother has a 2% rate and the infant of a diabetic father has a 6% rate. Interestingly the risk of type 2 diabetes in the child of a type 2 mother is much higher at 15–30%, rising to 50–60% if both parents have type 2 diabetes.

Known diabetics and pregnancy

Most ♀ with diabetes have normal deliveries and normal babies. In most instances these are ♀ with type 1 diabetes, although in some ethnic groups type 2 patients may make up a sizable group. In both groups it is of utmost importance to have pre-conception glycaemic control optimized, e.g. preferably an HbAlc in the non-diabetic range or <7.0% if that is not possible. The congenital malformation and spontaneous abortion rates are significantly higher when the HbA1c is elevated. Once the HbA1c is 4–6 standard deviations above the normal non-diabetic range there is a 4-fold ↑ in the malformation rate; at over 6 standard deviations above normal, this rises to a 12-fold risk. In the type 2 patients converting from oral agents to insulin is important. If not possible prior to conception it should be done as soon as a ♀ is found to be pregnant. Oral agents are potentially teratogenic and because of their ability to cross the placenta can further stimulate fetal β cells.

Pre-conception management

Pre-conception and post-conception advice is similar to that given to non-diabetic ♀, namely stopping smoking, reducing alcohol intake, avoiding unpasteurized dairy products, and adding oral folate supplements (5mg/day). Reviewing the need for any.potentially teratogenic drugs they may be taking (e.g. antihypertensive agents usually), and what they can be swapped to, is also advised.

Ideally all patients who have diabetes and are pregnant should be managed in a combined clinic with an interested obstetrician. Reviews are initially 2–4 weekly then 1–2 weekly in the last 1/3 of pregnancy. Screening and monitoring for conditions such as associated thyroid disease at these reviews is also advisable.

Maintain good glycaemic control

This is not just because of the risk of ketoacidosis which occurs in <1% of diabetic pregnancies and is associated with fetal loss in 20% of episodes, but also because of macrosomia in the fetus and both an ↑ fetal mortality (up to 2.2% of births in diabetic mothers) and an ↑ intervention rate at delivery. Aim to keep the glucose and HbAlc in the non-diabetic range to try to reduce the morbidity and mortality associated with pregnancy and diabetes. It should be remembered, however, that even with perfect control there is a small but significant excess of major congenital malformations in these children and an unexplained risk of late stillbirths.

Box 118.1 Monitoring during pregnancy

- Capillary blood glucose monitoring is performed at least 4 × /day.
- Monitor thyroid function.

Target glycaemic control

- Fasting glucoses of <5mmol/L.
- Postprandial glucoses of <7mmol/L.
- Keep the HbA1c in the non-diabetic range.

Treatment regimen

A basal bolus regimen gives greatest flexibility and is commonly used to achieve this target. In type 1 patients insulin requirements often fall in the 1st trimester, increase slightly in the second and then continue to rise until about 36 weeks, falling back to pre-pregnancy levels after delivery. In type 1 ♀ remember early pregnancy is a cause of falling insulin requirements and recurrent hypoglycaemia. It has been suggested up to 40% of ♀ with type 1 diabetes will experience significant hypoglycaemic episodes when pregnant and that hypoglycaemic awareness may alter. Advice regarding care with driving and other potentially hazardous pursuits is therefore needed early in pregnancy, if not before conception. Type 2 ♀ requiring insulin usually need 0.9 units/kg per day initially and 1.6 units/kg per day later in the pregnancy.

Monitoring of diabetic complications during pregnancy

Certain diabetic complications are known to worsen during pregnancy, and screening for nephropathy and retinopathy in particular is advised at least each trimester.

Fetal monitoring

Scanning of the fetus is performed at 10–12 weeks looking for congenital abnormalities and to confirm dates. Repeat scanning to check for excessive growth/macrosomia at 18–20 weeks, 28 weeks, 32 weeks, and 36 weeks, although the exact timing and frequency can vary between centres.

Management of delivery

At delivery, most units have set protocols but, in general, induction soon after 38 weeks' gestation (or not later than expected delivery date) and the use of a continuous insulin infusion with a separate dextrose and potassium infusion to maintain stable blood glucose levels is advisable. This is important as maternal hyperglycaemia during delivery can be associated with neonatal hypoglycaemia and an adverse neurological outcome in the infant, the infant responding to a hyperglycaemic environment in utero by ↑ its own insulin production.

After delivery

Monitoring of the infant with capillary blood glucoses post delivery is also often performed. The ↑ potential for hypoglycaemia in the mother and the baby if breast-feeding also needs watching out for, and extra carbohydrate snacks for the mother are often needed along with a 20–25% reduction in pre-conception insulin requirements. One day's worth of breast milk contains about 50g of carbohydrate. Oral hypoglycaemic agents should not be recommenced until after breast feeding has stopped.

Also consider monitoring thyroid function at 3 and 6 months post delivery.

Box 118.2 Treatment regimen for labour/delivery

- If labour is induced, omit the previous evening's long acting insulin.
- Infuse 10% glucose at 75–125mL/h (with 20mmol potassium per 500mL bag). Infuse via a syringe driver 2–4 units/h of soluble insulin initially (usually made as 50mL soluble insulin in 50mL of 0.9% saline in a 50mL syringe).
- Monitor capillary blood glucose levels hourly and adjust the infusion rate of the insulin to keep blood glucose levels in the 6–8mmol/L range.
- Monitor fluid balance carefully (especially if oxytocin is also being given).
- Check serum sodium if labour lasts over 24h (or 8h with oxytocin)

After delivery

- Halve the IV insulin infusion rate.
- Continue to monitor capillary blood glucose hourly for at least 4h then 2–4-hourly until the mother is eating normally.
- Return to pre-pregnancy regimen when eating normally but be careful as insulin requirements can be low for the first 24h.

Gestational diabetes

Epidemiology

Pregnancy potentially induces a state of insulin resistance with increases in the levels of growth hormone, progesterone, placental lactogen, and cortisol. This can therefore result in altered glucose handling. Impaired glucose tolerance during pregnancy occurs in up to 2–3% of pregnant ♀ and may be associated with an ↑ risk of subsequent type 2 diabetes in 20–50% of patients. Worsening maternal insulin resistance and associated hyperglycaemia usually becomes evident from the 2nd trimester onwards if it is going to occur.

As with ♀ previously known to have diabetes, there is an association with worsening carbohydrate intolerance and a worse maternal and fetal outcome. Untreated gestational diabetes has been shown to have a perinatal mortality of 4.4–6.4% compared to 0.5–1.5% in a similar ethnic normoglycaemic population. Intensive insulin treatment has been shown to reduce such complications. This is the rationale for careful multidisciplinary care of these patients.

Treatment

Initial treatment is with dietary advice and in 10–30% insulin is also required. Insulin therapy should be considered if fasting blood glucoses are >6.0mmol/L or post prandial levels are >8mmol/L. Obesity is not uncommon and the importance of post-delivery dietary modification and weight reduction, to reduce the risk of future type 2 diabetes, should also be reinforced. The varying insulin requirements during pregnancy occur as in those with previously known diabetes, and most (but not all) will not need insulin treatment following delivery. Monitoring is with home capillary blood glucose measurements, daily if on diet alone and more frequently if on insulin therapy. The frequency needed depends on the results obtained with the aim to keep all readings <7.0mmol/L. If diet alone fails, a basal bolus insulin regimen as used in the known diabetic is usually required. Decide on the total initial daily dose on the basis of the degree of hyperglycaemia present; 4–6 units per bolus is usual.

As with the previously known diabetic mother, the aim is to have a normal delivery, more often at 38 weeks to term depending on fetal growth. An OGTT 6 weeks after delivery is needed in all patients not requiring insulin post-delivery to confirm a return to normal glucose metabolism. A further reinforcement of diet and weight advice at this time is also usual practice. Whether these patients should be followed up in view of their ↑ risk of diabetes is unclear at this time, but annual fasting blood glucose levels in asymptomatic ♀ with a normal 6-week postpartum OGTT is often advised and more careful review is suggested in those with abnormal OGTTs.

Box 118.3 Methods of screening

- Urine dip testing for glucose should be performed on every pregnant woman at every antenatal visit.
- If glycosuria is found a fasting glucose is performed and if >6.0mmol/L a 75g OGTT is needed.
- Routine screening at 28–32 weeks is also often performed, either with random blood glucoses or a fasting blood glucose and if a fasting level is >6.0mmol/L or a postprandial level is >7.0mmol/L an OGTT is required.
- The diagnostic criteria for diabetes are no different from those in the non-pregnant population. A diagnosis of gestational diabetes or gestational IGT is made if the fasting glucose is 6.0–7.8mmol/L and/or the 2h postprandial level is 9.0–11.0mmol/L by the UK/St. Vincent definition. The WHO definition has a fasting level of 7.8mmol/L and/or a 2-h postprandial level of 7.8–11.1mmol/L.

Table 118.1 Interpretation of the 75g oral glucose tolerance test during pregnancy

	Plasma glucose (mmol/L)	
	Fasting	2h proprandial level
Diabetes	>7.0	>11.0
Gestational IGT	6.0–7.8	9–11
Normal	<6.1	9

High risk groups

Most ♀ with gestational diabetes are found on routine screening at about 30 weeks, but certain high risk groups should be screened earlier. These risk factors include:

- Previous gestational diabetes.
- A large baby in their last pregnancy, e.g. >4.0kg at term.
- A previous unexplained stillbirth/perinatal death.
- Maternal obesity.
- Family history of diabetes (1st-degree relatives).
- Polyhydramnios.

Contraception and diabetes

Oral contraceptives

The early combined oral contraceptive pills (OCP) impaired glucose tolerance and so were not advised in patients with diabetes. The use of 3rd-generation low-dose oestrogen-containing combined OCPs (e.g. 20mcg ethinylestradiol) is safe in ♀ <35 years of age. 3rd-generation OCPs are advised as they have a better risk profile for arterial disease and only occasionally increase insulin requirements.

As in the non-diabetic population, standard advice regarding the pill should be given and its avoidance in at-risk groups such as overweight smokers with a family history of thromboembolism and coronary heart disease is sensible. There is an ↑ risk of cerebral thromboembolism in type 1 patients, but the OCP dose not increase this.

In those with microvascular disease or coronary risk factors, the progesterone-only 'mini-pill' (POP) is safer than the combined OCP as it has no significant adverse effects on lipid metabolism, clotting, platelet aggregation, or fibrinolytic activity. It has been suggested that levonorgestrel- and norethisterone-containing POPs may reduce HDL_2 cholesterol subfractions. The avoidance of POPs in those with established arterial disease is advised.

Barrier methods

The sheath and the diaphragm were historically the contraceptive method of choice in people with diabetes, and do not have the metabolic risks of the oral contraceptives described above. But, both are less effective forms of contraception with a failure rate of 0.7–3.6/100 couple years for the sheath and 2/100 couple years for the diaphragm, compared to nearly 0.2/100 ♀ years with the combined OCP. In a population in which pregnancy carries significant risks, other forms of contraception are therefore now more often advocated.

Intrauterine contraceptive devices (IUD)

There is a concern that diabetes might make a pelvic infection associated with an IUD more severe and may render both copper containing and inert IUDs less effective, but not all studies have confirmed these worries. Nevertheless, if an IUD is used in a ♀ with diabetes a progestagen-releasing variety or a small copper device with regular use of spermicides are the current favourite options.

Hormone replacement therapy (HRT)

As with the OCP, diabetes itself is not a contraindication to the use of HRT. The oestrogens in HRT differ from those in the OCP and may actually reduce insulin resistance and also protect against coronary disease, although they may not actually reduce cardiovascular events in those with established coronary artery disease.

Further reading

Confidential Enquiry into Maternal and Child Health Report. ⌐ www.cemach.org.uk

Dornhorst A anc Chan SP (1998). The elusive diagnosis of gestational diabetes. *Diabet Med* **15**, 7–10.

Garner P (1995). Type 1 DM and pregnancy. *Lancet* **346**, 157–61.

Ilkova H (1995). Screening for gestational diabetes. *Diabet Rev Int* **3**(3), 1–2.

NICE (2008). Interpartum care. Clinical guidance CG63. Diabetes in Pregnancy. ⌐ www.nice.org.uk/guidance

NICE (2008). NICE guidelines. Diabetes in Pregnancy. NICE: London. ⌐ www.nice.org.uk/guidance

(2002). *Pregnancy and diabetes mellitus*. In Pickup J, Williams G (eds.) *Textbook of Diabetes*, *3rd* edn, Blackwell Science: Oxford. Chapter 65 Pregnancy and diabetes.

Intercurrent events or disease

Surgery

Preoperative assessment

Careful preoperative assessment is essential because of an ↑ risk of death and complications such as fluid overload from coronary heart disease and diabetic nephropathy. Any preoperative assessment in a patient with known diabetes should therefore include:

- An adequate history of diabetic complications.
- A full examination looking for evidence of peripheral vascular disease, peripheral neuropathy, and lying/standing BPs in case of autonomic neuropathy.
- Assessment of current and overall diabetic control using blood glucose measurements in all patients and glycated haemoglobin.
- General investigations should include serum urea + electrolytes/creatinine, FBC, urine dip testing for protein, and an ECG (in anyone >45 years old).

Any further investigation will be based on problems found in the history or examination such as foot ulceration and potential osteomyelitis which may give a source for infection such as an MRSA.

Attempts should be made to improve diabetic control, either on the ward or in a diabetic clinic, for any patient undergoing an elective procedure whose control is inadequate. An HbA1c <7.2% is considered good control, but an acceptable levels for most procedures would be <9%. Even with a good HbA1c level the preoperative glucose level (and if >11mmol/L the urine ketones) should always be measured as the perioperative treatment is based on this and some stabilization before administration of an anaesthetic may be required, particularly in the emergency situation.

Perioperative management

Ideally patients with diabetes are best operated on in the morning at the start of the list.

Patients normally on diet alone should have their capillary blood glucose levels checked hourly and avoid IV dextrose, and often need no other modification to their treatment. Patients taking oral agents should stop metformin for at least 48h preoperatively and miss their other agents on the morning of the procedure. If on chlorpropamide it should be missed the day before as well. Capillary blood glucose levels are again monitored regularly (1–2-hourly) and if >7.0mmol/L start a dextrose + insulin regimen as detailed in Box 119.1 and aim to keep the glucose in the 7–11mmol/L range.

In patients taking insulin undergoing a morning operation, miss the morning insulin dose and start on a dextrose + insulin regimen as shown in Box 119.1. If on an afternoon list give half the normal morning dose of soluble insulin with a light breakfast and start the dextrose + insulin regimen at midday. Again aim to keep the blood glucose in the 7–11mmol/L range.

Suitable insulin regimens
These come in 2 forms, the current favourite being a continuous IV insulin infusion adjusted on the basis of blood glucose measurements with a fixed dextrose infusion. The other is a single bag containing dextrose, insulin, and potassium known as the *Alberti regimen* or the *GIK (glucose insulin potassium) regimen* (📖 see Box 119.1)

Box 119.1 Insulin regimens

Continuous IV insulin infusion regimen/'sliding scale' insulin
50 units of soluble insulin in 50mL 0.9% saline (giving 1 unit/mL) are placed in a 50mL syringe and run through an automated syringe driver at a predetermined rate depending on regular capillary blood glucose measurements. Most units now have written guidelines for this type of regimen and each will need to be tailored to an individual patient, e.g. in insulin-resistant patients much larger amounts of insulin are needed. One such regimen is:

Blood glucose (mmol/L)	Insulin infusion rate (units/h or mL/h)
0–4.0	0.5 (+ recheck in 30min)
4.1–7.0	1.0
7.1–11.0	2.0
11.1–17.0	4.0
>17.1	6.0–8.0 (+ review regimen)

IV insulin regimens such as this should never be given without IV fluids and potassium to avoid hypoglycaemia or hypokalaemia, e.g. start with 100 mL of 5% dextrose containing 5mmol of potassium per hour. The postoperative rotating of dextrose and non-glucose containing IV fluids can increase the risk of hypoglycaemia, especially if there is not careful monitoring of the blood glucose. Initially hourly capillary blood glucose levels are needed, moving to 2-hourly measurements postoperatively once stable results are obtained. An attempt at keeping the IV dextrose infusion rate relatively constant makes this sort of regimen slightly safer. A preoperative potassium and daily repeat measurements are also required.

Postoperatively, once the patient has started eating adequately aim to revert back to a standard SC insulin regimen with a pre-meal dose of insulin 30min before food and the infusion stopping once this is working, i.e. when the food arrives. Patients previously on oral agents who require an IV insulin regimen may have an ↑ insulin demand due to infection or the stress of the procedure and may require SC insulin initially rather than just reverting to their preoperative oral agent(s), so be especially careful in this group.

The GIK regimen

Although not as popular as the above 'sliding scale' continuous regimen, this method does have the advantage of everything being given together so reducing the risk of insulin being given on its own. Into a 500mL bag of 5% dextrose add 8 units of soluble insulin and 5mmol of potassium. Run this mixture at 100mL/h and measure capillary blood glucoses hourly initially, aiming for levels of 7–11mmol/L ideally and 5–15mmol/L at worst. If >15mmol/L, swap this infusion for one with 10 units of insulin but also check the serum potassium level to see if that also needs adjusting. If blood glucose is <5mmol/L reduce the insulin to 6 units/500 mL of 5% dextrose. After each alteration recheck blood glucose levels after 1h and adjust further if required. Once stable reduce the capillary blood glucose levels to 2-hourly. As with the other IV regimen, convert to regular therapy once the patient is eating.

Certain situations may require further modification of this regimen, such as open heart surgery where the use of glucose-rich solutions and hypothermia can mean that higher doses of insulin are required initially.

Skin/connective tissue/joint disease

Skin

Diabetes results in an ↑ occurrence of infections such as vaginal candida, candida balanitis, and *Staphylococcus aureus* folliculitis. Ulceration in the feet due to neuropathy and peripheral vascular disease should also be considered. Other skin features to look for include the following.

Conditions specific to diabetes

- *Pretibial diabetic dermopathy*—'shin spots'.
- *Diabetic bullae*—bullosis diabeticorum, very rare tense blistering on feet/lower legs classically.
- *Diabetic thick skin*—cleroderma of diabetes seen in 2.5% with type 2 diabetes.
- *Periungual telangectasia*—venous capillary dilatation at the nail fold seen in up to 50% of people with diabetes.

Conditions seen more commonly in those with diabetes

- Necrobiosis lipoidica
- Vitiligo (seen in 2% with type 1 diabetes)
- Granuloma annulare (though this association is not proven conclusively).

Conditions associated with the other biochemical features seen in diabetes

- Acanthosis nigricans—with insulin resistance.
- Eruptive xanthomata—with hypertriglyceridaemia.

The most common skin lesion in diabetes are shin spots or diabetic dermopathy. These occur more commonly in ♂ than in ♀ and affect up to 50% of people with diabetes. Their aetiology is uncertain. They present initially as red papules and progress to give well circumscribed atrophic areas, brownish in colour. Usually seen on the shins, they can also be found on the forearms and thighs. There is no effective treatment of these but they usually resolve spontaneously over 1–2 years.

Necrobiosis lipoidica is seen in 0.3–1% of people with diabetes, and 40–60% of those with necrobiosis also have diabetes. It is more common in ♀ than in ♂. Classically seen on the shins, it has an atrophic centre with telangiectasia around the edge of an oval or irregular lesion, although early lesions can be dull red plaques or papules. Treatment with topical or injectable steroids may help improve these lesions; skin grafting and cosmetic camouflage have also been used.

When looking at the skin do not forget to check injection sites for lipo-hypertrophy or lipoatrophy as these are often much more amenable to treatment or correction. In the past an insulin allergy rash was also commonly seen, but more recently a transient local reaction, thought to be an IgE-mediated reaction, is more often seen.

Connective tissue/joint disease

Diabetes is associated with an ↑ incidence of pseudogout and osteoarthritis, but the classical condition to consider is the 'stiff hand syndrome' or *diabetic cheiroarthropathy*. In this the skin thickens and tightens which, in association with sclerosis of the tendon sheaths, results in limited joint mobility in the hands and less commonly the feet. This reduced joint mobility gives an inability to place the palms of the hand flat together and make the 'prayer sign'. No specific treatment for this currently exists.

Social and practical aspects

Current regulations for fitness to drive motor vehicles

Diabetes is said to influence the ability to drive safely because of hypoglycaemia or complications such as a reduction in vision acuity or fields. It carries a similar risk of accidents to epilepsy (e.g. relative risk of 1.23–1.24 compared to standard drivers). The Driver and Vehicle Licensing Agency (DVLA) Drivers Medical Unit produced a revised set of guidelines in February 1999, which are outlined here, the DVLA website should however be checked for regular updates (www.dvla.gov.uk).

A group 1 licence is the standard motorcycle/motor car licence (e.g. categories A and B) which also allows you to drive a private minibus carrying up to 16 people (category D1) or a vehicle between 3.5 and 7.5 tonnes (category C1). A group 2 licence allows you to drive heavy goods vehicles (HGVs) and passenger carrying vehicles (PCVs), and all holders of these must inform the DVLA of their diabetes what ever their treatment:

- Any patient with uncomplicated diabetes who is on *diet alone* does not need to inform the DVLA unless they live in Northern Ireland, they develop complications which will interfere with their ability to drive, or their therapy changes.
- ♀ who develop *gestational diabetes* need to inform the DVLA and must re-inform them 6 weeks after delivery if still on insulin. They must also stop driving while pregnant if their control is poor and automatically lose their group 2 licence until after delivery.
- *Insulin-treated patients* are required to inform the DVLA if they are on insulin therapy and will need to renew their licences every 1–3 years. They must demonstrate satisfactory control, recognize warning symptoms of hypoglycaemia, and have acceptable eyesight for a standard group 1 licence. New applicants for a driving licence or existing drivers starting on insulin do not automatically get a C1 + D1 licence. From 11/9/98 some previous licence holders, subject to annual review, can keep their class C1 vehicle licence for 3.5–7.5 tonne lorries, but not for D1. Since 1991 they were also barred from driving HGVs or PCVs. Drivers licensed before 1/4/91 who are on insulin are reassessed annually and may still do so.
- *Patients managed with tablets* need to inform the DVLA and can normally continue to hold both a group 1 (until 70 years old) and a group 2 licence, subject to a satisfactory medical. If vision deteriorates, hypoglycaemia is a problem, or they require insulin therapy this may alter.

Travel

Travel across time zones, exposure to unaccustomed exercise, and new infections make this an important area for both patient and doctor education. It is common sense to take more insulin than is needed for any time away, in case of an accidental loss or breakage. If new insulin supplies are needed, remember not all countries use only the U100 strength and tell the patient travelling abroad to look out for this, e.g 30 units or 0.3 mL of U100 strength insulin equates to 0.75mL of the U40 form and 0.38mL of U80. A letter stating the need to carry insulin, needles, and syringes/pen devices will also make Customs formalities slightly easier.

Patients with diabetes need the same immunizations and malaria prophylaxis as other travellers. In case they acquire an infection or illness while travelling, standard 'sick day rules' should be reinforced. These suggest that:

- Insulin therapy should never be stopped and may actually need to be ↑, even when food intake is reduced.
- If the patient is unable to tolerate solid food, a liquid form of carbohydrate such as Lucozade® or Dioralyte® should be taken instead. A patient who is unable to tolerate adequate oral fluids should seek medical advice.
- If unwell monitor urine for ketones and, if present, seek medical advice.
- During any illness consider increasing the frequency of capillary glucose testing.

Travel and adjustments in therapy are usually more of a problem for insulin-treated patients as those on oral agents can adjust the timing of their tablets to the new time zone with less risk of significant deteriorations in control.

In the insulin-treated patient:

- On *short flights* where the differences in time zones is small no major insulin adjustments are needed, but make sure snacks and extra carbohydrate are packed with hand luggage as the timing, quality, and quantity of airline food is rather variable.
- On *longer flights* where time zones are crossed the adjustments eeded will depend on their initial regimen and the direction of travel. If travelling east to west the day is longer and extra doses are needed; west to east gives a shorter day and so a reduction in therapy is required. With a basal bolus regimen take soluble insulin with each meal given and intermediate acting insulin given to fit in with the evening at the destination. In a twice-daily mixed regimen give an extra dose of soluble when going east to west and miss the evening isophane when going west to east.

Exercise

Non-diabetic people initially breakdown muscle glycogen for 5–10min, then use circulating glucose and non-esterified fatty acids. Hepatic glucose production increases, but free fatty acids are the main fuel used after 1–2h of exercise and without some form of energy intake most people become hypoglycaemic after 2–3h of strenuous exercise. Insulin sensitivity also decreases the day after severe exertion.

Type 1 diabetes

Insulin requirements are reduced during exercise. To reduce the risk of hypoglycaemia with acute exercise decrease the pre-exercise insulin dose, which would have its peak during the exercise, by 30–50%. If the exercise is due to last >2h also take 20–40g of extra carbohydrate before and hourly during exercise.

If the site of the insulin injection is the area being exercised absorption may be accelerated, especially if exercise is undertaken soon after the injection of an insulin analogue, so inject into an area that won't be exercised. With extreme exercise it may take several hours, if not until the next day, to fully replenish muscle glycogen stores and care is needed to avoid hypoglycaemia during this period.

Type 2 diabetes

Exercise increases peripheral glucose uptake and reduces endogenous insulin secretion. Physical training can increase insulin sensitivity which in type 2 patients can result in a reduction in HbA1c, BP, weight, and a better lipid profile. Hypoglycaemia is not usually a problem unless the patient is taking sulfonylureas, so extra carbohydrate is not normally indicated. In those using these agents a reduction in dosage may however be advisable.

Complications from diabetes and driving

Loss of hypoglycaemic awareness will result in permanent loss of an HGV/PCV licence and a temporary loss of a standard licence until specialist reports can confirm that awareness has returned. Any doctor making this diagnosis must tell the patient they are legally obliged to inform the DVLA of this diagnosis. If the patient refuses to do so the medical adviser at the DVLA should be informed once the patient has been informed in writing of the intention to do so. Avoiding all hypoglycaemic episodes for at least a month will help to regain hypoglycaemic awareness in some patients. A patient who is unable to regain this awareness *must* stop driving.

In a patient with frequent hypoglycaemic episodes or with poor control it seems sensible to advise them not to drive until things are better, and the DVLA should be contacted. As part of their regular checks the DVLA asks a doctor to complete a Diabetes III form which asks if control of the diabetes is satisfactory/stable and how long this has been for. This should help to pick up many of these patients. If you say their control is poor or unstable, do not forget to tell the patient what you have done and arrange to see them to improve this problem as reports to that effect will be needed by the DVLA before their licence is renewed.

Visual requirements are that you can read a number plate with 79.4mm high letters at 20.5m with glasses/contact lenses if worn. This equates to a visual acuity of between 6/9 and 6/12 on a Snellen chart. Group 2 licence holders must have an acuity of 6/9 or better in their good eye and not worse than 6/12 in the bad, but will not be licensed if they have an uncorrected acuity worse than 3/60 in either eye. Visual field defects of any sort, especially if bilateral, result in loss of HGV/PCV licences and may affect a standard licence.

Other complications such as limb amputations can alter the ability to drive, but driving is still possible if the vehicle is suitably modified.

Useful resources

Diabetes U.K, Macleod House, 10 Parkway, London NW1 7AA. Tel: 020 7424 1000 or Diabetes UK Careline: 08451202960 ☝ www.diabetes.org.uk

Driver and Vehicle Licensing Agency (DVLA), Drivers Medical Unit, Longview Road, Morriston, Swansea SA99 1DA. Tel: 01792 783795. Fax: 01792 783687 ☝ www.dvla.gov.uk

Emergencies in diabetes

Diabetic ketoacidosis

Diabetic ketoacidosis has a mortality of 2–5%. Many deaths occur due to delays in presentation and initiation of treatment, with a mortality rate of up to 50% in the elderly.

Diagnosis

This is usually based on a collection of biochemical abnormalities, namely:
- *Hyperglycaemia* >11.1mmol/L.
- *Acidosis* arterial pH <7.3, serum bicarbonate <15mmol/L, base excess <−10.
- *Ketonuria* Some dip testing methods only check for acetoacetate and acetone but not β-hydroxybutyrate. Captopril can also give a false +ve test for urinary acetone. Ketones may also interfere with some creatinine assays and give falsely high readings.

There is an uncommon condition of *euglycaemic ketoacidosis* (in 1–3% of cases at most) when ketones are produced early on in patients with a reduced carbohydrate intake. Blood glucose is <17mmol/L, acidosis is marked, and dehydration is not usually severe. Treatment is to initiate oral carbohydrate intake and monitor the need for IV insulin/fluids as in full-blown hyperglycaemic ketoacidosis.

Epidemiology

Diabetic ketoacidosis is common in patients with type 1 diabetes, with 1 in 11 subjects in the European IDDM complications study (EURODIAB) reporting hospitalization for this over a 12 month period. The incidence is 5–8/1000 diabetic patients per year, usually patients with type 1 diabetes but up to 25% of cases are patients with newly diagnosed/presenting diabetes some of whom subsequently obtain adequate control with oral agents or diet alone. In up to 50% of cases an infection is the precipitant and in 10–30% of cases it is their 1st presentation with diabetes.

Pathogenesis

Diabetic ketoacidosis occurs as a result of insulin deficiency and counter-regulatory hormone excess. Insulin deficiency results in excess mobilization of free fatty acids from adipose tissue. This provides the substrate for ketone production from the liver. Ketones β-hydroxy-butyrate, acetoacetate, and acetone) are excreted by the kidneys and buffered in the blood initially, but once this system fails acidosis develops. Hyperglycaemia also occurs as the liver produces glucose from lactate and alanine which are generated by muscle proteolysis. The reduced peripheral glucose utilization associated with insulin deficiency exacerbates this.

Hyperglycaemia and ketonuria cause an osmotic diuresis and hypovolaemia with both intracellular and extracellular dehydration. Glomerular filtration is reduced and blood glucose levels therefore rise even further as do the levels of counterregulatory hormones such as glucagon. The metabolic acidosis due to ketone accumulation leads to widespread cell death which combined with hypovolaemia is fatal if untreated.

Box 121.1 Clinical features

Polyuria, polydipsia, and weight loss are often seen. Muscle cramps, abdominal pain, and shortness of breath (air hunger or Kussmaul's breathing, with deep regular rapid breaths, suggesting acidosis) can also occur. Subsequent nausea and vomiting can worsen both the dehydration and electrolyte losses which often precede the onset of coma (occurring in about 10% of cases). Remember to consider other causes of coma and a raised blood glucose such as head injury, alcohol, and drug overdoses.

On examination the breath can smell of ketones (like nail-varnish remover) with postural hypotension (exacerbated by peripheral vasodilatation due to acidosis) and hypothermia also frequently seen. Infection and trauma can precipitate this problem and should be carefully looked for, especially in the unconscious patient.

Hypovolaemia at presentation is usually at least 5L with electrolyte losses of 300–700mmol of sodium, 200–700mmol of potassium, and 350–500mmol of chloride accompanying this. The daily intake of both sodium and potassium is 60mmol, so the severity of this is apparent

Management

Having first assessed the need for immediate resuscitation, and commenced a 0.9% saline IV infusion, take a history and examine the patient to look for obvious precipitants such as surgery, trauma, sites of infection, or myocardial infarction. Initial investigations will be modified by the history and examination and suggested site of infection but should at least include:

- Blood for urea/electrolytes (note ketone/creatinine assay interaction).
- FBC (a leukocytosis can occur without infection).
- Arterial blood gases ($P_a CO_2$ will be low due to hyperventilation with a metabolic acidosis, check pH and bicarbonate).
- Cultures of blood and urine.
- Chest radiograph and ECG.
- In the older patient (>40 years) also include an ECG and cardiac enzymes, even if asymptomatic.

Replacement of fluids, electrolytes, and insulin is the mainstay of treatment, along with treating any precipitant, such as infection. To monitor this treatment central venous access and urinary catheterization are often necessary and a NG tube may be useful, especially in the unconscious patient. In elderly people, those with a cardiac history, or those with autonomic neuropathy central venous access is imperative.

Monitoring

Once treatment has commenced, monitor fluid balance carefully and avoid fluid overload. Check capillary blood glucose hourly with serum potassium, sodium, and glucose 2 hourly and arterial blood gases 2–4-hourly depending on response. Reduce the frequency of tests once stabilized but check electrolytes at least daily for the 1st 72h. Continuous ECG monitoring will aid the detection of hypo- and hyperkalaemia in the acute phase. Magnesium and phosphate levels should also be checked as these can occasionally require replacement therapy.

Additional therapies

- *IV bicarbonate* is only rarely indicated as it can cause hypokalaemia and paradoxically worsen intracellular acidosis. If used, give only when the pH is <6.9 using 250mL of 1.26% bicarbonate given over 30–60min initially and monitor arterial blood gases to assess response, aiming for pH no greater than 7.1. This should probably only be used in an intensive care setting. Do not use 8.4% bicarbonate as its high sodium load can too rapidly alter electrolyte levels and precipitate pulmonary oedema as well as causing local tissue necrosis if it extravasates.
- In severe hypotension unresponsive to colloids and crystalloids inotropes may be required but agents such as *dopamine*, *dobutamine*, and *adrenaline* will all exacerbate insulin resistance necessitating a more aggressive sliding scale regime.
- *Heparin* in SC prophylactic doses can be given in the unconscious or immobile patent.
- Cover with *IV broad-spectrum antibiotics* should be used if no obvious precipitant is found and appropriate antibiotics if a site of infection is found.
- Cerebral oedema typically presents 8–24h after starting IV fluids with a declining conscious level and may have a mortality as high as 90%. If this occurs *dexamethasone* (12–16mg/day) and *mannitol* (1–2g/kg body weight) may be given.

Subsequent treatment

Once the blood glucose is stable in the 10–15mmol/L range, the ketoacidosis has settled, and the patient is eating and drinking normally consider swapping on to a SC insulin regimen but overlap the IV and the first SC dose by 2h. Stabilize on this therapy before discharge from hospital. Once the IV potassium supplements have stopped, give oral supplements for at least 48h with regular serum monitoring.

Patient education to determine the cause and so avoid a further occurrence, or for earlier presentation if it does occur, should also ideally be performed before discharge.

Box 121.2 Precipitants of diabetic ketoacidosis

• Infection	30–40%.
• Non-compliance with treatment	25%.
• Inappropriate alterations in insulin (i.e. errors by patient or doctor)	13%.
• Newly diagnosed diabetes	10–20%.
• Myocardial infarction	1%.

Initial treatment of ketoacidosis

IV 0.9% saline

- 2L in 2h then 1L over 2h, 2L in next 8h and 4L/day thereafter until blood glucose <11mmol/L. Then convert to dextrose saline or 5% dextrose.
- If the patient is profoundly shocked (e.g. systolic BP <80mmHg with severe dehydration or sepsis) or oliguric, this may need to be given more rapidly and colloids may also be needed. If elderly or there are signs of heart failure or cerebral oedema this may need to be given more slowly.

Potassium

Once the serum potassium is known the 0.9% saline has potassium added with the dose adjusted based on hourly serum potassium measurements until stable and measured 2–4-hourly over the next 12–24h. Add:

- 40mmol/L if K^+ <3.0mmol/L.
- 30mmol/L if K^+ 3.0–4.0mmol/L.
- 20mmol/L if K^+ 4.1–5.0mmol/L.
- 10mmol/L if K^+ 5.1–6.0mmol/L.
- None if K^+ >6.0mmol/L.

Insulin (via a continuous IV infusion)

- 50 units of soluble insulin in 50mL of 0.9% saline given at 6–8 units/h to drop glucose by about 5mmol/L per h and adjusted to keep blood glucose 10–14mmol/L until after ketoacidosis has cleared (usually need 3–6 units/h).
- Alternatively use 50 units of insulin in 500mL of 0.9% saline with added potassium infused at 80–100mL/h initially with a maintenance dose of 30–60mL/h once blood glucose is adequately controlled. IM regimens should be avoided and used only as a last resort. Give 20 units of soluble insulin initially with 10 units hourly until blood glucose falls and then 20 units 6-hourly until control is achieved.

Hyperosmolar, non-ketotic hyperglycaemia

This is a more sinister complication than ketoacidosis with a mortality as high as 50% and is said to be found in 11–30% of adult hyperglycaemic emergencies. It affects an older population than ketoacidosis (middle aged or elderly), 2/3 of cases are in patients with previously undiagnosed diabetes, and its insidious onset can be mistaken for many other conditions including a stroke.

Diagnosis

This is again a biochemical diagnosis:
- *Hyperglycaemia* (usually 30–70mmol/L).
- Serum osmolality *high* (> 350mmol/kg).
- *No acidosis* arterial pH 7.35–7.45, serum bicarbonate >18mmol/L, but remember lactic acidosis with infection or a myocardial infarction may alter this.
- *No ketonuria* + on urine dip testing can occur with starvation and vomiting.

Serum osmolality (in mosmol/kg) can be calculated if not available from the laboratory using the following equation:

Osmolality = 2(sodium + potassium) + glucose + urea

Epidemiology

This occurs in an older age group of insulin-producing type 2 patients, a large proportion of whom will not previously be known to have diabetes. Ingestion of high-sugar-containing drinks, intercurrent infection, and myocardial infarction are all commonly seen as precipitants of this condition. Drugs such as glucocorticoids, cimetidine, phenytoin, thiazide, and loop diuretics have all been implicated in the pathogenesis of this problem.

Pathogenesis

This occurs from a combination of insulin deficiency and counter-regulatory hormone excess with the insulin present stopping ketone production but in insufficient quantities to prevent worsening hyperglycaemia.

Box 121.3 Clinical features

There is normally an insidious onset with several days of ill-health and profound dehydration at presentation (equivalent to a 9–10L deficit). Confusion is not uncommon, nor is coma (especially once serum osmolality >440) and occasionally fits occur. Gastroparesis and associated vomiting with gastric erosions and subsequent haematemesis can occur. These patients are also hypercoagulable, and venous thromboses and cerebrovascular events are important to exclude.

Management

Initial investigation and treatment is the same as for ketoacidosis with fluid, electrolyte, and insulin replacement, although there are a few important exceptions as these are older patients:

- The fluid regimen should be less rapid/vigorous. Central venous access for monitoring is more often required. e.g. 1L of 0.9% saline over the first hour, 1L 2-hourly for the next 2h, then 1 L 4–6-hourly.
- If hypernatraemic (serum sodium >155mmol/L) consider 0.45% saline, rather than 0.9% although this may increase the risk of cerebral oedema if serum sodium or osmolality is altered too rapidly as it has a mortality as high as 70%.
- Prophylactic SC heparin should be considered, although recent evidence suggests more formal anticoagulation carries a high risk of upper gastrointestinal bleeding.
- A gentler insulin regimen is needed with 3–6 units/h of soluble insulin IV aiming to reduce the blood glucose by a maximum of 5mmol/h to avoid precipitating cerebral oedema.
- A more aggressive use of IV antibiotics is encouraged.

Subsequent treatment

Continue IV fluids and insulin for at least 24h after initial stabilization and then convert to maintenance therapy such as SC insulin or oral hypoglycaemic agents. Patient education to avoid further episodes is also advisable.

Hypoglycaemia

This complication of the treatment of diabetes should be excluded in any unconscious or fitting patient. If prolonged it can result in death. Most insulin-treated patients can expect to experience hypoglycaemic episodes at some time, with up to 1/7 having a more severe episode each year and 3% suffering recurrent episodes. The 25% of people on long-term insulin who lose their hypoglycaemic awareness are of particular concern. Nocturnal hypoglycaemic episodes with a hyperglycaemic response the next morning (due to ↑ counter-regulatory hormones—the Somogyi phenomenon), which tend to occur in younger insulin-treated patients, should not be forgotten and may only present with morning headaches or a drunken feeling.

Diagnosis

This is a biochemical diagnosis from a blood glucose <2.5mmol/L but is often first picked up by the patient, their family, or their doctor from the clinical features below. Saving serum before treatment for blood glucose, insulin, and C-peptide levels will confirm the diagnosis and may help determine the cause.

Pathogenesis

Hypoglycaemia results from an imbalance between glucose supply, glucose utilization, and insulin levels resulting in more insulin than is needed at that time. A reduced glucose supply occurs when a meal or snack is missed, or as a late effect of alcohol. It can also be due to delayed gastric emptying with autonomic neuropathy or be associated with coeliac disease, Addison's disease, or an acute illness, such as gastroenteritis. ↑ utilization occurs with exercise and high insulin levels mostly with sulfonylurea or exogenous insulin therapy. The net result of this imbalance is hypoglycaemia.

Human insulins have a slightly faster onset of action and a shorter duration of action than their animal predecessors, and a lot of patients report alterations in hypoglycaemic awareness when they switch from one to the other. Even so, no definite evidence of specific hypoglycaemic alterations due to human insulin itself has been reported.

Sulfonylurea therapy can cause hypoglycaemia due to β cell stimulation. This is most commonly seen from *glibenclamide*, especially in the elderly and those with reduced renal excreting ability, but can occur in anyone who takes this therapy and fasts, especially with longer acting agents such as *chlorpropamide*.

The biguanide *metformin* and the α-glucosidase inhibitor *acarbose* are unlikely to precipitate hypoglycaemia, but insulin-sensitizing agents such as the ACEIs and newer agents such as the thiazolidinediones (e.g. *rosiglitazone*) may do so.

Box 121.4 Clinical features

The features of hypoglycaemia can be divided into 2 main groups: *autonomic* symptoms and *neuroglycopenic* symptoms, as shown in Box 121.5.

The autonomic symptoms usually occur first (when the blood glucose <3.6mmol/L), but some drugs such as the non-selective β-blockers and alcohol may mask these with neuroglycopenia (at blood glucose <2.6mmol/L) then causing confusion with no warning. Some patients lose these predominantly autonomic warning symptoms and are therefore at higher risk of injury.

Management

In the conscious patient, oral carbohydrate (20–30g) is often sufficient to resolve the problem. This can be given as 5–6 glucose tablets or as a glass of milk or orange juice. Having raised the sugar rapidly then give something to maintain a normal blood glucose level such as 2 digestive biscuits. In the confused patient a buccal gel (e.g. GlucoGel®, a 30% glucose gel) is an alternative although this should not be used in the unconscious patient as there is a risk of aspiration.

In the unconscious patient, once a blood sample has been taken for glucose estimation, treat with 25–50mL of 50% glucose IV or 1 mg of IM or deep SC glucagon. Glucagon mobilizes glycogen from the liver and will not work if given repeatedly or in starved patients with no glycogen stores. In this situation or if prolonged treatment is needed, IV glucose is better (50% initially then 10%). The worry with 50% glucose is tissue necrosis if extravasation occurs.

Subsequent management

Having corrected the acute event determine why it happened and, if possible, alter treatment or lifestyle to stop it recurring. Extreme exercise may require an alteration in insulin doses for 24h, and alcohol causes not only initial hyperglycaemia but also a degree of hypoglycaemia 3–6h after ingestion, and may alter insulin requirements the next morning. Education to avoid precipitating hypoglycaemic episodes in these situations is advisable. Recurrent hypoglycaemic events may also herald a deterioration in renal or liver function and these should be excluded.

Patients on long-acting sulphonylureas who experience hypoglycaemia will need careful monitoring as the drug may last longer than the glucose or glycogen given to correct it and repeated hypoglycaemic episodes may occur. A continuous IV glucose infusion is therefore often needed in this situation, particularly in overdose with these agents.

Box 121.5 Signs and symptoms of hypoglycaemia

Autonomic
- Sweating.
- Pallor.
- Anxiety.
- Nausea.
- Tremor.
- Shivering.
- Palpitations.
- Tachycardia.

Neuroglycopaenia
- Confusion.
- Tiredness.
- Lack of concentration.
- Headache.
- Dizziness.
- Altered speech.
- Incoordination.
- Drowsiness.
- Aggression.
- Coma.

Further reading

Amiel SA, Tamborlane WV, and Sherwin RS (1987). Defective glucose counterregulation after strict glycaemic control of insulin-dependent DM. *New Engl J Med* **316**, 1376–84.

Cranston ICP and Amiel SA (1995). Hypoglycaemia. In Leslie RDG, Robbins DC, (eds). *Diabetes: Clinical Science and Practice*. Cambridge University Press: Cambridge, pp.375–91.

Hepburn D, Deary IJ, Frier BM *et al.* (1991). Symptoms of acute insulin induced hypoglycaemia in humans with and without IDDM. *Diabet Care* **14**, 949–57.

Krentz AJ and Nattrass M (1997). Acute metabolic complications of DM: diabetic ketoacidosis, hyperosmolar non-ketotic syndrome and lactic acidosis. In Pickup J, Williams G, ed. *Textbook of Diabetes*, 2nd edn. Blackwell Science: Oxford, pp.1–23.

Lebovitz HE (1995). Diabetic ketoacidosis. *Lancet* **345**, 767–72.

Pickup JC, Williams G (ed) (2003). Hypoglycemia in diabetes. In: *Textbook of Diabetes*, 3rd edn. Wiley-Blackwell Science: Oxford.

Part 12

Lipids and hyperlipidaemia

Lipids and coronary heart disease

Physiology

The two main circulating lipids, triglycerides and cholesterol, are bound with phospholipid and lipoproteins to make them more water soluble for transportation throughout the body. The apoproteins on the surface of these soluble masses help the body to recognize each of the different transport complexes:

- *Chylomicrons* Contain 85% triglycerides and 4% cholesterol. Made in the mucosa of the small intestine, they are broken down in the liver and peripheral tissues by lipoprotein lipase. Initially they contain apoprotein B-48 (apo B-48) but also acquire apo E and apo C-II from circulating HDL. Following metabolism by lipoprotein lipase in capillary endothelial cells, which is activated by apo C-II, chylomicron remnants are then removed by specific apo B and apo E receptors in the liver.
- *Very low density lipoproteins (VLDLs)* Contain 50% triglyceride, 15% cholesterol, and 18% phospholipid. They are the main carrier of triglycerides in circulation. Made with triglycerides synthesized in the liver, they also contain apo B-100 and apo E. VLDLs are broken down by lipoprotein lipase in peripheral tissue to give IDLs, or other remnants which are removed by the liver.
- *Intermediate density lipoproteins (IDLs)* These VLDL remnants contain mostly cholesterol and phospholipid and are either removed by the liver or metabolized to form LDLs.
- *Low density lipoproteins (LDLs)* Contain 45% cholesterol, 10% triglycerides, and 20% phospholipid. LDL has apo B-100 in its surface and transports most of the cholesterol in circulation. The liver has specific LDL receptors to extract it from the circulation. Half of the body's circulating LDL is removed from the plasma each day, mostly by the liver. Small dense or oxidized LDL (usually only 15% of the LDL pool) is not so easily recognized by these receptors and a scavenger pathway in macrophages and liver sinusoidal endothelial cells removes these via an acetyl-LDL receptor. Accumulation of oxidized LDL in macrophages produces the foam cells seen in atheromatous plaques.
- *High density lipoproteins (HDLs)* Made in the liver and gut contain 17% cholesterol, 4% triglycerides, and 24% phospholipid. HDL transports 20–50% of circulating cholesterol.

In practice, patients are managed by their levels of cholesterol (total, LDL, HDL) and triglycerides. Elevated total or LDL cholesterol with normal triglycerides is hypercholesterolaemia. Isolated elevation of triglyceride is hypertriglyceridemia and both together is combined or mixed hyperlipidaemia.

There is a direct linear relationship between hypercholesterolaemia and coronary heart disease (CHD). A man with a TC of 6.5mmol/L has double the risk of CHD of a man with a TC of 5.2mmol/L, and half the risk of a man with a cholesterol of 7.8mmol/L. Intervention studies show that reductions in total and LDL cholesterol reduce coronary and cerebrovascular events as well as mortality.

HDL cholesterol has an inverse relationship with CHD, i.e. increased levels are beneficial. A low HDL cholesterol may be due to lack of physical exercise, obesity, or the presence of hypertriglyceridaemia, and occurs in smokers. Whether isolated hypertriglyceridaemia causes vascular disease is still debated.

Mixed hyperlipidaemia is clearly associated with CHD. The Helsinki Heart study showed a 4-fold greater risk of cardiac events if the LDL:HDL ratio was >5.0 and the triglycerides >2.3mmol/L compared to those with lower levels of triglyceride. Hypertriglyceridaemia is associated with a low HDL cholesterol as well as small dense LDL particles. The aim of keeping triglycerides <1.5mmol/L is to indirectly increase the HDL cholesterol as well as for the small dense LDL to revert to the more benign, less dense LDL. Small dense LDL has a lower binding affinity for the LDL receptor, resulting in a longer t½ as well as greater susceptibility to oxidation.

Pathogenesis

Hyperlipidaemia is due to a combination of genetic factors and dietary intake, and as 2° to other conditions. It is a major risk factor for atherosclerosis.

- 1° *hyperlipidaemias*—usually genetically determined.
- 2° *hyperlipidaemias*—due to a combination of other diseases, drugs, and dietary anomalies.

Atherosclerosis

In atherosclerosis subintimal plaques start in medium-sized blood vessel walls when LDL cholesterol accumulates. A cholesterol-rich necrotic core surrounded by smooth muscle cells and fibrous tissue then develops. These plaques can calcify. If the surface of the plaques ulcerates, thrombosis occurs which can obliterate the lumen of a blood vessel.

Plaques may result from diffusion of elevated LDL cholesterol, a qualitative abnormality of LDL cholesterol, endothelial cell damage, or a combination of these. Endothelial cell damage may be due to:

- Physical trauma e.g. with hypertension.
- Toxins e.g. tobacco or alcohol.
- Low grade infection or inflammation e.g. chlamydia.
- Immune complex damage.

CHD/atherosclerosis risk factors

♂ sex, ↑ age, and a +ve family history are all linked with a greater risk for atherosclerosis, but they are beyond our control. Several modifiable risk factors are, however, recognized:

- *Cigarette smoking* >10 cigarettes/day increase the CHD odds ratio by 6.7-fold, while stopping smoking reduces risk of myocardial infarct (MI) by 50–70% within 5 years.
- *Hypertension* Increases the CHD odds ratio by 2.7-fold. Each 1 mmHg drop in diastolic blood pressure reduces the MI risk by 2–3%. But remember aspirin reduces MI risk by 33%.
- *Diabetes mellitus* (📖 see Epidemiology, p.636).
- *Hyperlipidaemia* A 10% fall in total cholesterol (TC) results in a 25% decrease in CHD risk, and plaque regression with reducing lipids is well documented.
- *Other* Less strongly associated factors include type A personality, hyperuricaemia, lack of exercise/sedentary lifestyle, and obesity.

Assessment of CHD risk

Risk assessment tables for CHD are now available such as the Sheffield tables, the New Zealand tables, and the Joint British Societies Coronary Risk Prediction Chart (Fig. 122.1). These calculate the likelihood of the patient's absolute risk of CHD over a period of years and/or the individual's relative risk assuming CHD is not present at this time. The data used for assessment include sex, age, blood pressure, presence of left ventricular hypertrophy, smoking, diabetes mellitus, and the measured values of total cholesterol (TC), HDL cholesterol, or the ratio of TC:HDL cholesterol. The tables give a prediction which is useful for estimating the need for treatment. Recently a new cardiovascular risk scoring program, QRISK, using data from British subjects, may prove to be more useful as it appears to be better at predicting outcome. The other risk assessment tables are calculated based on data of the Framingham study which appears to over-estimate the risk in the UK.

How to use the Coronary Risk Prediction Chart for 1° prevention (Fig. 122.1)

These charts are for estimating CHD risk (non-fatal MI and coronary death) for individuals who have not developed symptomatic CHD or other major atherosclerotic disease.

The use of these charts is not appropriate for patients who have existing disease which already puts them at high risk. Such diseases include:
- CHD or other major atherosclerotic disease.
- Familial hypercholesterolaemia or other inherited dyslipidaemia.
- Established hypertension (systolic BP >160mmHg and/or diastolic BP >100mmHg) or associated target organ damage.
- Diabetes mellitus with associated target organ damage.
- Renal dysfunction.
- To estimate an individuals absolute 10-year risk of developing CHD find the table for their gender, diabetes (yes/no), smoking status (smoker/non smoker), and age. Within this square define the level of risk according to systolic blood pressure (SBP) and the ratio of TC to HDL cholesterol. If there is no HDL cholesterol result then assume this is 1.0 mmol/L and then the lipid scale can be used for TC alone.
- High-risk individuals are defined as those whose 10-year CHD risk exceeds 15% (equivalent to a *cardiovascular* risk of 20% over the same period). As a minimum those at highest risk (≥20% c) should be targeted and treated now, and as resources allow others with a risk of >15% (b) should be progressively targeted.
- Smoking status should reflect lifetime exposure to tobacco and not simply tobacco use at the time of risk assessment.
- The initial blood pressure and the first random (non-fasting) TC and HDL cholesterol can be used to estimate an individual's risk. However, the decision on using drug therapy should be based on repeat risk factor measurements over a period of time. The chart should not be used to estimate risk after treatment of hyperlipidaemia or BP has been initiated.

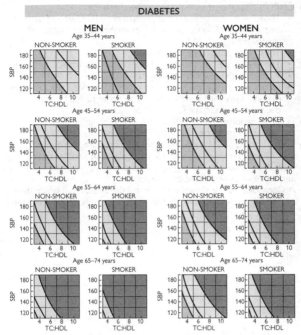

Fig. 122.1a Joint British Societies Coronary Risk Prediction Chart—individuals with diabetes. Reproduced and modified from *Heart* (1998), **80**, S1–S29. With permission from the BMJ Publishing Group.

- CHD risk is higher than indicated in the charts for:
  - Those with a family history of premature CHD (men <55 years and women <65 years) which increases the risk by a factor of approximately 1.5.
  - Those with raised triglyceride levels.
  - Those who are not diabetic but have impaired glucose tolerance.
  - Women with premature menopause.
  - As the person approaches the next age category. As risk increases exponentially with age the risk will be closer to the higher decennium for the last four years of each decade.
- In ethnic minorities in the UK the risk chart should be used with caution as it has not been validated in these populations.
- The estimates of CHD risk from the chart are based on groups of people and in managing an *individual* the physician also has to use clinical judgement in deciding how intensively to intervene on lifestyle and whether or not to use drug therapies.
- An individual can be shown on the chart the direction in which the risk of CHD can be reduced by changing smoking status, BP, or cholesterol.

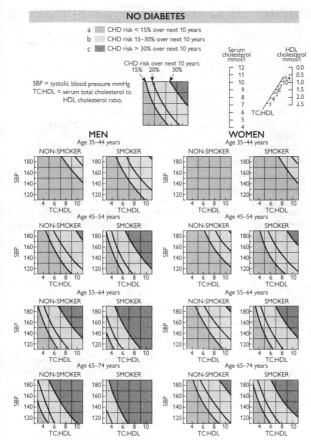

Fig. 122.1b Joint British Societies Coronary Risk Prediction Chart non-diabetic individuals. Reproduced and modified from *Heart* (1998), **80**, S1–S29. With permission from the BMJ Publishing Group.

Individuals at risk with hyperlipidaemia

- Those with premature CHD (<55 years in men, <65 years in women).
- Those with signs of other atherosclerotic disease (e.g. PVD, ischaemic cerebrovascular disease).
- Those with diabetes mellitus.
- Those with signs of insulin resistance such as acanthosis nigricans.
- Postmenopausal women not on HRT.
- Those with a high alcohol intake (♀ >14 units/week, ♂ >21).
- Those with a family history of hyperlipidaemia.
- Those with a family history of early CHD or other atherosclerotic disease.
- Those with known 2° causes of hyperlipidaemia (Ⓠ drugs and diseases as discussed in Causes, p.840).

Lipid measurements

Measurements should not be taken during an acute illness or during periods of rapid weight loss as these artificially lower the results. This is particularly important from 24h after a MI for up to 6 weeks (less if thrombolysed), as during this time the levels of TC and LDL cholesterol may be falsely reduced.

Pregnancy or recent weight gain will increase lipid levels. Following rapid weight gain or weight loss, leave at least a month before reassessing lipid levels.

Full lipid profile

Gives:
- TC.
- HDL cholesterol.
- LDL cholesterol.
- Triglycerides.

This needs to be a fasting sample, preferably after a 12h overnight fast (water is allowed). If non-fasting, only TC and HDL cholesterol measurements are accurate. Triglycerides rise postprandially and LDL is usually calculated with the formula below, so is inaccurate if not fasting. It is also invalid if triglycerides are >4.5 mmol/L:

$$\text{LDL (in mmol/L)} = TC - HDL - 0.45(\text{triglycerides})$$

The use of TC alone can be misleading as isolated HDL elevation can increase the value. Use of a TC:HDL or an LDL:HDL ratio is preferred, especially in ♀ and people with diabetes mellitus. Most risk calculation tables now use these ratios rather than total values alone.

Variations between assay method and different samples should not lead to more than a 3% variation, but more than one measurement should be used to decide on initial pharmacological intervention.

Conversion factors

American studies are often given in mg/dL rather than the SI units of mmol/L. A conversion of mmol/L × 38.8 gives mg/dL of cholesterol and mmol/L × 88.5 gives mg/dL of triglycerides.

Primary hyperlipidaemias

Background

There are two distinct elements in the diagnosis of 1° hyperlipidaemias: the genotype and the phenotype. At present the family history and the phenotypic findings in other family members are used as a surrogate for a genetic diagnosis. DNA-based technology currently employed in research can be clinically useful not just for initial diagnosis but also for family screening.

Polygenic hypercholesterolaemia

This is the most common cause of isolated hypercholesterolaemia. LDL clearance appears to be reduced by a variety of mechanisms, and the E4 allele of apo E is a common association. Patients do not have the characteristic xanthelasmata or extensor tendon deposits (xanthomata) seen in familial hyperlipidaemia. It is usually diagnosed by 1° screening programmes or when investigating some manifestation of atherosclerosis.

Familial hypercholesterolaemia (FH)

FH is an autosomal dominant disorder. Its gene frequency is 1 in 500 in western Europe and North America. In FH, hypercholesterolaemia is mainly (>95%) due to an increase in LDL cholesterol because of an LDL receptor mutation (on the short arm of chromosome 19) reducing the number of high affinity LDL receptors by up to 50%, so reducing LDL clearance and thus prolonging the circulating time before catabolism from the normal 2.5 days to >4.5 days. >1000 mutations have so far been described. Less commonly it is due to familial defective apolipoprotein B-100 (3–4%) and proprotein convertase subtilisin/kexin 9 gene (*PCSK9*) mutation (<1%). These can lead to several situations causing elevation of circulating LDL cholesterol by:
- Not producing any LDL receptors.
- Failure of LDL receptors to move to the cell surface.
- Abnormal binding of the receptor to LDL.
- Inability to adequately internalize LDL for metabolism.

Patients with FH have premature CHD (i.e. ♂ <55 years old, ♀ <65 years old) and must be treated vigorously as their standardized mortality ratio is at least 9 × greater than normal.

Clinical characterization

- TC >7.8mmol/L (>12.5 in homozygotes), LDL high from birth.
- Normal triglycerides.
- Clinical stigmata: xanthelasmic deposits around the eyes and on the tendons (i.e. fingers, hands, elbow, knee, and the Achilles tendon). Tendon xanthoma is more specific for FH than corneal arcus or xanthelasma. 7% of heterozygote FH (aged >19 years of age) have tendon xanthomas, although 75% of their parents exhibit this feature with separate studies suggesting 75% of ♂ and 72% of ♀ with homozygous FH have tendon xanthomas. It is important to note that tendon xanthomata may not be present until after 40 years of age.
- Early onset of a corneal arcus (in the 30–40 year age group).
- Achilles tendinitis may be the first clue to the presence of this condition in childhood.
- Homozygotes can have CHD presenting in childhood and certainly before the age of 30.
- Heterozygotes usually present after 30 years of age.
- A strong case can be made for FH where there may not be clinical stigmata but there is a strong family history and 1st-degree relatives with early onset CHD, e.g. before 50 years of age.

It is estimated that >50% of heterozygous FH patients will die from CHD before reaching 60 years of age if left untreated. 1 in 20 patients under 60 years old surviving a MI are FH heterozygotes. FH patients need to have their families investigated and the homozygous FH may need non-pharmacological therapies, such as plasmapherisis or surgical procedures such as ileal bypass, portocaval shunts, or liver transplatation. These treatments are not readily available and, along with pharmacological treatments, may be superseded by gene therapy in the future.

Screening at present is by measurement of blood lipids and looking for clinical stigmata or signs. It should involve immediate family members and can be done at any age. In newborn infants cord blood has been used to look at LDL cholesterol levels, but this screening method may be unreliable especially in heterozygote FH. Screening children is best carried out before 10 years of age, and then again at adolescence and early childhood. Between the ages of 1–16 years heterozygotes will have a 2-fold higher cholesterol level than unaffected siblings, so standard lipid profiles can be used. Over 16 years of age, use a full fasting lipid profile and clinical examination.

Familial defective apolipoprotein B-100 (FDB)

FDB is an autosomal dominant trait where a genetic defect of apo B-100 results in the delayed clearance of cholesterol. It is due to a single point mutation on apo B (e.g. Arg 3500—>Gln). This condition affects 1/600 people. All lipids originating from the liver are bound to apo B-100. 2 different mutations have also been described which result in ↑ levels of an LDL more prone to oxidation, causing delayed receptor pathway clearance of LDL which overloads the scavenger pathways so ↑ circulating cholesterol levels.

The diagnosis is made on slowly rising cholesterol levels and DNA studies for the point mutation. The management is similar to that of FH. 2% of cases previously described as FH are estimated to be due to FDB. Protease inhibitors have been reported to exacerbate this condition which may present with eruptive xanthomata.

Familial hypertriglyceridaemia

- This affects up to 1/300 people, often as an autosomal dominant trait with elevated VLDL levels, and is frequently accompanied by hypercholesterolaemia.
- Eruptive xanthomata (red and painful) and lipaemia retinalis can accompany massive triglyceridaemia, as can pancreatitis.
- Exacerbating factors include alcohol and drugs such as thiazide diuretics, glucocorticoids and the oral contraceptive pill.
- Adherence to a low-fat, alcohol-free diet with weight reduction usually helps.

Rare genetic hypertriglyceridaemias

2 rare but important familial causes of gross hypertriglyceridaemia are *lipoprotein lipase deficiency* and *apolipoprotien C-II deficiency*. Both are autosomal recessive conditions which present in childhood and are characterized by the presence of hyperchylomicronaemia.

- *Lipoprotein lipase* is the enzyme needed to metabolize chylomicrons; complete absence of this enzyme or production of an inactive form are both recognized defects. Usually heterozygous, but a much rarer and more severe homozygous form is also seen.
- *Apo C-II* is needed for the activation of lipoprotein lipase, and its deficiency results in hyperchylomicronaemia. Patients do not have premature CHD but can have recurrent abdominal pain due to pancreatitis.

Familial combined hyperlipidaemia (FCHL)

- FCHL is a definite risk factor for CHD.
- It occurs in 1/250 people.
- Patients usually present around 10 years later than those with FH.
- The aetiology is not yet known.
- It is the most common type of inherited dyslipidaemia, estimated to cause 10% of cases of premature CHD.
- It has no unique clinical manifestations and the diagnosis is based on raised lipids (>95th centile for age) and a family history of premature CHD in 1st-degree relatives.

Familial dysbetalipoproteinaemia

- Also known as *type III hyperlipidaemia* or *broad beta disease*.
- It is associated with early onset CHD.
- It is an uncommon disorder affecting 0.01–0.04% of people, with elevated IDL and chylomicron remnants.
- A characteristic clinical feature is the presence of palmar striae xanthoma.
- Tuberous xanthomata, found over the tuberosities of the elbows and knees, may also be present.
- The xanthomata of this familial disease can also be found in pressure areas, e.g. heels.
- In this condition, there is accumulation of IDL.
- Apo E is a constituent lipoprotein of IDL which has 3 genetically determined isoforms, E_2, E_3, and E_4.
  - E_3/E_3 occurs in 55% of people, E_2/E_2 occurs in 1%.
  - E_2 has the lowest binding affinity to the apo receptors and is therefore cleared from serum mostly slowly.
  - Apo E_4 has the greatest affinity and is more rapidly cleared.
  - Patients with familial dysbetalipoproteinaemia are phenotype E_2/E_2.

Rare familial mixed dyslipidaemias

These should be considered in any patient with unexplained neurology, organomegaly, or corneal opacities.

2 inborn metabolic disorders associated with atherosclerosis are:
- *Apolipoprotein A1-CIII deficiency* Should be suspected if hyperlipidaemia is corrected within 24 h of infusing 500mL of normal fresh frozen plasma.
- *Familial lecithin: cholesterol acyltransferase (LCAT) deficiency* In this recessively inherited disorder an enzyme necessary for intravascular lipoprotein metabolism is deficient resulting in elevated cholesterol and triglycerides. Clinically corneal lipid deposits result in visual disturbances and renal deposits in glomerular damage, proteinuria, and often renal failure.

The following disorders are not linked to the occurrence of premature atheroma formation:
- *Tangier disease (analphalipoproteinaemia or familial alphalipoprotein deficiency)* In this autosomal recessive condition apo A-I, which is found on HDL, is deficient. HDL level is low, as is TC while triglycerides are normal or high. Cholesterol accumulation gives enlarged orange coloured tonsils, hepatosplenomegaly, polyneuropathy, and corneal opacities.
- *Fish eye disease* A rare disorder from northern Sweden with high VLDL levels, low HDL, and a triglyceride rich LDL. As well as hypertriglyceridaemia, dense corneal opacities occur giving visual impairment.

- *Abetalipoproteinaemia* Results in fat accumulation due to failure of apo B-100 production. Cholesterol levels are low with no LDL and VLDL in many cases which results in fat accumulation in the gut and nerves. Vitamin E injections may prevent some of the neurological abnormalities observed (ataxia, nystagmus, dysarthria, and motor plus sensory neuropathies) but usually not the retinitis pigmentosa and acanthocytes which also feature.
- *Hypobetalipoproteinaemia* This autosomal dominantly inherited condition gives a TC of 1–4 mmol/L and can be associated with organomegaly and neurological changes in middle age due to fat deposition and abnormal red cell morphology. The homozygous state is similar to abetalipoproteinaemia.
- *Hyperalphalipoproteinaemia or HDL hyperlipoproteinamea* Results in mildly elevated HDL and TC; and may be beneficial. No treatment is needed; raised HDL can also occur with exercise, exogenous estrogen, phenytoin and phenobarbital use, or from alcohol.

Secondary hyperlipidaemias

Background

2° dyslipidaemias are relatively common, accounting for 10–20% of hyperlipidaemic adults. These can give a mixed hyperlipidaemia or a lone increase in cholesterol or triglycerides. There are multiple causes and treatment is based upon managing the 1° disease before making a further decision on the raised lipids. Often >1 cause is apparent in 2° hyperlipidaemias.

Causes

Include those below and in Table 124.1.
- *Diet* Due to excessive consumption of saturated fats and carbohydrate. Anorexia nervosa can also cause hypercholesterolaemia as a strict low fat, low calorie diet results in reduced cholesterol and bile acid turnover so ↑ circulating levels.
- *Obesity* (🕮 see Clinical features p.748)
- *Diabetes mellitus* (🕮 see Lipid abnormalities found in patients with diabetes, p778)
- *Hypothyroidism* Estimated to occur in 4% of those with hyperlipidaemia and compensated (subclinical) hypothyroidism in a further 10%. Usually resulting in hypercholesterolaemia with a TC of 9–20mmol/L. It also worsens genetic dyslipidaemias due to ↓ synthesis of hepatic LDL receptors.
- *Chronic renal disease* ↓ creatinine clearance is accompanied by hypertriglyceridaemia and a reduction in HDL cholesterol. Proteinuria, in the nephrotic syndrome, is associated with hypercholesterolaemia. Peritoneal dialysis may increase gut glucose load and worsen hypertriglyceridaemia. Remember—ciclosporin increases LDL cholesterol.
- *Liver disease* Especially with cholestasis resulting in abnormal LDL cholesterol. 1° biliary cirrhosis may elevate TC to >12mmol/L. Severe hepatocellular damage may lower LDL cholesterol by ↓ production of its component parts and the enzymes which metabolize it.
- *Cushing's syndrome* Glucocorticoids increase VLDL production thus hypertriglyceridaemia. The associated weight gain and glucose intolerance can make this effect more pronounced.
- *Lipodystrophies* A very rare group of disorders, hallmark of which is regional, partial, or generalized fat loss associated with hyperlipidaemia, especially unusually raised triglycerides. Also associated with glucose intolerance.
- *Glycogen storage diseases* Can have elevated lipids (triglycerides, cholesterol and mixed hyperlipidaemia) quite commonly, but usually only in type I (Von Gierke disease), type III (Forbes disease), and type IV (Hers disease).
- *Gout* Hypertriglyceridaemia occurs in about one-third of those with gout. Alcohol excess plays a part but it is not the sole cause.

- *Drugs* Medications commonly implicated are:
  - β-blockers, especially the non cardioselective ones.
  - Thiazide diuretics.
  - Exogenous oestrogens.
  - Anabolic steroids.
  - Glucocorticoids.
  - Isotretinoin.
  - Protease inhibitors (said to cause hyperlipidaemia in 50% after 10 months of treatment).
- *Excessive alcohol consumption* There is a J-shaped relationship between alcohol consumption and CHD. The ideal seems to be 2–3 units/day, maximum 14 units/week in women, 21 units/week in men.
- *Pregnancy* Cholesterol rises throughout pregnancy, mostly in the 2nd trimester. Triglycerides also rise, but in the final trimester and mostly in those with underlying genetic abnormalities. Both return to normal by 6 weeks post partum.

Table 124.1 Potential causes of 2° hyperlipidaemia

Elevated LDL cholesterol	Elevated triglycerides	Reduced HDL cholesterol
Diet (high saturated fats, high calories, anorexia)	Diet (weight gain + excess alcohol)	Diet (some low fat diets)
Drugs (glucocorticoids, thiazide + loop diuretics, ciclosporin)	Drugs (glucocorticoids, β-blockers, estrogens, isotretinoin)	Drugs (anabolic steroids, tobacco, beta adrenergic blockers)
Hypothyroidism	Hypothyroidism	Type 2 diabetes
Nephrotic syndrome	Type 2 diabetes	Insulin resistance syndromes/obesity
Chronic liver disease	Insulin resistance syndromes	Chronic renal failure
Cholestasis + biliary obstruction	Cushing's syndrome	
Pregnancy	Chronic renal failure	
	Peritoneal dialysis	
	Pregnancy	

Management of dyslipidaemia

Background

The emphasis will depend on the cause of the hyperlipidaemia and is aimed at reducing cardiovascular, peripheral vascular, and cerebrovascular risk. There are now recommended target values when treating patients.

Primary and secondary prevention

It is universally accepted that tackling hypercholesterolaemia in 2° prevention works. We now have solid evidence to support this, especially in the context of CHD, where a 10% fall in TC is estimated to result in a 25% decrease in CHD risk. Fatty lesion regression has also been clearly demonstrated. The gain is within 2 years of lowering the cholesterol, whether by diet or a combination of diet and drugs. There are 2 groups that need special mention, in patients with type 2 diabetes mellitus and in the acute coronary syndrome (high dose atorvastatin 80mg) show early benefit with statin treatment. In post-MI patients omega-3 fatty acids are recommended as it reduces the incidence of sudden death due to arrhythmias.

Tackling cholesterol in 1° prevention is controversial. There have been 1° prevention trials which show benefit from lowering cholesterol. The financial burden of this has to be confronted. An approach to this is to use the available risk assessment tables (🕮 see Fig. 122.1, p.829). An example would be to definitely treat if the risk of CHD is >2% per annum after a trial of dietary intervention. It has been argued that we should aim to treat if the risk is 1.5% per annum, but presently the economic argument against this holds sway.

Specific interventions

Dietary advice

All patients should see a dietitian. Fats should constitute <30% of energy consumed and saturated fats must be <30% of the total fat content. Vegetable and marine mono- and polyunsaturated fats should be ↑ in the diet. Total dietary cholesterol should not exceed 300mg per day. Foods advocated include fresh fruit and vegetables, which are also important sources of antioxidants. 4 months should be given to see if dietary manipulation will work. It is unusual to see more than a 15% fall in cholesterol from dietary measures, a reduction of 5% is more likely in free-living individuals on a diet.

Alcohol should be <14 units/week for a ♀ and <21 units/week for a ♂. Alcohol intake, at this level, confer CHD protection in men >40 and postmenopausal women.

Plant sterols and stanols, 2–3g daily, can reduce blood cholesterol by 10–15%. They are available commercially in enriched margarine spreads, yoghurt, and milky drinks.

Weight control

All overweight patients must be encouraged to lose weight. Weight reduction is closely attuned to dietary advice and physical exercise. Most weight is lost in the first 4 months of a regimen. A 10kg weight loss in an obese subject can reduce LDL cholesterol by 7% and increases HDL cholesterol by 13%.

Physical activity

Physical activity, especially aerobic exercise, is recommended. This should involve becoming breathless and be performed for 30–40min at least 3–5 times per week. Acute exercise will transiently change lipoprotein levels and increase lipoprotein lipase activity. These effects become more permanent with regular training. Triglyceride levels fall, HDL cholesterol levels rise, especially the HDL_2 subfraction with more vigorous exercise, and the LDL cholesterol is of the less dense variety which is not so atherogenic. The changes are dose dependent with ↑ exercise and a 20% alteration in each variable is achievable after 6 weeks.

Modification of other risk factors

Other risk factors such as hypertension, smoking, and diabetes mellitus must be addressed.

Drug therapy

Numerous agents can be used for both 1° and 2° prevention in patients in whom diet has been ineffective.

HMG CoA reductase inhibitors (statins)

- *Indications* High LDL or VLDL ie. 1° hypercholesterolaemia, heterozygous + homozygous FH, mixed hyperlipidaemia. Not all these medications are licensed for use in children and should be used with caution in ♀ of childbearing age because of insufficient safety data in pregnancy and potential teratogenicity. The medication should be stopped for at least 3 months before pregnancy is planned. Women must be warned about pregnancy when on these drugs.

- *Mechanism of action* Competitive inhibition of 3-hydroxy-3-methylglutaryl coenzyme A (HMG CoA) which is the rate-limiting enzyme in cholesterol synthesis. Its activation increases hepatocyte LDL receptor numbers and reduces VLDL synthesis while enhancing its hepatic clearance. 📖 See Table 125.1 for comparative lipid lowering profile and Table 125.2 for dosage.

- *Side-effects* Statins are usually very well tolerated but are known to cause headaches, nausea, and some abdominal discomfort, the main concerns are a hepatitis like picture and myositis. LFTs and creatine kinase should be measured before they are prescribed and used with caution in those with an excessive alcohol intake. It is recommended that the medications should be discontinued if the liver enzymes aspartate transaminase (AST) and/or alanine transaminase (ALT) show more than a 2–3-fold elevation above the upper limit of normal. LFTs should therefore be checked every 3–4 months initially and at least annually in the long term. Myositis is rare and tends to occur when prescribed with other medications, e.g. ciclosporin, fibrates, or when renal impairment or untreated hypothyroidism are present. Clinically there is a picture of swollen tender muscles and creatine kinase being >10 × the upper limit of normal. Rhabdomyolysis is even rarer.

- *Interactions* All statins can interact with *ciclosporin, nicotinic acid,* and are used with caution with *fibrates*. *Warfarin* interacts with atorvastatin, simvastatin and rosuvastatin. *Erythromycin* interacts with all statins. *Digoxin* interacts with atorvastatin and simvastatin. *Rifampicin* interacts with fluvastatin and pravastatin. Atorvastatin and rosuvastatin may also interact with the *oral contraceptive pill, antacids,* and some *antifungals.*

- *Costs* In 1992 it was estimated that CHD prevention by a cholesterol-lowering program using a statin calculated as cost per quality adjusted life year (QALY) was £400–£550 compared with hip replacement (£1100), coronary artery bypass surgery (£1300), breast screening (£5000), and hospital haemodialysis (£17 500). In the same year (1992) about £500 million was spent in the NHS for CHD, of which more than a half was for inpatient hospital care. In 1997 the Standing Medical Advisory Committee issued guidelines on the use of statins and, based on that advice, Warwickshire Health Authority calculated that it would cost them 20% of their drug budget, some £100 000 per practice, to implement. These costs do not include diagnostic tests as well as time to detect, counsel, and treat the patients. These costs are enormous and are very relevant in the context of limited NHS resources. There is no case against 2° prevention, but screening and 1° prevention are economically still a very sensitive issue.

Table 125.1 Comparative lipid lowering profile of statins

Statin	% fall in LDLc	% fall in triglycerides	% rise in HDLc
Atorvastatin	38–54	13–32	3–7
Fluvastatin	17–34	8–12	3–6
Pravastatin	18–34	5–13	5–8
Rosuvastatin	50–63	10–28	3–14
Simvastatin	26–48	12–38	8–12

Fibrates

- *Indications* High VLDL, triglycerides, or IDL, i.e. mixed hyperlipidaemias which have not responded adequately to diet or other therapy. These medications are less effective than the statins at lowering cholesterol but better at ↑ HDL cholesterol and more effective in lowering triglycerides. Reduce triglycerides by 20–60%, increase HDL by 15–30%, and reduce LDL by 5–25%.

- *Mechanism of action* Alter lipoprotein metabolism to reduce VLDL triglyceride synthesis by ↑ lipoprotein lipase activity and LDL-receptor mediated LDL clearance while ↑ HDL synthesis. The effect on LDL cholesterol may vary in isolated hypertriglyceridaemia to increase LDL cholesterol. 📖 See Table 125.2 for dosage

- *Side-effects* Occasionally cause nausea, anorexia, or diarrhoea and precipitate gallstones (mostly clofibrate). Also pruritus, rashes, hair loss, and impotence. They should not be used in patients with severe liver disease (AST/ALT>2–3 × upper limit of normal) and renal dysfunction (creatinine >150micromol/L) as they are conjugated in the liver prior to excretion by the kidney. Myopathy, although rare, is the main concern, and the risk of this increases if used with statins.

- *Interactions* Use with caution in combination with *statins*. Can enhance the effects of *warfarin* and *antidiabetic agents* and is contraindicated in those on *orlistat*.

Table 125.2 Dosage of lipid lowering drugs

Drug	Dose/day
Statins	
Atorvastatin	10–80mg
Fluvastatin	20–80mg
Pravastatin	10–40mg
Rosuvastatin	10–40mg (5–20 mg in patient of Asian origin)
Simvastatin	10–80mg
Fibrates	
Bezafibrate	400–600mg
Ciprofibrate	100mg
Clofibrate	50–65kg, 1.5g; >65kg, 2g
Fenofibrate	67–267mg
Gemfibrozil	0.9–1.2g
Anion-exchange resins	
Colestyramine	12–36g (in single dose or up to 4× /day)
Colestipol hydrochloride	5g 1–2× /day (max 30g/day)
Nicotinic acid group	
Acipimox	500–750mg in divided doses
Nicotinic acid MR	375–2000mg
Nicotinic acid	300mg–6g in divided doses
Omega-3 fatty acids	
Omacor®	1–4g
Maxepa®	Up to 10g
Cholesterol absorption blocker	
Ezetimibe	10mg

Anion exchange resins (bile acid sequestrants)

- *Indications* High LDL, i.e. hypercholesterolaemia. Largely superseded by statins, these are now best used as adjuncts when LDL has not fallen enough with a statin alone. They are also the only drug licensed for use during pregnancy.
- *Mechanism of action* Bind to bile acids in the gut so reducing their enterohepatic circulation and ↑ bile acid excretion. This increases hepatocyte cholesterol requirements which increases LDL receptor production so reducing circulating LDL levels. Under optimum conditions, LDL cholesterol can be reduced by 20–30%, triglycerides rise by 10–17%, and HDL increases by 3–5%.
- *Side-effects* These agents remain in the gut, so constipation, bloating, nausea and abdominal discomfort are not uncommon. Constipation, found in 35–40% of those on these agents, can be helped with bulking laxatives. Less often a bleeding tendency due to vitamin K malabsorption can be seen. These agents can also exacerbate hypertriglyceridaemia but HDL cholesterol is often ↑ slightly. To reduce the side effects start with low doses and build up gradually over the next 3–4 weeks while maintaining a good fluid intake.
- *Interactions* These agents can reduce the absorption of *warfarin*, *digoxin*, β*-blockers*, *pravastatin*, *fluvastatin,* and *hydrochlorothiazide*. Many other agents such as *simvastatin* have not been checked so to avoid any potential interaction advise patients to take all other drugs 1–3h *before* or 4–6h *after* the resin.

Nicotinic acid and acipimox

- *Indication* High LDL, VLDL, IDL, or triglycerides. Nicotinic acid is the most effective medication for ↑ HDL-cholesterol. In practice, however, their use is limited by the side-effect profile, especially flushing. A new preparation, Niaspan®, a modified release nicotinic acid product is now available and does seem to cause fewer unwanted side effects and should be first choice. Acipimox is not commonly used in clinical practice.
- *Mechanism of action* Work by inhibiting lipolysis in adipocytes so altering fatty acid flux and reducing VLDL synthesis and HDL clearance. VLDL levels fall, as do triglycerides (by 20–50%) and LDL (by 5–25%) while HDL levels rise (by 10–50%).
- *Side-effects* Common, with 30% unable to tolerate these agents. Vasodilatation giving cutaneous/facial flushing occurs in most patients but tends to improve after 2–3 weeks of therapy or if given prostaglandin inhibitors such as aspirin in combination with it. Avoid taking with hot drinks as these increase its absorption and so worsen the flushing. Gastritis is also a common problem but the more severe hepatitis occurs in only 3%. Tachycardias, dry skin, and exacerbations of gout and precipitation of acanthosis nigricans and retinal oedema are also recognized side effects. *Nicotinic acid* can adversely affect glucose control in diabetes mellitus. *Acipimox*, a nicotinic acid analogue, seems to be less problematic but is also less potent.
- *Interactions* Potentiate the effects of antihypertensive therapies.

Omega-3 fatty acids (Omacor®, Maxepa®)

- *Indications* Severe hypertriglyceridaemia.
- *Mechanism of action* Inhibit the secretion of VLDL due to ↑ intracellular apo B-100 destruction. Normal patients see both a fall in VLDL and LDL but LDL may rise in the hypertriglyceridaemic individual.
- *Side-effects* As high doses are needed, this is a high calorie load and may increase obesity. More commonly gives nausea and belching. Omacor® produces fewer unwanted effects and is less calorific as it is used in a smaller dose.
- *Interactions* None significant.

Cholesterol absorption blocker

This is a new class of cholesterol-lowering medication. Presently only one preparation, ezetimibe, is available, and is now the 2nd line of treatment after a statin.

- *Indications* LDL cholesterol-lowering in patients who are intolerant of statins or in combination with a statin in those that are not adequately controlled with a statin alone. Also in the very rare condition of sitosterolaemia, where there is an ↑ absorption of plant sterols.
- *Mechanism of action* Dietary and biliary cholesterol absorption is selectively inhibited. Ezetimibe (10mg) monotherapy produces an 18% fall in LDL cholesterol, an increase in HDL cholesterol of 1–3%, and triglycerides are not affected. In combination therapy with a statin, ezetimibe reduces levels by an additional 22% to that obtained by statin alone.
- *Interactions* None significant.

Which drug to use when (for diet-resistant dyslipidaemias)

Elevated LDL cholesterol only

- 1st choice:
  - Statins.
- 2nd choice:
  - Cholesterol absorption blocker.
  Then:
  - Bile acid sequestrants.
  - Nicotinic acid.
  - Fibrates.

Combination therapy if the above fail to reduce LDL adequately includes:

- Statin + bile acid sequestrant (can give 50% fall in LDL + 10–15% rise in HDL).
- Statin + cholesterol absorption blocker (can give an additional 22% fall in LDL + 3% rise in HDL).
- Statin + nicotinic acid (can give a 50% fall in LDL + 25–50% rise in HDL).
- Nicotinic acid + bile acid sequestrants (can give 35% fall in LDL + 25–50% rise in HDL).
- Statin + bile acid sequestrant + nicotinic acid (can give 66% fall in LDL + 25–50% rise in HDL).

Elevated triglycerides only
- 1st choice:
  Fibrates.
- 2nd choice:
  Omega-3 fatty acids.
- 3rd choice:
  Nicotinic acid

All three groups can occasionally be used together if 1 or 2 of the above groups are insufficient.

Mixed hyperlipidaemia
- 1st choice:
  Fibrate.
- 2nd choice:
  Fibrate + statin (but needs close monitoring).
  Fibrate + nicotinic acid.

As with elevated LDL alone, combination therapy may sometimes be useful with emphasis on avoiding side effects and interactions as above.

Further reading

American Diabetes Association (2004). Position statement, Dyslipidaemia management in Aduts with diabetes. *Diabetes Care Supplement*, **21**: s68–s71.

Bhatnagar D (2006). Diagnosis and screening for familial hypercholesterolaemia: finding the patient, finding the genes. *Annals of Clinical Biochemistry* **43**, 441–56.

Cannon CP, Braunwald E, McCabe CH, et al. (2004). Intensive versus moderate lipid lowering with statins after acute coronary syndromes. *New England Journal of Medicine* **350**, 1495–504.

Colhoun H, Betteridge DJ, Durrington PN et al. (2005). Rapid emergence of effect of atorvastatin on cardiovascular outcomes in the collaborative atorvastatin diabetes study (CARDS). *Diabetelogia* **48**, 2482–5.

De Backer G, Ambrosioni E, Borch-Johnsen K, et al. (2003). European guidelines on cardiovascular disease prevention in clinical practice. *European Heart Journal* **24**, 1601–10.

Downs JR, Clearfield M, Wies S, et al. (1998). Primary prevention of acute coronary events with lovastatin in men and women with average cholesterol levels: results of AFCAP/TexCAPS. Air Force/Texas Coronary Atherosclerosis Prevention Study. *JAMA* **299**, 1615–21.

Durrington P (2003). Dyslipidaemia. *The Lancet* **362**, 717–31.

Dyslipidaemia Advisory Group, on behalf of the Scientific Committee of the National Heart Foundation of New Zealand (1996). 1996 National Heart Foundation guidelines for the assessment and management of dyslipidaemia. *New Zealand Medical Journal* **109**, 224–32.

Hippisley-Cox J, Coupland C, Vinogradova Y, et al. (2007). Derivation and validation of QRISK, a new cardiovascular disease score for United Kingdom: prospective open cohort study. *British Medical Journal* **335**, 136–41.

International Atherosclerosis Society (1996). *Clinician's Manual on Hyperlipidaemia*, 4th edn. London: Science Press.

JBS 2 (2005). Joint British Societies' Guidelines on prevention of Cardiovascular Disease in clinical practice. *Heart* **91** (Suppl 5), 1–52.

National Institute for Health and Clinical Excellence (2006). Statins for the prevention of cardiovascular events. *Technology Appraisal* **94**. www.nice.org.uk/TA094

Reckless, JPD (1996). Economic issues in coronary heart disease prevention. *Current Opinion in Lipidology* **7**, 356–62.

Royal College of General Practitioners (1992). *Guidelines for the Management of Hyperlipidaemia in General Practice.*

Sacks FM, Pfeffer MA, Moye LA, *et al.* (1996). The effect of pravastatin on coronary events after myocardial infarction in patients with average cholesterol levels. *New England Journal of Medicine* **335**, 1001–9.

Scandinavian Simvastatin Survival Study Group (1994). Randomized trial of cholesterol lowering in 4444 patients with CHD: the Scandinavian Simvastatin Survival Study. *Lancet* **334**, 1383–9.

Shepherd J, Cobbe SM, Ford I, *et al.* (1995). West of Scotland Coronary Prevention Study Group. Prevention of CHD with pravastatin in men with hypercholesterolaemia. *New England Journal of Medicine* **333**, 1301–7.

Aims of treatment

In general the aim in asymptomatic patients (1° prevention) should be to achieve:
- TC <5.2mmol/L.
- LDL cholesterol <4mmol/L.
- HDL cholesterol >1mmol/L in ♂; >1.2 in ♀ (TC:HDL ratio <6).
- Triglycerides <1.7mmol/L.

For patients with CHD or post MI (2° prevention) and diabetes mellitus, the target should be:
- TC of <4mmol/L.
- LDL cholesterol <2mmol/L.
- HDL cholesterol >1.0mmol/L in ♂. > 1.2mmol/L in ♀.
- Triglycerides <1.5mmol/L.

If these optimal levels are not achievable, at least a 25% fall from pre-treatment serum TC concentration or 30% reduction in LDL cholesterol is acceptable, whichever gets to the lowest

Endocrine and diabetes nursing and dietetics

Endocrine and diabetes nursing

Insulin regimens

In type 1 diabetes a patient's insulin dose can be changed and adjusted depending on the carbohydrate food eaten. This was assessed by the DAFNE group in the context of structured education. This type of education teaches skills to replace insulin by matching it to carbohydrate, in a free diet on a meal-to-meal basis. This flexible type of insulin therapy has lead to improved physical health and well being.

Further reading

Pickup J, Mattock M, and Kerry S (2002). Glycaemic control with continuous subcutaneous insulin infusion compared with intensive insulin injections in patients with Type 1 diabetes: meta-analysis of randomized controlled trials. *BMJ* **324**, 705.

Injection technique: practical advice

To ensure the most reliable absorption of insulin, injections must be made into the SC tissue and not the muscle or dermis layer. IM injections can accelerate insulin absorption and increase the risk of hypoglycaemia. ID injections can lead to leakage, pain, or an enhanced immune response.

To reduce the risk of IM injection a skin fold should be obtained using the thumb and index or middle finger, taking up the dermis and SC tissue but leaving the muscle behind. The hold on the skin should be maintained throughout the injection and released once the needle has been removed. Releasing the hold on the skin before this can lead to IM injection.

To reduce the risk of IM injections thinner and shorter insulin needles are available. Pen needles are available in 5mm, 6mm, 12mm, and 12.7mm lengths. Smaller needles can also reduce the anxiety of injections. 📖 See Table 126.1

Absorption

Insulin absorption differs from one body region to another.
- Abdomen: fast.
- Arms: fast to medium.
- Thighs: slow.
- Buttocks: slow.

Exercising a limb in which an injection has been given increases the absorption rate.

Table 126.1 Use of different needle lengths in various patients with diabetes

Needle length	Injectors profile	Comments
5–6mm	Children, adolescents, thin to normal weight adults	Children, adolescents, thin adults, use a lifted skin fold.
8mm	Normal weight adults	Most people should be able to use a 8mm needle
12–12.7mm	Overweight adults	

Further reading

Smuss K, Hannet I, McGonigle J, et al. (1999). Ultra short (5mm) needles: Trial results and clinical recommendations. *Practical Diabetes International* **16**, 22–25.

Continuous subcutaneous insulin infusion (CSII)

CSII (pump therapy) is becoming more popular in the UK. Short-acting insulin is infused from a small portable pump at one or more basal rates, with boosts in the doses activated by the patient at mealtimes.

The cannula is changed every 2–3 days, it is connected to the body usually at the abdominal site.

Patient education for CSII must include programming the pump, carbohydrate counting, blood glucose monitoring frequency, (at least 4 times per day), and what to do in the event of a pump breakdown.

NICE Guidelines published in 2003 recommend CSII as one option for people with type 1 diabetes for whom multiple dose insulin therapy has failed: those with marked dawn phenomenon or hypoglycaemic unawareness. Recommendations include children, adolescents, and pregnant women. It is not recommended for people with type 2 diabetes.

Further reading

DAFNE Study Group (2002). Training in flexible, intensive insulin management to enable dietry freedom in people with type 1 diabetes: dose adjustment for normal eating (DAFNE) randomised controlled trial. *BMJ* **325**: 746.

NICE (2003). Guidance on the use of continuous subcutaneous insulin infusion for diabetes (NGL-4913). Technology appraisal guidance; no. 57. London, UK.

Shearer A, Bagust A, Sanderson D, *et al.* (2004). Cost-effectiveness of flexible intensive insulin management to enable dietry freedom in people with type 1 diabetes in the UK. *Diabet Med* **21**(5): 460–7.

Travel

It is important that the patient carries some form of identification. Diabetes UK produce an ID card that has a photograph of the person alongside their name and the words 'I have diabetes' translated into French, German, Greek, and Spanish.

International flights eastwards or westwards involve crossing time zones and days will be shortened or lengthened. On flights where time zones are crossed, people will need an approximate increase/decrease in their insulin that equates to the change in hours. Extra insulin is taken with the appropriate meal.

For time zone changes <4 hours no changes are usually necessary. Diabetes UK Care line offers information on aspects of travelling with diabetes.

Insulin syringes abroad

Some countries are still using U40 insulin and syringes, these are identified by colour. U40 has a red coloured syringe cap and dose markings. U100 has orange.

Insurance

Comprehensive travel insurance is necessary. The policy should not rule out pre-existing health conditions.

Climate

Insulin is stable for approximately 1 month up to temperatures of 25°C. In higher temperatures use of a cool bag is advised or a Frio® insulin cool wallet. In cooler temperatures insulin needs to be kept above 2°C.

Hot weather can increase peripheral circulation and can speed up insulin absorption. If the patient becomes cold this can slow the absorption rate and result in higher blood glucose levels.

Hypoglycaemia

Box 126.1 An easy to remember treatment plan is the rule of 15

- l5g of quick acting carbohydrate e.g. glucose/lucozade followed by
- 15g of long acting carbohydrates e.g. biscuits/bread/cereal followed by
- 15min wait and retest.

Pituitary function: dynamic tests

Before any patient undergoes dynamic testing it is imperative that they are properly prepared to ensure the test can be performed safely and reliably. It is the doctor's responsibility to explain to the patient the reason for a specific test or tests and what the test involves.

The patient may need to stop certain medication which would interfere with the test i.e. oral oestrogen therapy must be stopped for 6 weeks if cortisol levels are to be assessed.

> **Box 126.2**
>
> When booking an appointment for a patient to attend the testing it is important to check:
> 1. The medication they are taking does not interfere with the test.
> 2. They fulfil the testing criteria e.g. contraindication for ITT, epilepsy, or unexplained blackouts.
> 3. If a test requires specific baseline blood tests or EGG to ensure patient safety, only those taken within 3 months of the test are acceptable (with the exception of potassium levels in the assessment of Conn syndrome, where a potassium of 3.6 or above must be proved biochemically as near to the test date as possible).

An information sheet outlining the test and the preparation required may be sent to the patient with the appointment date.

The day of the test
- The patient must have the test fully explained by the Endocrine Specialist Nurse who must outline the risks and contraindications, ensuring the patient is able to make a fully informed consent.
- Written consent must be obtained before any patient proceeds to testing, this must be filed in the patients notes.
- Each test has a precise protocol which must be adhered to, but it is worth mentioning that before patients are discharged there are certain discharge criteria which must not be overlooked. (In Oxford following an ITT it is our practice for the patient to stay for 2 hours on completion of the test. This ensures the patient has lunch, promoting normal serum glucose, and is rested following the stress of the procedure.)

▶To ensure patient safety and reliable interpretation of the results, the Endocrine Specialist Nurse must be familiar with not only the test protocol but the preparation and discharge criteria.

Education of the patient

Box 126.3 Emergency pack contents
- 100mg vial hydrocortisone sodium succinate
- Water for injection 5mL
- 2mL syringe
- 1 green needle
- 1 blue needle
- Cotton wool
- Plaster

NB Always check expiry date of both hydrocortisone and water

Instructions for administration of emergency hydrocortisone injection

▶ Please note that you should *always* obtain medical advice alongside the administration of this injection so that the cause of illness can be identified and treated. We do not expect a relative or friend to give this injection under normal circumstances, only in an emergency whilst awaiting medical assistance.

Administration
1. Place green needle on end of syringe.
2. Draws 2mL of water into syringe.
3. Inject water into hydrocortisone powder to dissolve and shake gently.
4. Draw up hydrocortisone liquid into syringe.
5. Use upper outer quadrant of buttock.
6. Insert needle at 90° to the skin.
7. Inject solution.
8. Remove needle and press with cotton wool, cover with plaster.

Box 126.4 Information far patients receiving long-term steroid replacement (an example)

Patients taking: hydrocortisone, dexamethasone, prednisolone

- You should carry on your person a 'Steroid Card' giving details of your current dose of steroid tablets and the names, addresses, and telephone numbers of your family and hospital doctor.
- If advised to do so, you should be wearing a permanent bracelet or necklace stating that you are receiving steroids and giving a telephone number so that, if necessary, further relevant information can be obtained. This is so that if you are unconscious and in need of medical attention, this vital information is immediately available.
- The 1st dose of steroids of the day should be taken immediately on waking, before getting out of bed. They should be left by the bedside together with a glass of water on the preceding night. The evening dose should be taken no later than 6 pm.

What to do if you are unwell

- If you have a mild illness (e.g. head cold) with little or no fever, you do not need to change your medication.
- If you have a fever and are feeling unwell (e.g. influenza or an infection) then you should double the dose of steroid, by taking twice your normal number of tablets, until you are well again, usually 48–72 hours. During this period **you must inform your GP that you are unwell.**
- If you are seriously ill, especially with vomiting or diarrhoea, the steroids may not be effective. You must **contact your GP as soon as possible** and arrange for medical review and administration of an IM injection of steroids. We have given you an ampoule of hydrocortisone (100mg) for your GP to use in this circumstance. Please show this letter to your GP.
- If in doubt or if you have any queries don't hesitate to contact us. However you should contact your GP first if you are unwell.

Think ahead and don't run out of tablets. Always keep a spare supply with you.

Developed by Prof. J Wass and Dr N Karavitaki, Department of Endocrinology, Churchill Hospital, Oxford, January 2003.

Nutrition

Dietary treatment of endocrine disorders

Lifestyle factors, especially changes in diet and physical activity, have a part to play in the treatment of many endocrine disorders.

Diabetes

It is recommended that all people diagnosed with diabetes have an individual consultation with a state-registered dietitian within 4 weeks of diagnosis and that follow-up is offered as appropriate and includes an annual review. Dietary advice must take account of the individual's wishes and willingness to change and should address personal, cultural, and religious preferences and take into account the individual's beliefs and lifestyle.

Aims of dietary treatment
- To maintain or improve health through appropriate food choices
- To achieve and maintain optimal biomedical outcomes, including maintenance of blood glucose levels, lipid levels, and BP within the normal range and reducing risks of microvascular and macrovascular disease
- To optimize outcomes in established diabetic nephropathy and any concominant disease e.g. coeliac disease.

Dietary recommendations
There is now broad consensus on the type of diet which is most beneficial for people with diabetes and this conforms to the idea of a healthy diet for the non-diabetic population:
- Reduction in total fat intake (<35% total energy intake) and saturated fat intake (<10% total energy intake).
- Reduction in total sucrose intake to 10% of dietary energy intake.
- Salt intake <6g/day.
- 5 servings of a variety of fruit and vegetables daily.
- Moderate alcohol intake, in line with national recommendations of 2–3 units/day for ♀ and 3–4 units/day for ♂ and 2–3 days without alcohol weekly.

Diabetes UK publish nutritional recommendations for people with diabetes, but state that these are consensus rather than evidence-based guidelines. The latest recommendations are:
- Greater emphasis on the benefits of regular physical activity and weight management, especially for the 80–90% of people with type 2 diabetes who are either overweight or obese (📖 p.866).
- More flexibility in the proportion of monounsaturated fat and carbohydrate in dietary intake.
- Sucrose no longer restricted to a specific amount.
- Selection of carbohydrate-containing foods of low glycaemic index e.g. pasta, oat-based foods like porridge and muesli, and pulses like lentils, baked beans, and kidney beans.

Hyperlipidaemia

(📖 See p. 842)

Dietary interventions have been shown to lower serum blood cholesterol levels by 10%, although this effect is difficult to achieve in free-living populations. People with severe hyperlipidaemia e.g. familial hyperlipidaemia will need referral to a state-registered dietitian, but those individuals with mildly or moderately raised lipid levels may be offered lifestyle advice in primary care.

Aims of dietary treatment

To achieve blood lipid levels within the normal range by appropriate food choices.

Dietary recommendations

Cardioprotective dietary recommendations for those with raised cholesterol and LDL cholesterol:

- If obese, weight reduction is the priority.
- ↑ moderate physical activity for 20–30min for 5–7 days/week.
- Reduction in total fat (<30% total energy intake).
- Reduction in saturated fat (<10% total energy intake) or substitution of mono-unsaturated fat for saturated fat.
- ↑ intake of soluble fibre—fruit, vegetables, oats, and pulses.
- Reduction in salt intake to <6g/day.
- Moderate alcohol intake, in line with national recommendations.
- Reduction in dietary cholesterol if excessive.

Raised triglycerides

- Weight loss is the treatment priority.
- Reduction or avoidance of alcohol.
- Replace refined carbohydrates with those of low glycaemic index.

Other dietary factors

Fish and omega-3 fatty acids

There is conflicting evidence for the role of fish and fish oils. Some studies show omega-3 oils reduce total cholesterol, LDL cholesterol, and triglycerides, but recent meta-analyses have shown no benefit of fish oil consumption on mortality.

Plant sterols and stanols

Some plant extracts have been shown to lower cholesterol. Specialist food products e.g. margarine, milk, yogurt, have been manufactured to include plant sterols and stanols and these will lower cholesterol if eaten in sufficient quantities. The lipid-lowering effect is dose-dependant and these foods are relatively expensive.

Polycystic ovary syndrome

The optimal diet for women with polysytic ovary syndrome is not yet established, but there is evidence for the effectiveness of both weight reduction and increased physical activity (📖 p.866). At present, recommendations are based upon a low fat diet with moderate carbohydrate intake of low glycaemic index. There have been some reports of improvements in insulin resistance in women who adopt a low carbohydrate diet, but the long-term benefits are unclear.

Aims of dietary treatment

- To achieve and maintain optimal biomedical outcomes including reduction of hyperinsulinaemia and hyperandrogenaemia by appropriate food choices.
- To achieve and maintain body weight within the normal range for overweight or obese individuals.
- To reduce the long-term risks of type 2 diabetes, cardiovascular disease, and some cancers.

Dietary recommendations

- If obese, weight reduction is the priority.
- ↑ moderate physical activity for at least 20–30min on 5–7 days/week.
- Reduction in total fat (<30% total energy intake).
- Moderate carbohydrate intake of low glycaemic index.
- Salt intake <6g/day.
- 5 servings of a variety of fruit and vegetables daily.
- Moderate alcohol intake, in line with national recommendations of 2–3 units daily for ♀ and 2–3 days/week without alcohol.

Amenorrhea

2° amenorrhea may be caused by polycystic ovary syndrome or by low body weight associated with either excessive exercise or anorexia nervosa. It is frequently seen in ballet dancers and professional gymnasts. Dietary treatment should be undertaken in conjunction with a specialist dietitian.

Aims of treatment

- The main short-term goal is to achieve a body weight at which menstruation returns.
- The long-term goals include restoring bone density and fertility.

Diets adopted by those attempting to maintain a low body weight tend to be low in fat and animal protein (often vegetarian), resulting in inadequate iron, B vitamins, and calcium intake and some trace elements e.g. zinc and selenium.

Treatment has to address the psychological issues surrounding restriction of dietary intake and to recommend an energy-dense diet with sufficient minerals and vitamins to promote maintenance of body weight within the normal range.

Reactive hypoglycaemia

(📖 See p. 644)

This is often associated with insulin resistance and is frequently reported by ♀ with polycystic ovary syndrome. There is no evidence for the most effective treatment, but some anecdotal evidence exists for adoption of a low glycaemic index diet. Advice should promote small, regular meals and snacks as appropriate and include a recommendation for inclusion of moderate portions of carbohydrates of low glycaemic index.

Physical activity

Regular daily physical activity (as opposed to sessions of formal exercise) is of benefit to people with both type 1 and type 2 diabetes, those with hyperlipidaemia, and ♀ with polycystic ovary syndrome, regardless of body weight. Physical activity aids weight control, improves insulin sensitivity and lipid levels, and maintains muscle mass. ↑ daily exercise also has a role in the prevention of type 2 diabetes.

Recommendations

- Moderate activity (brisk walking, jogging swimming, dancing) should be taken on most days of the week for at least 20–30min.
- Aerobic exercise (running, rowing, aerobic classes) offers most cardioprotection and should be taken 2–3 times weekly for at least 30min.

Weight management

Weight management and weight loss is of importance in many endocrine disorders. Realistic targets for weight loss should be agreed, as many people with endocrine disorders are unable to reduce their body weight to within the normal range. This appears to be due to both genetic and environmental factors. Modest weight loss (5–10%) of body weight has been shown to improve both insulin sensitivity and diabetes control. Weight losses of 11% reduce mortality in type 2 diabetes by 25%.

Weight reduction is recommended through a combination of diet and ↑ physical activity. A reduction in energy-dense foods, especially those containing large amounts of fat and sugar is advised. Alcohol should be restricted or avoided. There is no convincing evidence for the most effective method of weight loss and the best strategy is that which matches the individual's food preferences and lifestyle. These include:

- Energy restriction/calorie counting (calculated as daily energy requirements less 500kcal/day).
- Commercial weight-loss groups.
- Low carbohydrate diets—these have been shown to be effective in the short-term, but there are no long-term data.

Diets which exclude major food groups or which rely on a limited range of foods e.g. cabbage soup diet and grapefruit diet are nutritionally unsound and are not recommended.

Behavioural programmes have been shown to increase success for lifestyle change and the most effective strategies for weight loss include these elements:

- Reduction of daily energy intake of 500–1000kcal/day.
- At least 3 hours of physical activity/week.
- Self-monitoring, including food and exercise diaries.
- Setting realistic goals.

Part 14

Laboratory endocrinology

Pitfalls in laboratory endocrinology

Introduction

The previous issue of this handbook contained a chapter entitled 'Normal ranges' for endocrine-related laboratory tests. The purpose of this chapter is to explain why this compendium of data needs to be viewed with a degree of caution and why you, as a clinical endocrinologist, should be actively liaising with your laboratory service about the assays that they provide, their reference ranges, and the performance of these assays. Laboratory methods are complex and are affected by a number of factors which can often only be considered and explored if information is shared by frequent liaison between clinicians and laboratory scientists. Uncritical use of numbers obtained from the literature may lead to errors and bad management decisions.

Box 128.1 Factors to be considered for laboratory investigations

- Pre-analytical factors:
  - Sample timing.
  - Which tube?
  - Sample transport factors.
  - Biological variation.
  - Which stimulation test?
- Analytical factors:
  - Assay specificity.
  - Assay standardization.
  - Analytical performance.
  - Hook effects.
  - Antibody interference.
  - Particularly problematic assays.
- Post analytical factors:
  - Reference ranges.
  - Units.
  - Interpretation.

Pre-analytical factors

Half of all errors in the diagnostic process are due to pre-analytical factors and 20% of errors are related to sample collection. Even in hospitals where there is a heightened awareness of these problems, there is a prevalence of 1% pre-analytical errors. These effects can be of sufficient magnitude to alter the analysis enough to create situations for clinical errors. Most problems can be prevented by clear instructions and documented policies for sampling.

Some issues are relatively straightforward such as collecting the sample into the correct blood tube and ensuring that samples are transported to the laboratory fast enough at the correct temperature. If in doubt a comprehensive list can be found at ⌂ http://www.diagnosticsample.com/

In order to be certain whether 2 or more samples taken from an individual are different, it is important to consider the biological variation that naturally occurs. A comprehensive list can be found at ⌂ http://www.westgard.com/intra-inter.htm. In addition, the clearance t½ of each analyte should be considered: endogenous hormones and tumour markers like pharmaceuticals and 90% of the change occurs after $4.5 \times t½$.

Many endocrine function tests require stimulation tests. What is the evidence for the one you plan to use? How much difference exists for different stimulants? For examples of the effects of different stimulants of GH see Rahim *et al*, *Clin Endocrinol* 1996;45:557–62.

Box 128.2 Examples of pre-analytical errors

- Incorrectly or unlabelled samples.
- Undefined or inappropriate sample timing.
- Wrong tubes.
- Haemolysis.
- Lipaemia.
- Delayed transport.
- Incorrect transport temperature.

Box 128.3 Examples of within person (biological) variation

Aldosterone	29%
Androstenedione	16%
CA125	36%
CA153	5.7%
CEA	10.6%
DHAS	3.4%
Prolactin	24%
SHBG	9%
Testosterone (♂)	10%
TSH	20%

Variation expressed as cv(%) [Coefficient of variation = (standard deviation/ mean)*100]

Analytical factors

Most endocrine assays are immunoassays which rely on binding of an analyte by a diagnostic antibody. The binding specificity will depend on the care and attention with which the manufacturer has chosen the reagents. Typical interferences in small molecules are due to slightly different molecular forms and typically occur with steroid and digoxin assays. Peptide hormones are more complex because so many differently glycosylated forms of those peptides exist.

Standards for pituitary hormones are generally derived from purified pituitary extracts which contain a mixture of peptides. This leads to different assays having quite marked biases between each other due to different binding affinities of the antibodies to the different isoforms. A similar situation exists with hCG for which many multiple molecular forms co-exist. Attempts to find international consensus for standards which can be used in diagnostic systems are being made, particularly for growth hormone and glycated haemoglobin at the present time.

Analytical performance or assay reproducibility is important in determining the critical differences between patient samples. A significant difference between consecutive samples at 95% confidence will require a difference of 1.96 × the method standard deviation at the appropriate concentration.

The hook effect occurs when very high analyte concentrations flood the available antibody *in vitro* and this leads to artefactually low results. It is less common nowadays as assays have large dynamic ranges but new cases continue to be reported, and there are published case reports for all hormones and tumour markers.

Antibody interference is a widespread problem that affects approximately 1% of immunoassays. It is insidious and is due to endogenous antibodies which interfere with analyte binding *in vitro*. Most importantly, they cannot be detected by usual quality control mechanisms. There are a number of laboratory techniques that can be used to clarify whether such interference is present but it is inherent on the clinician to alert the laboratory to a potential clinical mismatch.

Some assays can only be classified as problem assays. These include thyroglobulin and low concentrations of oestradiol (<300pmol/L) and testosterone (<5nmol/L). The former is due to the high prevalence of endogenous anti-thyroglobulin antibodies which are particularly prevalent in patients with thyroid disease. The latter are due to antibody specificity; however, it is hoped that this will be resolved with the introduction of mass spectrometry into routine clinical practice.

Post-analytical factors

Interpretation of assay results is made in relation to reference ranges provided by the laboratory. These usually represent the 95th centiles of a population of healthy individuals. However, the definition of normality is subjective and reference ranges are affected by such factors as age, gender, and in some cases by ethnicity. Moreover, for hormones, time of day, month, and season will be important. For some analytes, it is difficult to obtain appropriate samples to construct ranges such as in children and circumstances that are difficult to obtain in health e.g. following pharmacological stimulation or samples of CSF.

If the central 95th centile reference ranges are used, there is a 5% chance that a result will be out-of-range due to chance. As the number of tests taken are ↑, so will the risk of a chance abnormality. The increase will be x% (where $x = 1 - 0.95^a$ and a is the number of tests performed).

Literature from the USA and European journals may use different units— beware! SI units use molar or mass (g) and volumes reported in litres.

Most assays are standardized with international preparations. These are usually the molecular forms that are most prevalent when basal samples are taken. However, following stimulation non-standard molecules are released into the circulation which have different clearance rates and different binding characteristics to the diagnostic antibodies *in vitro*. This can lead to marked differences between methods. For example, following stimulation by ACTH corticosteroid precursors are released which will compete with cortisol for binding in the assay; similarly following stimulation of GH release different isoforms of GH are secreted and the most abundant 20 and 22kDa isoforms clear at different rates leading to variations in recognition by the diagnostic antibodies at different times during the test.

Box 128.4 Disastrous outcomes

- *Assay interference*: a series of patients has been described in whom aggressive therapy for chorioncarcinoma was instituted for diagnoses that were based on assays affected by *in vitro* artefacts.
- *Antibody specificity*: a patient has been described who had prolactin measured by 3 different assays giving 3 different answers. The solution awaited a clinical answer when the hyperprolactinaemia resolved after stopping the offending medication.
- *Interference by insulin auto-antibodies*: a patient has been described with recurrent hypoglycaemia due to insulin auto antibodies caused by myeloma. This patient demonstrated *in vivo* interference by endogenous antibodies as well as *in vitro* interference.
- *Hook effect*: a patient presents with a large pituitary tumour that appears to be non-functioning as the prolactin is normal and the patient is treated surgically. The following day the blood sample is reassayed after dilution and the high prolactin is uncovered when the antibody is no longer flooded by excess prolactin.

Reference intervals

Introduction

All values are for serum unless specified otherwise.

Box 129.1 Definitions

- *Serum* A serum sample is collected in a plain tube, left to permit clotting, then centrifuged and separated.
- *Plasma* A plasma specimen is collected in a tube containing EDTA or lithium heparin, centrifuged immediately and separated.

Box 129.2 Table notes

[a] Lithium heparin tube cold spun immediately and frozen.
[b] Serum, cold spun, flash frozen.
[c] Fasting sample collected into 10mL plastic lithium heparin tube containing 200mcL Trasylol® (aprotinin – proteolytic enzyme inhibitor), cold spun and flash frozen.
[d] Acid-containing container (20ml 6M HCl).

Thyroid function

Table 129.1

Analyte	SI units	Traditional units	Conversion factor
TSH	0.35–5.50mU/L	0.35–5.50mU/L	1
Total T_4	60–140nmol/L	4.5–11.0mcg/dL	12.9
Free T_4	11.5–22.7pmol/L	0.9–1.8ng/dL	12.9
Total T_3	0.9–2.8nmol/L	60–190ng/dL	0.015
Free T_3	3.5–6.5pmol/L	2.3–4.3pg/mL	1.54

Adrenal and gonadal function

Table 129.2

Analyte		SI units	Traditional units	Conversion factor
Cortisol (9 a.m.)		180–620nmol/L	6.5–22.5ng/dL	27.6
Aldosterone	Supine	100–500pmol/L	3.6–18ng/dL	27.7
	Erect	600–1200pmol/L	21.5–43.3ng/dL	27.7
Plasma renin activity	Supine	0.5–2.2nmol/h/L	N/A*	
	Erect	1.2–4.4nmol/h/L	N/A	
DHEAS	♀	1.9–9.4micromol/L	5.1–25.4pg/mL	0.0027
	♂	2.8–12micromol/L	7.6–32.4pg/mL	0.0027
Androstene-dione	♀	3–9.6nmol/L	8.5–27.5mcg/L	3.49
	♂	2.6–7nmol/L	7.5–20mcg/L	3.49
17–hydroxy-progesterone	Follicular	1–10nmol/L	3.3–33mcg/L	3.3
	Luteal	1–20nmol/L	3.3–66 mcg/L	3.3
Oestradiol	Follicular	17–260pmol/L	61–936pg/mL	3.6
	Mid-cycle	370–1470 pmol/L	1332–5290pg/mL	3.6
	Luteal	180–1100pmol/L	648–3960pg/mL	3.6
	♂	0–191pmol/L	0–688pg/mL	3.6
Progesterone	Follicular	<3nmol/L	<9.6ng/mL	3.2
	Luteal	14–89nmol/L	45–285ng/mL	3.2
	♂	0.9–4.0nmol/L	2.9–13ng/mL	3.2
Testosterone	♂	8.4–28.7nmol/L	29–100ng/mL	3.5
	♀	0.5–2.6nmol/L	1.7–9ng/mL	3.5
Dihydro-testosterone	♂	1–2.6nmol/L	29–76ng/dL	0.034
	♀	0.3–0.8nmol/L	8.7–23ng/dL	0.034
Sex hormone binding globulin	♀	18–114nmol/L	18–114nmol/L	1
	♂	13–71nmol/L	13–71nmol/L	1

* a variety of different units are used by non-UN labs

Pituitary hormones

Table 129.3

Analyte		SI units	Traditional units	Conversion factor
FSH	Follicular	0.5–5U/L	0.5–5mU/mL	1
	Mid-cycle	8–33U/L	8–33mU/mL	1
	Luteal	2–8U/L	2–8mU/mL	1
	Post-menopausal	>30U/L	>30mU/mL	1
	♂	1.4–18.1U/L	1.4–18.1mU/mL	1
LH	Follicular	3–12U/L	3–12mU/mL	1
	Mid-cycle	20–80U/L	20–80mU/mL	1
	Luteal	3–16U/L	3–16mU/mL	1
	Post-menopausal	>30U/L	>30mU/mL	1
	♂	3–8U/L	3–8mU/mL	1
Prolactin	♀	60–620mU/L	3–31ng/mL	20
	♂	45–375mU/L	2.2–19ng/mL	20
Growth hormone (basal)		0–20mU/L	0–10ng/mL	3
IGF-1	20 years	16–118nmol/L	120–885ng/mL	7.5
	40 years	14–47nmol/L	105–353ng/mL	
	60 years	10.5–35nmol/L	79–263ng/mL	
	>60years	7.0–28nmol/L	52–210ng/mL	
ACTH[a]		2.2–17.6pmol/L	10–80ng/L	0.22
Inhibin B		80–150pg/mL		

[a] Lithium heparin tube cold spun immediately.

Bone biochemistry

Table 129.4

Analyte	SI units	Traditional units	Conversion factor
Parathyroid hormone[b]	1.0–6.1pmol/L	10–60pg/mL	0.1
Total 25-hydroxy-cholecalciferol[b]	25–125nmol/L	10–50ng/mL	2.5
25-hdroxy calcitriol (sunlight dependent)	25–75nmol/L	10–30ng/mL	Winter (Nov–April)
	37–150nmol/L	15–60ng/mL	Summer (May–Nov)
25-hydroxy calcidiol (dietary)	<25nmol/L	< 10ng/mL	Winter
	< 25nmol/L	< 10ng/mL	Summer
1, 25-dihydroxy-cholecalciferol[b]	48–125pmol/L	20–50pg/mL	2.4
Calcitonin[a]	<0.08mcg/L		
P1NP[b] procollagen extension peptide	26–110mcg/L		

[a] Lithium heparin tube cold spun immediately
[b] Serum, cold spun, flash frozen
[c] Fasting, Trasylol® tube, lithium heparin, cold spun and flash frozen

Plasma gastrointestinal and pancreatic hormones

Table 129.5

Analyte	SI units	Traditional units	Conversion factor
Insulin (fasting)[c]	21.5–115 pmol/L	3.1–17mU/L	6.9
C-peptide (fasting)	0.17–0.5nmol/L	0.5–1.5ng/mL	0.33
Gastrin[c]	0–40 pmol/L	0–89pg/mL	0.45
Glucagon[c]	0–50 pmol/L	0–179pg/mL	0.28
Vasoactive intestinal polypeptide (VIP)[c]	0–30 pmol/L	0–71pg/mL	0.42
Pancreatic polypeptide[c]	0–300 pmol/L	0–1250pg/mL	0.24
Somatostatin[c]	0–150 pmol/L		
Chromogranin A[c]	0–60 pmol/L		
Chromogranin B[c]	0–150 pmol/L		
Neurotensin[c]	0–100 pmol/L		

[c] Fasting, Trasylol® tube, lithium heparin, cold spun and flash frozen

Tumour markers

Table 129.6

Analyte	SI units
βhCG	0–5 U/L
Carcinoembryonic antigen (CEA)	0–2.5U/L
Prostate specific antigen (PSA)	0–4mcg/L
Alphafetoprotein	0–7 IU/mL

Urinary collections

Table 129.7

Analyte	♂ SI units (micromol/24h)	♀ SI units (micromol/24h)
Normetadrenaline		
20–40 years	3.6	3.0
40–60 years	4.25	3.45
60–80 years	4.5	3.65
Metadrenaline		
20–40 years	1.9	1.4
40–60 years	1.9	1.4
60–80 years	1.9	1.4
3-methoxytyramine		
20–40 years	3.3	2.75
40–60 years	3.1	2.55
60–80 years	2.8	2.3

Table 129.8

Urinary analyte	SI units (mmol/L)	Traditional units	SI units mmol/24h	Conversion factor
Cortisol			0–280	
Calcium	1.25–3.75	50–150mg/L	2.5–7.5	0.025
Phosphate	7.5–25	0.2–0.8mg/L	12.9–42	32.3
Potassium	20–60	20–60mmol/L	♂: 37–139 ♀: 34–103	1.0
Sodium	50–125	50–125mmol/L	♂: 83–287 ♀: 61–214	1.0
5-hydroxyin-doleacetic acid		1.9–8.1mg/24h	10–42Umol/L/24h	5.2

Appendix

Patient support groups and other endocrine organizations

Useful addresses (UK)

Addison's Disease Self Help Group*

Androgen Insensitivity Syndrome Support Group
PO Box 269, Banbury, Oxfordshire OX15 6YT

CAH Support Group*

Carcinoid Syndrome Support Group*

Conn's Syndrome*

Diabetes UK
10 Queen Anne Street, London, W1M 0BD

The Gender Trust*
PO Box 3192, Brighton, BN1 3WR

Child Growth Foundation*

Kleinfelter's Syndrome Association*

British Menopause Society*

National Osteoporosis Society
Camerton, Bath, BA2 OPJ

National Association for the Relief of Paget's Disease*

Polycystic Ovaries Research and Support Group*

Kallmann's Syndrome
The Pituitary Foundation, PO Box 44,
Bristol BS99 2UB

The Pituitary Foundation
PO Box 44, Bristol BS99 2UB

British Thyroid Foundation
PO Box 97, Weatherby, West Yorkshire, LS23 6XD

Thyroid Eye Disease Association*

The Turner Syndrome Society*

* Contact Group via Society for Endocrinology, 17/18 The Courtyard, Woodlands, Bradley Stoke, Bristol BS32 4NQ.

Useful addresses overseas

American Diabetes Association
1701 North Beauregard Street,
Alexandria, VA 22311, USA

American Thyroid Association
Montefiore Medical Centre,
111 East 210th Street, Room 311, Bronx,
New York 10467, USA

Australian Pituitary Foundation
PO Box 4792, North Rocks, NSW 2450,
Australia

Australian Thyroid Association
PO Box 186, Westmead, NSW 2134,
Australia

Brain and Pituitary Foundation of America
1360, Ninth Avenue, Suite 210,
San Francisco, USA

The Endocrine Society
4350 East West Highway
Suite 500
Bethesda, Maryland 2084–4426
USA

European Federation of Endocrine Societies
Medizinische Poliklinik der Universitat Wurzburg
Klinische Forschergruppe
Rontgenring 11
D 97070 Wurzburg
Germany

National Osteoporosis Foundation
1150 17th Street NW, Suite 500,
Washington DC 20036, USA

Pituitary Tumour Network Association
16350 Ventura Boulevard, Encino, CA
91436, USA

The Pituitary Foundation
TMP 532.333 Ceder Street, Newhaven,
CT 06510, USA

Thyroid Foundation of Canada
96 Mack Street, Kingston, Ontario,
Canada

Useful web sites

Diabetes UK   www.diabetes.org.uk

American Diabetes Association   www.diabetes.org

American Thyroid Association   www.thyroid.org

National Institutes of Health   www.nih.gov

Polycystic Ovarian Syndrome Association   www.pcosupport.org

Society for Endocrinology (UK)   www.endocrinology.org

European Federation of Endocrine Societies   www.euro-endo.org

British Thyroid Association   www.british-thyroid-association.org

The Association for Multiple
Endocrine Neoplasia Disorders   www.amend.org.uk

The Endocrine Society   www.endo-society.org/pubaffai/factsheet.htm

Index